Viral Loads

EMBODYING INEQUALITIES: PERSPECTIVES FROM MEDICAL ANTHROPOLOGY

Series Editors
Sahra Gibbon, UCL Anthropology
Jennie Gamlin, UCL Institute for Global Health

This series charts diverse anthropological engagements with the changing dynamics of health and wellbeing in local and global contexts. It includes ethnographic and theoretical works that explore the different ways in which inequalities pervade our bodies. The series offers novel contributions often neglected by classical and contemporary publications that draw on public, applied, activist, cross-disciplinary and engaged anthropological methods, as well as in-depth writings from the field. It specifically seeks to showcase new and emerging health issues that are the products of unequal global development.

Viral Loads

Anthropologies of urgency in the time of COVID-19

Edited by

Lenore Manderson, Nancy J. Burke and Ayo Wahlberg

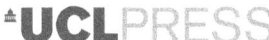

First published in 2021 by
UCL Press
University College London
Gower Street
London WC1E 6BT

Available to download free: www.uclpress.co.uk

Collection © Editors, 2021
Text © Contributors, 2021
Images © Contributors and copyright holders named in captions, 2021

The authors have asserted their rights under the Copyright, Designs and Patents Act 1988 to be identified as the authors of this work.

A CIP catalogue record for this book is available from The British Library.

This book is published under a Creative Commons Attribution Non-Commercial 4.0 International licence (CC BY-NC 4.0). This licence allows you to share and adapt the work for non-commercial use providing attribution is made to the author and publisher (but not in any way that suggests that they endorse you or your use of the work) and any changes are indicated. Attribution should include the following information:

Manderson, L., Burke, N.J. and Wahlberg, A. (eds). 2021. *Viral Loads: Anthropogies of urgency in the time of COVID-19*. London: UCL Press. https://doi.org/10.14324/111.9781800080232

Further details about Creative Commons licences are available at http://creativecommons.org/licenses/

Any third-party material in this book is published under the book's Creative Commons licence unless indicated otherwise in the credit line to the material. If you would like to reuse any third-party material not covered by the book's Creative Commons licence, you will need to obtain permission directly from the copyright holder.

ISBN: 978-1-80008-025-6 (Hbk.)
ISBN: 978-1-80008-024-9 (Pbk.)
ISBN: 978-1-80008-023-2 (PDF)
ISBN: 978-1-80008-026-3 (epub)
ISBN: 978-1-80008-027-0 (mobi)
DOI: https://doi.org/10.14324/111.9781800080232

Contents

List of figures	ix
List of tables	xi
List of contributors	xiii
Acknowledgements	xxi

1 Introduction: stratified livability and pandemic effects 1
   Ayo Wahlberg, Nancy J. Burke and Lenore Manderson

Part I: The power of the state

2 Care in the time of COVID-19: surveillance, creativity and *sociolismo* in Cuba 27
   Nancy J. Burke

3 Militarising the pandemic: lockdown in South Africa 47
   Lenore Manderson and Susan Levine

4 Rights, responsibilities and revelations: COVID-19 conspiracy theories and the state 67
   Elisa J. Sobo and Elżbieta Drążkiewicz

Part II: Exclusion and blame

5 The 2020 Los Angeles uprisings: fighting for Black lives in the midst of COVID-19 91
   Hanna Garth

6 The biopolitics of COVID-19 in the UK: racism, nationalism and the afterlife of colonialism 108
   Jennie Gamlin, Sahra Gibbon and Melania Calestani

7 The shroud stealers: coronavirus and the viral vagility of prejudice 128
   Aditya Bharadwaj

8 Unprecedented times? Romanian Roma and discrimination during the COVID-19 pandemic   147
Cristina A. Pop

9 Turkey's Diyanet and political Islam during the pandemic   162
Oğuz Alyanak

10 Citizen vector: scapegoating within communal boundaries in Senegal during the COVID-19 pandemic   181
Ato Kwamena Onoma

Part III: Unequal burdens

11 Pandemic policy responses and embodied realities among 'waste-pickers' in India   201
Surekha Garimella, Shrutika Murthy, Lana Whittaker and Rachel Tolhurst

12 The amplification effect: impacts of COVID-19 on sexual and reproductive health and rights in Indonesia   222
Linda Rae Bennett and Setiyani Marta Dewi

13 Vulnerabilities within and beyond the pandemic: disability in COVID-19 Brazil   243
Claudia Fonseca and Soraya Fleischer

14 'You are putting my health at risk': genes, diets and bioethics under COVID-19 in Mexico   260
Abril Saldaña-Tejeda

15 Scarcity and resilience in the slums of Dhaka city, Bangladesh   281
Sabina Faiz Rashid, Selima Kabir, Kim Ozano, Sally Theobald, Bachera Aktar and Aisha Siddika

Part IV: The reach of care

16 Making do: COVID-19 and the improvisation of care in the UK and US   303
Ellen Block and Cecilia Vindrola-Padros

17 Carescapes unsettled: COVID-19 and the reworking of 'stable illnesses' in welfare state Denmark   324
Sofie Rosenlund Lau, Marie Kofod Svensson, Natasja Kingod and Ayo Wahlberg

18 Care within or out of reach: fantasies of care and
    connectivity in the time of the COVID-19 pandemic   344
    Earvin Charles Cabalquinto and Tanja Ahlin

19 Pandemic times in a WhatsApp-ed nation: gender
    ideologies in India during COVID-19   362
    Haripriya Narasimhan, Mahati Chittem and Pooja Purang

20 Purity's dangers: at the interstices of religion and
    public health in Israel   384
    Tsipy Ivry and Sarah Segal-Katz

Part V: Lessons for a future

21 Fracturing the pandemic: the logic of separation and
    infectious disease in Tanzania   409
    Rebecca Marsland

22 Living together in precarious times: COVID-19 in the
    Philippines   427
    Gideon Lasco

23 COVID-19 in Italy: a new culture of healthcare for future
    preparedness   443
    Chiara Bodini and Ivo Quaranta

Index   456

List of figures

3.1	Land invasion	59
6.1	Handmade banner supporting the National Health Service (NHS)	114
11.1	Sifting and collection of recyclables	202
11.2	Policy screening flow	208
14.1	Caricature about obesity	268
14.2	Caricature about obesity	269
14.3	Caricature designed to educate children	269
14.4	Caricature designed to educate children	270
15.1	An adolescent prepares snacks in Dhaka	290
17.1	Health Minister Magnus Heunicke urging Danes to 'flatten the curve'	325
19.1	When ur maid comes back after lockdown	368
19.2	With wives burdened, men want helpers back	369
19.3	When your mother is not cooking various dishes during lockdown	371
19.4	Work from home	373
19.5	Dear Tummy	374
19.6	After three months of quarantine	374
19.7	The lockdown is to keep everyone safe and healthy	375
19.8	The social distance	375
20.1	Immersion pool in a mikveh in Haifa	390

List of tables

11.1 Inclusion and exclusion criteria   207

List of contributors

Tanja Ahlin is a Lecturer in Anthropology and Science and Technology Studies at the University of Amsterdam. For her doctoral research, she conducted fieldwork in India and Oman on how digital technologies shape care at a distance in Indian transnational families of nurses. She is currently examining how communication technologies influence deaf and hard-of-hearing people's belonging and socialities. http://tanjaahlin.com/

Bachera Aktar is Assistant Director, Center of Excellence for Gender, Sexual and Reproductive Health and Rights in the James P. Grant School of Public Health, BRAC University, Dhaka, Bangladesh, and has particular interest in food and nutrition, health inequity and the social determinants of health. She has over 11 years of experience of implementing public health programmes and research in rural and urban areas in Bangladesh.

Oğuz Alyanak is Volkswagen Foundation Postdoctoral Fellow at the University of Göttingen, Germany, and editorial assistant of social media for *Medical Anthropology*. His dissertation was on Muslim men's night lives at the Franco-German borderland. He is now exploring occupational injuries and illnesses among Turkish immigrants in Europe.

Linda Rae Bennett is a medical anthropologist and Associate Professor at the Nossal Institute for Global Health, the University of Melbourne, with 25 years of ethnographic experience researching sexual and reproductive health and rights, gender-based violence and health inequities in Indonesia.

Aditya Bharadwaj is Professor of Anthropology and Sociology at the Graduate Institute of International and Development Studies, Geneva. His current research examines infertility, childlessness and healthcare seeking in resource-poor settings in Nepal and India.

Ellen Block is an Associate Professor of Anthropology in the Sociology Department at the College of St Benedict and St John's University in

Minnesota. Her work focuses on the intersections of health, kinship and care in sub-Saharan Africa and the United States. Her current project examines the professional and interpersonal effects of COVID-19 on healthcare providers in the US. She is co-author of *Infected Kin: Orphan care and AIDS in Lesotho* (2019).

Chiara Bodini is at the Centre for International and Intercultural Health, University of Bologna, and specialises in infectious diseases and in public health. Her work focuses on health inequalities and the social determinants of health, and on the role of social movements and community participation in health promotion and healthcare delivery.

Nancy J. Burke is Professor of Public Health and Anthropology and John D. and Catherine T. MacArthur Foundation Endowed Chair, University of California, Merced. She also serves as Co-Director of the UC-Cuba Academic Initiative. Her current research includes projects focused on ageing in Cuba, syndemic care for high-cost, high-utilising safety-net patients in the United States, and cancer patient navigation programmes in US public hospitals.

Earvin Charles Cabalquinto is a Lecturer in Communication in the School of Communication and Creative Arts at Deakin University, and a member of the Alfred Deakin Institute for Citizenship and Globalisation. He is interested in mobile intimacy and the digitalisation of both domestic and public spaces. He is currently investigating how elderly people from Culturally and Linguistically Diverse (CALD) backgrounds in Melbourne, Australia, forge and sustain relationships among their close and distant support networks. http://www.ecabalquinto.com.

Melania Calestani is Senior Lecturer at Kingston and St George's, University of London. She has carried out fieldwork on social/cultural constructions of wellbeing and health in Andean Bolivia with indigenous communities. In the UK, she has conducted ethnographic research on processes of decision-making in the NHS. https://www.kingston.ac.uk/staff/profile/dr-melania-calestani-871/.

Mahati Chittem is an Associate Professor of Health and Medical Psychology in the Department of Liberal Arts at the Indian Institute of Technology Hyderabad (IITH), Hyderabad, India. Her research interests lie in chronic disease management, including doctor–patient–family communication, end-of-life decision-making, and adherence to doctors' recommendations, and in cultural contexts of health behaviours, primarily diet, exercise and sex.

Setiyani Marta Dewi is a sexual and reproductive health (SRH) practitioner with 12 years of experience in SRH education and service provision for vulnerable populations including female sex workers, street youth, LGBTQI+ individuals and school-based adolescents in Indonesia.

Elżbieta Drążkiewicz is a Senior Research Fellow at the Slovak Academy of Sciences, and specialises in organisational, political and economic anthropology. Her research includes studies of foreign aid and development management, public health governance and education systems. She is an author of *Institutionalised Dreams: The art of managing foreign aid*.

Soraya Fleischer is a Professor in the Department of Anthropology, University of Brasília, Brazil, currently studying the aftermath of the Zika epidemic in northeast Brazil. She hosts Mundaréu (https://mundareu.labjor.unicamp.br), a podcast aimed at bringing anthropology to a wider public. http://lattes.cnpq.br/4854939558671572.

Claudia Fonseca is Professor of Anthropology at the Federal University of Rio Grande do Sul, Brazil. She has conducted research on leprosy, including questions of care, patient activism, stigma and deficiency. She is presently engaged with lower-income urban families, examining the interaction between community, kin networks and public policies for the care of dependent members of the household.

Jennie Gamlin is Associate Professor at the UCL Institute for Global Health and deputy director of the Centre for Gender and Global Health. She teaches Critical Anthropology of Global Health and Gender and Global Health. Jennie's current research explores the coloniality of gender and maternal health in Mexican Wixárika communities. She has lived and worked in Mexico for extended periods. https://iris.ucl.ac.uk/iris/browse/profile?upi=JBGAM46.

Surekha Garimella is a Senior Research Fellow leading the Accountability for Informal Urban Equity Hub (ARISE) at The George Institute for Global Health India (TGI). Her interdisciplinary background is in nutrition, applied economics and public health; her present research includes gendered health systems, ethics of research practice, political economy and accountability.

Hanna Garth is a sociocultural and medical anthropologist at Princeton University, specialising in the anthropology of food. Her work addresses issues of inequality and structural violence, with regional interests in Latin America, the Caribbean and the United States. She is the author of *Food in*

Cuba: The pursuit of a decent meal, and co-editor of *Black Food Matters: Racial justice in the wake of food justice*. http://www.hannagarth.com.

Sahra Gibbon is Associate Professor of Medical Anthropology in the Anthropology Department at UCL, convenor and founder of the programme in Biosocial Medical Anthropology at UCL, and co-editor with Jennie Gamlin of the 'Embodied Inequalities' book series with UCL Press. She has carried out research in the UK, Cuba and Brazil examining the interface between genomics, public health and inequalities. https://www.ucl.ac.uk/anthropology/people/academic-and-teaching-staff/sahra-gibbon.

Tsipy Ivry is Senior Lecturer and Chair of the graduate programme in medical and psychological anthropology in the Anthropology Department, University of Haifa. She is author of a comparative ethnography, *Embodying Culture: Pregnancy in Japan and Israel* (2010). Since 2006, she has studied the intersections of religion and reproductive biomedicine, and most recently, pregnancy and childbirth following the 11 March 2011 disasters in Eastern Japan. https://sites.google.com/hevra.haifa.ac.il/tsipy-ivry/home.

Selima Kabir is an Assistant Research Coordinator at the BRAC School of Public Health, BRAC University, Bangladesh, where she uses her different skills at work in collaboration with her passion for anthropological research. She is overseeing a project on Gender and COVID-19, and has experience working on gender, sexual and reproductive health and migration.

Natasja Kingod is a Postdoctoral Researcher at the Steno Diabetes Center in Copenhagen, Denmark. Her research focuses on diabetes self-management, patient knowledge, praxiography and online and offline peer-to-peer support in Denmark.

Gideon Lasco is a Senior Lecturer at the University of the Philippines Diliman's Department of Anthropology and Research Fellow at the Ateneo de Manila University's Development Studies Program. He obtained his medical (MD) and master's degrees (MSc in Medical Anthropology) from the University of the Philippines and his PhD from the University of Amsterdam. His research interests include contemporary issues including the drug wars in Asia and the COVID-19 pandemic.

Sofie Rosenlund Lau is a social pharmacist, whose doctoral dissertation concerned the routinisation of cholesterol-lowering medicines for the prevention of cardiovascular disease in Denmark. She is a Postdoctoral Researcher at the Center for Research and Education in General Medicine,

University of Copenhagen, and is examining the reasons for and consequences of the massive use of pharmaceuticals among frail seniors.

Susan Levine is Associate Professor of Anthropology in the School of African and Gender Studies, Anthropology and Linguistics, University of Cape Town. Her research interests include critical pedagogy, child labour and child health, and she is the author of *Children of a Bitter Harvest: Child labour in the Cape winelands* (2013).

Lenore Manderson is Distinguished Professor of Public Health and Medical Anthropology in the School of Public Health, University of the Witwatersrand, South Africa, and holds appointments also with Brown University, US, and Monash University, Australia. Her current work on inequality includes a major study of the complexity of informal caregiving for Alzheimer's disease and related dementias in rural South Africa. http://www.lenoremanderson.com.

Rebecca Marsland is a Senior Lecturer in Social Anthropology at the University of Edinburgh. She has carried out research on malaria, HIV/AIDS and funerals in Tanzania. She is currently combining medical anthropology with multispecies ethnography to think about insect health and veterinary medicine.

Shrutika Murthy is a research assistant at The George Institute for Global Health India (TGI), and works in the Accountability for Informal Urban Equity Hub (ARISE). Her work and research interests revolve around issues pertaining to caste, gender, urban poverty and health systems and policy.

Haripriya Narasimhan is an anthropologist and Associate Professor in the Department of Liberal Arts, IIT Hyderabad, India. She is currently involved in two independent research projects that look at the world of Hindi television soap operas, and the discourse on diabetes. She has fieldwork experience in Tamilnadu and Mumbai, Maharashtra.

Ato Kwamena Onoma is a Senior Program Officer at the Council for the Development of Social Science Research in Africa (CODESRIA) and author of *The Politics of Property Rights Institutions in Africa* (2009) and *Anti-Refugee Violence and African Politics* (2013). His current work explores mobility, belonging and intercommunal relations in Africa primarily through the prisms of epidemics and interment practices.

Kim Ozano is a social scientist working in the Accountability for Informal Urban Equity Hub (ARISE) at the Liverpool School of Tropical Medicine. Her research focusses on participatory paradigms, health inequity, inclusion and health systems strengthening. She is currently working on generating quality criteria for participatory action research approaches that aim to strengthen health systems.

Cristina A. Pop is an Assistant Professor of Medical Anthropology and Medical Humanities at Creighton University, Nebraska. Her research interests are reproductive health and healthcare, vaccination anxieties, post-communist transformations and discourse analysis. She is currently working on a book about cervical cancer in Romania.

Pooja Purang is a Professor of Psychology at the Department of Humanities and Social Sciences, Indian Institute of Technology, Bombay. Her areas of research include organisational justice, culture, diversity and gender-related issues in the workplace.

Ivo Quaranta is Professor of Cultural and Medical Anthropology at the University of Bologna, where he is current director of the Centre for International and Intercultural Health. His main interests focus on the analysis of the social production of suffering and the cultural elaboration of illness experience; he has worked in northwest Cameroon, the UK and Italy.

Sabina Faiz Rashid is Dean and Professor at the BRAC School of Public Health, BRAC University. A medical anthropologist by training, she has over 25 years of work experience in Bangladesh. Her areas of expertise are ethnographic and qualitative research, with a focus on urban populations, adolescents and marginalised groups. She is particularly interested in examining the impact of structural and social factors on the ability of these populations to realise their health and rights.

Abril Saldaña-Tejeda is Associate Professor of Sociology at the Department of Philosophy, Universidad de Guanajuato, Mexico, and focuses on the social determinants of health, genomics and postgenomics. She is currently exploring bioethical principles, practices and regulations on human genome editing and stem cell research in Latin America.

Sarah Segal-Katz is a certified Halachic instructor from Beit Morasha. She holds an MA in Jewish Philosophy and Kabbalah from Revivim Honors program in Jewish Studies at the Hebrew University. Segal-Katz is an activist in the fields of feminism, religion and state, currently taking part in an appeal to the High Court of Justice regarding women's right to take state rabbinical exams. She is founder of Gluya Center. https://sarahsegalkatz.com/

Aisha Siddika has a master's in Gender Studies and worked at the BRAC School of Public Health, BRAC University for one year (2019–2020).

Elisa J. Sobo is Professor and Chair of Anthropology, San Diego State University. Her recent work concerns parents' use of cannabis-based therapies for children with intractable epilepsy, ethnomedical understandings about healthy child development in relation to alternative education and paediatric vaccination. She is currently part of a nationwide participatory action research initiative focused on community-based capacity building for an equitable and effective COVID-19 vaccination rollout.

Marie Kofod Svensson is a Postdoctoral Research Fellow at the Danish Heart Association. Her doctoral research was on how children and their families in Denmark experience life following diagnosis of congenital heart disease (CHD). In her current research, she is exploring how couples experience prenatal screening for congenital heart disease.

Sally Theobald has a Chair in Social Science and International Health at the Liverpool School of Tropical Medicine, and a background of geography and development studies. Her research focuses on gender, health, and health systems strengthening in different contexts, including in fragility and in informal urban settlements, in Africa and Asia. Sally is PI for the GCRF Accountability for Informal Urban Equity Hub (ARISE).

Rachel Tolhurst is a Reader at the Liverpool School of Tropical Medicine and Research Director of the GCRF Accountability for Informal Urban Equity Hub (ARISE). Her research interests centre on social drivers of inequities in health and wellbeing, including intersections between gender equity, poverty and disability.

Cecilia Vindrola-Padros is a medical anthropologist interested in applied health research and the development of rapid approaches to research. She co-directs the Rapid Research Evaluation and Appraisal Lab (RREAL) with Ginger Johnson, works as a Senior Research Fellow in the Department of Targeted Intervention, University College London, and is a Social Scientist at the NIAA Health Services Research Centre (HSRC), Royal College of Anaesthetists (RCoA).

Ayo Wahlberg is Professor MSO at the Department of Anthropology, University of Copenhagen. His research has focused on reproductive and genetic technologies (in China and Denmark), traditional herbal medicine (in Vietnam and the United Kingdom) and health. He currently leads a five-year European Research Council (2015–2020) project 'The Vitality of Disease'.

Lana Whittaker is a Postdoctoral Research Associate, working in the GCRF Accountability for Informal Urban Equity Hub (ARISE) at the Liverpool School of Tropical Medicine. She is a human geographer, whose research focusses on inequality, poverty and food insecurity, and the interventions and policies that seek to address these issues.

Acknowledgements

In the early months of 2020, the SARS-CoV-2 virus spread from Wuhan to Tehran, Islamabad, Milan, Madrid, New York, New Delhi, Johannesburg and Rio de Janeiro. Within weeks, lockdowns and border closures had been strictly enforced. It soon became evident that the COVID-19 pandemic was impacting especially those who were already living precarious lives. As medical anthropologists based in South Africa and Australia, the US West coast and Denmark, respectively, we were captivated by this unfolding and its impact, and the value to us, in sense-making, of our own knowledge of anthropology. We reached out to our colleagues throughout the world with a call for anthropologies of urgency: the results of this outreach are found in the chapters in *Viral Loads*. We are grateful to all contributors who responded unreservedly and worked so meticulously on their chapters through the very difficult months of 2020, juggling caring duties at home, work, home-schooling and sometimes health crises with their commitment to the people and places with whom they have been ethnographically engaged for years. The results are a testament to their scholarship and provide important ethnographic accounts and compelling analyses of the disturbing effects of the pandemic.

We would like to thank Sahra Gibbon and Jennie Gamlin, editors of the series 'Embodying Inequalities: Perspectives from Medical Anthropology' at UCL Press, for welcoming our call to mobilise medical anthropologists and for working with us to sharpen our vision and objectives. We thank too very much our editor at the press, Chris Penfold, for steadfastly guiding us through peer review and subsequent production, helping us ensure the quality and relevance of *Viral Loads*. Likewise, we would like to thank our production team, Jaimee Biggins, Melody Dawes and Linda Mellor, for expeditiously bringing *Viral Loads* to print. And we thank Margaret Ramsay for her superb indexing skills.

Viral Loads has truly been a cross-continental effort. Taking turns to stay up late or rise early, we Zoomed across three, roughly equidistant world time zones in California, Melbourne and Copenhagen. In realising this book, Ayo Wahlberg would like to thank colleagues at the Department of Anthropology, University of Copenhagen, all of whom have been engaged in efforts to ethnographically examine the many consequences of COVID-19. Ayo would like to acknowledge the European Research Council project 'The Vitality of Disease – Quality of Life in the Making' (grant no. ERC-2014-STG-639275), as the Viral Loads project ended up becoming a crucial part of the intellectual work that this project aimed for. Nancy Burke would like to thank Raul Fernandez for raising questions that led to this work; Niurca Acosta Hernández, Xiomara Hernández Pérez and Elba Capote for their keen insights; and colleagues at the University of California, Merced, for their intellectual community. Lenore Manderson thanks the radio, TV and press journalists who early engaged her to reflect on the pandemic as it came to be; and her colleagues at the University of the Witwatersrand, Johannesburg, and friends throughout South Africa, the US and Australia, whose accounts of the effects of COVID-19 were a reminder of the tragedy to which we were witness.

1
Introduction

Stratified livability and pandemic effects

Ayo Wahlberg, Nancy J. Burke
and Lenore Manderson

On the streets of Mumbai, in the favelas of Rio de Janeiro, in South Africa's informal settlements and in overflowing hospital corridors in Milan, Madrid and New York, the unfolding COVID-19 pandemic and efforts to 'flatten the curve' laid bare and amplified, viscerally, failures of government and healthcare governance. The pandemic exposed gross variations in access to healthcare, and showed glaring disregard for the lives of the majority of people, deeply rooted inequalities and uneven co-morbidities. Thriving on human sociality, commensality and intimacy, the SARS-CoV-2 virus raced through a globally connected world, disproportionately infecting those compelled to live and work in constricted conditions. Laboratories around the world hurried to understand how this virulence might be stopped – to develop treatments to inhibit COVID-19's potentially life-threatening progression, and to develop vaccines to prevent transmission and further infection. As we write in February 2021, vaccines are being rolled out. Even so, questions of production and distribution globally have yet to be resolved, not least in less-resourced parts of the world, and for those most vulnerable among 'frontline' workers, those living without legal documentation and those with limited or no rights to healthcare. Meanwhile, morbidity and mortality continued to rise at a staggering pace in the second wave, with hospitals in Los Angeles, Stockholm, London, Manaus and Lisbon teetering. The only strategy for most governments, when coronavirus surfaced in humans in late 2019 and throughout 2020, was for individuals to be compelled and responsibilised to do their part: stay at home, maintain physical distance, wash their hands and self-quarantine. The first months of 2021 suggest that this will likely remain the primary strategy of control among most populations.

The exhortatory measures of preventive action and isolation had little regard for the limits to the capacity of many people to 'shelter in place', observe hand hygiene and ensure physical distancing. As numerous anthropologists and others have insisted (Iskander 2020, 1, 15; Kochhar 2020), these are luxuries of the few in a grossly uneven world where millions live on the streets, in crowded quarters, without adequate water and sanitation, making do. Further, people already living with (multiple) chronic illnesses – the so-called 'underlying conditions' of COVID-19 – have been asked by health authorities to take extra care by self-isolating, again with little regard for their ability to do so, not least because such chronic conditions disproportionately affect those who are least well off (Manderson and Wahlberg 2020), and the accumulation of chronic conditions places increasing economic pressure on them (Manderson and Warren 2016). As the first year closed, the effects of the pandemic and of efforts to contain it continued to be unevenly experienced in racialised, disabling and discriminatory ways. As contributing authors in this volume demonstrate, the COVID-19 pandemic loaded onto already existing socio-economic inequalities, racial discrimination and uneven access to healthcare, exacerbating what we call *stratified livability*. Exigent temporalities have laid bare and amplified disadvantage. These reverberations across disease risk, control, containment and care call for anthropologies of urgency.

Over the past few decades, anthropologists have shown how epidemics of HIV/AIDS, SARS, H1N1 influenza, cholera and Ebola are all 'mirrors held up to society' (Lindenbaum 2001, 380). These are seen to follow and produce 'cycles of shame and blame, stigmatising discourses, isolation of the sick, fear of contagion, and end-of-the-world scenarios' (Herring and Swedlund 2010, 4), as 'an "outbreak narrative" is often pushed by international agencies and governments in northern settings' (Leach et al. 2010, 371). At the same time, Charles Briggs has illustrated how communicability itself is infectious, with narratives of epidemics that typically naturalise socio-economic, racial and sexual inequalities 'as if bacteria and viruses gravitate toward populations and respect social boundaries' (2005, 274). Through the designation of 'risk groups', representations of epidemics are transformed into self-knowledge and self-regulation while also intensifying stigmatisation and discrimination. Most recently, in *The Anthropology of Epidemics*, Ann Kelly, Frédéric Keck and Christos Lynteris have argued that:

as a mode of constitution of social life that has been cast anew by recent conceptions of virality, information, and communication … epidemics necessitate not simply the study of the disease itself and the way it affects social relations, but also the study of its modes of anticipation, visualisation, fictionalisation, and materialisation (2019, 1, 15).

In *Viral Loads*, we draw on such anthropological insights and ethnographic evidence gleaned from other diseases, conditions and times, and use this archive to illuminate the circumstances and effects of COVID-19. This is the anthropology of urgency. Anthropologists have the responsibility to bring knowledge of other infections and other disasters, structures and systems, to anticipate and interpret responses to the pandemic. At the same time, we carry a responsibility to chronicle such viral loads and their social impact (Herring and Swedlund 2010; Kelly et al. 2019). This is not ethnography conducted in haste as an alternative to the slow research that is a hallmark of our discipline (Adams et al. 2014), although rapid ethnographic assessment surely has its place in times of crisis. Nor is it a pathography of the disease itself (MacPhail 2015). Rather, as we analyse the particularities of this novel coronavirus and the social and political responses that it has elicited, our prior work and long-term engagements shape our interpretive lens.

On 3 April 2020, in the *Financial Times*, Arundhati Roy (2020) argued that '(h)istorically, pandemics have forced humans to break with the past and imagine their world anew. This one is no different. It is a portal, a gateway between one world and the next'. In this volume, we illustrate how COVID-19 serves as a portal to rethink and reimagine health and medical care, health systems and welfare throughout the world. It is also a portal to rethink the structures, systems and ideologies that shape health and wellbeing. Like those involved in the front line of social movements in 2020, we attend to the social and racialised unevenness and gross economic disparities exposed in the uneven distribution of illness and death, and in the limits of global and local responses to the pandemic. The pandemic demands that we revisit and sharpen our understandings of state power, public health and citizenship. COVID-19, like any disease, is a social and political as well as a biological fact, grinding against the lived realities of everyday life. Its examination is a launching pad to draw out how any disease is implicated in and might impact on social life.

In *Viral Loads*, the contributing authors mobilise anthropological concepts to analyse how these developments interrupt daily lives, state infrastructures and healthcare systems, and, in turn, how these structures, systems and everyday flows shape the course of the pandemic. This interplay of biology and society finds form on all continents. COVID-19 instantiates anthropological theory and layers our evidence base. In *Viral Loads*, we illustrate how the COVID-19 pandemic has exposed the stratified livability that medical, social and cultural anthropologists have ethnographically documented over decades.

Lockdown: the power of the state

In Part I of this volume, 'The power of the state', we begin by considering institutionalised and governmental responses to the pandemic as it gained momentum and took shape and form throughout 2020. People looked to the state for quick intervention as health crises unfolded, even if they were surprised and sometimes resistant to the crude measures available. Countries faced the deadly combination of a highly contagious 'stealth' virus, host populations with no immunity, decades of austerity, the neglect of healthcare systems and an all too obvious lack of 'preparedness' (Benton and Dionne 2015; Caduff 2015; Lakoff 2017). With this toxic mix, governments worldwide drew on nineteenth-century tactics of infection control to contain infection and head off its exponential transmission. Nation-states and the power structures within them mandated curfews and lockdowns, closed borders, and tested and quarantined people in more or less coercive and authoritarian ways. Within six months, over half the world's population was affected by restrictions of movement, checking both global and local flows of goods and populations. Physical distancing requirements and self-isolation recommendations halted the habitual busyness of everyday life. Flights were grounded, stay-at-home measures were enforced, movement in public spaces was limited. The capacity to maintain these measures fluctuated, in some cases, monitored through digital technology, a viral network to ensure viral containment. Countries like Vietnam and Finland managed to keep infection rates low by enforcing lockdown and responding to localised outbreaks, but more widely, nation-states responded to the economic, political and human costs of the virus very differently. In countries like Brazil and the US, where political leaders downplayed and even dismissed coronavirus, rates soared early; through to the end of 2020, they continued to do so.

Box 1 COVID-19: a timeline

- Late December 2019: Doctors in Wuhan, capital of China's Hubei province, raise concerns about a SARS-like virus in patients presenting with pneumonia symptoms and are initially censured by State authorities.
- 7 January 2020: Chinese health authorities rule out SARS and race to subtype what media are calling a 'mystery virus'.
- 12 January: WHO confirms that 'a new type of coronavirus (novel coronavirus, nCoV)' has been identified.
- 23 January: Wuhan city goes into lockdown, closing airports, train stations and highways in an effort to contain the outbreak, but hundreds of thousands of people had already fled the city by air, rail and road. International air travel out of Wuhan becomes a key pandemic vector.
- 3 February: Built in 10 days, Huoshenshan Hospital opens for coronavirus patients to alleviate overwhelmed hospitals in Wuhan city.
- 11 February: The International Committee on Taxonomy of Viruses (ICTV) names the novel coronavirus 'severe acute respiratory syndrome coronavirus 2 (SARS-CoV-2)', which the WHO promptly shortens to 'COVID-19'.
- 9 March: Doctors in Bergamo, part of Italy's northern Lombardy region, warn of overwhelmed hospitals and critical shortages in personal protective equipment, leading Prime Minister Giuseppe Conte to impose a national quarantine. A week later, military trucks are filmed moving coffins from Bergamo to neighbouring provinces.
- 10 March: Schools are closed down in Iran, which has become a COVID-19 epicentre, as hospitals are overwhelmed and numerous senior government officials fall ill.
- 11–23 March: European countries follow suit announcing lockdowns and/or restrictions: Denmark (11 March), Spain (14 March), France (17 March), Germany (22 March), UK (23 March).
- 23 March: President Cyril Ramaphosa of South Africa announces a 21-day lockdown which would be enforced by the military, disproportionately impacting those living in informal settlements.
- 24 March: Prime Minister Narendra Modi announces a complete lockdown in India, leading to frantic scenes and protests as

migrant labourers try to return from major cities to their towns of origin.
- 26 March: Under fire for mixed messaging and also downplaying the seriousness of the pandemic, UK Prime Minister Boris Johnson tests positive for COVID-19, eventually requiring intensive care before recovering.
- Early April: New York becomes the first epicentre of the US as the city runs out of respirators and personal protection equipment, leading to tensions between governor Andrew Cuomo and the Federal Government as President Donald Trump downplays the virus. Field hospital units are set up in parks and refrigeration trucks are brought in to store bodies.
- April: In Ecuador and Peru, bodies pile up in hospital corridors and on streets as healthcare officials struggle to keep up with the pandemic.
- End April: Brazil becomes Latin America's epicentre as hospitals are overwhelmed and mass graves are dug to cope with the growing numbers of dead. Meanwhile, President Jair Bolsonaro insists that COVID-19 is a minor disease.
- May–June: Throughout the world (US, Germany, Qatar, Singapore and more) workers in meat plants and other factories with cramped working and dormitory living conditions are exposed to COVID-19 through workplace outbreaks.
- 8 July: President Jair Bolsonaro of Brazil tests positive for COVID-19 while continuing to deny the seriousness of the pandemic as Brazil sees infection and mortality rates soar.
- 20 July: Researchers at the University of Oxford report that a vaccine they are developing has triggered an immune response in 1,000 test persons.
- 2 October: President Donald Trump of the US tests positive for COVID-19 and is transported from the White House to the Walter Reed National Military Medical Center for treatment.
- 9 November: Pfizer and BioNTech announce by press release that the mRNA vaccine they have been developing 'was found to be more than 90 per cent effective in preventing COVID-19' in Phase 3 trial participants.
- 8 December: 90-year-old Margaret Keenan from Coventry in the UK becomes first person to receive a vaccine for COVID-19 outside of trials.

- 15 December: The US surpasses 300,000 deaths from COVID-19 as a surge in infections following Thanksgiving holiday gatherings takes hold, while Brazil with the second largest tally of deaths surpasses 180,000. Hospitals throughout the world struggle to keep up with the 'second wave' and countries close borders in attempts to contain new viral strains.
- 31 January: Globally, the reported number of infections was close to 108 million, and the death toll directly associated with COVID-19 had reached 2.1 million. Hospitals in the US, Sweden, the UK, Brazil, Japan and Portugal struggled to keep up with a 'second wave' of patients.

Restrictive measures were near universally applied; these tended to reinforce existing spatial inequalities. In many countries, the rich were able to 'escape' to their holiday cottages, and middle-class workers juggled home-schooling responsibilities while setting up home offices in their living rooms. But so-called 'essential workers', often living in dense city quarters, continued to work so that supermarkets and convenience stores were open and home delivery available. Others – living on the fringes of cities, in mobile homes and shelters, and on the streets – continued working to maintain basic services – street cleaning, garbage collection, and cleaning hospitals and hotels. Still others worked in unsafe yet essential industries, including meat packing plants, which became super spreader sites (Shultz 2020; Zhou 2020). Spatial inequality, characteristic of cities worldwide, meant that those already disadvantaged and discriminated were at much greater risk of exposure to COVID-19. Low income, precarious employment and, for many, the challenges associated with 'illegal status', further compromised their access care. These people were also least able to take time off work to care for themselves and avoid infecting others, and were at greatest risk of severe symptoms, sequelae and death.

As a twenty-first-century pandemic, COVID-19 was shaped by and is shaping contemporary social life, through forms of virtual communication, global and regional political economies, the shifting nature of nation-states, and the role of governments and supragovernment entities. In the first substantive chapter of *Viral Loads*, Nancy J. Burke describes how an app, Pesquisador Virtual, was designed and introduced by the Universidad de las Ciencias Informáticas, with the Ministerio de

Salud (MINSAP) of Cuba, to provide real-time identification of people symptomatic of COVID-19. The app served as a tool in the country's arsenal against infection, along with brigades of physicians and medical students going door-to-door to screen residents, population-based testing, school and border closures, and mask-wearing enforced through fines. These interventions were largely adapted from prior effective efforts in controlling infectious disease (Whiteford 2000); the app enhanced rather than displaced them. Meanwhile, as across the globe, new WhatsApp groups began to promote food delivery for a fee, although in Cuba restaurants also brought food to elderly residents for free. Nancy J. Burke describes the systems of surveillance and governance enacted by the Cuban state under the guise of care – along with official recognition of tension between public health measures and cultural practices – and creative moves among individuals and groups to support each other while earning incomes as tourist revenue receded. These practices could coexist as a result of Cuba's particular form of post-Soviet socialism; their intersections suggest one way in which care was produced and enacted during the pandemic as in other crises, in the context of geopolitical isolation. Even so, as several authors illustrate, these responses were not atypical nor limited to a particular ideology or system of government. Everywhere, people adapted to the convergence of seeming totalitarian control with extraordinary kindness and expressions of solidarity.

Stringent lockdowns early in the pandemic were enforced in other countries too, including South Africa, India and Bangladesh, as we illustrate. Maintaining or reinstating total lockdowns became near impossible, however, given the devastating socio-economic and personal consequences of these measures for most people. Responding to the emerging direct costs of lockdown, restrictions often loosened – but too early, only to be tightened again regionally or nationally when spikes of new infections occurred. The Australian city of Melbourne was one of the few able to reinstate and – for three months – sustain harsh lockdown to virtually eliminate all community transmission.

Viral transmission escalated rapidly in early 2020, in Wuhan, Lombardy, Madrid and throughout the US, notably New York. This fuelled a sense of urgency. Field hospitals were erected in parks and convention centres were converted; military vehicles were requisitioned to transport corpses; and political messaging centred on the metrics of COVID's spread and toll. Public health campaigns rolled out to exhort people to physically distance, wash hands, wear masks, cough into elbows, monitor symptoms, self-isolate and quarantine. Posters reiterating these messages were plastered across cities. Plexiglass shields were introduced into shops and public institutions, and, with symbolic payoff as much as protection against infection, between drivers and pillion riders on motorcycles in Indonesia, the Philippines and Vietnam. Distancing lines and standing spots were painted on footpaths to organise queuing. Home living rooms and kitchen tables were turned into offices where possible. And, as we have already noted, so-called 'essential services' continued, such that people in the lowest-paying jobs remained at risk – cleaners, couriers, rickshaw drivers, bus drivers, fast food eatery staff, food production workers and more (see Chapter 15 by Rashid and colleagues, and Garimella and colleagues, Chapter 11). It is still too early for the epidemiological data to demonstrate the price of this segregation between those who serve and those able to continue to live within bubbles of protection (Manderson and Veracini 2020).

Additional limitations on movement to contain viral spread slowed the return of citizens living abroad. Governments grappled with imported cases, from Italian tourists in Cuba to returning citizens in Senegal (see Onoma, Chapter 10), then the inevitable shift to community spread. Such measures to control contagion exacerbated the economic effects of the pandemic for those most precariously employed. From street peddlers in Bangladesh to bed and breakfast entrepreneurs in Havana, the lack of access to potential customers has had devasting effects, increasing hunger, indebtedness and fear. Countries like Australia and New Zealand, because they are islands, simply closed their border to outsiders to the cost of the travel and tourism industries. At the same time, the seeping of infection into the community as a result of breaches in infection control from quarantine hotels, via security guards and cleaning staff, highlighted as vectors of disease not returning citizens but the marginalised workers charged with containing them. Border control shifted in Australia from nation to individual states, as the military moved in to prevent people from crossing state boundaries. Lockdown contained and controlled populations, overriding modes of everyday living that for many, until then, had operated across borders for medical care, education, employment and family connections (Ormond and Lunt 2020; Whittaker et al. 2010). While the tensions and personal costs of containment were patent in some countries, the to and fro across borders elsewhere slipped past, or continued to warrant levels of militarisation that predated COVID-19 (De León 2015). COVID-19 opened up questions of the role of the state in caring for citizens, in contrast to the lesser regard of stateless people, those living marginal lives (and marginalised experiences of COVID-19) and those who, because of their pathways of mobility, were not even in the record.

As suggested above, lockdown measures were often enforced not by virtual technology, but by deploying troops, in ways reminiscent of population containment during other wars on infection – Ebola is the most recent – and wars against populations and political interests (Benton and Dionne 2015; Lynteris and Poleykett 2018). Viruses are micro-guerrillas, moving across surfaces and from person to person with stealth and subterfuge, and militarisation was (and is) always about containing populations. Microbes are less easily contained.

In Chapter 3, Lenore Manderson and Susan Levine describe South Africa's early and temporary success to contain transmission through stringent lockdown, enforced by police, defence troops and private security employees. Soldiers in camouflage and masks strong-armed homeless residents into camps and broke into homes in informal settlements, brandishing arms to threaten and kill particular citizens; they patrolled shopping malls and apprehended those escaping to beaches and parkland. Drawing on technologies that had been the hallmark of apartheid, South Africa effected lockdown with relatively little violence and resistance. Under apartheid, citizens were brutalised by house arrests, curfews, detention, torture and imprisonment. But with a backdrop of chronic and systemic poverty, the massification of debility through TB and HIV/AIDS, and a robust public health infrastructure for coping with chronic disease, the country largely accommodated rules around lockdown and its militant surveillance, and the racial inflections of social hierarchy contained in their imposition. In South Africa, political authority was sufficiently robust to remain unchallenged even while COVID-19 deepened poverty, unemployment and hunger. Viral spread eventually outran the measures to contain it.

South Africa was only one of many countries to introduce lockdown through emergency regulations, enabling law enforcement as if it were wartime. In countries like Malaysia and South Korea too, lockdown, isolation and quarantine were presented as necessary measures and military personnel ensured their strict adherence. Elsewhere, as in Italy, the earliest days of self-isolation were novel and anxiously romanticised, with social media busy with clips of balcony concerts to rally public support and confidence; this technology of support was echoed in various ways, including in the UK, and as Aditya Bharadwaj describes in this volume, in India. At the same time, individuals and collectivities flayed the World Health Organization and United Nations and found in the spread of the virus proof of 'deep state' conspiracy. In Chapter 4, Elisa J. Sobo and Elżbieta Drążkiewicz take on this tendency toward conspiracy, and the emergence of collectives of seemingly incongruous groups purporting conspiracy theories in the face of public health challenges. They contend that such conspiracy theories serve as powerful tools to express the tensions that arise between governance and freedom as individual rights are pitted against state-defined visions of the public good.

Exclusion, blame and consequence

Public responses to coronavirus took their cues from other viral outbreaks and illnesses in the late twentieth and first decades of the twenty-first century: HIV and AIDS, SARS-CoV-1, MERS, dengue, H1N1 (swine flu), Ebola and Zika (MacPhail 2015; Mason 2016; Niehaus and Jonsson 2005; Williamson 2018). Scapegoating and increasing vitriol were directed at governments, populations and communities associated with likely spread of infection; to countries perceived as central to the pandemic (notably China); and to questions of capacity to case find, prevent and contain.

In Part II of the volume, 'Exclusion and blame', we attend to the familiar ways in which the pandemic kindled scapegoating and conspiracy theories, rumour, blame and stigma. Medical anthropologists have documented at length the stigmatising power of infection, most markedly in relation to HIV and AIDS, as viral spread was threaded into other stigmatising identities, affiliations and activities – same-sex relationships, injecting drug use, sex work and place (Parker and Aggleton 2003; Patton 1991; Rhodes et al. 2005). The stigma of these alliances flowed to other identities linked to HIV infection, such that haemophilia and particular ethnicities were also initially subject to powerful discourses of blame. COVID-19 has been spared considerable stigma because its spread, airborne, was less predictable and unassociated with perceived breaches in morality. Even so, as the pandemic unfolded, we have witnessed scapegoating towards populations who have long been subject to discrimination.

COVID-19 brought to the surface the ways in which global inequality is welded into the colonial past, underpinning racist regimes in the present. Being Black quickly proved to be the best predictor of infection and death from COVID-19 in countries like the US and UK. Being a person of colour otherwise was weighted to risk of infection and poor outcome, with this in turn tied to poverty, unemployment, food and housing insecurities, chronic disease and comorbidities. Exposing these links between the social and the biological, anthropologists have drawn on and foregrounded decades of work on structural violence, structural vulnerability, syndemics and comorbidity, as well as colonialism, neocolonialism, globalisation and their ugly legacies (Farmer 2001; Fassin 2007). But in 2020 there was a global eruption of outrage against racism, and COVID-19 spurred the Black Lives Matter movement against institutionalised and personalised racism, and propelled insistence on transformation. Hanna Garth makes this personal for us all. In her account of outrage in Los Angeles following George Floyd's murder on 25 May, Garth brings structural violence to the fore: not just because of the concurrence of protests against violence and COVID-19 but because the pandemic illustrated how racism determines health outcomes. Some of the most striking mass-mediated images from 2020 were of mask-wearing protestors on the streets in various cities in the US, at a time where COVID-19 was disproportionately lethal for people of colour. COVID-19 might have been less virulent in the US had there been less violence, structural and literal, from racism.

At the societal level, everywhere, viral loads are disproportionately shouldered by the disadvantaged and discriminated. Jennie Gamlin, Sahra Gibbon and Melania Calestani in their chapter explore how legacies of colonialism in the UK are experienced in populations placed in high exposure roles as frontline health and social care providers. The naming of these 'essential workers' ensuring food, amenities and care as BAME (Black, Asian and Minority Ethnic) highlights the 'nostalgic nationalism' underlying pandemic preparedness and public health response. Gamlin and colleagues connect the roles of EU migrants, caring for the ill and dying, with ongoing isolationism arising in post-Brexit UK. The government's refusal of EU offers of personal protective equipment for these caregivers, for example, left many unsafe and contributed to the overrepresentation of Black and ethnic minority populations in coronavirus death toll figures, again highlighting the continuity of present inequalities to colonialism and its racial hierarchies.

Writing on the forms of discrimination that Dalit groups endured as the pandemic unfolded in India, Aditya Bharadwaj introduces the figure of the 'shroud stealer' from the writings of twentieth-century poet and scholar Ahmed Ali, as an allegory for caste-based violence and inequality. He discusses Dalit activists' observation that the term 'social distancing' as a safety measure simply bled into established upper caste prejudice and practices of 'untouchability'. In this way pandemic responses in India reinforced the dehumanisation of poverty and its stratification. 'Shroud stealers' who dug up graves to recover and resell burial shrouds as part of a macabre economy during the 1918 influenza pandemic, Bharadwaj argues, can help us reflect on the unfolding pandemic, and better apportion responsibility, including our own.

Cristina A. Pop extends an examination of caste and related age-old hierarchies in her analysis of how singling out the Roma in Romania during the H1N1 flu pandemic (2009–10), and a recent measles epidemic (2016–18), help explain Roma reactions to confinement measures during the early months of the COVID-19 pandemic. As Pop shows, Romania's responses brought into public visibility old and new assumptions about the need to purify the 'social body' from 'corruption', 'superstition' and 'civil disobedience', thereby setting the ground for continued discrimination against Roma.

The pandemic has also provided opportunities for publics to question the legitimacy of the state, and for alternative congregations and alliances to test their power against the state. Oğuz Alyanak addresses this in his analysis of the ways Turkey's ruling party, Adalet ve Kalkınma Partisi (Justice and Development Party, AKP), retained its legitimacy despite mounting criticism. Alyanak considers scholarly conversations on moral authority and politics, with a particular emphasis on political Islam, to explain how a moral discourse on COVID-19 (which validated stigma against LGBT communities) enabled new configurations of state power. As he illustrates, the Diyanet, the Turkish religious authority, weighed heavily in conversations on the pandemic during its first phase peak in mid-April, and through this, the AKP was able to divert attention from its own mishandling of the situation. The use of political Islam, however, was a dangerous manoeuvre, for it risked the lives of the very people whom the Turkish state is meant to protect.

Pandemics call into question who falls inside and outside the boundaries of state protection and belonging. Ato Kwamena Onoma takes up questions of boundary maintenance, referencing the scapegoating of Peul migrants from Guinea during the 2013–16 Ebola epidemic to explore current reactions to nationals returning to Senegal. Blame on these returning citizens for the spread of the virus, expressed on radio, social media and in news outlets, Onoma argues, illustrates the limitations of citizenship and the porousness of communal boundaries in public health crises. Tense relations between migrants and home communities informed recent discourses, so demonstrating how configurations of blame are always shaped by particular histories and socio-economic realities.

Unequal burdens

Anthropologists and others have documented how poverty and racial discrimination are always 'underlying conditions' impacting health, healthcare, vulnerability and poor outcomes (Benjamin 2020; Crane and Pascoe 2020). Given how coronavirus spreads, housing and housing conditions emerged as 'hot spot' sites for transmission, so exposing the unequal distribution of space. In India, migrant workers fled their cramped urban living conditions to return home during lockdown, often travelling by foot for hundreds of kilometres. In Singapore, known for its futuristic, modernised cityscapes, the living conditions of thousands of migrant workers came to light as their crowded dormitories turned into transmission hotspots (Kathiravelu 2020). In Melbourne, people in social housing were criminalised with a second wave outbreak on 4 July 2020, stimulating debate on state housing policies. In Cuba, the call to shelter-in-place exposed the precarity of crumbling buildings, whose modifications to create extra rooms to meet the government's commitment to housing for all inhibited airflow in sweltering tropical heat.

The realities of lockdown and threat of COVID-19 infection for those precariously housed and marginalised, as Surekha Garimella, Shrutika Murthy, Lana Whittaker and Rachel Tolhurst illustrate, were experienced as yet another of a series of insults and injuries to body and mind. Garimella and colleagues mobilise the concept of 'debility' to drive home the endemic versus exceptional nature of the pandemic on those who live by waste-picking in India. In controlling COVID-19 and ensuring critical care as needed, resources have been diverted from other public health programmes, patient needs and vulnerable populations. Linda Rae Bennett and Setiyani Marta Dewi illustrate how COVID-19 has amplified pre-existing challenges to sexual and reproductive health and rights, with potential long-term consequences due to interrupted services. They show how a clear 'amplification effect' from COVID-19 and responses to it is discernible in Indonesia and beyond, as everyday lives routinely marked by deprivation of resources, access to healthcare and the denial of human rights, are disproportionally vulnerable to COVID-19.

This cutback and suspension of services, with resources redirected to address urgencies related to COVID-19, occurred widely. Claudia Fonseca and Soraya Fleischer illustrate the impact of COVID-19 on disability support for lower income Brazilians caught in the crossfire of physical or mental disability, poverty and minimal state services. Their focus is on children born with microcephaly and other disabilities associated with maternal infection of the Zika virus in 2015–16. Such childhood disabilities precipitated a range of interventions supporting both individual children and their families. COVID-19 deflected this attention. Yet, as Garimella and colleagues also illustrate for India, COVID-19 was a disaster neither new nor untoward. For populations who are habitually without basic sanitation, steady employment or regular housing, COVID-19 may be just one more misery, or the 'last straw' that cuts off the meagre gains of the past few decades.

In Mexico, the challenge seems less about the diversion of resources and more the strategic amplification of individual blame to obfuscate underlying structural inequalities fuelling pandemic spread. Abril Saldaña-Tejeda details the state's continual attention to individual bodies, diets and genetic make-up that place the responsibility for 'risk', 'vulnerability' and poor outcomes on individuals. Blaming and fat-shaming became a focal point for infection, diverting public attention from structural inequalities to individual bodies and personal (ir)responsibility. Saldaña-Tejeda argues that attention must be given to other forms of vulnerability and 'underlying conditions' such as police brutality, pre-existing negligence and poverty if we are to understand the disproportionate impact of COVID-19 in Mexico.

Sabina Faiz Rashid, Selima Kabir, Kim Ozano, Sally Theobald, Bachera Aktar and Aisha Siddika draw on their collaborative research to describe the devastating impact on vulnerable and impoverished populations of measures to contain COVID-19 in Bangladesh. The nationwide lockdown initiated in Bangladesh in late March shut down public transport, shops and all institutions (education, business, partial government, etc.); millions of informal sector workers (street peddlers, domestic workers, rickshaw drivers, construction workers, day labourers, etc.) lost their only income source. As the authors illustrate, for adolescents and young adults, the pandemic and resultant lockdown magnified pre-existing instability, uncertainty, social suffering and neglect.

The reach of care

Shifts of resources and priorities to address COVID-19 everywhere came at the cost of the already stretched capacity of health systems to diagnose and treat endemic and chronic conditions such as diabetes and heart disease, cancers and malaria. In countries with constrained resources, 'normal capacity' is limited at the best of times, vulnerable to austerity, neoliberalism, countless 'structural adjustment' and global health projects. Here, medicine is unstable, access triaged and care practices improvised on an everyday basis (Livingston 2012; Nguyen 2010; Street 2014).

While lockdowns slowed infection and transmission, they were also used initially to 'buy time' in the context of woeful lack of preparedness. Few places, it turned out, had adequate infection control measures, laboratory services, personal protection equipment, intubators and mechanical ventilators to manage large numbers of acute cases. This was so despite decades of public health warnings, particularly from 2003 (with SARS-CoV-1), and years of multilateral and regional investment to develop and implement local pandemic preparedness plans (Caduff 2015; Sambala and Manderson 2018).

Early efforts were designed to control the pandemic and so avoid overwhelming healthcare systems, as had happened in Wuhan as the novel coronavirus took hold in January 2020. With speed, however, Milan, Bergamo, Madrid, New York and New Delhi were overwhelmed; with the onset of winter in the northern hemisphere, again municipal governments erected tented field hospitals, appropriated other spaces, and (in Europe) sent patients across national borders for hospital care. Everywhere, healthcare systems were overwhelmed by an influx of patients requiring intensive respiratory care, and often had to reprioritise resources in anticipation of such influxes during first, second and third peaks of infection. By January 2021, as the second wave of infection peaked, intensive care unit capacity reached zero percent in major cities in Europe, the US and elsewhere in the Americas, South Africa and increasingly in countries across Asia. Rural hospitals struggled to cope, and everywhere, exhausted healthcare workers struggled, yet again, to locate beds and resources. The necessity of improvisation (Livingston 2012), and the hopelessness of such efforts, was by this time no longer an index of national poverty, and systems in which shortages of supplies and staff are common.

Ellen Block and Cecilia Vindrola-Padros illustrate how healthcare workers in the UK and US grappled with an unknown disease while working with massive shortages of personal protective equipment and, at times, hospital beds and respirators. Forms of triage and improvisation became a daily reality of 'frontline' healthcare workers in European and American cities with surges of critically ill patients. Block and Vindrola-Padros, in demonstrating how healthcare staff worked to adapt to circumstances, overcoming often obdurate bureaucratic obstacles, reinforce what anthropologists have long shown to be the case in situations of (chronic) crisis (Samuelsen 2020; Street 2014; Livingston 2012).

In writing on people living with (multiple) chronic conditions, Sofie Rosenlund Lau, Marie Svensson, Natasja Kingod and Ayo Wahlberg illustrate how established and institutionalised forms of care were abruptly disrupted as resources shifted from welfare services and routine prioritisations of care towards COVID-19. In Denmark, the political decision to 'postpone … all forms of outpatient surveillance of patients with stable illnesses' generated instability and uncertainty, especially for people living with multiple conditions and in need of extensive social support; Fonseca and Fleischer (this volume) also illustrate this for families with children with disabilities in Brazil. Those living with 'underlying conditions' were asked to self-isolate, and the care provided to them in the past was constrained. Care workers warned that isolation would affect people with cognitive decline who could not understand why loved ones had stopped visiting them. Lockdown worsened loneliness that was already a burden, and exposed disease hierarchies within Denmark's universal healthcare system. At the same time, the intervention kept COVID-19 mortality rates low through 2020.

COVID-19 has, in many ways, been the first digital pandemic, although mobile phone coverage and internet connectivity have increased dramatically over the past two decades. Notwithstanding a wide digital divide, for millions of people, digital forms of communication and social media platforms have made it possible for people to work from home, participate in distance learning, shop online to avoid supermarket visits, and socialise and provide care virtually. New technologies such as Zoom and Teams flourished along with established social media such as Facebook and WhatsApp to allow people to connect with colleagues, friends and loved ones. Earvin Charles Cabalquinto and Tanja Ahlin show how media platforms like Google, Facebook and YouTube came to capitalise on 'their moment', partnering with organisations like the WHO to 'promote care at a distance'. These efforts, the authors show, generated 'fantasies of caregiving', allowing multinational social media giants to amplify profits through advertisements and online engagements. Meanwhile, the difficulties and struggles of people whose marginality and vulnerability left them without the social networks, support systems or technologies of care, were largely overlooked.

Haripriya Narasimhan, Mahati Chittem and Pooja Purang show how, in India, living in an extended lockdown of over seven weeks (25 March to 18 May) presented an existential crisis for the middle classes. Worried about getting essential commodities, a highly mediated class struggled with sudden changes in their daily lives. These anxieties were attenuated by coronavirus-related statistics appearing on their mobiles in this highly WhatsApp-ed nation (Agrawal 2018). With the highest number of WhatsApp users in the world, the Indian middle classes constantly chat with family or friends, forward jokes and memes, and participate in serious debates on any number of 'groups'. Narasimhan, Chittem and Purang show how through the circulation of jokes and memes, 'traditional' gender roles in the home were challenged not by globalisation or feminism but by the virus. And while these media satirised the revision of gender roles, they also illustrated how COVID-19 enforced changes as working men and women struggled to find order in upended home and working life.

The challenges of a healthcare system under pressure pre-pandemic, and the opportunities that the crisis afforded to review social conventions, are also addressed in Tsipy Ivry and Sarah Segal-Katz's chapter, this time with pressure from religious authorities. Ivry and Segal-Katz describe how women rabbinic scholars engaged in efforts to raise awareness of the problematic interstices between institutional religious and health services, and in doing so, turned COVID-19 into an opportunity. The pandemic exposed contradictions between public health messages about hygiene and risks of infection, and the mandated use of public ritual bath houses on the cessation of menstrual bleeding. This contradiction at a time of crisis allowed women to reclaim authority in rabbinic debates on intimacy, and highlighted how religious authority overstepped and underperformed in assuring hygienic conditions. In both these examples – of India and the redistribution of domestic labour, and of Israel and halachic laws on purity – the pandemic created opportunities to reflect on the institutionalisation of gender and its inequalities.

Lessons for a future

When global media were still reporting on a 'mystery virus' in Wuhan in January 2020, researchers and conspiracy theorists alike pondered its origins. With the first confirmed cases linked to the Huanan Seafood Market, scientists speculated about how and at which point the novel coronavirus SARS-CoV-2 zoonotically jumped species, and so to the pandemic. Culprits included horseshoe bats and pangolins – species that evoke Mary Douglas's (1966) analysis of anomaly and danger. While some believed the spillover can be pinpointed to the seafood market, others argued that given its 'stealth' nature, COVID-19 was likely already in circulation much earlier. Whatever the origins, COVID-19 intensified global concerns about the effects of humanity's encroachment on ever greater swathes of forest and land. A year on, it continues to provoke reflection.

Rebecca Marsland draws upon her many years of research on malaria in Tanzania to illustrate not only the challenges that epidemics and pandemics create in resource poor settings, but also the complexity of interventions contingent on human/insect separation in contexts better characterised by co-existence. She argues that despite many calls for global solidarity in pandemic times, we are certainly not all 'in it together'. Marsland chronicles how viruses, bacteria and insect/animal vectors intervene in human socialities. As efforts to control malaria have consistently shown, interventions depend on a logic of separation in a world where farming, urbanisation and industrialisation continue to trouble nature/culture boundaries. Marsland makes a strong case for thinking in terms of 'multidemics' rather than the singular experience implied by the term pandemic.

Gideon Lasco carries these ideas into his argument that the coronavirus pandemic has drawn attention to the necessity, for social scientists and other publics, of an ecological, non-anthropocentric view of the world. Noting that humans grapple with microbes, surround themselves with plants and engage with non-human animals, Lasco reflects on the Philippine experience of COVID-19, offering illustrative examples, sketching tentative insights and concluding with a research agenda for future work. Lasco argues that as the pandemic unfolds, we need to ask how humans and non-humans can live together in precarious times. He offers a way forward to think about environments and ecologies, with implications for anthropological teaching, research and practice.

Finally, in their chapter, Chiara Bodini and Ivo Quaranta show how the pandemic drew attention to market-oriented reforms which undermine the capacity of healthcare systems, with attention to Italy as one of the regions outside of China which very early experienced exponential infection rates. The collapse of hospitals in the north of Italy in early 2020 was in some ways not surprising, given cuts during preceding years; in this context, families lost loved ones and were unable to say goodbye to them. Bodini and Quaranta emphasise that future preparedness should not be reduced to maintaining medical supplies and their adequate storage, of sufficient virological testing and contact tracing capacities. They call for a culture of health and healthcare capacity built up around local participatory action. Together, the chapters in this section point to a rethinking of 'preparedness' and 'response', away from a biomedical focus on how to extinguish an outbreak and towards thinking about the building of more resilient and balanced societies.

Past, present, future

Viruses are famously not fully alive; rather 'they verge on life' (Villareal 2004). For decades, virologists have sought to understand the mechanisms by which viruses parasitise host cells in order to multiply and spread. There are thousands of viruses, their pathogenic effects on human hosts range from 'mild flu-like symptoms' to deadly organ failure. The effect of COVID-19 on those who contract it spans this spectrum of severity: extremely virulent for some (especially those who are elderly, those with certain 'underlying medical conditions'); less virulent for others (Wahlberg 2020). While media reporting has focused on infection and mortality rates, a growing number of people who contract COVID-19 live with its debilitating sequelae months after their infection. Initially invisible by the focus on mortality, hundreds of thousands of 'Long COVID' patients have found each other through social media to insist that they be counted (#CountLongCovid) (Callard and Perego 2021). To this day, we know little of the virus and its natural and social history. It has simply not been around long enough. While many currently use 'Long COVID' to describe extended symptoms and drawn-out periods of recovery, we do not know yet whether there might also emerge post-viral syndromes or other debility or life-threatening conditions, as occurs with other viral infections: shingles following chicken pox; post-polio syndrome decades after poliomyelitis; immune-compromised conditions after dengue infections; cervical cancer following human papillomavirus. COVID-19's lethality has not unfolded. Equally, it is unclear how often people get second or even third COVID-19 infections. There are questions about terminology, clinical features, epidemiology, the natural history and the social life of the disease/diseases. There are also questions about how the disease is monitored, how we factor in underreporting, and how we might best model and manage its continued spread. The new directions of research in coming years, and the translation of this into interventions and models of care, are matters of thoughtful speculation.

In the twenty-first century, if it ever did, it no longer makes sense to think in terms of epidemiological transition. Globally, multiple forms of infectious disease, noncommunicable disease and related disability co-circulate, often with cascading co-morbidities (Manderson and Warren 2016). As COVID-19 burst on to the global health agenda, it joined a long list of medical conditions which continue to affect millions of people around the world. For over a century, medical anthropologists have ethnographically studied how individuals, families and loved ones perceive, live with and respond to medical conditions. COVID-19 is yet another communicable condition that now syndemically interacts with various other biological, social, economic and political conditions. The virus itself, and the responses to it ethnographically documented in this volume, have all too lucidly accentuated the stratified livability that results when poverty, racial discrimination and disability are permanent 'underlying conditions'.

While countless medical questions remain, as the chapters in *Viral Loads* show, anthropologists have been at the forefront, alongside epidemiologists and virologists, documenting, monitoring, analysing and interpreting patterns of transmission, and tracking the social life of the COVID-19 as it reshapes lives. It is essential that we remain so engaged. As we document, the pandemic has exposed how, worldwide, livability remains stratified and entrenched as lockdowns, viral infections and (access to) medical care are experienced and lived in racially, socio-economically and globally uneven ways. The biopolitical distinctions between 'making live' and 'letting die', of *bios* and *zoē*, are insufficient if we are to capture and account for the vast differences and divides that separate, for example, the lives of India's migrant labourers stranded by lockdown, with little access to medical care, from the lives of those who live in spacious, serviced residences that keep the outside world at bay. Stratified livability calls for anthropologies of urgency if we are to document and account for the far-reaching consequences of a twenty-first-century pandemic in Africa, Asia, Europe, Latin America and North America. This anthropology of urgency underscores the need for our voices in other concurrent crises that threaten our lives: crises of racism, violence, inequality and climate change. The comparative analysis that the chapters in *Viral Loads* enables is essential. It sharpens our understanding of the racialised, disabling and discriminatory ways in which the pandemic and responses to it came to impact on people around the world throughout 2020 and beyond. At the same time, it demonstrates the strength of anthropological theory, rich ethnography and critical engagement to make sense of a world that seems to be imploding, and to reveal intersections, strategies and structures that map possibilities.

References

Adams, Vincanne, Nancy J. Burke and Ian Whitmarsh. 2014. 'Slow research: Thoughts for a movement in global health'. *Medical Anthropology: Cross-Cultural Studies in Health and Illness* 33(3): 179–97.

Agrawal, Ravi. 2018. *India Connected: How the smartphone is transforming the world's largest democracy*. Oxford and New York: Oxford University Press.

Benjamin, Ruha. 2020. 'Black skin, white masks: Racism, vulnerability & refuting black pathology'. Accessed 8 December 2020. https://aas.princeton.edu/news/black-skin-white-masks-racism-vulnerability-refuting-black-pathology.

Benton, Adia and Kim Yi Dionne. 2015. 'International political economy and the 2014 West African Ebola outbreak'. *African Studies Review* 58(1): 223–36.

Briggs, Charles L. 2005. 'Communicability, racial discourse, and disease'. *Annual Review of Anthropology* 34: 269–91.

Caduff, Carlo. 2015. *The Pandemic Perhaps: Dramatic events in a public culture of danger*. Berkeley, CA: University of California Press.

Callard, Felicity and Elisa Perego. 2021. 'How and why patients made Long Covid'. *Social Science & Medicine* 268: 113426.

Crane, Johanna T. and Kelsey Pascoe. 2020. 'Becoming institutionalized: Incarceration as a chronic health condition'. *Medical Anthropology Quarterly*. https://doi.org/10.1111/maq.12621.

De León, Jason. 2015. *The Land of Open Graves: Living and dying on the migrant trail*. Berkeley, CA: University of California Press.

Douglas, Mary. 1966. *Purity and Danger: An analysis of concepts of pollution and taboo*. London: Routledge.

Farmer, Paul. 2001. *Infections and Inequalities: The modern plagues*. Berkeley, CA: University of California Press.

Fassin, Didier. 2007. *When Bodies Remember, Experiences and Politics of HIV in South Africa*. Berkeley, CA: University of California Press.

Herring, D. Ann and Alan C. Swedlund, eds. 2010. *Plagues and Epidemics: Infected spaces past and present*. London: Routledge.

Iskander, Natsha. 2020. 'Qatar, the coronavirus, and cordons sanitaires: Migrant workers and the use of public health measures to define the nation'. *Medical Anthropology Quarterly* https://doi.org/10.1111/maq.12625.

Kathiravelu, Laavanya. 2020. 'COVID-19 exposes the Singapore migrant worker experience'. East Asia Forum: Economics, Politics and Public Policy in East Asia and the Pacific, 11 November 2020. Accessed 11 November 2020. https://www.eastasiaforum.org/2020/11/11/covid-19-exposes-the-singapore-migrant-worker-experience/.

Kelly, Ann H., Frédéric Keck and Christos Lynteris, eds. 2019. *The Anthropology of Epidemics*. London: Routledge.

Kochhar, Rijul. 2020. 'Disability and dismantling: Four reflections in a time of COVID-19'. *Anthropology Now* 12(1): 73–5.

Lakoff, Andrew. 2017. *Unprepared: Global health in a time of emergency*. Berkeley, CA: University of California Press.

Leach, Melissa, Ian Scoones and Andrew Stirling. 2010. 'Governing epidemics in an age of complexity: Narratives, politics and pathways to sustainability'. *Global Environmental Change* 20(3): 369–77.

Lindenbaum, Shirley. 2001. 'Kuru, prions, and human affairs: Thinking about epidemics'. *Annual Review of Anthropology* 30: 363–85.

Livingston, Julie. 2012. *Improvising Medicine: An African oncology ward in an emerging cancer epidemic*. Durham, NC: Duke University Press.

Lynteris, Christos and Branwyn Poleykett. 2018. 'The anthropology of epidemic control: Technologies and materialities'. *Medical Anthropology: Cross-Cultural Studies in Health and Illness* 37(6): 433–41. https://doi.org/10.1080/01459740.2018.1484740

MacPhail, Theresa. 2015. *The Viral Network: A pathography of the H1N1 influenza pandemic*. Ithaca, NY: Cornell University Press.

Manderson, Desmond and Lorenzo Veracini. 2020. 'Bubbles: Covid and its metaphors'. *Meanjin* Spring. Accessed 8 December 2020. https://meanjin.com.au/essays/bubbles-covid-and-its-metaphors/.

Manderson, Lenore and Ayo Wahlberg. 2020. 'Chronic living in a communicable world'. *Medical Anthropology* 39(5): 428–39. https://doi.org/10.1080/01459740.2020.1761352

Manderson, Lenore and Narelle Warren. 2016. '"Just one thing after another": Recursive cascades and chronic conditions'. *Medical Anthropology Quarterly* 30(4): 479–97. https://doi.org/10.1111/maq.12277

Mason, Katherine A. 2016. *Infectious Change: Reinventing Chinese public health after an epidemic.* Palo Alto, CA: Stanford University Press.

Nguyen, Vinh Kim. 2010. *The Republic of Therapy: Triage and sovereignty in West Africa's time of AIDS.* Durham, NC: Duke University Press.

Niehaus, Isak and Gunvor Jonsson. 2005. 'Dr Wouter Basson, Americans, and wild beasts: Men's conspiracy theories of HIV/AIDS in the South African Lowveld'. *Medical Anthropology: Cross-Cultural Studies in Health and Illness* 24(2): 179–208. https://doi.org/10.1080/014597405909

Ormond, Meghann and Neil Lunt. 2020. 'Transnational medical travel: Patient mobility, shifting health system entitlements and attachments'. *Journal of Ethnic and Migration Studies* 46(20): 4179–92.

Parker, Richard and Peter Aggleton. 2003. 'HIV and AIDS-related stigma and discrimination: A conceptual framework and implications for action'. *Social Science & Medicine* 57: 13–24.

Patton, Cindy. 1991. *Inventing 'African AIDS'.* London: Routledge.

Rhodes, Tim, Merrill Singer, Philippe Bourgois, Samuel R. Friedman, and Steffanie A. Strathdee. 2005. 'The social structural production of HIV risk among injecting drug users'. *Social Science & Medicine* 61: 1026–44.

Roy, Arundhati. 2020. 'The pandemic is a portal'. 3 April 2020. Accessed 4 June 2020. https://www.ft.com/content/10d8f5e8-74eb-11ea-95fe-fcd274e920ca.

Sambala, Evanson Z. and Lenore Manderson. 2018. 'Ethical problems in planning for and responses to pandemic influenza in Ghana and Malawi'. *Ethics & Behavior* 28(3): 199–217.

Samuelsen, Helle. 2020. 'Accelerated fragility: Exploring the supply-demand nexus at health facilities in rural Burkina Faso'. *Africa* 90(5): 934–51.

Shultz, Hannah. 2020. 'Share Public Health. Transcript: COVID-19 impact on meatpacking workers'. 20 May. Accessed 4 June 2020. http://www.mphtc.org/share-public-health-transcript-covid-19/.

Street, Alice. 2014. *Biomedicine in an Unstable Place: Infrastructure and personhood in a Papua New Guinean hospital.* Durham, NC: Duke University Press.

Villareal, Luis P. 2004. 'Are viruses alive?' *Scientific American* 291: 100–05.

Wahlberg, Ayo. 2020. 'Healthcare systems overcome – the virulence of COVID-19'. *The Viral Condition: Identities Virtual Symposium*, R. Kaur, ed. Accessed 2020. https://www.identitiesjournal.com/the-viral-condition-virtual-symposium/healthcare-systems-overcome-the-virulence-of-covid-19.

Whiteford, Linda M. 2000. 'Idioms of hope and despair: Local identity, globalization and health in Cuba and the Dominican Republic'. In *Global Health Policy, Local Realities: The fallacy of the level playing field*, edited by Linda M. Whiteford and Lenore Manderson, pp. 57–78. Boulder, CO: Lynne Rienner Publishers.

Whittaker, Andrea, Lenore Manderson and Elizabeth Cartwright. 2010. 'Patients without borders: Understanding medical travel'. *Medical Anthropology* 29(4): 336–43. https://doi.org/10.1080/01459740.2010.501318

Williamson, K. Eliza. 2018. 'Care in the time of Zika: Notes on the "afterlife" of the epidemic in Salvador (Bahia), Brazil'. *Interface-Comunicação, Saúde, Educação* 22: 685–96.

Zhou, Jie Jenny. 2020. 'Meatpacking was already dangerous for workers. COVID made it worse'. *Los Angeles Times*. 8 September 2020. Accessed 8 December 2020. https://www.latimes.com/politics/story/2020-09-04/meatpacking-was-already-a-dangerous-job-for-california-workers-the-pandemic-made-it-worse

Part I
The power of the state

2
Care in the time of COVID-19
Surveillance, creativity and sociolismo *in Cuba*
Nancy J. Burke

On 19 April, the Universidad de las Ciencias Informáticas in Cuba, in collaboration with the Ministerio de Salud (MINSAP), announced the launch of Virtual Screen, *Pesquisador Virtual*, an app designed to provide 'real time identification of those with COVID-19 symptoms'. Users were told 'it is simple', and instructed to download the app, input their personal information, and, if they display symptoms, record their location, their interactions over the previous week and any contact with COVID-19 patients (Redaccion OnCuba 2020a). Along with brigades of physicians and medical students going door to door to actively screen residents, administer tests and provide symptomatic treatment as needed, the app was seen as another tool in Cuba's arsenal for controlling the spread of the virus that built on decades of effective infectious disease control. At the same time, police handed out fines to those not wearing masks. New services were promoted on WhatsApp groups, such as the delivery, for a fee, of fresh vegetables to the homes of those unable or unwilling to wait in long lines for daily provisions. *Paladars* (small, privately owned restaurants) adapted delivery services to bring food to elderly residents for free. Daily communications on state TV from the president and minister of public health, while reiterating the importance of social distancing, acknowledged how hard it was not to kiss people hello and to maintain six feet between each other, especially for Cubans for whom physical closeness is a part of daily life.

    I explore the productive tensions inherent in the expansive forms of surveillance and governance enacted by the Cuban state under the guise of caring for the population since the arrival of the novel coronavirus SARS-CoV-2, and the creative moves among individuals and groups to support each other while earning an income as revenues from the tourist sector disappeared. I propose that the co-existence and intersection of these practices are made possible by Cuba's particular form of post-Soviet bureaucratic socialism (Hoffmann 2016) and are conditioned by multiple forms of social and physical infrastructure. Analysis of these forms of care is useful for understanding how care is enacted and experienced in a time of crisis and geopolitical isolation.

Arundhati Roy (2020) posited the pandemic as a portal through which to imagine new futures, but others have argued that pandemic responses reveal what was already there (Whitacre et al. 2020). In the United States, this has taken the form of revealing the gross generational inequities that have led to disproportionate burdens of chronic illnesses and persistent poverty in black and brown populations, and the consequent disproportionate burden of death from complications linked to COVID-19 (Garth, Chapter 5). In Cuba, the reforms and slight changes that have occurred since the mid-2000s were revealed as just that – slight. The pandemic response re-instantiated the value of what had been lauded as the key triumphs of the Cuban Revolution – universal healthcare, investment in education, and commitment to addressing inequality and injustice throughout the world as operationalised in international medical missions. It highlighted the bureaucratic nature of the government's approach to population health, using punitive means of enforcement, and the valuable experience gained from participation in international and local responses to prior epidemics (e.g. dengue, HIV/AIDS, Ebola). It also created an opening for the re-assertion of comprehensive, coordinated and centralised state power in the interest of the public's health. At the same time, the pandemic response afforded the creation of new forms of relational care and entrepreneurism utilising online platforms and cellular data. Such responses were made possible by Cuba's socialist and *social* infrastructure, including training a deep and expansive public health workforce, and the changes, albeit complicated, that occurred with the opening of the economy since the 1990s. These forms of connectedness enabled creative approaches to *resolver*, or meet daily needs, in a context where the combination of US sanctions, crumbling municipal and housing infrastructures, loss of tourist revenue and the pandemic made it more and more difficult to do so.

At the time of this writing (November 2020), Cuba has 8,110 cases and 133 deaths.[1] This equates to 12 deaths per million. Compared with comparably sized nations such as Bolivia, the Dominican Republic and Belgium, ranked 44, 46 and 18, respectively, with cases ranging from 144,390 to 567,532, Cuba's pandemic response has resulted in impressively low numbers. In the following, I detail the Cuban government's swift and early response as part of a professional ethos of care, and highlight key aspects of the island's socialist infrastructure that underlie and pose challenges to this public health response and its enforcement. I follow this with a description of individual acts of community support, particularly on behalf of those most vulnerable. I conclude with a reflection on what this convergence of humanitarian intervention and governmentality reveals in this moment on the island.

Biopolitics and the anthropology of care

Anthropologists studying Cuba's healthcare system have highlighted the strong arm of the state in the maintenance of extraordinary health outcomes with few financial resources, the techniques the government has employed to engage citizens in the production of these metrics, and their subsequent influences on subjectivity (Andaya 2013, 2014; Brotherton 2005, 2012). Conducting research in the 1990s, Sean Brotherton described the deprivations of what is referred to on the island as the Special Period in a Time of Peace (*el Periodo Especial*), a time of extreme economic scarcity that severely impacted living standards, led to rising unemployment, and witnessed the plummeting of the value of national currency and further deterioration of already faulty housing and municipal infrastructures. This was seen as a state of exception (Agamben 2005) in which a well-educated population, 'inundated with biomedical knowledge', developed 'state fostered expectations and feelings of entitlement' to a level of wellbeing and healthcare that the socialist government could no longer provide (Brotherton 2005, 360). Faced with incomes insufficient to meet basic needs, Cubans relied more and more on their networks of *socios*,[2] friends and acquaintances connected to resources, including accessing care and prescribed and necessary medications (Brotherton 2012). Brotherton looked to Foucault's concept of biopolitics to theorise the production of 'governable subjects' (Burchell et al. 1991) on the island, arguing that strategies underlying the establishment of the Cuban healthcare system required increasing degrees of state intervention, management and protection, resulting in a Cuban form of biological citizenship. Biopolitical strategies, according to Foucault (1990, 139), seek to understand and regulate 'the level of health, life expectancy, and longevity' of population groups. Care for the health of the population is clearly a biopolitical endeavour, and one that infers both intimate and disciplinary processes.

As anthropologists have illustrated, physicians and nurses play essential biopolitical roles within Cuba's socialist health infrastructure (Andaya 2014; Brotherton 2012; Burke 2013). Having been declared 'symbols of the Revolution' by Fidel Castro (Rojas 1986), they are positioned within neighbourhoods and communities to reinforce the values of the Revolution through their continuous contact with the population, and their attention to lifestyle factors as elemental to health. Most recently, oncology clinical trials have been inserted into Cuban primary care practice, suggesting an extension of this biopolitical role into experimental treatments (Graber 2018; see also Livingston 2012). Within what Graber (2018) identifies as a professional ethos of care, physicians build upon their intimate relationships with patients in their neighbourhoods and health areas to incorporate palliative care and clinical research into their primary work of disease prevention and chronic disease management. In so doing, they engage in everyday practices that transform their work (e.g. incorporating experimental trials into clinical care) and their relationships with patients (normalising cancer as a chronic illness). Graber illustrates how the contours of individual care in the context of Cuba's neighbourhood clinics serve as an extension of the state's commitment to care for the population. Responses to pandemics, as we shall see, require a biopolitical approach that benefits from the trust established in these micro-interactions.

Medical institutions have worked to direct humanitarian resources to situations and places of extreme need (Farmer 2005), while they have played a regulative role imposing coercive norms of behaviour through conceptualisations of health and security (Foucault 1990; Ong 2003; Rose 2009). Lisa Stevenson's historical analysis of the mid-twentieth century tuberculosis outbreak in Northern Canada provides some insight into the complex tacking back and forth between the individual and population, or between Foucault's *anatomo-* and *bio-* politics, in the context of epidemics (Garcia 2010; Livingston 2012; Stevenson 2014). In her juxtaposition of the 1940s–1960s tuberculosis outbreak with the more recent suicide epidemic among Northern Canadian Inuit (in the 1980s), Stevenson (2014) aligns government efforts to provide care to a population through forced removal with the pain and suffering such separations wrought on individuals and families. As she describes, this 'anonymous care', directed toward population groups rather than toward named and known individuals and members of families and communities, met bureaucratic ends but was experienced as a form of genocide by those 'cared for'. This suggests important differences between 'anonymous care' aimed at population health, such as a population group experiencing a pandemic, and relational care provided to individuals, 'the way that someone comes to matter' (Garcia 2010).

Reflections on the Cuban response to the HIV/AIDS epidemic raise similar concerns. Rather than approaching HIV/AIDS transmission as an individual behavioural challenge within a human rights/individual choice framework, as occurred in much of the world, the Cuban government in the 1980s responded to the return of 40,000 troops from highly infected parts of Central Africa with classic public health strategies. The government implemented routine testing, contact tracing with partner notification, close surveillance and isolation of all seropositive individuals. This swift population level disciplinary response was possibly due to the socialist government's willingness to do so, despite likely opposition, and because of the comprehensive health system already in place. While the government was largely successful in controlling viral spread, especially compared with neighbouring Haiti and Puerto Rico, this was achieved at the cost of the forced isolation of people who tested positive in AIDS sanatoria. The approach was criticised as a violation of human rights (Scheper-Hughes 1994, 2020).

Perhaps more prescient to the current pandemic response, was the Cuban experience with the dengue outbreak of the 1980s, which also involved a 'massive and military' response (Whiteford 2000, 63) that resulted in the eradication of the source of the virus – the *Aedes aegypti* mosquito – three months after the epidemic reached its highest peak (Kouri et al. 1986). This response, explored further below, was multilevel, coordinated across sectors, and required the mobilisation of thousands of community health workers tasked with entering homes, assessing vector control compliance and imposing fines if necessary. The epidemic, recognised in May and brought under control by August, resulted in 0.46 deaths per 1,000 cases, the 'lowest lethality index reported until then for a dengue epidemic involving confirmed dengue haemorrhagic fever (DHF)' (Kouri et al. 1986). In the unfolding response to the COVID-19 pandemic, Cuba again employed traditional public health strategies designed to contain, control and manage the population, and, through them, the virus. At the same time, Cuban individuals worked through their social networks – *socios* – to provide forms of relational care.

Heeding early warning signs

Cuba's first cases of COVID-19 were confirmed on 11 March 2020 – three Italian tourists visiting the town of Trinidad, a World Heritage Site. The tourists were immediately isolated, as were the 11 people with whom they had come into contact. But the government had been preparing well before this. In January 2020, the National Action Plan for Epidemics, last revised during the Ebola outbreak in West Africa in 2014, was updated and activated, surveillance commenced at all ports, and immigration officials were trained in COVID-19 response (e.g. immediate testing and quarantine of those suspected of being infected). In February, polyclinics were reorganised across the island, and beds identified for potential patients. Staff were trained in COVID-19 symptoms, testing and quarantine, and in March meetings across Cuba's 15 provinces started to coordinate responses across sectors, identify and activate testing labs and began research into diagnostics and treatments. Daily briefings from the Ministry of Public Health on state TV began; tax payments were suspended for all small businesses; and protections were put in place for worker salaries and social security. Before the first case was confirmed, deans from medical schools across the country had already called for volunteers to participate in administration of active screening. Over 28,000 medical students responded (MEDICC 2020). In mid-March, 155 workshops turned their attention to manufacturing masks, schools were closed and outbound travel by Cuban citizens was limited to humanitarian reasons. By the end of the month, Camilo Cienfuegos, in Pinar del Rio, was the first community put under quarantine.

On 1 April, face coverings were made obligatory, and by 5 April, all police stations were staffed with someone from the district attorney's office, placed there to charge those in violation of COVID-19 regulations according to Article 87 of the penal code (crimes against health). Alcohol sales were limited, and drinking was prohibited in public; restaurants were closed or limited to take-out. By 15 April, 20 communities in six provinces were under total or partial quarantine and by 23 April, over nine million of the island's total 11.4 million population had been visited in their homes or places of work as part of the active screening programme (Gorry 2020; MEDICC 2020). At the end of the month, through primary care case detection and contact tracing, the sources of infection for 85.7 per cent of active cases had been identified (Gorry 2020).

Mobilisation of the public health system

As in prior epidemics, Cuba's readiness to act builds on the socialist infrastructure of free and universal healthcare and education established as a core tenet of the post-1959 Revolutionary state. Trained infectious disease specialists, microbiologists, laboratory technicians, epidemiologists and over 13,000 family doctors and nurses serving neighbourhoods across the island positioned the country well for a quick response. This density of trained health professionals was made possible by the 13 medical universities and 25 medical faculties across the country that confer six-year medical degrees at no cost to students. Medical training has been prioritised since Fidel Castro came into power in 1959, at which time over 3,000 of the island's 6,286 doctors migrated to the United States (Gómez 2019), leaving the country with a dearth of trained physicians equipped to build a new national healthcare system envisioned to reflect socialist values and the principle of health as a human right.

Cuba's public health infrastructure took shape over time, first in 1965 with the integral polyclinic programme (*policlinico integral*), and in 1974, with the 'Medicine in the Community' programme (*policlinicos comunitarios*). In the 1980s, the healthcare system was re-envisioned to become the well-known Family Doctor and Nurse programme, *Medico y Enfermera de la Familia* (MEF). Elemental to this, physician and nurse pairs were placed in every neighbourhood, thus creating *consultorios* (neighbourhood clinics) responsible for the population of a 'health area', usually of about 120 households. Physicians and nurses retain detailed health histories of individuals embedded in families and social networks and serve as a hub for referral to the next levels of care in the polyclinic and hospital (Burke 2013). The achievements of Cuba's health system, which build upon this structure, are important not only for their impacts on the population, but also because the government has used them to gain international prestige, respect (Feinsilver, 2008, 1993) and, at times, hard currency (Briggs and Mantini-Briggs 2009; Brotherton 2013). The strength of Cuba's health statistics has become a significant source of Cuban nationalism and 'global empowerment' (Eckstein 1994, 128). The MEF programme, central to the production of these health statistics, has also been criticised for its potential role in neighbourhood level surveillance (Brotherton 2012, 2008).

In the midst of the scarcities of the Special Period of the 1990s, the public health system – like all industry on the island – was threatened. While the government made a commitment to retain investments in public health, education and biotechnology, the geopolitical isolation resulting from the continuing US Trade Embargo and loss of the Soviet Union greatly impacted access to externally produced medicines, basic materials for local pharmaceutical production and clinical supplies. In addition, vegetables, fruit and other basic elements of the Cuban diet were difficult to find in urban centres due to lack of fuel. Building initiatives designed to deliver on the state's commitment of housing for all slowed to a halt, leaving the crumbling housing inherited by the Revolution to continue to decay (Coyula-Cowley 2000). Municipal infrastructures including water and wastewater plants built over 50 years previously were left to deteriorate (Cueto and de Leon 2010; Randal 2000; Westbrook and de Freitas Alves 2016).

Economic reforms enacted to stimulate the economy and bring in much needed hard currency included continued investment in biotechnology and expansion of patents (Reid-Henry 2010), investment in tourism (recreational, educational and medical), introduction of a dual currency and opening to entrepreneurism (Burke 2013). While the scarcities experienced in the 1990s have to varying degrees continued into the present, the strength of Cuba's socialist public health infrastructure has been identified as the reason behind continuously robust health indicators (Spiegel and Yassi 2004). A core element of this infrastructure is the *libreta*, or ration book. Despite the scarcities imposed by the US Embargo and geopolitical shifts, Cuba is known as a place where *nadie se muere de hambre* (no one dies from hunger) (Garth 2019) due to a national food ration system which provides about half of an individual's monthly nutritional requirements, with additional rationed items for children, the elderly and those with certain chronic conditions (e.g. diabetes, cancer), at very low cost.

Since Fidel Castro fell ill and turned over power to his brother Raul in 2006 and Raul to Miguel Díaz-Canel in 2018, Cuban politics have undergone major transformations largely in the interest of continuity (Hoffmann 2016). While scholars have argued over how to characterise this period, referring to it as post-Soviet, post-socialist and post-Soviet/post-socialist, some have suggested that the transition is most appropriately described as a shift from a charismatic socialism characterised by mass mobilisation to a more depersonalised bureaucratic socialism which has brought with it a diversification of Cuba's public sphere, particularly through the liberalisation of access to digital media and data, liberalisation of travel and migration, and more moderate foreign policy (Hoffmann 2016). In the 2000s this transition led to centralisation and efficiency campaigns that began to reshape the healthcare system yet again, largely in response to the burden on the system placed by Cuba's robust and extensive medical missions (Briggs and Mantini-Briggs 2009; Brotherton 2013; Feinsilver 2008).

In 2016, Cuba's foreign policy opening resulted in rapprochement with the United States. US President Obama's visit to the island in March that year symbolised hope and possibility for many and resulted in a reinvestment in tourism with the expectation of an onslaught of US visitors. The 2016 election of Donald Trump as the 45th president of the United States quashed this hope. With his election, the US Embargo tightened, locked in by the Helms–Burton law passed in 1996, which curtails foreign trade and investment on the island. In 2019, the Trump administration imposed 86 new punitive measures including full implementation of the Helms–Burton Act. From September 2019, this has resulted in reductions in oil imports from Venezuela, which left Cuba functioning with 50 per cent of its required fuel (Rodriguez 2020a). Economic challenges were exacerbated by a regional drought that reduced agricultural production over the prior year. In the context of the pandemic, the Cuban government faced difficulty in procuring much-needed respirators, and medical donations from China were stymied by US intervention (Granma 2020; Rodriguez 2020a). The Jack Ma Foundation's donation of facemasks, diagnostic kits, ventilators and gloves, for example, was thwarted because a major shareholder of the Avianca Airlines cargo carrier set to bring the materials was a US-based company, subject to the trade restrictions set by the US embargo (Weissenstein 2020). As Cuban economist Jose Luiz Rodriguez argued, 'At this point, no one questions that the pandemic is not just a health crisis. It is what the social sciences describe as a "total social fact," in the sense that it convulses all social relations, and shocks all the actors, institutions and values' (2020b).

Prior epidemic experiences

In addition to Cuba's robust primary care system, the healthcare workforce's experience with prior epidemics influenced the island's ability to respond. In Cuba these include dengue outbreaks (1981, 1997), a neuropathy epidemic[3] (1990s), cholera outbreaks (2012–13), and Zika (2019). The 1980s dengue epidemic provides the clearest precedent for the current pandemic in terms of response. Prior to 1981, dengue haemorrhagic fever (DHF) had not been seen in the Caribbean region; it was limited to Southeast Asia and the western Pacific (Kouri et al. 1986). But in the summer of 1981, when infestations of the mosquito vector *Aedes aegypti* were recorded in almost all the island's urban centres, Cuba was hit by a major dengue epidemic that included DHF cases and fatalities. The Ministry of Health reported 344,203 cases between May and August 1981, with 116,151 hospitalised and 158 deaths. The last case was reported in October 1981. Similar to the swift response to

COVID-19, once the epidemic was recognised in June 1981, the government launched an intensive national campaign to eradicate the *Aedes aegypti* mosquito, initially managed by the Cuban civil defence and later the Ministry of Public Health (Kouri et al. 1989). The government's response included 15 provincial directors, 60 entomologists, 27 general supervisors, 729 team leaders, 2,801 inspectors and 1,947 vector controllers (Whiteford 2000). On the ground, approximately 15,000 health workers were mobilised to conduct house-to-house inspections, during which they identified potential mosquito larvae breeding grounds, treated disposal containers with insecticides, and treated the insides of apartments and buildings with portable blowers. The insecticide Malathon was sprayed from planes, sanitary laws regarding treatment of containers were enforced and health education about the mosquito and its ability to transmit the virus intensified (Gessa and Gonzalez 1987; Kouri et al. 1986; Whiteford 2000). All available resources were marshalled to quell the epidemic; the government spent close to US$43 million on the campaign, mainly on insecticides. But like the current COVID-19 response, the Cuban government relied largely on existing human capital. Household inspections and breeding ground removal were conducted by community members who, after being trained, became 'vector controllers' organised into brigades with the power to fine those who failed to comply with regulations designed to reduce breeding sites (Kouri et al. 1986; Whiteford 2000; Gessa and Gonzalez 1986). The similarities with the current behavioural challenges associated with reducing the spread of COVID-19 are clear, as is the role of infrastructure – social and physical – in the state's response. Neighbours surveilled each other's homes to ensure that they complied with eradication efforts and could be fined if not. Those who failed to comply put others in danger, as now those who fail to wear face coverings or maintain social distance may put others at risk. Crumbling buildings and inadequate water supply influenced, in the 1980s, the maintenance of water containers in households; in 2020 these conditions make sheltering in place and hygienic hand washing challenging.

Internationally, Cuban healthcare professionals have responded to epidemics and natural disasters as part of a long tradition of international humanitarianism begun in post-quake Chile in 1960. Since just 2005, the Henry Reeve Brigade[4] has provided free medical services in nearly 30 post-disaster and epidemic situations, including the cholera outbreak following the 2010 earthquake in Haiti and the 2014 Ebola epidemic in West Africa (Ubieta 2019). Especially following the expulsion of Cuban physicians from formerly allied states in Brazil, Ecuador and Bolivia, a robust cadre of doctors on the island with excellent field experience were poised to support the pandemic response. When 28,000 students responded to the medical school deans' call for volunteers, they needed to be supervised and their case findings evaluated and communicated to clinicians. Family doctors in each neighbourhood, many of whom had returned from international missions, filled this supervisory role.

Cuban doctors were the first to arrive in Wuhan, China (Granma News Staff 2020). On 26 March, the first team to go abroad began treating COVID-19 patients in Lombardy, Italy, and since this time over a thousand health professionals have worked in 18 countries on three continents. Of note is the number of women serving as part of the nurse brigade working in Barbados (95 of the 101 are women). As mentioned previously, Cuba's international missions serve a symbolic as well as financial role (Bernstein 2013; Briggs and Mantini-Briggs 2009; Brotherton 2013).

The state is back

The government's immediate response to the looming global pandemic included both international support and, as mentioned above, the re-instantiation of paternalistic controls on the population. In April, six people confined to an isolation centre in Sancti Spiritus escaped. Isolation centres, established in March 2020, are adapted schools and hotels in which those either diagnosed with or suspected to have been exposed to COVID-19 are housed, with the supervision of medical personnel. News reports detail the limitations on movement for individuals in quarantine, and the high degree of medical attention they receive including temperature checks and PCR testing (Curbelo 2020). The escapees were found in their own homes; upon their arrest only 24 hours later, they were subject to three months to a year in prison (Redaccion OnCuba 2020b). Police started imposing fines of 300 pesos (the equivalent of a month's salary) in April under the supposition of Article 87 of the penal code,[5] but the specific decree enforcing face covering was not published until 12 May. The state began limiting alcohol sales in May, and drinking in public became a finable offence in the same month. Those criticising the state's approach to the pandemic or deemed to spread false information on social media were subject to fines and arrest (Alemán 2020), a return, in some senses, to the pre-transition mode of response to dissidence (Hoffmann 2016). As noted by Amalia Peréz, 'along with the amplifying effects of inequality and precarity associated with this crisis, the expansion of authoritarianism, hidden in the justification of health management and prevention, is also a risk' (Pérez and Correa 2020).

State provisions were also reinstated, fostering a return to what had been a slow loosening of dependency with the burgeoning of the private sector under Raul Castro's reforms. The ration book, thought to be on its way out just months prior, was restored and reinvigorated in April 2020 in attempts to keep Cubans from traveling far from home to different grocery stores in search of basic goods, and to minimise long lines as potential sources of infection. Cubans pay less than the equivalent of US$2 for their monthly rations, which is estimated as 12 per cent of the food's real value (Benjamin n.d.). With the recognition of increasing unequal access to hard currency between those living on a state salary or pension and those working in the tourist sector or receiving remittances from abroad over the last decade, government subsidisation of every citizen regardless of income at the cost of approximately one billion/year has been a point of contention. In 2011, for example, Raul Castro stated that the ration system distributes food at 'laughable prices' and that a system introduced in a time of shortages had turned into 'an unbearable burden for the economy and a disincentive to work' (Benjamin n.d.). Raul Castro's reforms included a gradual reduction in the items included in *la libreta*. But during the pandemic, the offerings expanded. In recognition of the economic hit that citizens, especially those in the tourist sector, have taken with the closure of the island in response to COVID-19, the state began to pardon taxes for entrepreneurs and to ensure salaries for state workers, including artists and musicians, in March 2020.

Care (and humour)

Among ordinary citizens, pandemic response revealed the creativity and care Cubans have for each other, including via the well-known Cuban turn to humour. Anthropologists working on the island in the 1990s and since have chronicled the pivotal role of humour, jokes and laughter in coping on a daily basis with scarcities and insecurities – food, water, electricity and fuel – during and following Cuba's *Periodo Especial*. Jokes recorded included one popular in the 1980s mocking that the Revolution had eradicated capitalism's three classes (upper, middle and lower) only to replace them with three new socialist ones: the *dirigentes* (few communist officials at the top), the *diplogente* (the fewer diplomats and foreigners in the middle) and the *indigentes* (the indigent masses at the bottom). The egalitarianism of socialism made everyone equal by making everyone poor (Henken 2007). During the Special Period, another group was added, the *delincuentes* (delinquents, people who survived by breaking the law). As a Cuban blogger commented, 'there seems to be a direct relationship between the seriousness of the problems and the ingenuity of our humour, so in times of crisis hilarity wins. The nineties were marked by scarcities and abundant jokes; prodigious in both problems and humour' (Sanchez 2012).

Nadine Fernandez (2010) reminds us of this humour in her account of the affectionate name many had for their white 1950s model refrigerators in the 1990s: *el coco* – white on the outside and only water on the inside. At the same time, she highlighted the sharp edges of this humour when addressing race and difference. Other popular jokes of the time include: 'What are the three successes of the Cuban Revolution? Medicine, education and athletics. What are the three failures of the Cuban Revolution? Breakfast, lunch and dinner'. Tanuma (2007) argues that such jokes indicate a post-utopian irony reflecting ambivalence toward the status quo and the state. This ironic stance enabled criticism in a somewhat acceptable manner.

Humour emerging in the context of the pandemic includes the song by Virulo, *Dale Candela*, which critiques US President Trump's suggestion of injecting bleach as a means to kill the coronavirus. The recurring refrain of '*dale candela para que el virus se muera*' (heat it up so that the virus dies) refers to uncooked bats as a source of the virus (insomne 2020). Other jokes include those referring to the refrigerator as a great place to store clothing (because there is no food), and finally understanding what good *la libreta* serves, as a passport to leave the house, since it is no longer useful for accessing food in empty state-run bodegas.

Jokes like these are told while Cubans wait in long lines for groceries, not adequately social distancing and fumbling with wearing masks as the temperature continues to rise. Streets in Central Havana became a hot spot for spreading the virus (OnCubaNews 2020), given their crowding due to the state of the buildings, rising temperatures and the need to *resolver* (meet daily needs). Nearly 80 per cent of the city was built between 1902 and 1958, and a large proportion of this housing stock was already in disrepair at the onset of the Revolution in 1959 (Kerr 2009). In central Havana, 85 per cent of housing is over 80 years old, and the remainder between 40 and 80 years old (Coyula 2010). Much of this housing is crumbling, overcrowded and in dire need of repair; there has been little renovation of existing structures. In addition, municipal utilities, including electricity and water, continue to breakdown. In

April 2020 residents of Havana were asked to reduce their electricity use and preserve water in anticipation of the kinds of blackouts and brownouts that characterised the Special Period.

Prior to the pandemic, Cubans expressed concern about how President Trump's crackdown on trade was impacting the availability of prescription drugs – particularly hypertension medication, which many people take daily – and food. As a result, people were traveling across the city at the rumour of one store having canned tomatoes in order to get them before they disappeared, and turning to the black market for medications no longer available on pharmacy shelves. Since the onset of the pandemic, these sanctions, resulting from the Helms–Burton Act, have also impacted the availability of personal protective equipment (PPE) and real time reverse transcription polymerase chain reaction (PCR) tests on the island, both acquired through donations from the Pan American Health Organization (PAHO) and trade with China (Duran 2020). In response to the lack of PPE, 'makers' started to construct face masks and shields out of recycled plastic bottles. They created a network of collectors across neighbourhoods and towns, and shared patterns and methods via social media to enable individuals across the island to join in. Their makeshift masks are worn by medical personnel throughout Cuba (Cabrera 2020).

In addition to waiting in lines and shopping for each other, Cubans established WhatsApp groups to facilitate grocery delivery to the elderly, and the state created online shopping options that were less successful (Boza 2020). These groups were made possible by the increased access to cellular data Cubans have had since 2016, and high speed internet in homes and public spaces since 2017. With the quick adaptation of the long Cuban tradition of *sociolismo*, the use of social networks and friendships to meet daily needs, WhatsApp also facilitated entrepreneurial endeavours such as gyms offering free classes and renting out bicycles. Restaurants and cafeterias started using WhatsApp for pizza, dinner, pastry and fresh juice delivery. Cuber, Cuba's version of Uber, expanded to deliver groceries and other products. *Paladares* such as *cafeteria Jaunky's Pan* repurposed their delivery service to ensure that elderly Cubans could receive groceries at home at no cost (Lima 2020). Some of these adaptations were expansions on or adaptations of pre-existing entrepreneurial projects; others – particularly those designed to provide support and social connections to older Cubans living alone – were collective and creative responses to a recognised need, a way to minimise suffering among the most vulnerable.

Conclusions

Cuba's pandemic response reveals the value of a deep and available public health workforce, trained and experienced in epidemic response, and the continued power of the state to mobilise across sectors in the context of an emergency. Vietnam has also had success in keeping the pandemic at bay through similar early closure of borders, multisector coordination, healthcare system mobilisation, extensive monitoring and investigation of potential cases, strict quarantine enforcement and massive health education and communication campaigns. These endeavours, as in Cuba, are made possible by a government willing to enforce containment measures. The strong arm of the state was evidenced in Vietnam, for example, in the quick quarantine of a community of 10,000 residents near Hanoi when four cases were reported in February 2020. In April, the country entered a heavily enforced nationwide 14-day lockdown (Minh Hoang et al. 2020). Similar to the Cuban response, the Vietnamese government developed several apps to facilitate case reporting and contact tracing but took things a step further by making declarations of health status and travel history via apps compulsory (Trevisan and Le 2020). At the end of April 2020, the country had only 270 cases; in early December, it still had only 1,361 reported cases and 35 deaths. As noted in a recent editorial in the *American Journal of Public Health*, 'the Vietnamese experience suggests the need for a strong public health infrastructure and good coordination among the government agencies dealing with the emergency' (Trevisan and Le 2020). It also suggests, as does the Cuban response, the value of biopolitics to pandemic control.

In the context of the pandemic, Cuban health professionals have worked to 'adapt biomedicine to people's needs, and, by doing so, ensure continuity of care' (Graber 2018, 276). In this case, continuity refers to everything from meeting basic needs to enforcing public health measures to limit spread. The response to the pandemic highlights paternalistic and egalitarian roles of the state (in the delivery of social goods per the mass mobilisation model) as well as the space within this biopolitical regime for individuals and communities' 'capacities to reshape and transform health politics' (Graber 2018, 277) through local interpretations and enactments of care. Thus, the Cuban pandemic response contributes to emerging trends in the anthropology of care that elaborate connections between everyday practices, the inter-relational and intersubjective aspects of care, and the regimes and hierarchies of governance. As Buch so aptly describes in her review on anthropology and care, '(w)ithin these discussions, care remains a shifting and unstable concept – alternately referring to everyday practices, engagements with biomedicine, biopolitics, affective states, forms of moral experience and obligation, structures of exploitation, and the relationships between these various things' (2015, 279).

The Cuban pandemic response also reveals the value of the daily practices of survival, captured in the term *resolver*, that Cubans have in their back pocket, honed from prior and continuous experiences of economic uncertainty. These include extensive networks of *socios* through which needs for medicines and food might be met, and care for the most vulnerable delivered. These networks have been characterised elsewhere as essential infrastructure for urban living, filling in where public services fail (Simone 2004). Challenges to shelter in place orders on the island reveal the effects of persistent poverty and geopolitical isolation on individuals' ability to stay in lockdown in the midst of neglected housing, electrical and sanitary infrastructure. As the images of crowded streets and long lines on blogs and online newspaper sites attest, people find it difficult to stay inside crumbling buildings with little to no air flow and at times intermittent water and electricity.

The multiple forms of care emergent in the Cuban response to the pandemic – bureaucratic approaches to population health which take the form of anonymous care (Stevenson 2014) accompanied by new forms of relational care facilitated by cellular data – take place within contexts of social, public health and physical infrastructures in varying levels of decay (buildings, water pipes and treatment plants, electrical conduits), maintenance and transition (see also Cabalquinto and Ahlin, Chapter 18). All are active participants conditioning Cuba's pandemic response (Appel et al. 2018; Larkin 2013).

In October 2020, Cuban airports re-opened to tourists, and entrepreneurs on the island who had thrived pre-pandemic with full bed and breakfasts and tour groups breathed a sigh of relief. Since then, the number of new infections have started creeping up. For example, on 27 November 2020, MINSAP reported 35 new cases of COVID-19. Twenty-eight of these were tourists (Redaccion OnCuba 2020c). How the country will continue to maintain pandemic control while opening up to international tourism – an essential form of revenue on the island – remains to be seen.

Notes

1. https://oncubanews.com/cuba/cuba-casi-la-mitad-de-los-contagios-por-coronavirus-esta-semana-fueron-importados/. Redaccion OnCuba. 2020c.
2. *Socios* are friends or acquaintances through which one accesses business advantages/opportunities or resources needed for daily living. *Socios* are a key part of *sociolismo*, a strategy Cubans employ to *resolver*, or get what they need, in a context of scarcity.
3. Over 50,000 cases of optical and peripheral neuropathy were diagnosed between 1991 and 1994, out of a population of 10.8 million. According to MINSAP, likely causes include nutritional deficiencies stemming from the deprivations of the Special Period complicated by alcohol and tobacco use (Centers for Disease Control and Prevention 1994).
4. Group of Cuban health professionals, established in 2005 in response to Hurricane Katrina, regularly deployed to provide humanitarian support in response to disasters throughout the world.
5. This article refers to crimes against health.

References

Agamben, Giorgio. 2005. *State of Exception*, 1st ed. Chicago, IL: University of Chicago Press.

Alemán, Dario Alejandro. 2020. 'Decreto 370: Tribulaciones de Camila ante la Ley'. *El Estornudo*, 11 May 2020. Accessed 20 August 2020. https://revistaelestornudo.com/camila-acosta-decreto-370-periodismo-independiente-cuba/.

Andaya, Elise. 2013. 'Conceiving statistics: The local practice and global politics of reproductive health care in Havana'. In *Health Travels: Cuban health(care) on and off the island*, edited by Nancy J. Burke, pp. 205–30. Berkeley, CA: University of California Medical Humanities Press.

Andaya, Elise. 2014. *Conceiving Cuba: Reproduction, women, and the state in the post-Soviet era*. New Brunswick, NJ: Rutgers University Press.

Appel, Hannah, Nikhil Anand and Akhil Gupta. 2018. 'Introduction: Temporality, politics, and the promise of infrastructure'. In *The Promise of Infrastructure*, edited by Nikhil Anand, Akhil Gupta and Hannah Appel, pp. 1–40. Durham, NC: Duke University Press.

Benjamin, Medea. n.d. 'Dividing the pie: Cuba's ration system after 50 years'. CODEPINK. Accessed 7 February 2020. https://www.codepink.org/dividing_the_pie_cuba_s_ration_system_after_50_years.

Bernstein, Alissa. 2013. 'Transformative medical education and the making of new clinical subjectivities through Cuban-Bolivian medical diplomacy'. In *Health Travels: Cuban health(care) on and off the island*, edited by Nancy J. Burke, pp. 154–78. Berkeley, CA: University of California Medical Humanities Press.

Boza, Glenda. 2020. '¿Cómo no fracasar con TuEnvio? Un tutorial para comprar en Cuba'. *Periodismo de Barrio*. Accessed 2 October 2020. https://www.periodismodebarrio.org/2020/05/como-no-fracasar-con-tuenvio-un-tutorial-para-comprar-en-cuba/.

Briggs, Charles L. and Clara Mantini-Briggs. 2009. 'Confronting health disparities: Latin American social medicine in Venezuela'. *American Journal of Public Health* 99(3): 549–55.

Brotherton, P. Sean. 2005. 'Macroeconomic change and the biopolitics of health in Cuba's Special Period'. *Journal of Latin American Anthropology* 10: 339–69.

Brotherton, P. Sean. 2012. *Revolutionary Medicine: Health and the body in post-Soviet Cuba*. Durham, NC: Duke University Press Books.

Brotherton, P. Sean. 2013. 'Fueling la Revolucion: Itinerant physicians, transactional humanitarianism, and shifting moral economies in Post-Soviet Cuba'. In *Health Travels: Cuban health(care) on and off the island*, edited by Nancy J. Burke, pp. 129–54. Berkeley, CA: University of California Medical Humanities Press.

Buch, Elana D. 2015. Anthropology of aging and care. *Annual Review of Anthropology* 44: 277–93.
Burchell, Graham, Colin Gordon, and Peter Miller, eds. 1991. *The Foucault Effect: Studies in governmentality*, 1st ed. Chicago, IL: University of Chicago Press.
Burke, Nancy J., ed. 2013. *Health Travels: Cuban health(care) on and off the island*. Berkeley, CA: University of California Medical Humanities Press.
Cabrera, Mónica Rivero. 2020. 'Tecnologías resilientes para esta y otras crisis'. *Periodismo de Barrio*. Accessed 28 July 2020. https://www.periodismodebarrio.org/2020/07/tecnologias-resilientes-para-esta-y-otras-crisis/.
Centers for Disease Control and Prevention. 1994. 'International notes epidemic neuropathy – Cuba, 1991–1994'. *Morbidity and Mortality Weekly Report* 43(10): 183, 189–92.
Coyula, Miguel. 2010. 'Havana: Aging in an aging city'. *MEDICC Review* 12: 1–4.
Coyula Cowley, Mario. 2000. 'Housing in Cuba'. *Designer/Builder* 7(7): 29–35.
Cueto, Jose Enrique and Omar de Leon. 2010. 'Evaluation of Cuba's water and wastewater infrastructure including high-priority improvements and order-of-magnitude costs'. Accessed 10 September 2020. https://www.ascecuba.org/asce_proceedings/appendix-b-evaluation-cubas-water-watershed-infraestructure-student-paper-presented-annual-meeting-not-included-printed-version-proceedings/
Curbelo, Jesus Jank. 2020. 'En aislamiento'. *Periodismo de Barrio*. Accessed 28 July 2020. https://www.periodismodebarrio.org/2020/05/en-aislamiento/.
Duran, Francisco. 2020. 'Stemming COVID-19 in Cuba: Strengths, strategies, challenges'. Accessed 10 November 2020. *MEDICC Review*. https://europepmc.org/article/med/32478709.
Eckstein, Susan. 1994. *Back from the Future: Cuba under Castro*. Princeton, NJ: Princeton University Press.
Farmer, Paul. 2005. *The Uses of Haiti*. Monroe, ME: Common Courage Press.
Feinsilver, Julie M. 1993. *Healing the Masses: Cuban health politics at home and abroad*. Berkeley, CA: University of California Press.
Feinsilver, Julie M. 2008. 'Oil-for-doctors: Cuban medical diplomacy gets a little help from a Venezuelan friend.' *Nueva Sociedad* 2016: 14.
Fernandez, Nadine T. 2010. *Revolutionizing Romance: Interracial couples in contemporary Cuba*. New Brunswick, NJ: Rutgers University Press.
Foucault, Michel. 1990. *The History of Sexuality, Vol. 1: An introduction*, Reissue ed. New York: Vintage.
Garcia, Angela. 2010. *The Pastoral Clinic: Addiction and dispossession along the Rio Grande*. Berkeley, CA: University of California Press.
Garth, Hanna. 2019. *Food in Cuba: The pursuit of a decent meal*. Palo Alto, CA: Stanford University Press.
Gessa, J. and R. Gonzalez. 1987. 'Ordenamiento del medio en el programa de erradicacion de Aedes aegypti. Cuba, 1984'. *Boletín de la Oficina Sanitaria Panamericana* 102: 237–45.
Gómez, Enrique Ubieta. 2019. *Red Zone: Cuba and the fight Against Ebola in Western Africa*. New York: Pathfinder Press.
Gorry, Conner. 2020. 'COVID-19 case detection: Cuba's active screening approach'. *MEDICC Review* 22(2): 58–63. https://mediccreview.org/covid-19-case-detection-cubas-active-screening-approach/.
Graber, Nils. 2018. 'An alternative imaginary of community engagement: state, cancer biotechnology and the ethos of primary healthcare in Cuba. *Critical Public Health* 28(3): 269–80.
Granma 2020. 'El bloqueo impide el envio de respiradores artificiales a Cuba'. Accessed 10 November 2020. http://www.granma.cu/cuba/2020-04-11/empresa-estadounidense-compra-compania-proveedora-de-respiradores-artificiales-y-suspende-envios-a-cuba-por-causa-del-bloqueo-11-04-2020-15-04-54?page=3.
Granma News Staff. 2020. 'Cuban doctors in China to reinforce medical command center established in our embassy'. Accessed 21 December 2020. http://en.granma.cu/mundo/2020-02-03/cuban-doctors-in-china-to-reinforce-medical-command-center-established-in-our-embassy.
Henken, Ted. 2007. *Dirigentes, Diplogente, Indigentes, and Delincuentes: Official corruption and underground honesty in Today's Cuba*. Commissioned by the Cuban Research Institute. Florida International University, Miami, FL. Accessed 10 August 2020. https://cri.fiu.edu/research/commissioned-reports/dirigentes-henken.pdf.
Hoffmann, Bert. 2016. 'Bureaucratic socialism in reform mode: The changing politics of Cuba's post-Fidel era'. *Third World Quarterly* 37: 1730–44.
insomne, L. pupila. 2020. 'Virulo le canta al Coronavirus … y a Trump: Dale candela (letra y audio). La pupila insomne'. Accessed 30 July 2020. https://lapupilainsomne.wordpress.com/2020/05/06/virulo-le-canta-el-coronavirus-y-a-trump-dale-candela-letra-y-audio/.

Kerr, Robert. 2009. *The Metamorphosis of Cuban Architecture: Development, decay, and opportunity*. Edinburgh, UK: University of Edinburgh.
Kouri, Gustavo P., Maria G. Guzmán and José R. Bravo. 1986. 'Hemorrhagic dengue in Cuba: History of an epidemic'. *Bulletin* of the Pan American Health Organization (PAHO) 20(1): 24–30.
Kouri, Gustavo P., Maria G. Guzmán, José R. Bravo and C. Triana. 1989. 'Dengue haemorrhagic fever/dengue shock syndrome: Lessons from the Cuban epidemic, 1981'. *Bulletin of the World Health Organization* 67(4): 375–80.
Larkin, Brian 2013 'The politics and poetics of infrastructure'. *Annual Review of Anthropology* 42: 327–43.
Lima, Leydis Hernández. 2020. 'La cafetería Juanky's Pan y otros proyectos ayudan a ancianos vulnerables'. *Periodismo de Barrio*. Accessed 5 October 2020. https://www.periodismodebarrio.org/2020/04/la-cafeteria-juankys-pan-se-une-a-otros-proyectos-para-ayudar-a-ancianos-en-situacion-vulnerable/.
Livingston, Julie. 2012. *Improvising Medicine: An African oncology ward in an emerging cancer epidemic*. Durham, NC: Duke University Press.
MEDICC. 2020. Cuba's COVID-19 strategy: Main actions through April 23, 2020. Accessed 27 July 2020. https://mediccreview.org/cubas-covid-19-strategy-main-actions-through-april-23-2020/.
Minh Hoang, Van, Hong Hanh Hoang, Quynh Long Khuong, Ngoc Quang La and Thi Tuyet Hanh Tran. 2020. 'Describing the pattern of the COVID-19 epidemic in Vietnam'. *Global Health Action* June 2020: 13.
OnCubaNews. 2020. 'Reforzarán aislamiento social en La Habana por expansión de la Covid-19'. Accessed 30 July 2020. https://oncubanews.com/cuba/reforzaran-aislamiento-social-en-centro-Zhabana-por-expansion-de-la-covid-19/.
Ong, Aihwa. 2003. *Buddha Is Hiding: Refugees, Citizenship, the New America*. Berkeley, CA: University of California Press.
Pérez, Amalia and Ahmed Correa. 2020. 'COVID-19, derechos y estado de emergencia en Cuba'. elTOQUE. Accessed 29 November 2020. https://eltoque.com/covid-19-derechos-y-estado-de-emergencia-en-cuba/.
Randal, Judith. 2000. 'Does the U.S. embargo affect Cuban health care?' *Journal of the National Cancer Institute* 92: 963.
Redaccion OnCuba. 2020a. 'Pesquisas desde el celular en Cuba'. Accessed 28 July 2020. https://oncubanews.com/cuba/pesquisas-desde-el-celular-en-cuba/.
Redaccion OnCuba. 2020b. 'Seis personas escaparon de un centro de aislamiento en Cuba y fueron capturadas'. Accessed 12 December 2020. https://oncubanews.com/cuba/seis-personas-escaparon-de-un-centro-de-aislamiento-en-cuba-y-fueron-capturadas/.
Redaccion OnCuba. 2020c. 'Cuba: casi la mitad de los contagios por coronavirus esta semana fueron importados'. Accessed 29 November 2020. https://oncubanews.com/cuba/cuba-casi-la-mitad-de-los-contagios-por-coronavirus-esta-semana-fueron-importados/.
Reid-Henry, Simon M. 2010. *The Cuban Cure: Reason and resistance in global science*. Chicago, IL: University of Chicago Press.
Rodriguez, José Luis. 2020a. 'La Batalla Económica y Frente a la COVID en la Cuba Actual (I). OBELA Observatoria Económica Latinamericano'. Accessed 12 December 2020. http://www.obela.org/documento/la-batalla-economica-y-frente-a-la-covid19-en-la-cuba-actual.
Rodriguez, José Luis. 2020b. 'La Batalla Económica y Frente a la COVID en la Cuba Actual (II). OBELA Observatoria Económica Latinamericano': Accessed 15 November 2020. http://www.obela.org/documento/la-batalla-economica-y-frente-a-la-covid19-en-la-cuba-actual.
Rojas, Marta. 1986. *El medico de la familia en la sierra maestra*. La Habana, Cuba: Editorial Ciencias Medicas.
Rose, Nikolas. 2009. *The Politics of Life Itself: Biomedicine, power, and subjectivity in the twenty-first century*. Princeton, NJ: Princeton University Press.
Roy, Arundhati. 2020. 'The pandemic is a portal'. *Financial Times*, 3 May 2020. Accessed 30 July 2020. https://www.ft.com/content/10d8f5e8-74eb-11ea-95fe-fcd274e920ca.
Sanchez, Yoani. 2012. 'Really? Cubans never joke about the revolution?' *Translating Cuba*. Accessed 29 November 2020. https://translatingcuba.com/really-cubans-never-joke-about-the-revolution-yoani-sanchez/.
Scheper-Hughes, Nancy. 1994. 'An essay: AIDS and the social body'. *Social Science & Medicine* 39: 991–1003.
Scheper-Hughes, Nancy. 2020. 'Epidemics and containment: Cuba and the HIV/AIDS epidemic'. *Anthropology Today* 36: 22–4.

Simone, AbdouMaliq. 2004. 'People as infrastructure: Intersecting fragments in Johannesburg'. *Public Culture* 16: 407–29.
Spiegel, Jerry and Annalee Yassi. 2004. 'Lessons from the margins of globalization: Appreciating the Cuban health paradox'. *Journal of Public Health Policy* 25(1): 85–110. https://doi.org/10.1057/palgrave.jphp.3190007.
Stevenson, Lisa. 2014. *Life Beside Itself: Imagining care in the Canadian Arctic.* Berkeley, CA: University of California Press.
Tanuma, Sachiko. 2007. 'Post-utopian irony: Cuban narratives during the "Special Period" decade'. *PoLAR: Political and Legal Anthropology Review* 30: 46–66.
Trevisan, Maurizio and Linh Cu Le. 2020. 'The COVID-19 epidemic: A view from Vietnam'. *American Journal of Public Health* 110(8): 1152–3.
Ubieta, Enrique. 2019. *Red Zone: Cuba and the battle against Ebola in West Africa.* Atlanta, GA: Pathfinder Press.
Weissenstein, Michael. 2020. 'Cuba: US embargo blocks coronavirus aid shipment from Asia'. Associated Press. Accessed 22 December 2020. https://apnews.com/article/2858fbaa2dd5460fa2988b888fc53748.
Westbrook, Alexandra and Nayara Sabrina de Freitas Alves. 2016. 'Havana's wastewater treatment plants: Changes over time and estimate of replacement cost'. ASCE. Accessed 29 November 2020. https://www.ascecuba.org/asce_proceedings/havanas-wastewater-treatment-plants-changes-over-time-and-estimate-of-replacement-cost/.
Whitacre, Ryan P., Liza Stuart Buchbinder and Seth M. Holmes. 2020. 'The pandemic present'. *Social Anthropology*, 19 May. https://doi.org/10.1111/1469-8676.12829.
Whiteford, Linda M. 2000. 'Local identity, globalisation, and health in Cuba and the Dominican Republic'. In *Global Health Policy, Local Realities: The fallacy of the level playing field*, edited by Linda M. Whiteford and Lenore Manderson, pp. 57–79. Boulder, CO: Lynne Rienner Publishers.

3
Militarising the pandemic
Lockdown in South Africa
Lenore Manderson and Susan Levine

Until mid-2020, South Africa controlled the transmission of coronavirus and avoided a heavy toll from COVID-19 by an early and stringent lockdown enforced by police and defence troops. The iconic images of the pandemic were of soldiers in camouflage and masks, strong-arming homeless residents and populations in informal settlements. Such images are redolent of South Africa's long history of police, soldiers and private security employees enforcing civil obedience; significant numbers of citizens live with the memory of their own house arrests, detention and imprisonment (Ross 2003). Consistent with apartheid's deployment of the military to curtail social movement, arms were used to threaten and kill particular citizens at the height of South Africa's aggressive COVID-19 response, so underlying the violence of class and race hierarchy. For those old enough to have lived through the worst years of apartheid curfews, passbooks, military surveillance, torture and house arrests, the sudden arrival of COVID-19 not only deepened poverty, unemployment and hunger, but it also unveiled the thin veneer of South Africa's transition to democracy. Having already endured chronic and systemic poverty, the massification of debility through TB and HIV/AIDS, and an uneven public health infrastructure to address chronic disease, the country has accommodated rules governing lockdown and its different forms of militant surveillance. The deadly experience of chronic pandemics created the conditions under which citizens across the country, in both urban and rural settings, complied to a much larger extent with public health protocols than in other parts of the world where we continue to witness the tragic results of anti-masker campaigns and COVID-19 denialism. That said, the spatialisation of poverty in the form of insecure and densely populated black townships has militated against the possibility of adequate social distancing (Manderson and Levine 2020).

How and why did South Africa manage with so little violence and resistance to enforce lockdown, and what counter factors came into play to address what might have been the catastrophic transmission of the virus in its early months? In this chapter, we show how lockdown in South Africa was enforced through its militarisation, drawing on the techniques and technologies of apartheid. We reflect on the unevenness of the risk and outcomes of infection from early in the pandemic, including in relation to the economic and social conditions of everyday life and access to care. We draw inspiration from a diverse range of theoretical directions and concepts to analyse South Africa's lockdown. Derrida's 'hauntology' allows us to apprehend the structural legacies of apartheid; Goffman's 'total institution' provides understanding of how the military works; Habermas (1975) allows us to comprehend the responsibility of the state to its population, and so to question state shortfalls, not only in South Africa but also in other settings. As we show, racism and capitalism converge and co-exploit to sharpen the inequalities of the pandemic.

Lockdown

South Africa's lockdown was initiated on 26 March, at the time one of the strictest lockdowns to be imposed globally. It continued to be extended thereafter at different levels, with the rise and fall of infections. Yet, even by the time the lockdown was introduced, schools and universities had already taken the first steps to deliver courses online, and retail, personal services and other industries had contracted in scope and engagement. Entry into corporate spaces and public buildings was limited; social distancing and hand sanitisation were pervasive. Armed security guards and police were far more visible along city streets and malls than they might have been under ordinary circumstances; bank tellers and shop assistants stepped back from customers; and television and radio news and magazine programmes consistently attended programmes to the sanitary requisites of prevention and the risks inherent in everyday life. The lockdown reinforced these practices, with strict Stage 4 constraints to movement that initially prohibited and later limited the hours of outdoor exercise, walking dogs and other recreational uses of public space, and mandated the use of masks when outside the home. The sale and purchase of cigarettes was prohibited, most likely to obviate excursions to shops, although also because smoking increased the risk associated for respiratory infection. Alcohol was also prohibited to limit what are, under any circumstances, painfully high levels of intimate partner violence (Friedman 2020), and as a measure to limit car accidents and injuries due to inebriation, which might lead to hospitalisations that would take up beds and medical services needed for patients with respiratory distress. The lockdown and associated measures constraining social life arguably contained the transmission of coronavirus for a time; in theory, they enabled hospitals, laboratories and health services to reorient to manage growing numbers of people with COVID-19. Some of the constraints were subsequently judged unconstitutional and irrational by the High Court of South Africa on 2 June 2020, by which time, 37,525 cases of coronavirus infection had been reported. And this was only the beginning of what became a shocking escalation of cases that fed on poverty, immiseration and civil unrest.

Even before lockdown had been declared, disinfectant dispensers were handheld by guards at shop doors; within three months, pedal dispensers had been installed in some premises to further minimise human contact. At upmarket establishments, temperatures were taken upon entry and contact details logged for tracking and tracing. Only a few people at a time were (and, in November 2020, still were) allowed into shops and government offices, including police stations and social security offices; the remainder stood spaced out to observe social distancing regulations, in South Africa as in the global north. Our social skin expanded to accommodate distance in contexts of privilege where social distancing is possible. In his May address to the nation, President Cyril Ramaphosa said that 'hugging and kissing is a thing of the past' (Tembo 2020). Self-surveillance, the regulation of others through citizen arrests and public shaming through social media platforms, assisted state response. Although the use of social media to 'sting' people recalcitrant or wilfully disobeying the law is not unique to South Africa (Sundaram 2015), the incremental encouragement of citizen surveillance pushed Michel Foucault's (2012) panopticon to its limit.

The temporary nature of this containment did not prepare South Africans for the scale and speed of viral spread. At the first lockdown, there were 927 reported cases; on 22 April, there were 4,546 cases and a total of 65 deaths; these low numbers, relative to infections and death rates elsewhere in the world, suggested that continued extreme state measures were unnecessary. But the effectiveness of such measures to avert a catastrophe were overestimated. By mid-July, South Africa was number five in the global league stakes that no one wanted to win; the number of cases and deaths continued to rise and viral transmission continued to accelerate across provinces and from urban to rural areas. By mid-November 2020, there were 750,000 cases of infection and over 20,000 deaths, with rural areas and the poorest states increasingly affected.

From the beginning of lockdown, the heightened presence of private security forces, citizen arrests,[1] the police, newly empowered national park rangers and the massification of South Africa's military response to enforce COVID-19 lockdown regulations contributed to a highly differentiated reality along the well-worn lines of class, race and gender. Two key questions emerged from these events and the continued repercussions of the pandemic: the extent to which social and economic inequality results in vulnerability to infection; and, as discussed below, the processes and consequences of militarisation in enforcing adherence to lockdown. By mid-July, the top 10 countries globally in terms of total reported cases of coronavirus were mostly countries with relatively large populations. The unequal impact of COVID-19, however, reflected not population density nor health systems factors alone, despite the fact that these factors surely influenced patterns and risks of transmission and infection. Rather, these countries, all high and middle-income countries, were among the most unequal countries in their regions and in the world (using World Bank Gini coefficients and government reports). We had, in the early weeks of the pandemic, argued that COVID-19 would track social fault lines and disproportionately infect and affect poor people (Manderson and Levine 2020). COVID-19 did not 'track' such fault lines: it fed on, burned into and abraded them. While vaccine development proceeded at remarkable pace through 2020, with research groups and pharmaceutical companies in the UK, Australia and the US fiercely competing, questions of its production at scale, and its stability, affordability, distribution and delivery, especially in countries with weak health systems and limited human and other resources, have yet to be addressed. In this respect, COVID-19, like HIV before it, will continue to impact unevenly in ways that penalise both the individuals and countries who are poorest and with the least power.

The one sure means we have to limit risk is to manage proximity, but proximity is also a scarce resource for people who live in the insanitary and crowded conditions that prevail in informal settlements, tenement buildings, workers' dormitories, high-rise apartments and public housing estates, slums and favelas in cities like Cape Town, Mexico City, New York, London, Delhi and Sao Paulo. People with low incomes, some without formal papers that allow them free access to services, routinely live with their families and others in makeshift shelters, often confined to single rooms. These are places with limited municipal services and poor social care, areas that typically lack sewage, drainage and waste disposal. They are characterised by extreme poverty and endemic unemployment, property and intimate partner violence, drug and alcohol abuse, and gang rule. The people in these environments live with disproportionate rates of chronic disease, the outcome of a calculated necropolitics (Mbembe 2008). In South Africa, this includes especially HIV; in India and South Africa, TB; and everywhere high rates of cardiometabolic disease, poor nutrition and poor mental health. Poor people do not have enough food, and lockdown has stripped many of even the most precarious and poorly remunerated income-generating activities such as recycling, flower markets and informal food stands. In some cases, in acknowledging this, state and NGO entities have extended grants and food relief; in other cases, they have not.

On 11 May, the South African Social Security Agency (SASSA) introduced a programme – the Special COVID-19 Social Relief of Distress Grant – which would provide 350 rand (c. US$20) per month for six months to people who were unemployed, were receiving no other benefits, and met other conditions relating to age and residence (South African Government 2020). Applications had to be electronic. Clearly, the intervention was unlikely to assist people whose employment was always precarious, who lacked access to basic virtual communication technology or who could not afford to pay for data. Moreover, people living in impoverished conditions without resources cannot adhere to the rules of social distance. They may not have reliable or clean water, and they may not be able to buy soap to wash their hands regularly, nor afford to make or purchase masks (Ross 2020). Further, despite little acknowledgement of this in dominant discourse in relation to COVID-19, poor populations everywhere have access to fewer health and medical services, are least often insured, may have no right to care, may be unwilling to present for care because of prior experiences of violence, disrespect and abuse, and often lack transport and cash to access and pay for advice or medication. COVID-19 magnified inequalities as it exploited them. Structural violence, discrimination and fear feed into understandings of the pandemic and everyday interactions, and were exploited by troops and police overseeing adherence to lockdown in informal settlements. The assertion of military power and the extension of police rights to punish caused as much fear – if not more – than the virus itself.

Theorising militarisation

In South Africa, as noted above, in order to enforce lockdown, there was increased use of police, military and militia deployed from private security companies and armed response teams, many of them soldiers from civil wars and insurgencies in neighbouring countries. The outsourcing to militarised forces to ensure public health compliance, rather than to social or healthcare workers, centralised state power and consolidated the uneven distribution of force along the lines of class and race. Likewise, it deepened fear in the social context of collective grief, loss and growing hunger and unemployment. The 1.5-metre rule of interaction and social distance became a mnemonic of risk and its embodiment in race and class. Such is the dystopic if not myopic landscape of COVID-19.

The rationale for military engagement is perhaps obvious yet it is useful, for our purposes, to reiterate this. The military is a highly organised and tightly regimented institution – a 'total institution' (Goffman 1961) – comprising a large number of people trained to operate without question, as part of a group, in unpredictable, volatile and dangerous settings. The scenarios of future violence for which defence forces are trained include terrorism with highly technical weaponry that might include chemical and biological warfare, explosive devices, and armed drones and guided missiles, and, on the other hand, low intensity and low-technology warfare such as that characteristic of recent civil wars and episodic resistance in countries in southern and central Africa, including Angola, Mozambique, Zimbabwe, DR Congo and Rwanda. Many of the troops and security officers involved in enforcing lockdown have had experience in such settings. South African soldiers are also trained to work alongside civilian entities in disaster management, including to rescue affected populations, reduce population risk and run disaster management centres. The laws that define these roles were invoked in 2020 to meet the emergent needs of taming and containing the pandemic.[2]

Contemporary democracies, including South Africa after apartheid, are meant to balance the lives of individuals and families with the collective interests related to social, economic and public life. Habermas (1975), among other theorists, has argued that by protecting contemporary democracy, the public sphere allows for mediation between family and the state, in ways that might temper the arbitrary exercise of power. The methods of governance for this include both formal and informal public institutions that enable debate, dissent and consensus. The ensuing debates, and power and authority, flow through political parties and parliamentary processes, trade unions and associations, and different structures of authority (including those associated with formal religion and traditional authority structures). The media, which in South Africa has a strong tradition and enduring practice of directly engaging in public life, also plays a significant role in governance in civil society. But the state also controls the military (excluding those militarised states where the reverse is true) and exercises power through it. COVID-19 has empowered the military in many contexts to reassert state domination over civilian populations under the guise of protection and care, while the military has taken advantage of the virus to subvert attempts to protest against and address systemic injustices and human rights abuses. COVID-19, like other global pandemics, has laid bare the myth of democracy as outlined by Habermas (1975). Let us take this moment to revisit the patriarchal and racist foundations of democracy as established by an elite class of white men to the exclusion of all others (Pateman 1989), and we will be better equipped to understand the uneven distribution of care in societies masquerading as egalitarian.

In South Africa after apartheid, the political rights of all people were guaranteed in the constitution, one of the most liberal, and clear, worldwide. The judicial system was established to assess claims between individuals and communities or groups in the private sphere, and to establish justice where points of contestation existed between specific populations and the state. At the core of these structures and the principles that underlie them are ideas of public good and the role of the state to ensure this. The legitimacy of a welfare state, even with a truncated active contribution to welfare, derives from its capacity to protect civil liberty and allow for democratic debate, protect the general population against sectarian interests (while allowing, within limits, their articulation consistent with commitment to democracy) and to provide a range of services essential for everyday life. The mandate to ensure and protect public health derives from this: specific state entities have a responsibility to guarantee conditions of public safety and wellbeing, including through the provision of infrastructure and services. These change with time. At present, they might include potable water, electricity, drainage, sewerage and garbage collection, and adherence to environmental and occupational health and building standards, although not all of these exist in all places, and although what is considered an infrastructural right might also change (clean energy, for example). Public health includes these services insofar as breaches in these areas might indirectly or directly infringe on health, as has been long documented in the case of bacterial disease outbreaks. In certain circumstances, the capacity of the state to maintain these conditions is undermined, as might occur in the case of an extreme weather event such as flood or drought or unprecedented local disaster (an explosion in a crowded inner city area, for instance, or a fire in a high-rise block or tearing through a suburb). Under such conditions, one can imagine the value of a reserve army of workers, as a defence force not engaged in active warfare might be regarded. How an army might be deployed in the case of infectious disease not transmitted as a result of the breakdown of infrastructure or social structure is less obvious. The use of the military in previous epidemics, not in South Africa but elsewhere on the continent – as occurred with Ebola – suggests that states are prepared to use exceptional measures under exceptional circumstances and to suspend usual protocol, as mandated by the constitutional responsibility of a state to declare an emergency. The coronavirus pandemic was one such moment.

In this context, discussion and debate about lockdown did not relate to options, but were centrally concerned with the threat of escalating infection and its venality. This extended to talk-back radio sessions on the implications of closing institutions, to the way in which isolation might impact on everyday life, to risks for specific activities. A week before the initial lockdown, one of us (LM) led a 90-minute webinar and Q & A session with the Institute of Plumbing South Africa, with hundreds of workers sharing computers and cell phones at service points and workshops to discuss the risks of infection as a result of using portable toilets on building sites, or accepting calls to attend to plumbing problems at people's homes. These media, word of mouth, WhatsApp, Facebook and press reports all allowed for the travel of information, of variable quality, about viral risk, spread and encounters, in ways that facilitated citizen's engagement in and reinforced the lively quality of South Africa's democratic institutions.

However, perhaps influenced by a rising mood of fear and anxiety, there was limited discussion of the ways that state acts of care – instantiated by advice about social distancing and hand washing and institutionalised through strictly enforced lockdown – might affect different populations. Although radio, television and social media provide venues for critical and oppositional voices in South Africa, these were unevenly distributed, and the most vocal concerns about lockdown related to monetary impact – an inevitability as the economy shuttered – and paid relatively limited attention to those whose lives were already precarious. With the easing of restrictions across the country there was an easing of draconian measures to curb the virus, but the easing of the military and police response was also attributed to ordinary citizens and activist journalists who rendered visible the violence of the state and the deepening of chaos at a moment that called for epistemic and ethical generosity.

Ebola occurred, as anthropologists illustrated, in the context of highly fragmented societies where the ghosts of colonial domination seeped into the management of bodies and communities during the crisis (Parker, et al. 2019; Sams, et al. 2017). In South Africa, with its specific history of militarisation, the response to COVID-19 was remarkably if uncomfortably accommodated, even as questions of race, racism and structural violence gained purchase. It was tolerated too despite the assumed impossible return of apartheid era curfews, lockdowns and the use of the military to contain populations and the movement across (internal) borders (Levine 2020).

The upscaling deployment of police and militia to urban and rural South Africa distorts the temporal imaginary of the past as it animates the present. The collapse of linear time is best indexed by Derrida's illuminating idea of 'hauntology', where the ghosts of the past enflesh the present (see Davis 2005). In South Africa, the specific history of militarisation to impose apartheid and enact gross human rights abuses might suggest that this response would be intolerable. And yet, the mass use of surveillance technologies to enforce COVID-19 lockdown regulations and curfews in South Africa, as elsewhere, seem largely to have been tolerated to a far greater extent than might be anticipated, with limited capacity to oppose these measures when set against the immediate threat of viral invasion and its effects on human lives. The increased presence of force, via the bodies of armed security guards, police and soldiers, consolidated fear along the lines of class and race, and sharpened the fear of the consequences of disease in terms of growing hunger, unemployment and localised violence. Without addressing questions of inequality, South Africa is likely to face similar problems in containing future unfolding crises in health and wellbeing. The uncomfortable trinity of class, race and gender remains in South Africa – as elsewhere – a prism through which an ontology of inequality surfaces at different intersectional axes, each of which requires further elaboration with the unfolding COVID-19 pandemic.

Enforcing isolation

The initial and continued lockdowns depended, increasingly, on enforcement. The informal settlements of South Africa, the slums of Mexico and the favelas of Brazil have long been characterised by gun rule and the venal power of street gangs, but in mid-2020, these spaces were equally sites of soldiers and police, using terror and the occasional display of force to maintain social distancing, curfews and isolation. In South Africa, on 26 March, 2,820 soldiers were mobilised to work with police to enforce Stage 5 lockdown and its strict regulations to stave off catastrophic levels of infection and death (Anon 2020). On 22 April 2020, 73,180 regular, reserve and auxiliary personnel of the South African National Defence Force were deployed for nine weeks – until 26 June – in an operation that cost around 4.5 billion rand (US$2.4 million). Even before this decision, anecdotal accounts of unnecessary and at times gratuitous use of force and police brutality were emerging; troops dressed in army fatigues, in military formation, weapons at the ready, descended on townships to disperse populations and enforce shelter in place. Local municipalities commissioned armoured personnel carriers – the Casspirs, Buffels and Hippos used to repress black populations under apartheid – to round up people without homes and reinforce lockdown.[3] People who were homeless in Johannesburg and Pretoria were rounded up and confined in sports stadiums and ovals. By late April, armed soldiers, municipal police, private security forces (including former militia) and national park rangers were being deployed to 'fight' the virus by fighting those at risk of infection. The war on COVID-19 was claimed to be one of the largest army deployments in the country's history. Consistent eye-witness accounts and reports of police brutality and abuse went beyond the levels of violence, already endemic, that mimic the enforcement of law as applied to race and place under apartheid, and that continue to the present as reactions to and a result of extreme inequality, deprivation and xenophobia. While not on the same scale as apartheid era violence, and with very different political groups in power, the muscle memory of militia deployment and the unapologetic abuse of police power signals the distinct failure of South Africa's democratic transition to upturn the ghosts of apartheid. The Marikana massacre for instance, in 2012, left 42 mine workers dead after then President Jacob Zuma ordered police to shoot at unarmed mine workers who were fighting for a living wage. Rather than an ethics of care in the face of grave adversity, the mining tycoon resorted to apartheid-era murder. The elasticity of history keeps looping back to this default response rather than more imaginative, or at the very least, less violent approaches to deploying care in time of crisis.

The confluence of science, medicine and the army is not new; direct links between the military and medical and surgical practice are well established historically and in the present (Chua 2018; Cooter et al. 1999; Harrison 2001; Pickstone 1992; Terry 2017). The matrix of South Africa's response to COVID-19 follows the use of police to enforce vaccination during the 2009 avian flu epidemic in Malawi (Sambala and Manderson 2017; 2018); the earlier use of surveillance and quarantine as a method to stem the spread of HIV/AIDS in Cuba (Scheper-Hughes 1993); and the controversial deployment of the military in Liberia during the height of the epidemic of Ebola virus disease (EVD) (Aizenman 2020). The Ebola epidemic was the largest of its type ever seen, characterised by its rapid transmission and terrifying case fatality, with almost 30,000 people infected and 11,000 fatalities, mainly in Guinea, Liberia and Sierra Leone. Kelley Sams and colleagues (2017) point out that this was the first time that anthropologists were early involved in relatively large numbers, although along predictable lines: to help ensure that public health interventions were locally relevant (Wilkinson et al. 2017). The measures of militarisation and policing that characterised the response to COVID-19 – to identify and quarantine cases – were amplified by (and amplified the power of) the iatrogenic impact of war metaphors for patients surviving or succumbing to illness (Sontag 2001). Further, in the race for a vaccine, the United States launched Operation Warp Speed in partnership with the US Defence Force and leading virologists. Its mission was to defeat the enemy because 'winning matters ... a massive scientific, industrial, and logistical endeavor unlike anything our country has seen' (National Public Radio 2020). Since then, the language of war has extended to reinvoke Cold War politics, with accusations of biological warfare and cyber espionage of scientific research increasingly redolent of the 1950s.

At the same time, the global upscaling of troops and other armed personnel as frontline forces to combat the spread of coronavirus was unprecedented. Far from the lexicon of war as metaphor to describe battles against illness, actual militia were tasked with implementing lockdown regulations to fight this viral enemy. Armed soldiers and police were not the metaphorical fighter cells of the human immune system under siege in bodies with HIV (Martin 1994); rather, as already described, in South Africa, armed soldiers in camouflage and police with masks were tasked to combat the virus by controlling population mobility, density and interaction even while equally vulnerable to infection. This militarised response was not unique; globally, defence forces and technologies were deployed at unprecedented levels to combat the spread of coronavirus. The first use of war infrastructure that captured global media attention was, arguably, army vehicles carrying coffins in Bergamo, Italy, in mid-March, when with hindsight, the number of deaths was enviably low. In Malaysia, also in March, army forces with protective face masks joined police to enforce border control and national lockdown.⁴ In the US, some 2,000 defence reserve personnel from the National Guard were called up on 19 March, and by 24 March, 9,000 troops were providing transportation, engineering, and planning and logistics, including administering tests and supporting medical personnel, as part of state efforts to control the spread of infection (Lengyel 2020). Field hospitals were erected to manage expanding caseloads and the need for hospitalisation. In Belgrade from 9 July, police used tear gas, armoured vehicles and horses to disperse people protesting against renewed lockdown conditions implemented in an effort to manage the impact of increased cases on Serbia's health system. In Australia, from early July, armed forces were patrolling the highways, truck routes and border tracks dividing the states of Victoria, New South Wales and South Australia. And over this time, countries worldwide, including those with the greatest numbers of infections and others (Peru, Mexico, Chile, India, Nigeria, Turkey, UK) militarised their responses to the pandemic. And while the rhetoric of the deployment of defence forces has not surprisingly tilted towards the care of the public, this 'care' has extended to patrol stores and protect looting, forcibly transfer people believed to be infected to hospital – in Nigeria, for example – and constrain everyday movement. In Nigeria, military personnel did not receive training to carry out policing functions, and this has been linked to reports of the systematic harassment and brutalisation of the population, including the deaths of violators of lockdown measures in Lagos, Abuja, Warri and elsewhere in the country (Iweze 2020).

The murder of George Floyd by policemen in Minneapolis on 25 May 2020, and the consequent roll-out of protests across the US and worldwide, extended the role of the military; troops increasingly complemented armed police to constrain protests against systematic racism and violence. The deployment of the military to 'fight' coronavirus provided states with growing opportunities to demonstrate their capacity to exercise physical control over members of the population for political as well as biological purposes. At the same time, COVID-19 provided a reason (or an excuse) for states to roundup and detain unregistered migrants and refugees (e.g. in Malaysia and in South Africa).⁵ By using the military to do this, states illustrated how the war on coronavirus might serve a dual purpose: containing viral spread and rooting out people, too, who were seen to be undesirable.

Thus the war on coronavirus interlocked with and enabled not a war against poverty, but a war against people who were poor. Throughout 2020, as people were evicted from houses for which they could no longer

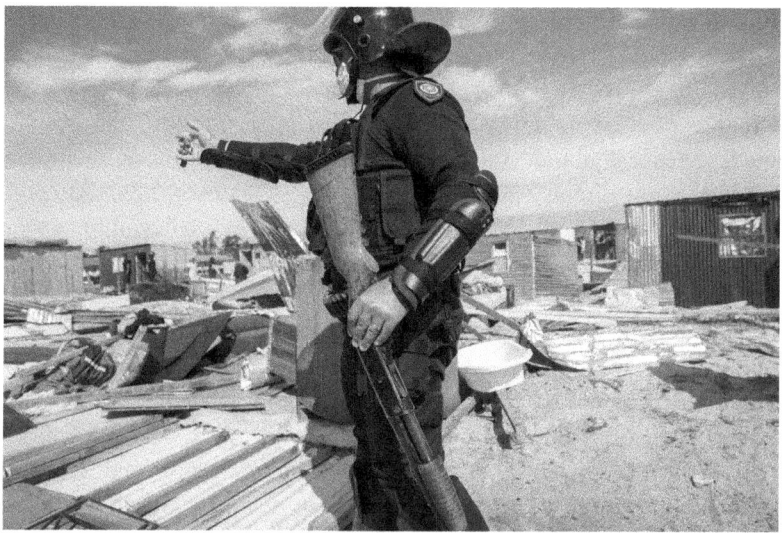

Figure 3.1 Land invasion. On an otherwise quiet Sunday in August, the Anti-Land Invasion Unit arrived at the settlement next to the new area called Covid, and, without warning to the community, proceeded to tear it down. Contract workers employed by the city carried the big pieces of tin to two waiting trucks. Photo: Samantha Reinders/NPR

pay rent, new informal settlements sprang up. Three settlements in the Cape Flats, on the periphery of the City of Cape Town – 'Covid', 'Sanitizer' and '19' (as in COVID-19) – are named as wry mnemonics of their history. But the tin shacks that people built for shelter were destroyed as quickly as they were built, torn down by contract workers and employees of the city's Anti-Land Invasion Unit, donned in riot gear and armed (Reinders 2020; see Figure 3.1).

The world was already lethal

The murder of George Floyd – suffocated under the force of a police officer's knee – ignited the massification of protestors in cities across the United States and, with speed, worldwide. President Donald Trump deployed armed forces to disperse peaceful protesters with tear gas and rubber bullets in the name of implementing curfew regulations put in place to limit the duration of public protest. Outside the White House, ostensibly to protect a photo shoot of the president, protestors were denied their constitutional right to peaceful protest. Floyd was the latest link in a tragic (and continuing) chain of brutal deaths and injuries involving police, again, in the US and worldwide – Australia, United Kingdom, France, Belgium, South Africa: Rodney King, Malice Wayne Green, Abner Louima, Amadou Diallo, Eric Garner, Michael Brown, Freddie Gray, Philando Castile, Ahmaud Arbery and Breonna Taylor, among them (Allman 2020; Stott et al. 2020; Taskinsoy 2020). Greater public scrutiny of police brutality of Black South Africa began to appear on Facebook posts. In a world battling with two forms of breath restriction – the suffocating effects of COVID-19 and the 'I can't breathe' movement triggered by Floyd's murder – Black people around the world not only fear and die from the virus; they also fear and are killed by security officers (see Garth, Chapter 5). Thus the pandemics of racism and COVID-19 are aligned and solicit similar militarised responses.

Troops deployed by President Cyril Ramaphosa to maintain the nationwide lockdown to contain infection, as described above, were extended from an initial three weeks and continued until 30 September. As noted, armed private security companies were also granted the right to enforce COVID-19 regulations. The police were able – as before – to issue fines, and to strong-arm, arrest and remove 'disobedient' members of the public. As radical new modes of sociality were introduced to diminish the wanderlust of the virus and its multiple forms of transmission, President Ramaphosa praised the courage, resilience, responsibility and sacrifices of ordinary South Africans. He failed, however, to be precise about the shape of these sacrifices, and he failed to condemn officers who abused their power by contributing to the 'economy of terror' that brought together the toxic combination of a militarised state apparatus with a deathly virus (for a comparison with Haiti, see James 2010).

As noted, deeply reminiscent of curfews that constrained the movement of dehumanised populations by criminalising black Africans as 'vagrants' under apartheid, the police enforced COVID-19 curfews in overcrowded areas, especially in informal settlements that lack the most basic necessities – always and particularly during COVID-19 – of running water, indoor toilets and electricity (Manderson and Levine 2020). The Minister of Cooperative Governance and Traditional Affairs Nkosaaana Dlamini Zuma is partly responsible for the declaration of a curfew that became established in law as: 'Every person is confined to his or her place of residence from 8:00 pm until 05:00 am daily, except where a person has been granted a permit'. Surveillance technologies returned with the ease of muscle memory, and thus the haunting. The pandemic had been militarised. An SMS message from a friend living in Athlone – a mostly coloured neighbourhood in Cape Town – read:

My brother in Knysna passed away today at noon due to a stroke. The police kept us behind walls. I was even sprayed by pepper spray on my way to get airtime … I can't even go to his funeral, I'm just very sad … I couldn't see for a couple of days because of the pepper spray … wish this lockdown was over, but hey I'm not taking any chances now, too afraid of the cops and army … A young mom that was still breastfeeding was shot on her boob with a rubber bullet, an elderly man was shot with a Taser, some people got fines for standing behind their gates in their own yards, as much as R1500. Oh my God, there's so much to tell, but my airtime will not make it. … they really treat us like animals, and that's the part the President doesn't see (Mara).

Against the opportunity to radically change South Africa's default position in times of crisis that leans into the logic of militarised force aimed at the poor, cities across the country afforded even greater power to law enforcement officers. In the Western Cape, the province initially hardest hit by the pandemic, the Cape Metro Police were backed by the City of Cape Town's traffic services, the latter reported to operate a 'heavily armed municipal militia' (Farr and Green 2020). Defence Minister Nosiviwe Mapisa-Nqakula justified the use of military force in terms of tightening regulations, and to 'make sure that our people understand fully the dangers of getting this virus'. The return of apartheid-era military tanks including iconic Casspirs, renamed by the Democratic Alliance (DA), the ruling party in the province, as 'hardened vehicles' (Farr and Green 2020), offers obvious material and symbolic links between the past and present moment that continues to violate black lives. This violation corroborates videos and stories circulating via social media and personal communication of police abuse, killing and humiliation of members of the public during national lockdown. This includes most recently the eviction of Bulelani Qolani, dragged naked from his shack, which the police ripped apart before his eyes (Lali and Stent 2020). Greg Nicolson, a journalist with the South African newspaper the *Daily Maverick*, had written, nine weeks earlier: 'I have a strong feeling that we may see a rise in incidents of what we regard as abuse simply because the police and the soldiers out there are not quite clear how to enforce the curfew arrangements' (Nicolson 2020).

Reports in local newspapers and social media indicate that whether or not the laws and regulations protected people from the virus, or slowed its spread, the police and others granted exceptional authority grossly abused their power. After Collins Khosa was verbally assaulted by police for standing outside his house, his parents report that police chased him into the house, ripped his shirt, broke their door down, swore and fired rubber bullets (Lali and Stent, 2020). The racism of criminalisation during COVID-19 regulations ricocheted against the tide of global forms of dehumanisation captured locally in Collins Khosa's murder and globally in George Floyd's. In his exceptional reporting on the murder of Khosa, Kneo Mokgopa (2020) wrote:

> The killing of Floyd sparked global protests under the hashtag, 'Black Lives Matter'. The death of George Floyd gathered international outrage, including from our own government, and protests around the globe. So many of us have tried to figure why it is that Collins Khosa's death, and the litany of other black people killed by South African law enforcement, could not ignite the same outrage and protests, even within our borders.

Mokgopa's response to reports that 12 people were killed in the first few weeks of lockdown signals that no impoverished person was shocked by the fact that in South Africa the police kill more than three times the number of people killed by the police in the United States. It instantiates Derrida's idea of hauntology and the normalisation of systemic violence that the pandemic revealed. Mokgopa's conclusion was this:

> If you are poor and black your life does not count to this society. It is often the state that will come to you with a gun. Your home can be destroyed, you can be assaulted, tortured and killed with impunity. This is the experience of impoverished people across South Africa. Our dignity is continuously vandalised by the state (2020).

Conclusion

In acknowledging the hardship that such extreme measures placed on the majority of the population, in April 2020 President Ramaphosa announced a '500 billion rand (around US$26 billion) package to shore up an economy devastated by the fallout from the coronavirus pandemic and support those who've been worst affected' (Naidoo 2020). This massive relief package was intended to support the economy and vulnerable people, in recognition that efforts to contain COVID-19 would result in increased homelessness, destitution and mass unemployment. In this respect and in terms of scale, COVID-19 was reminiscent of the 1918

H1N1 pandemic (the so-called 'Spanish Flu'), the most devastating pandemic of modern times (Philips 2020). Then, a century ago, South Africa was one of the five worst-hit parts of the world, with about 300,000 dead within six weeks. After it had finally ebbed, a doctor reflected in the *South African Medical Record* in January 1919: 'It has truly been an irreparable calamity which has fallen on South Africa' (Philips 2020).

The 1918 flu was not the only experience of pandemic in South Africa. More people have been infected and died from HIV and AIDS in South Africa than anywhere else in the world; in 2017, 7.7 million people were living with HIV. In the early twenty-first century, under the leadership of President Thabo Mbeki, when deaths from AIDS were escalating, the police curbed protest action by the Treatment Action Campaign (TAC) demanding access to antiretroviral treatment (Robins 2004). Looking back, one wonders how infection rates and the immense social and individual suffering in Sub-Saharan Africa could have been limited if governments had been as pro-active as the present moment (Heywood 2009; 2020). And yet with 2020 hindsight, the lockdown has only intensified poverty, hunger and unemployment, and led to the further curtailment of rights among the country's most vulnerable residents. It has yet to flatten the curve.

A healthcare intervention of the magnitude raised by the South African government needed a strong infrastructure based on an economy of compassion, not terror. Diseases of poverty including HIV, tuberculosis, hypertension and diabetes, plus the additional public health crises of gender-based violence, drug and alcohol dependence and food insecurity, co-mingle with vices of power, systemic racism and privilege. In the context of these multiple layers of vulnerability, the presence of the state in the form of curfews and surveillance technologies, however violent and punitive, has also been greeted by some as a form of state care and concern. Especially among middle and upper class South Africans who feared the fates of the US, Italy, the UK, Belgium and other countries with waves and second wave spikes, the strong arm approach deployed by the president has been largely well received. Unlike the tenor of this general praise, for the poor and dispossessed the COVID-19 pandemic was less of a rupture than a deepening of social fragility.

Jake Skeets (2020) writes that the world before COVID-19 'was already lethal', and that systemic disaster capitalism has diminished the possibility of hope, for there is no past to which we would wish to return: 'If we yearn for a time before the pandemic, what do we yearn for?' What indeed, do we yearn for? If we could answer this question, it might be possible to remake a world beyond COVID. This would be a world that would dismantle the machinery of force that deepens public suffering in the face of pandemic. It would fuel modes of care that require the total abolition of racial capitalism, and the global forces of colonial pillage that render some lives more valuable than others.

Notes

1. In terms of Section 42 of the Criminal Procedure Act of 1977, a South African Citizen has the right to arrest the following persons: Trespassers; Persons engaged in an affray (Public Fighting); and Persons who he (sic) has a reasonable suspicion have committed a Schedule One Offence.
2. South Africa, Disaster Management Act, 2002 (Act no. 57 of 30 December 2002).
3. See this for example: https://edition.cnn.com/2020/04/02/africa/homeless-community-south-africa-coronavirus-intl/index.html.
4. There are links here to the police use of pepper balls to disperse people protesting the death of George Floyd in Washington DC on 1 June, and the consistent oppositional force to resist #BlackLivesMatter protests worldwide.
5. Al Jazeera reporters have been arrested and interrogated and there are reports of sustained online abuse (13 July 2020).

References

Allman, Kate. 2020. 'Police state or safety net?: How NSW entered a strange "new normal"'. *SJ: Law Society of NSW Journal* 66: 30.
Anon. 2020. 'South Africa to deploy 73,000 more troops to enforce COVID-19 lockdown'. *Defence Post*, 22 April 2020. Accessed 4 June 2020. https://www.thedefensepost.com/2020/04/22/south-africa-deploy-73000-troops-covid-19-lockdown/.
Chua, Jocelyn Lim. 2018. 'Fog of war: Psychopharmaceutical "side effects" and the United States military'. *Medical Anthropology* 37(1): 17–31.
Cooter, Roger, Mark Harrison and Steve Sturdy, eds. 1999. *Medicine and Modern Warfare*. Amsterdam, The Netherlands: Rodopi.
Davis, Colin. 2005. 'Hauntology, spectres and phantoms'. *French Studies* 59(3): 373–9.
Derrida, Jacques. 1994. *Specters of Marx: The State of the Debt, the Work of Mourning, and the New International*. Abingdon, UK: Routledge.
Farr, Vanessa and Lesley Green. 2020. 'Amid escalating gang violence, the city of Cape Town wages war on the poor'. *Daily Maverick*, 8 July 2020. Accessed 10 July 2020. https://www.dailymaverick.co.za/author/vanessa-farr-and-lesley-green/#gsc.tab=0.
Foucault, Michel. 2012. *Discipline and Punish: The birth of the prison*. New York: Vintage.
Friedman, Steven. 2020. 'South Africa's lockdown: A great start, but then a misreading of how society works'. *The Conversation*, 4 June 2020. Accessed 10 July 2020. https://theconversation.com/south-africas-lockdown-a-great-start-but-then-a-misreading-of-how-society-works-139789.
Goffman, Erving. 1961. *Asylums: Essays on the social situation of mental patients and other inmates*. New York: Anchor.
Habermas, Jürgen.1975. *Legitimation Crisis*. Boston, MA: Beacon Press.
Harrison, Mark. 2001. *The Medical War: British military medicine in the First World War*. Oxford, UK: Oxford University Press.
Heywood, Mark. 2009. 'South Africa's treatment action campaign: Combining law and social mobilisation to realize the right to health'. *Journal of Human Rights Practice* 1(1): 14–36.
Heywood, Mark. 2020. 'Coronavirus: Why protecting human rights matters in epidemics'. *Daily Maverick*, 24 February 2020. Accessed 4 June 2020. https://www.dailymaverick.co.za/article/2020-02-24-covid-19-why-protecting-human-rights-matters-in-epidemics/#gsc.tab=0.

Iweze, Daniel Olisa. 2020. 'Covid-19 and Nigeria's counterinsurgency operations in the northeast.' *Kujenga Amani*, 4 June 2020. Accessed 20 May 2021. https://kujenga-amani.ssrc.org/2020/06/04/covid-19-and-nigerias-counterinsurgency-operations-in-the-northeast/.

James, Erica Caple. 2010. 'Ruptures, rights, and repair: The political economy of trauma in Haiti'. *Social Science & Medicine* 70(1): 106–13.

Lali, Vincent and James Stent. 2020. 'Bulelani Qolani: What happened before he was dragged naked from his shack?' *GroundUP*, 9 July 2020. Accessed 10 July 2020. https://www.groundup.org.za/article/bulelani-qolani-what-happened-he-was-dragged-naked-his-shack/.

Lengyel, Joseph J. 2020. 'Air Force Gen. Joseph L. Lengyel, Chief of the National Guard Bureau, holds a news conference at the Pentagon'. *Transcript*, 24 March 2020. Washington DC: US Department of Defense. Accessed 4 June 2020. https://www.defense.gov/Newsroom/Transcripts/Transcript/Article/2124943/air-force-gen-joseph-l-lengyel-chief-of-the-national-guard-bureau-holds-a-news/.

Levine, Susan. 2020. 'South Africa's response to Covid-19 and the ghosts of apartheid'. *Corona Times*, 21 May 2020. Accessed 4 June 2020. https://www.coronatimes.net/south-africa-covid-19-ghosts-of-apartheid/.

Manderson, Lenore and Susan Levine. 2020. 'COVID-19, risk, fear, and fall-out'. *Medical Anthropology* 39(5): 367–70.

Martin, Emily. 1994. *Flexible Bodies: Tracking immunity in American culture from the days of polio to the age of AIDS*. Boston, MA: Beacon Press.

Mbembe, Achille. 2008. 'Necropolitics. In *Foucault in an Age of Terror: Essays on biopolitics and the defence of society*, edited by Stephen Morton and Stephen Bygrave, pp. 152–82. Basingstoke, UK: Palgrave Macmillan.

Mokgopa, Kneo. 2020. 'Unthere: Blackness is where language comes to die.' *Daily Maverick*, 22 June 2020. Accessed 20 May 2021. http://www.dailymaverick.co.za/article/2020-06-22-unthere-blackness-is-where-language-comes-to-die/.

Naidoo, Ravi. 2020. 'The pandemic's economic devastation has created a rare opportunity for a New Deal in South Africa.' *Daily Maverick*, 29 April 2020. https://www.dailymaverick.co.za/opinionista/2020-04-29-the-pandemics-economic-devastation-has-created-a-rare-opportunity-for-a-new-deal-in-south-africa/.

National Public Radio. 2020. 'Coronavirus update: President Trump announces "Operation Warp Speed"'. 15 May 2020. Accessed 4 June 2020. https://www.npr.org/2020/05/15/857105042/coronavirus-update-president-trump-announces-operation-warp-speed

Nicolson, Greg. 2020. 'Eight witnesses saw soldiers assault Collins Khosa – IPID report'. *Daily Maverick*, 10 June 2020. Accessed 10 July 2020. https://www.dailymaverick.co.za/article/2020-06-10-eight-witnesses-saw-soldiers-assault-collins-khosa-ipid-report/#gsc.tab=0.

Parker, Melissa, Tommy Matthew Hanson, Ahmed Vandi, Lawrence Sao Babawo and Tim Allen. 2019. 'Ebola and public authority: Saving loved ones in Sierra Leone'. *Medical Anthropology* 38: 440–54.

Pateman, Carole. 1989. *The Disorder of Women: Democracy, Feminism, and Political Theory*. Palo Alto, CA: Stanford University Press.

Philips, Howard. 2020. 'South Africa bungled the Spanish flu in 1918. History mustn't repeat itself for COVID-19'. *The Conversation*, 10 March 2020. Accessed 4 June 2020. https://theconversation.com/south-africa-bungled-the-spanish-flu-in-1918-history-mustnt-repeat-itself-for-covid-19-133281.

Pickstone, John, ed. 1992. *Medical Innovations in Historical Perspective*. New York: St Martin's Press.

Reinders, Samantha. 2020. 'Photos: Why South Africans built an illegal settlement called Covid'. *Goats and Soda: Stories of Life in a Changing World*, 15 November 2020. Accessed 8 December 2020. https://www.npr.org/sections/goatsandsoda/2020/11/15/934003088/photos-why-south-africans-built-an-illegal-settlement-called-covid.

Robins, Steven. 2004. 'Long live Zackie, long live': AIDS activism, science and citizenship after apartheid'. *Journal of Southern African Studies* 30(3): 651–72.

Ross, Fiona. 2003. *Bearing Witness: Women and the truth and reconciliation commission in South Africa*. London: Pluto Press.

Ross, Fiona. 2020. 'Of soap and dignity in South Africa's lockdown'. *Corona Times*, 8 April 2020. Accessed 4 June 2020. https://www.coronatimes.net/soap-dignity-south-africa-lockdown/.

Sambala, Evanson Z. and Lenore Manderson. 2017. 'Anticipation and response: Pandemic influenza in Malawi, 2009'. *Global Health Action* 10: 1341225.

Sambala, Evanson Z. and Lenore Manderson. 2018. 'Ethical problems in planning for and responses to pandemic influenza in Ghana and Malawi'. *Ethics & Behavior* 28(3): 199–217.

Sams, Kelley, Alice Desclaux, Julienne Anoko, Francis Akindès, Marc Egrot, Khoudia Sow, Bernard Taverne, Blandine Bila, Michèle Cros, Moustapha Keïta-Diop, Mathieu Fribault and Annie Wilkinson. 2017. 'From Ebola to plague and beyond: How can anthropologists best engage past experience to prepare for new epidemics?' *Fieldsights, Member Voices*, 7 December 2017. Accessed 4 June 2020. https://culanth.org/fieldsights/from-ebola-to-plague-and-beyond-how-can-anthropologists-best-engage-past-experience-to-prepare-for-new-epidemics.

Scheper-Hughes, Nancy. 1993. 'AIDS, public health, and human rights in Cuba'. *The Lancet* 342(8877): 965.

Skeets, Jake. 2020. 'The other house. Musings on the Diné perspective of time'. *Emergence Magazine* 8. Accessed 4 June 2020. https://emergencemagazine.org/story/the-other-house/.

Sontag, Susan. 2001. *Illness as Metaphor and AIDS and its Metaphors*. London: Macmillan.

South African Government. 2020. Social Relief of Distress (SRD) grants. Accessed 4 June 2020. https://www.gov.za/covid-19/individuals-and-households/social-grants-coronavirus-covid-19.

Stott, Clifford, Owen West and Mark Harrison. 2020. 'A turning point, securitisation, and policing in the context of Covid-19: Building a new social contract between state and nation?' *Policing: A Journal of Policy and Practice*. Accessed 4 June 2020. https://doi.org/10.1093/police/paaa021.

Sundaram, Ravi. 2015. 'Publicity, transparency and the circulation engine: The media sting in India'. *Current Anthropology* 56:S297–305.

Taskinsoy, John. 2020. 'Diminishing dollar hegemony: What wars and sanctions failed to accomplish, COVID-19 has'. SSRN, 7 April 2020. Accessed 4 June 2020. http://dx.doi.org/10.2139/ssrn.3570910.

Tembo, Theolin. 2020. 'SA hit hard at news that kissing and hugging are a thing of the past'. DFA, 14 May 2020. Accessed 4 June 2020. https://www.dfa.co.za/south-african-news/sa-hit-hard-at-news-that-kissing-and-hugging-are-a-thing-of-the-past-65f94e6a-ec11-5520-9284-1757acb41db5.

Terry, Jennifer. 2017. *Attachments to War: Biomedical logics and violence in twenty-first-century America*. Durham, NC: Duke University Press.

Wilkinson, Annie, Melissa Parker, Frederick Martineau and Melissa Leach. 2017. 'Engaging "communities": Anthropological insights from the West African Ebola epidemic'. *Philosophical Transactions of the Royal Society B – Biological Sciences* 372(1721): 20160305.

4
Rights, responsibilities and revelations
COVID-19 conspiracy theories and the state
Elisa J. Sobo and Elżbieta Drążkiewicz

> This is what Bill Gates and George Soros want to do... Secretly stick you with a chip while testing you for the corona virus.... the Dems have a bill on the house floor ready to vote on it to require this .... House Bill 6666.... no bull.... look it up and WAKE UP !!!! (10 May 2020, Facebook post showing deeply inserted nasal swab, https://www.facebook.com/john.barno.1/posts/3216228888396817, original punctuation)

When the SARS-CoV-2 virus began its global spread, launching the COVID-19 pandemic, the race for a vaccine began. Simultaneously, authorities sought to reduce the novel coronavirus's propagation and lower the strain on hospitals and morgues. Around the world, governments began regulating not only where people could go and with whom but how to dress (with masks and gloves) and behave (no shaking hands, keeping 2 m distance from each other and so on). As epidemiologists turned to intensified contact tracing, private companies and governing bodies joined forces to create new technologies for scaling up surveillance, including virtual queuing tools, devices warning individuals should they get too close to others and contact tracing apps.

All this was discussed daily in households and on social media. In many instances, concerns over control, authority, transparency and freedom – fuelled by competition between officially sanctioned, expert knowledge and popular knowledge – supported the circulation of 'conspiratorial beliefs'. Around the world, fraught discussions ensued regarding COVID-19 cover-ups, pandemic geopolitics, bot and humanly driven disinformation floods on social media, and reporting bias in the press.

The rapid incorporation of COVID-19 into conspiratorial schemes worldwide (Freeman et al. 2020; Uscinski and Enders 2020) provides us with a useful set of cross-culturally comparable conspiracy theories involving the state, and thus a useful lens through which to enhance our thinking about how conspiracy theories work as sociocultural critiques – and what work they do for those who have built careers or identities promoting them, cynically or not (see Bailey 1994). Our project draws on ideas propagated in the first two-thirds of 2020. We focus on discourses circulated via platforms like Twitter and Facebook within Ireland, Poland and the US (where we have worked for many years). With this focus, we ask how the 2020 pandemic is loaded onto and used by those with vested interests to amplify, in the Global North, structure-agency, governance-freedom, responsibilities-rights tensions – tensions related to ideal visions of and for the state and, ultimately, for justice and liberty. To gain insight, we aim our investigation toward so-called conspiracy theories questioning state-sponsored health interventions including but not limited to vaccination. Because no approved COVID-19 vaccine existed at the time of our investigation, the prospect of vaccination provided a particularly viable projective screen for existential concerns: it was easily drawn into use as evidence for the central claims of those already backing a conspiratorial world view.

We are interested specifically in how, in Ireland, Poland and the US, and likely other democratic states, local conditions shape people's reception of, and by extension compliance with, governmental public health emergency efforts, and how conspiracy theories come into play in the process. We are interested in readings of disease threats that connect 'facts on the ground' in ways that differ from how authorised public health experts would have us connect them – readings thereby labelled as 'conspiracy theories'. After preeminent political anthropologist F.G. Bailey, we see this as a competitive process of 'claim and counterclaim … about the way our world is and the way it should be' (1991, 17). Such a focus affords us the opportunity to interrogate what COVID-19-related conspiracy theories might accomplish for those vested in broadcasting them, and how and why even seemingly similar conspiratorial ideas can vary in important local and historically particular ways.

Pandemic sense-making and dissent

We begin by observing that, in conspiratorial theorising, knowledge is not an end in itself (Boyer 2006; Briggs 2004). This view lines up with general anthropological thinking on knowledge as instrumental – as used to interpret and act in the world; consequently, it is not distinguishable from culture (Barth 2002; see also Bailey 1991, 17–18). Further, theorising about the world does not begin with knowledge but with how people know things, and so we must examine the processes by which people make connections in a fragmented world, how these reflect particular styles of reasoning and what can be known under particular historical circumstances (Hastrup 2004). This is especially relevant in the context of COVID-19, with all its unknowns and the ways these have been exacerbated by the diverse containment, communication and transparency strategies adopted by different governments.

Today's pandemic conspiracy theories are less contests regarding specific detailed facts (although they may be this overtly) than contests regarding values. Adopting Bailey's vantage, through COVID-19 conspiracy assertions, communities place their values 'onto the front stage' for affirmation (1994, 152). Their theories are testimonials to deep-rooted understandings about the state's role in relation to citizens and other stakeholders, corporations included.

Such visions of how society should function and of the prerogatives and limits of government vary across societies. If conspiracy theories are shaped by our worldviews (e.g. Harambam 2020), consequently, even when the contents of conspiracy theories appear similar across societies, their meanings must differ, at least to some degree.

Using case studies, we interrogate publicly propagated conspiratorial views on vaccination and other public health measures (social distancing, contact tracing, testing) related to the present pandemic. The anthropologist's task – the remit of all social theorists, in fact – is to 'find explanation beyond the truth of the events themselves' (Hastrup 2004, 468). As Engle-Merry and Coutin (2014) point out, to understand conflicts over knowledge we must understand the political dynamics of these conflicts – which may remain unseen to those embroiled in them (see also Bailey 1994). Taking political context seriously is crucial not only to fully grasping what various conspiracy theories have to tell us. It is paramount to diffusing harm-promoting aspects of COVID-19 denialism.

Conspiratorial thinking

So-called conspiracy theories are fluid networks of ideas deployed against the grain of accepted understandings to argue that specific events do not unfold at random or as the secondary fall-out of mundane social processes or day-to-day, disinterested bureaucratic decisions. Rather, agents work covertly and malevolently backstage, pulling strings. Often, conspiracy theories assume that conspirators act to harm others; they operate through dichotomous categorisations of 'us' vs 'them', good vs evil.

Although lay discourse tends to lump them together, disdainfully, conspiracy theories vary. Some have little more in common than their reliance on suspicions regarding secret operations. Further, conspiracy theories may contain multiple individually false claims; or they may spuriously connect substantively well-justified 'facts'. They may stand alone, or conjoin, or nest into 'superconspiracies' (Barkun 2013). The salience of conspiracy theories within group culture and their importance for social belonging also varies. Sometimes they are paramount to group identity. When such groups are put on the defensive they may close ranks; their ideas may become 'self-sealing' (Sunstein and Vermeule 2009, 204). That said, a group's members can hold richly diverse and sometimes contradictory positions in support of the same core concern (Harambam 2020).

Medical conspiracies and the state

Much of anthropology's conspiracy theory-related scholarship has appeared in medical anthropology, partly reflecting the subfield's longstanding involvement with health aid flows from the Global North to the Global South. Such programmes often provoke concerns related to sovereignty, exploitation and social coherence – i.e. perceived ruptures in the social contract. When voiced in local idioms these can be read as conspiracy theories (see Leach and Fairhead 2007; Fassin 2011).

Many cultures use blood-stealing and organ-thieving stories to index how they physically fuel the global economy. International medical research in sub-Saharan Africa provides a 'particularly prolific' matrix for such stories (Geissler and Pool 2006, 975). They express colonial trauma and critique both the non-democratic distribution of science's benefits, and the state's role in supporting this.

Epidemics also implore conspiratorial interpretations where the state has historically failed in its duties toward citizens. Take the 2008 cholera outbreak in Harare, Zimbabwe. When the government insisted that individual behaviour change (better handwashing and food hygiene) would stem transmission, residents pushed back. They pointed to structural drivers such as the dilapidated water and sanitation infrastructure, and condemned various arms of the state for victim-blaming and corruption. In challenging official discourses, they expressed 'an aspirational vision of citizenship based on political rights, social recognition, and access to high-quality public services delivered by a robust, responsible state' (Chigudu 2019, 415).

In Venezuela, cholera conspiracy theories directly addressed an 'economy of erasure' in which marginalised populations remained unheard (Briggs 2004; see also Mathur 2015). The theories embodied a bid to be seen – and a refusal to be reduced, for instance by epidemiology, which thrives by 'turning people into categories and numbers' (Briggs 2004, 167). They articulated local–global links in ways that questioned the discursive production and segregation of these domains in addition to highlighting their state's failures (p. 175).

Similar insights are seen in ideas regarding HIV/AIDS, widely rumoured initially to have been invented for nefarious genocidal purposes. State-backed corporate treachery did undergird the pandemic's hold in some ways in some locations, for instance, through machinations related to the construction of a dam in Haiti that destroyed various communities' livelihoods, pushing people into HIV-fostering survival strategies (Farmer 1992). In Eastern Indonesia, HIV/AIDS-related conspiracy theories reflected everyday experiences of 'inconsistent applications of policies, missing information, and omissions in formal practice' and colonisation, militarisation and racialisation in the study setting (Butt 2005, 432). South African men's conspiracy theories in Bushbuckridge linked HIV/AIDS-related suspicions to precarity wrought by job loss and, more broadly, deindustrialisation, itself subtended by the distribution of power and of racism in the globalised economy (Niehaus and Jonsson 2005, e.g. 182, 202). Conspiracy theories pervaded US HIV/AIDS discourses also, in ways similarly linked to social, political and economic marginalisation (Sobo et al. 1997).

A waiting matrix

COVID-19 emerged in the context of many already-circulating, conglomerate 'superconspiracies' (Barkun 2013). For instance, it was quickly fitted into, and helped amplify, conspiracy theories circulating regarding the health dangers of 5G networks – themselves rooted in much older worries about the profit-minded capitalist promotion of purportedly unsafe electromagnetic technologies, and worries about modernity itself (Tiffany 2020). 5G's initial roll-out in China, where COVID-19 was identified, seemed proof of a causal link. It also boosted antecedent chauvinistic prejudices, which situations of crisis intensify (see Butter and Knight 2020; Bovensiepen 2016).

In England, pre-existing anti-Semitic and antimuslim prejudice fed belief among 20 per cent of the population that 'Jews have created the virus [SARS-CoV-2] to collapse the economy for financial gain' and that 'Muslims are spreading the virus as an attack on Western values' (Freeman et al. 2020). Likewise, labelling SARS-CoV-2 as the 'Chinese Virus' or 'Kung Flu' drew upon already well-established jingoist and racist tropes. It also expressed pre-existing geopolitical tensions: as some in the US blamed its rival China for covering up a laboratory accident or worse in Wuhan, others on social media lauded China for besting the Global North via how efficiently they managed the pandemic. In these and related narratives, SARS-CoV-2 is cast not as coincidental but as part of larger conspiratorial machinations.

In addition to underwriting racist scapegoating and related brutalities, COVID-19 conspiracy theories entail other risks. Vaccination is, internationally, the desired 'magic bullet' in the fight against SARS-CoV-2. However, given that, for instance, about one in five members of a representative sample of English adults surveyed believe this vaccine 'will be used to carry out mass sterilization' or 'will contain microchips to control the people' (Freeman et al. 2020), mass vaccination promises to prove an uphill battle. (The vaccine rollout, which began well after this chapter was written, has, in fact, been challenged by those who question its ultimate aims; e.g. Sobo 2021.)

Contested expertise

The dominant way for establishment experts to deal with conspiracy theories is to try to 'debunk' them, often ineffectively. A rich social science literature explains that 'debunking' disregards people's extant knowledge (e.g. Leach and Fairhead 2007). Further, enhanced communications and computing technologies now support a subjective 'incredulity toward metanarratives' or 'grand narratives' (Lyotard 1984; Vine and Carey 2017). The technocultural environment of the internet intensifies the situation further in the Global North by democratising the 'knowledge-power hierarchy' (Kirmayer et al. 2013, 180), reinforcing expert-doubting overconfidence in one's capacities for discernment.

How this plays out varies across nations. In the US, for instance, idealised distaste for any concentration of power (Fenster 2008), an emphasis on free thinking, and the sanctity of free choice further deepen distrust of authority. The good citizen does not follow blindly. This is further supported in the realm of healthcare by institutionalised requests that patients self-educate and ask providers questions regarding treatment options, and the doubt-sustaining demand that patients (now, 'consumers') consent to and assume the risks even of biomedically-indicated procedures.

The debunking approach to conspiracy theories and other dissenting knowledge does sometimes work, for example, for hypocognised problems or those not already freighted with cultural meaning. But COVID-19 was for most people immediately associated with prior epidemic diseases, including not just HIV/AIDS and H1N1 influenza but the first SARS-COV panic (2003–04). Further, COVID-19 is characterised by a much higher degree of indeterminacy.

The uncertainty regarding specific origins, successful cures, prevention measures and risk for transmission expressed within the scientific community is exacerbated in the public mind by conflicting messages from different health authorities (regarding interactions with ibuprofen, who is vulnerable, etc.) – and from national and regional leaders. Belarusian president Alexander Lukashenko has touted washing with, and drinking, vodka as a cure; in the US Donald Trump has promoted hydroxychloroquine, a drug approved for malaria and rheumatoid arthritis; officials in Bolivia have distributed ivermectin, an anti-parasite drug, as an ostensible cure. None of these recommendations have authorised science's endorsement (O'Grady 2020). A good example of the doubt-reinforcing confluence of varied advice was seen in the dilemma masks posed for the public as the pandemic took hold (wear them, don't wear them, use special ones, homemade is fine, only health services professionals should wear them, etc.).

Negotiating boundaries between bogus and genuine claims is typical of the work done by people exploring alternative or dissenting perspectives (Pelkmans and Machold 2011; Mathur 2015). The plethora of positions the public has been provided by the state and others regarding COVID-19 supports doubt; doubt creates discomfort (Pelkmans 2013). Yet, an erosion of trust in authoritative and scientific knowledge does not extinguish the 'will to truth' (Aupers 2012). On the contrary, it opens a space for alternative forms of knowing. Lay investigation flourishes in publics already convinced of their own discernment and primed to express this by an ethos of wariness of expertise, and with reference to the oppositional forces of local and global governance, and of agency and structure.

Accordingly, COVID-19 conspiracy theories ask universally: what are governments trying to do through COVID-19? What information are governments hiding? What are they revealing? Why? And who is behind it all? Who profits? We explore some answers below, bearing in mind that beyond the theories described sit those vested in their propagation – those who leverage them as evidence of a priori claims, profiting themselves in various ways in the process.

New viral loadings: leveraging pandemic conspiracy theories

To explore the critiques of power conspiracy theories entail, and how they are deployed, we present three case studies. In each, interested parties actively characterised the pandemic counterfactually, for their own advantage.

Ireland: rejecting foreign rule and state corruption

Irish people expressing conspiratorial views on the pandemic questioned whether the risk was as severe as the authorities suggested. Many applied neologisms popular in the English-speaking world such as 'plandemic' or 'scamdemic' to suggest premeditated duplicity. For example, in May, member of parliament Mattie McGrath used this construction to imply that the lockdown regulations negatively affecting the Irish economy were a scam benefiting foreign corporations:

> It's a joke at this stage. We need to move on and get back to work. We are now at the stage where instead of having a pandemic it's becoming a scamdemic. Big businesses, the likes of [foreign superstores] Tesco and Aldi, and all the big places are flying, but all the small stores, small businesses, small retailers, they are being squeezed out of it by the two-metre social distancing. It just makes things totally unworkable (Farrell and Mooney 2020).

Gemma O'Doherty, once a celebrated investigative journalist, now best known for her fringe right-wing views and anti-vaccine statements, took a similar stance. O'Doherty is a founder of Anti-Corruption Ireland, which she defines as a 'formation devoted to ending this toxic culture of corruption that is ripping our republic to shreds'. Her agenda includes the 'fight against the threat of globalism' and its risk to 'national sovereignty, cultural and natural heritage, and endangering our independence'. Through social media, O'Doherty repeatedly implied that use of existing vaccines correlated with the COVID-19 death rate, and that COVID-19 vaccines would pose risks too when introduced. One of her widely circulated flyers claimed that 'Covid19 is no more serious than the flu', and that because 'we don't close the economy for [flu] and never quarantine the healthy … social distancing is fraudulent' (O'Doherty 2020a). In a leaflet, she argued:

> The state's draconian reaction to Covid19 has nothing to do with protecting health. It's an orchestrated ploy to implement the final phase of totalitarian 'one world' governance. This is the core objective of UN Agenda 2030, a plan to destroy nation states and depopulate our planet. It is also known as the New World Order. The State is forcing citizens to give up their fundamental rights, freedoms, and privacy using: orweallian [sic] surveillance via carcinogenic 5G, DNA-Altering mandatory vaccines, cashless society, control of media/end free speech (O'Doherty 2020b).

O'Doherty and her followers often share and recycle Twitter and Facebook posts originating elsewhere, and other conspiracy theory proponents around the world return the favour. However, conspiratorial views propagated by O'Doherty and her followers are more than recycled internationally circulating tropes. While almost every conspiracy theory propagated during the pandemic expresses concern over a loss of freedom, in Ireland this view resonates particularly strongly with the colonial legacy of, and national sentiments rooted in, the conflict with Britain (Moore and Sanders 2002). The painful memory of brutal foreign rule was particularly visible in the arguments made by O'Doherty and John Waters when they legally challenged Ireland's lockdown restriction, in the High Court, in April and May 2020. Their supporters perceived their actions as protective of the freedoms of Irish people. Those lauding O'Doherty's and Waters' legal efforts often spoke of them as courageous patriots ready to fight corrupt politicians and countering state efforts to suppress citizens. Frequently, they would draw parallels between the 1922 Irish civil war and the pandemic situation, describing the fight against lockdown measures as participation in the unfinished revolution.

O'Doherty and Waters, in their court statements and in public communications at the time, frequently referenced the new COVID-19 situation as 'the police state'. On 28 April, at the height of the court case dispute, O'Doherty tweeted, 'The words Irish and freedom are inextricably linked. No people fought harder for it throughout history than us. We're not going to give it away now to an unhinged police mob, an unelected government and their #fakenews who shamed themselves again today #LockdownIreland #Covid19' (O'Doherty 2020c).

In other communications, O'Doherty referred to Irish police (the Garda Síochána) as Gestapo or Nazi forces, and criticised COVID-19 laws that allowed for armed Gardaí at COVID-19 checkpoints. In Ireland, such use of force resonates specifically with memories of the colonial state and the brutal policing exercised by the British to control the Irish population (as one response, when the Garda Síochána was formed in 1923, it was purposefully primarily unarmed). When Irish conspirationists evoke the police state, they not only prey upon general concerns over the loss of freedom, but specifically Irish sentiments and fears.

In her pandemic communications, O'Doherty often referenced an 'unelected government' that is supposedly inflating death rates to frighten the public while using mass immigration to make the Irish a minority. For some, an 'unelected government' might refer to international organisations. In the Irish context, however, the phrase had additional inward-facing meaning.

Just before COVID-19 hit Ireland, in February 2020 parliamentary elections had been a three-way race, in which Sinn Féin, a left-wing party, received the most first-preference votes it had received since the 1970s. This was a big blow for the two dominant centre-right parties: Fine Gael (the governing party, led by Leo Varadkar), which came in third, and Fianna Fáil, which came in second. The votes clearly showed dissatisfaction with the establishment. However, before a new government was formed, infection began to spread. Emergency legislation was enacted by the outgoing rather than the incoming Senate, and state governance remained in the hands of Varadkar. In response, conspirationists such as O'Doherty and Waters cast COVID-19 as a plot to allow 'the establishment' to remain in power, disregarding the election's results. In line with this logic, the (old) government misled people into believing that their immune systems could not deal with the virus: it enforced a very strict lockdown, and introduced emergency laws (according to conspirationists) to 'buy more time' in power.

Seemingly universal conspiracy theories gain traction when they amplify or provide a fitting explanation for a story already being told locally. In the Irish context, resonance with the specific political situation coincident to the pandemic's outbreak fuelled their appeal.

Poland: retaining democratic desires

On 24 June 2020, six months into the pandemic and just days before the Polish presidential election, Poland's President Andrzej Duda made an official visit to Washington, DC. During the live broadcast of this bilateral meeting, Polish national television announced: 'Poland will be the first country that will be supplied by the USA with the coronavirus vaccine'. Given that this news came to Duda from Donald Trump, and was propagated by state-owned media managed by Duda supporters, its veracity was hard to assess. However, it was immediately picked up by 'scamdemic'-endorsing social media channels. On 25 June, a member of Facebook's *Nie wierzę w Koronawirusa – Grupa wsparcia/NIE JESTEŚ Sam* (I don't believe in Coronavirus – Support group/YOU ARE NOT ALONE), to which over 93,000 people belong, asked, '*I gdzie będą pierwsze testy?*' ('and where will they do initial testing?'). Answering herself, she implied Poland. Other members quickly echoed her concerns, suggesting sarcastically that their reward for friendship with the US was to be first in line for this. Interlocutors agreed that, just as during the world wars, the Polish nation would become a battlefield for all empires and '*mięso armatnie*' (cannon fodder) for the more powerful, who would force Polish citizens to receive vaccinations experimentally. Associating Duda with the 'Jewish lobby', some concluded that this was retaliation for when, in 2009, the country refused to buy vaccines from Big Pharma corporations (Nie wierzę w Koronawirusa 2020).

The views expressed by this group's members (mostly followers of alt-right presidential candidate Krzysztof Bosak, who was running against Duda) resemble the superconspiracies discussed above, their threads weaving pandemic worries into well-rehearsed anti-Semitic and Big Pharma tropes. However, as in the Irish case, here, too, 'universal' ideas need, for traction, to resonate with locally rooted sentiments and already-internalised culturally specific tropes. The Polish people endured struggles for independence from Russia, Prussia and the Austro-Hungarian Empire in the nineteenth century, from Fascist Germany and the Soviet Union during World War II, and from Communism in the 1940s–80s. These tropes are highly relevant to Bosak's followers.

However, conspiracy theories can be utilised by actors on all sides of the political spectrum when a nation is entangled in political rivalry, as is Poland: divided societies are particularly susceptible to conspiratorial thinking. Conspiracy theories help to simplify complex histories, enabling people to make sense of constant political changes and diverse perspectives (Boyer 2006). When a proliferation of groups occurs, and differences between factions are subtle and mostly entail boundary-making, conspiracy theories become central to identity, keeping group members alert to opponents' manipulations (Moore and Sanders 2002).

These processes are visible in the ways in which Poland's private media expressed concerns over governmental mismanagement of the pandemic. A recurring theme of their criticism was that the 'state is purposely hiding the numbers' to enhance its chances of winning the elections, in part by lifting the lockdown quickly. The state's rush to run elections at a time when health risks were still high only enhanced public suspicion of its motives.

The idea that the government was hiding the truth behind a façade caught on strongly. Healthcare professionals attested that unreliable COVID-19 counts simply reflected systematic failures and insufficiencies of the country's healthcare system. Regardless, the theory that 'the Government is lying to us' and 'hiding the truth' propagated in private media. It never was labelled as paranoid thinking in the way that alt-right candidate Bosak's followers' theories were labelled as such: conspiratorial ideas voiced by the opponents of the ruling party have retained their status as a justified form of political criticism.

Humphrey (2003) argues that, in the post-socialist Eastern European and Central Asian region, omnipresent conspiratorial thinking and a culture of suspicion is justified given the high number of actual conspiracies experienced in the last century (see also Carey 2017). The fact that a government with a known history of abusing democracy was managing this pandemic made many conspiratorial accusations highly plausible. However, the deep lack of trust in the Polish state is not just a result of this reality (Drążkiewicz 2016). It inheres in the political philosophy that underwrote Poland's post-1989 political culture – a philosophy born out of the struggle against communism and built on the assumption that true democracy cannot be realised in and by the state. This ideology presumes that government is the enemy of the people and so should never be trusted. Although since 1989 the government has changed often, Polish suspicion towards authority abides regardless of who is in power. In this context critical questions and theories that might be labelled as conspiracy theories are given space as a valid form of political engagement.

US: shoring up a dream

In the US, well-known tropes also are in play, but here they are linked to the crumbling American Dream of self-built prosperity, and to concerns regarding the freedoms meant to support it. Well before COVID-19, employment and wages for the US masses were declining. The notable uptick in suicides and drug and alcohol-related deaths among college-educated Whites, a demographic once favoured for economic mobility if not stability, demonstrates pervasive anxiety about achieving the American Dream (Krause and Sawhill 2018).

The nation's failure to protect citizens from predatory lenders (which led to the 2008 foreclosure crisis and subsequent recession) coupled with 'government bailouts' meant to shore up corporate wealth catalysed increasing cynicism regarding once-trusted institutions. The internet enabled disheartened citizens to engage with each other in ways heretofore impossible (see 'contested expertise', above). Yet as Bailey notes, culture entails 'lies that make life possible' through their capacity to both legitimise actions and 'neutralize despair' (1994, 4). So, rather than questioning the American Dream as myth, which would mean giving up on the prospect, many citizens found it more satisfying to blame their downward mobility on 'bad apples', favouring the proposition that a few (very powerful) bad actors in positions of power barred them from 'success'. This perspective fuelled populist desire for leadership from beyond 'the establishment'.

Enter Donald Trump, a self-proclaimed self-made man promising to 'drain the swamp' – the US federal government – of said bad actors (Bierman 2018). To gain followers, Trump courted and received the endorsement of an 'alternative media' superstar, far-right extremist and conspiracy theory monger Alex Jones. The ethos of suspicion long held strongly at the fringes of US society ripened with Trump's candidacy, throughout which he encouraged distrust of science and of the mainstream press. His presidency brought the phrases 'alternative facts' and 'fake news' squarely into the national and then international lexicon (see Glassner 2018) as he encouraged his base to blame downward mobility on those previously in power (the Democrats), and their elite allies.

Then, in 2017, an anonymous source purportedly named after the letter by which the government designates those with access to restricted information – Q – gained a following after bringing to light news of Trump's secret struggle on America's behalf to overthrow a 'deep state' during a soon-coming 'storm' or 'great awakening'. Q's proselytisers

(Jones included) use religious tropes and deploy in-group/out-group rhetoric to foster a sense of social belonging among adherents, who form a loose community active on social media. This millennialist conspiracy cult – QAnon – casts itself as a patriotic vanguard doing work of historic significance. It seems to appeal most to individuals feeling somewhat isolated or otherwise struggling (LaFrance 2020; Roose et al. 2020).

The vigilantism of a few acolytes aside, most adherents use the internet to do their own research into the often-cryptic messages Q 'drops', seeking to connect otherwise disparate dots. For instance, after a White House pandemic briefing on 14 March 2020, spurred by 'scamdemic'-type suspicions, some drew a connection between Trump's necktie colour choice (yellow) and the maritime flag signalling system, asserting that Trump thereby proclaimed the pandemic a hoax.

Amidst ideas circulating, some singled out White House coronavirus task force member Anthony Fauci, Director of the National Institute of Allergy and Infectious Diseases, as a deep state pawn. In this scenario, Fauci's contradiction of some of Trump's statements signalled his disloyalty (QAnon had already cast Fauci as a traitor, linking him to Hillary Clinton; LaFrance 2020). In addition to mounting calls to fire Fauci, some undertook a short-lived campaign to display hospitals as empty, despite media reports to the contrary (Nguyen 2020).

As Trump moved to 'reopen' the US economy 'by Easter' (12 April 2020), Fauci continued urging caution. His requests for social distancing, face masks and so on were seen by denialists as direct, tyrannical threats to various civil liberties, including not just the right to make a living in industries ordered shut, but how to live. Beginning in mid-April, anti-lockdown protests led by pre-existing right-wing militias (Wilson 2020) began in various states. Resentments were fitted into antecedent conspiracy theories regarding the state's ulterior motives. Further, in keeping with the way conspiracy theories function to affirm discernment, rally attendees self-identified as knowing the truth: the masses were being duped so that others could profit.

And here is a thread we wish to pull vigorously: a concern with corporate nefariousness, giving expression to a US-specific need for sustaining faith in one's chances to attain the American Dream despite increasing wealth inequity. Trump's base, cultivated from among the disaffected, preserves an imagined ladder to self-made success through faith in his leadership (not coincidentally, at his election convention Trump promised to 'save the American Dream'). In part from this loyalty, simultaneous to anti-lockdown protests, rumours linking Fauci to Big Pharma bourgeoned. But there was more to it than that. Fauci sees

COVID-19 squarely through the lens of authorised science – a lens discounted by Trump's base and consistently pelleted with 'alternative facts' by others drawn to conspiracy theories. Moreover, Fauci argues, again pointing to science, that COVID-19 will be vaccine preventable. This simple contention expanded the anti-Fauci, anti-lockdown faction, providing a dog whistle for so-called anti-vaxxers.

Although some would stereotype anti-vaxxers as liberals who favour alternative medicine, alternative schools and expensive organic food, a good proportion are fundamentalist homeschoolers and survivalists undesiring of any interaction with the state. Others are part of Trump's base. Beyond vaccination's purported health risks (which Trump has endorsed), these citizens worry that vaccine mandates disregard civil liberties – and many believe that they do so in support of profits for Big Pharma, in whose shadow the government works. In many minds, Big Pharma itself underwrote the creation and spread of SARS-CoV-2, or at least exaggerated its dangers, specifically to sell vaccines. Fauci, along with Bill Gates and others, supposedly invested in vaccines and so stands to profit immensely. Conjoined to this story is worry that vaccines will introduce into the body microchips to monitor the population and, in some renditions, sap free will.

Seeing common cause, anti-vaxxers not normally associated with Trump's vocal base have been motivated to speak up. As they do, it becomes clear that the liberal–conservative dichotomy is false. For one thing, both factions would replace the anti-vax label, and the extremism it implies, with a focus on informed choice. Both see themselves as freedom fighters. Both see Big Pharma as out to get 'us', its interest in profits potentially opening a door to mandatory vaccination or even to vaccine-fuelled enslavement by authoritarian states or a global regime. Although each group is somewhat differently anchored in terms of a priori social networks, and although the right-wing #FireFauci, 'reopen America' mandate is ultimately broader than that of the vaccination rights or the 'health/medical freedom' contingent, current confluences in their discourses illustrate how conspiracy theories are leveraged. They reveal how alt-right messaging is being deployed by an 'alt' alt-right – one for which personal freedoms, self-determination and anti-authoritarianism, are likewise more important than the social good writ large. In Krugman's words, for them, 'freedom' references a right to 'the untrammeled pursuit of self-interest' or 'sacralized selfishness' (2020).

Similarities don't stop there. Like many of QAnon's prominent proponents, many 'wellness entrepreneurs' promoting 'medical freedom' also have built enviable fortunes via conspiracy mongering, for instance through goods and services sold on their websites. Coming together to protest state handling of COVID-19 gives all parties access to crossover markets (Breland 2020; Satija and Sun 2019). As a key driver of success, avarice is a virtue, not a sin, so long as everyone is equally free to take a piece of the pie.

Big Pharma, in contrast, is cast in this narrative as wanting the pie for itself. Further, Big Pharma is seen as posing as if the final authority while, given their emphasis on self-sovereignty, those fusing anti-vax interests onto anti-lockdown rhetoric encourage followers to 'do their homework' and make up their own minds. Encouragement toward self-education also flows forth from many mainstream US organisations, including some corners of orthodox healthcare: savvy consumerism and self-determination are that central to US national consciousness. So are the concerns regarding corporate duplicity leveraged in conspiracy theories. These themes are played to different effect by different factions, but their deployment from all sides should not be surprising, given their cultural salience.

The world as seen through this conspiracy theory lens 'is not some bizarre parallel universe' (LaFrance 2020). It is the same universe in which most Americans live, shaped by and reinforcing of the national ethos. What appears as one conspiracy theory on the surface may contain several versions of something proximally the same, but different in terms of the ends desired and the lifestyles represented. When surface fusion brings separate interest groups closer to their aims, conjoined action will not represent a compromise.

Implications

The above conspiracy theories point to perceived ruptures in the social contract, sometimes directly articulating ideas regarding what that contract should be ('normative rules', as per Bailey; also, a collusive lie [1991, 35]). Social and political tensions inform these anxious counter-narratives in ways that 'put [political] relations to the test' (Fassin 2011, 48), giving voice to a demand to mend those tears in the social fabric or flouted rules that make the world feel unjust.

But the case studies showed more than political contests. They also spoke to political anthropology's concern with how 'true-believers' persuade others to forego reason and follow a 'jack o'lantern' (Bailey 2008, 5): crafting messages that resonate generatively with people's locally specific governance-related anxieties is central here (see Lepselter

2016). Health – being essential, fragile and fickle – serves exceedingly well as a projective screen for such concerns. The theories deployed in our case studies also gained leverage through their enmeshment with pre-existing superconspiracies (e.g. regarding Big Pharma, the Deep State).

This was no coincidence. Not only does history matter to a conspiracy's appeal (see Ryer 2015); known conspiracy theory advocates took an active role in ensuring the absorption of COVID-19-linked ideas into pre-existing frameworks, elaborating and endorsing the newer ideas as further evidence of prior claims against various state formation. They also deployed them for gain (e.g. for votes or to sell goods). Extending Bailey's observations regarding witchcraft accusations and other political transactions (1994, 1991), the case studies showed that conspiracy theories have instrumental utility in addition to expressive value.

Notwithstanding, the conspiracy theories contained some potentially hazardous counterfactual assertions, such as recommendations to shun COVID-19 vaccinations if and when they arrive. Addressing the existential concerns underwriting these directives and the alternative facts used to support them, rather than simply endeavouring to provide 'correct' information, may be helpful in lessening the prospect of harm.

Undesired governance

In our examples, four problematic expressions of state power served as focal points for dissent. First there was 'the *Nanny State*', which distrusts citizens to make appropriate health decisions, and so over-interferes through regulation. A *Corrupted Nanny State* further uses current crises, like COVID-19, for its own political gain. A Nanny State in either form transmutes into a *Police State* if force is conjoined to this aim.

Then there was the *Façade* or *Cardboard State* – terms borrowed from Polish politics. On the surface, a Cardboard State appears as a functioning democracy. Yet its façade hides a corrupt and broken system, which, while benefitting the elite, is at constant risk of collapse. Such an unsustainable state hides things because it cannot keep up; it pretends away COVID-19 because it does not have the resources to stem the pandemic or because admitting the problem would work against its self-presentation of successful governance.

We saw also the *Shadow State*. As Wedel (2011) argues, the Shadow State is made of 'flexians' – members of corporate boards and think tanks who pull governmental strings in service of capitalist profit-making. This state fails citizens not through patronising over-interference or ineptitude but because it is not calling the shots to begin with.

Corporations (for example Big Pharma) can run a Shadow State, and corrupt politicians can run the Corrupted Nanny or Cardboard State. The regular Nanny State is simply overbearing; the Police State, merely totalitarian. But the *Deep State* has highly developed, overtly sinister plans with occult origins – plans whose aims extend well beyond simple self-interest. Sometimes termed the New World Order, the Deep State is not tethered to actual government institutions. Instead, like smoke and mirrors, it exists to deflect attention from one's state and its shortcomings – but its invocation confirms that shortcomings do exist: government for the people is hobbled.

Not all states express themselves in all these ways; and other expressions likely exist. Further, expressions vary on the ground. Regardless, our comparative work shows that conspiracy theories are not a prerogative of some specific political system or a particular historical moment (Ryer 2015; contra Marcus 1999). Nor are they simply an expression of anxiety over the condition of modernity or globalisation, as some have suggested (for example Aupers 2012; Harding and Stewart 2003).

Their main purpose is articulation of social and political criticism. A state described by a conspiracy theory using any of the above guises, combined or alone, and however indirectly, has disappointed citizens, as our cases demonstrate. This explains how apparently universal tropes can express locally particular complaints about the state's failure to uphold its end of the governance bargain.

Fact and fiction

This brings us back to the boundaries between conspiracy theories and 'genuine' claims, an issue of concern for health and state authorities during this pandemic as well as for social scientists. As Hastrup (2004) points out, knowledge is always messy. It is reductive and selective; it turns empirical complexity into clear, but therefore limited, propositions, and we always disregard some information. Further, people like to doubt (Carey 2017). But individual activities in relation to knowledge do not occur in a vacuum. Our work helps illuminate the role of the state here, even beyond the typology offered.

For one thing, any emphasis on ascertaining the truth value of competing ideas forces people to take sides in polarised ways. This observation is particularly relevant in relation to ideas about COVID-19 because so much bureaucratic effort has been dedicated to prioritising certain truth claims over others. And, as Carey demonstrates, the more involved the state is with people's quotidian lives – the more it is 'experienced via its apparatus as a complex infrastructure', the more fertile the ground will be for conspiracy theories (2017, 98). The intensified structuring role that states have taken in this pandemic, coupled with the historical realities that we outlined for Ireland, Poland and the US, has helped COVID-19 conspiracy theories take wing. As Pelkmans (2013) warned, the collapse of trust in institutions and the absence of actual certainty gives the conspiratorial imagination free rein.

Moreover, knowledge is always political, and knowledge systems are always generating conflicts (Engle-Merry and Coutin 2014). As we have seen in the Polish case especially, the boundaries between conspiracy theories and legitimate (authorised) theories often blur (see also Bailey 1994). Further, the designation 'conspiracy theory' is always political, produced by people in positions of power. Pelkmans and Machold highlight the 'distorting effects of the fields of power through which theories travel' (2011, 77), noting that conspiracy theories begin in an unmarked state, as all theories do. The label's application – or not – imposes a definition of the situation favouring those who apply it; and if they have more power than conspiracy theory proponents, particularly if a conspiracy theory's truth claims are weak, the label is likely to stick. Consequently, the label 'conspiracy theory' is both a lumping device for dissenting narratives and a reciprocating technology for the production of doubt: it denounces as implausible the sceptical views a conspiracy theory promotes. It attempts to impose if not reinforce marginalisation (see Briggs 2004).

Yet, even labelled as such, conspiracy theories can affect the state, inhibiting for instance an effective pandemic response through the doubt they sow. Since trust is a relational issue (if you trust me, I trust you), the state is not a passive player here: the state's choice of governance strategies makes a difference, adding to or preventing the spread of conspiracy theories and further mistrust. Regardless, conspiracy theories can offer the disempowered 'a pretty satisfying approximation [of truth], demonstrating how in the modern interconnected world, people make sense of the actions and motives of powerful others with reference to old, familiar scripts' (Brown and Theodossopoulos 2003, 334). Particularly in regard to COVID-19, conspiracy theories reveal, in superficially universal but deeply local ways, that state systems are neither as they seem, nor as they should be.

References

Aupers, Stef. 2012. '"Trust no one": Modernization, paranoia and conspiracy culture'. *European Journal of Communication* 27(1): 22–34. https://doi.org/10.1177/0267323111433566.

Bailey, F.G. 1991. *The Prevalence of Deceit*. Ithaca, NY: Cornell University Press.

Bailey, F.G. 1994. *The Witch Hunt*. Ithaca, NY: Cornell University Press.

Bailey, F.G. 2008. *God-Botherers and Other True-Believers*. Ithaca, NY: Cornell University Press.

Barkun, Michael. 2013. *A Culture of Conspiracy: Apocalyptic visions in contemporary America*. Berkeley, CA: University of California Press.

Barth, Fredrik. 2002. 'An anthropology of knowledge'. *Current Anthropology* 43(1): 1–18. https://doi.org/10.1086/324131.

Bierman, Noah. 2018. 'Trump shifts meaning of "Drain the Swamp" from ethics to anything he objects to'. *Los Angeles Times*, 9 February 2020. Accessed 29 June 2020. https://www.latimes.com/politics/la-na-pol-swamp-20180209-story.html.

Bovensiepen, Judith. 2016. 'Visions of prosperity and conspiracy in Timor-Leste'. *Focaal: Journal of Global and Historical Anthropology* 75: 75–88. https://www.berghahnjournals.com/view/journals/focaal/2016/75/fcl750106.xml?rskey=7fCeIE&result=1

Boyer, Dominic. 2006. 'Conspiracy, history, and therapy at a Berlin "Stammtisch"'. *American Ethnologist* 33(3): 327–39.

Breland, Ali. 2020. 'Wellness influencers are spreading QAnon conspiracies about the Coronavirus'. *Mother Jones*, 15 April 2020. Accessed 28 July 2020. https://www.motherjones.com/politics/2020/04/wellness-qanon-coronavirus/.

Briggs, Charles L. 2004. 'Theorizing modernity conspiratorially: Science, scale, and the political economy of public discourse in explanations of a cholera epidemic'. *American Ethnologist* 31(2): 164–87. https://doi:10.1525/ae.2004.31.2.164.

Brown, Keith and Dimitrios Theodossopoulos. 2003. 'Rearranging solidarity: Conspiracy and world order in Greek and Macedonian commentaries on Kosovo'. *Journal of Southern Europe and the Balkans* 5(3): 315–35. https://doi.org/10.1080/14613190310001610760.

Butt, Leslie. 2005. '"Lipstick girls" and "fallen women": AIDS and conspiratorial thinking in Papua, Indonesia'. *Cultural Anthropology* 20(3): 412–42. https://doi.org/10.1525/can.2005.20.3.412.

Butter, Michael and Peter Knight. 2020. *Routledge Handbook of Conspiracy Theories*. Abingdon, UK: Routledge.

Carey, Matthew. 2017. *Mistrust: An ethnographic theory*. Chicago, IL: HAU Books.

Chigudu, Simukai. 2019. 'The politics of cholera, crisis and citizenship in urban Zimbabwe: "People were dying like flies"'. *African Affairs* 118(472): 413–34. https://doi.org/10.1093/afraf/ady068.

Drążkiewicz, Elżbieta. 2016. '"State bureaucrats" and "those NGO people": Promoting the idea of civil society, hindering the state'. *Critique of Anthropology* 36(4): 341–62. https://doi:10.1177/0308275x16654553.

Engle-Merry, Sally and Susan Bibler Coutin. 2014. 'Technologies of truth in the anthropology of conflict: AES/APLA Presidential Address, 2013'. *American Ethnologist* 41(1): 1–16. https://doi.org/10.1111/amet.12055.

Farmer, Paul. 1992. *AIDS and Accusation: Haiti and the geography of blame*. Los Angeles, CA: University of California Press.

Farrell, Craig and Ann Mooney. 2020. '"END THE SCAMDEMIC" Coronavirus in Ireland – McGrath calls for end to "scamdemic" as TDs demand lockdown eases to help kick-start economy'. *The Irish Sun*, 1 June 2020. Accessed 29 June 2020. https://www.thesun.ie/news/5490081/coronavirus-ireland-mcgrath-end-scamdemic-lockdown-eases/.

Fassin, Didier. 2011. 'The politics of conspiracy theories: On AIDS in South Africa and a few other global plots'. *The Brown Journal of World Affairs* 17(2): 39–50.

Fenster, Mark. 2008. *Conspiracy Theories: Secrecy and power in American culture*, 2nd ed. Minneapolis, MN: University of Minnesota Press.

Freeman, Daniel, Felicity Waite, Laina Rosebrock, Ariane Petit, Chiara Causier, Anna East, Lucy Jenner, Ashley-Louise Teale, Lydia Carr, Sophie Mulhall, Emily Bold and Sinéad Lambe. 2020. 'Coronavirus conspiracy beliefs, mistrust, and compliance with government guidelines in England'. *Psychological Medicine* 21: 1–13. https://doi.org/10.1017/S0033291720001890.

Geissler, P.W. and R. Pool. 2006. 'Popular concerns about medical research projects in sub-Saharan Africa – a critical voice in debates about medical research ethics'. *Tropical Medicine and International Health* 11(7): 975–82. https://doi.org/10.1111/j.1365-3156.2006.01682.x.

Glassner, Barry. 2018. *The Culture of Fear: Why Americans are afraid of the wrong things: Crime, drugs, minorities, teen moms, killer kids, mutant microbes, plane crashes, road rage, & so much more*. Revised ed. New York: Basic Books.

Harambam, Jaron. 2020. *Contemporary Conspiracy Culture: Truth and knowledge in an era of epistemic instability*. London: Routledge.

Harding, Susan and Kathleen Stewart. 2003. 'Anxieties of influence: Conspiracy theory and therapeutic culture in millennial America'. In *Transparency and Conspiracy: Ethnographies of suspicion in the new world order*, edited by Harry West and Todd Sanders, pp. 258–86. Durham, NC: Duke University Press.

Hastrup, Kirsten. 2004. 'Getting it right: Knowledge and evidence in anthropology'. *Anthropological Theory* 4(4): 455–72. https://doi.org/10.1177%2F1463499604047921.

Humphrey, Caroline. 2003. 'Stalin and the blue elephant: Paranoia and complicity in post-communist metahistories'. In *Transparency and Conspiracy: Ethnographies of suspicion in the new world order*, edited by Harry West and Todd Sanders, pp. 175–203. Durham, NC: Duke University Press.

Kirmayer, Laurence J., Eugene Raikhel and Sadeq Rahimi. 2013. 'Cultures of the internet: Identity, community and mental health'. *Transcultural Psychiatry* 50(2): 165–91. https://doi.org/10.1177/1363461513490626.

Krause, Eleanor and Isabel V. Sawhill. 2018. 'Seven reasons to worry about the American middle class'. Brookings Social Mobility Memos, 5 June 2020. Accessed 29 June 2020. https://www.brookings.edu/blog/social-mobility-memos/2018/06/05/seven-reasons-to-worry-about-the-american-middle-class/.

Krugman, Paul. 2020. 'The cult of selfishness is killing America'. *New York Times*, 27 July 2020. Accessed 27 July 2020. https://www.nytimes.com/2020/07/27/opinion/us-republicans-coronavirus.html.

LaFrance, Adrienne. 2020. 'The prophecies of Q: American conspiracy theories are entering a dangerous new phase'. *The Atlantic*, 14 May 2020. Accessed 29 June 2020. https://www.theatlantic.com/magazine/archive/2020/06/qanon-nothing-can-stop-what-is-coming/610567/.

Leach, Melissa and James Fairhead. 2007. *Vaccine Anxieties*. London: Earthscan.

Lepselter, Susan. 2016. *The Resonance of Unseen Things: Poetics, power, captivity, and UFOs in the American uncanny*. Ann Arbor, MI: University of Michigan Press.

Lyotard, Jean-Francois. 1984. *The Postmodern Condition: A report on knowledge*. Translated by Geoff Bennington and Brian Massumi. Manchester, UK: Manchester University Press.

Mathur, Nayanika. 2015. '"It's a conspiracy theory *and* climate change": Of beastly encounters and cervine disappearances in Himalayan India'. *HAU: Journal of Ethnographic Theory* 5(1): 87–111. https://doi.org/10.14318/hau5.1.005.

Marcus, George. 1999. *Paranoia Within Reason: A casebook on conspiracy as explanation*. Chicago, IL: University of Chicago Press.

Moore, Ronnie and Andrew Sanders. 2002. 'Formations of culture: Nationalism and conspiracy ideology in Ulster loyalism'. *Anthropology Today* 18(6): 9–15. https://doi.org/10.1111/1467-8322.00147.

Nguyen, Tina. 2020. 'How a pair of anti-vaccine activists sparked a #FireFauci furor'. *Politico*, 13 April 2020. Accessed 29 June 2020. https://www.politico.com/news/2020/04/13/anti-vaccine-activists-fire-fauci-furor-185001.

Nie wierzę w Koronawirusa Facebook Group. 2020. Comment, 15 June 2020. Accessed on 22 August 2020. https://www.facebook.com/groups/705623010178549/permalink/768392920568224/.

Niehaus, Isak and Gunvor Jonsson. 2005. 'Dr Wouter Basson, Americans, and wild beasts: Men's conspiracy theories of HIV/AIDS in the South African lowveld'. *Medical Anthropology* 24(2): 179–208. https://doi.org/10.1080/01459740590933911.

O'Doherty, Gemma. 2020a. *Anti-Corruption Ireland*. Accessed 29 June 2020. https://anti-corruptionireland.com/.

O'Doherty, Gemma. 2020b. 'COVID19 is a staged event to usher in a police state and a globalist "one world" government'. Anti-Corruption Ireland. Accessed 22 August 2020. https://anti-corruptionireland.com/downloads/.

O'Doherty, Gemma (@gemmaod1). 2020c. Twitter, 28 April 2020. Accessed 29 June 2020. https://twitter.com/gemmaod1/status/1255176537000873984?s=20.

O'Grady, Siobhán. 2020. 'Trump is not the only leader pushing unproven coronavirus remedies'. *Washington Post*, 5 May 2020. Accessed 29 June 2020. https://www.msn.com/en-nz/news/world/trump-is-not-the-only-leader-pushing-unproven-coronavirus-remedies/ar-BB14uPBD?li=BBqdg4K.

Pelkmans, Mathijs. 2013. *Ethnographies of Doubt: Faith and uncertainty in contemporary societies*. London: I.B. Tauris/Bloomsbury Academic.

Pelkmans, Mathijs and Rhys Machold. 2011. 'Conspiracy theories and their truth trajectories'. *Focaal: Journal of Global and Historical Anthropology* 59: 66–80. https://doi.org/10.3167/fcl.2011.590105.

Roose, Kevin, Andy Mills, Julia Longoria and Sindhu Gnanasambandan. 2020. 'Episode 7: Where we go one'. Rabbit Hole, *The New York Times*, 28 May 2020. Accessed 29 June 2020. https://www.nytimes.com/2020/05/28/podcasts/rabbit-hole-qanon-conspiracy-theory-virus.html.

Ryer, Paul. 2015. 'The Maine, the Romney and the threads of conspiracy in Cuba'. *International Journal of Cuban Studies* 7(2): 200–11.

Satija, Neena and Lena H. Sun. 2019. 'A major funder of the anti-vaccine movement has made millions selling natural health products'. *Washington Post*, 20 December 2020. Accessed on 29 June 2020. https://www.washingtonpost.com/investigations/2019/10/15/fdc01078-c29c-11e9-b5e4-54aa56d5b7ce_story.html.

Sobo, E., G. Zimet, H. Cecil and T. Zimmerman. 1997. 'Doubting the experts: AIDS conspiracy rhetoric and AIDS misconceptions among runaway adolescents'. *Human Organization* 56(3): 311–20.

Sobo, E.J. (2021). 'What does the American Dream have to do with the COVID-19 vaccine?' Sapiens.org, 25 February 2021. Accessed February 2021. https://www.sapiens.org/culture/covid-19-vaccine-protestors/.

Sunstein, Cass R. and Adrian Vermeule. 2009. 'Conspiracy theories: Causes and cures'. *Journal of Political Philosophy* 17(2): 202–27.

Tiffany, Kaitlyn. 2020. 'Something in the air'. *The Atlantic*, 30 April 2020. Accessed 11 September 2020. https://www.theatlantic.com/technology/archive/2020/05/great-5g-conspiracy/611317/.

Uscinski, Joseph E. and Adam M. Enders. 2020. 'The coronavirus conspiracy boom: Nearly a third of the people we polled believe that the virus was manufactured on purpose. Why?' *The Atlantic*, 30 April 2020. Accessed 29 June 2020. https://www.theatlantic.com/health/archive/2020/04/what-can-coronavirus-tell-us-about-conspiracy-theories/610894/.

Vine, Michael and Matthew Carey. 2017. 'Mimesis and conspiracy: Bureaucracy, new media and the infrastructural forms of doubt'. *Cambridge Journal of Anthropology* 35(2): 47–64. https://doi.org/10.3167/cja.2017.350205.

Wedel, Janine. 2011. *Shadow Elite: How the world's new power brokers undermine democracy, government, and the free market*. New York: Basic Books.

Wilson, Jason. 2020. 'The rightwing groups behind wave of protests against Covid-19 restrictions'. *The Guardian*, 17 April 2020. Accessed 27 July 2020. https://www.theguardian.com/world/2020/apr/17/far-right-coronavirus-protests-restrictions.

Part II
Exclusion and blame

5
The 2020 Los Angeles uprisings
Fighting for Black lives in the midst of COVID-19
Hanna Garth

On Memorial Day, 25 May 2020, George Floyd, a 46-year-old Black man was murdered by a white police officer in Minneapolis, Minnesota. Floyd was under arrest for allegedly using a counterfeit bill at a local market. A witness captured the murder on their phone and the video went viral. The officer killed Floyd with a carotid chokehold, pressing his knee into Floyd's neck as Floyd called out for his mama until his last breath. Protests began in Minneapolis on 26 May; as people gathered to pay their respects at a memorial that formed outside the Cup Foods store where Floyd was murdered, people began to demonstrate, and eventually a crowd of hundreds chanting 'I Can't Breathe' and 'Black Lives Matter' marched to the 3rd Precinct of the Minneapolis Police.

Floyd's murder took place a few months into the COVID-19 lockdowns and quarantines taking place across the United States where, by 26 May, there were over 1.6 million cases of COVID-19 and around 100,000 deaths. Reporters and media pundits speculated that after weeks stuck inside, the Memorial Day holiday weekend and the start of summer coalesced to draw people out of their homes and onto the streets to protest in greater numbers than ever before. This is a very different take from my own. In Los Angeles, I observed the ways in which the protests following Floyd's murder in the midst of the pandemic illuminated longstanding connections between white supremacy, structural inequality and poverty in Black and Brown communities. The racialised disparities of COVID-19 are an additional form of state sanctioned violence on top of police brutality that Black and Latinx people face, and these two forms of violence converged to push people to fight for something better. Months into the pandemic, it was clear that government leadership to control the pandemic would not come from the federal level, and increasingly local leaders were clear that opening up the economy, not saving lives, was their priority. A political system and general social ethos that favoured profits over lives would not eliminate the forms of white supremacy and structural inequality that undergird the plague of police violence in the US.

In Los Angeles, the protests began on 27 May, the day after they started in Minneapolis, beginning in downtown LA where protestors walked onto the 101 Freeway, blocking traffic. LA County Sheriff Villanueva tweeted that he 'shared the nation's outrage' and that 'police brutality is unacceptable under any circumstances'. Protestors returned to downtown LA the following day (Pierce 2020). The size and tone of these protests were relatively small and subtle. Organisers from the local chapter of Black Lives Matter and the Movement for Black Lives (M4BL) regularly gathered downtown to protest police misconduct, brutality, and ongoing killings and anti-Black violence perpetuated by the Los Angeles Police Department (LAPD). For years, organisations like the LA chapter of Black Lives Matter, Dignity and Power Now, and Reform LA Jails have been relentlessness in fighting against police violence and misconduct, and for the removal of the District Attorney Jackie Lacey. Since 2013, when the hashtag #BlackLivesMatter movement was created by three radical Black organisers in the Los Angeles area – Alicia Garza, Patrisse Khan Cullors and Opal Tometi, in response to the acquittal of George Zimmerman, the man who murdered 17-year-old Black boy, Trayvon Martin – the work of these organisations has been mainstream.

Beginning in Los Angeles in 2013, #BlackLivesMatter became a national and then a global movement. In 2013, as Garza, Cullors and Tometi joined thousands in the streets of Ferguson, Los Angeles, New York and beyond, 'they were armed with the statistic that in the U.S., a Black person is killed by a state sanctioned actor every 28 hours' (Burton 2015). #BlackLivesMatter, movements for prison abolition and police abolition, are not merely virtual mediatised movements; they are serious, organised movements that have made and continue to make significant progress to interrogate and eliminate anti-Blackness and racial inequality (Kelley 2016). 'The most effective Black political mobilisation since the civil rights era' (Castillo 2020), #BlackLivesMatter has grown into a global movement (Smith 2015; 2017; Kerrigan 2015; Vargas 2015). By 3 July 2020, the *New York Times* claimed, 'Black Lives Matter May Be the Largest Movement in U.S. History'.[1]

The scaled-up iteration of the Black Lives Matter movement in response to George Floyd's death occurred in the midst of the pandemic, but it seemed that the protests were not contributing to the spread of COVID-19. Instead, the powerfulness of the movement shed light not only on police brutality, but also on other racialised injustices, including the disproportionate number of cases and deaths from COVID-19.

In the BLM-LA podcast series entitled 'This is Not a Drill! The Power of Protest!' one of BLM's founders, Patrisse Khan Cullors, spoke of her motivation to continue fighting for Black life: 'It wasn't until I had a child that the urgency of changing this place felt almost like a desperation'. She had long been 'living with the terror of knowing how vulnerable I am, I feel like I could handle something happening to me, but if something were to happen to my child. Looking at my child and not ever ever ever imagining anyone harming him, no one but Black mothers know that kind of agony'. These thoughts and sentiments motivate many involved in the M4BL.

I have lived in Los Angeles since 2007, and since 2009 I have conducted research on the efforts of food justice organisations to increase access to healthy food in South and East LA (Garth 2020; Garth and Reese 2020). Although I lived and conducted research in these areas during the rise of the M4BL, I was not heavily involved in the movement. In July 2013, I watched Zimmerman's acquittal for the murder of Trayvon Martin, and the subsequent uprisings, unfold from my living room, my oldest son in my arms. He was six months old, and, without childcare, I decided not to join the protests with him. Instead, I donated money and was politically supportive of the cause. In May 2020, I gave birth to our third child, and with COVID-19 we had been strictly quarantining since the birth. So, seven years after the first, I sat in my living room, a baby in my arms, watching the uprisings unfold. I sought to keep my composure for the sake of my children, who were already under stress from the ways in which COVID-19 and quarantining had disrupted their lives. But I am not OK (Cox 2020). I fear for the lives and safety of my children and my family in the face of the virus, but from the day they were born until the day I die I will fear for their lives in the face of state-sanctioned police violence.

Following George Floyd's murder, the scale of protests grew significantly. By Saturday 30 May, organised protests had spread throughout Los Angeles. I received text messages from the M4BL and followed the calls for action on the Black Lives Matter – Los Angeles Facebook page. A protest at Pan Pacific Park, located next to one of LA's iconic shopping centres – the Grove – was set for noon on Saturday, and that day Governor Newsom declared a state of emergency and called in the National Guard. On 31 May, the city of Los Angeles set a 6 p.m. curfew; Santa Monica set its curfew for 4 p.m.; other cities followed with curfews at different times. A barrage of text messages came into our phones through the emergency notification services, advising of different curfew times.

Almost immediately, BLM-LA started organising around specific needs for the city and greater Southern California communities. BLM-LA set a Zoom meeting with Los Angeles Police commissioners on 2 June, demanding action for over 600 police murders committed by LAPD, calling for accountability and the prohibition of unnecessary force and violence on peaceful protestors. The meeting was open to the public and quickly hit the 500-person limit. Local-level organising in the city and greater region was well coordinated, with planned protests going out on social media accounts in tandem with other M4BL text message updates to anyone who had subscribed. The protests dovetailed with demands for specific changes to law and policy, including defunding the LAPD and eliminating police officers from schools in the Los Angeles Unified School District (LAUSD). Beyond the core Black Lives Matter group, organisations from across the city began posting statements and creating action plans in general support of Black Lives and antiracism, and calling for LAPD to be defunded or reformed.

In this chapter, I draw upon the Black radical tradition to analyse the links between the 2020 uprisings and the disparities of the COVID-19 pandemic in Los Angeles. I analyse the ways in which state-sanctioned police murder of Black people is linked to health disparities and the neglect of Black communities. As Black, Latinx and other Angelenos of colour are more likely to serve as essential workers, disproportionately exposed to the virus, they are also less likely to have adequate healthcare coverage or adequate access to testing. Ultimately, as the rapid spread of the virus threatens all Angelenos, the City of Los Angeles made efforts (and at the time of writing, is still doing so) to curb the COVID-19 spread in predominately Black and Latinx areas of the city, as part of a broader campaign to flatten the curve. While COVID-19 comes to the forefront, there has been insufficient attention to the problems caused by decades of divestment, loss of well-paying jobs and the relentless police violence that plague communities of colour. Lockdowns, protests, job loss, declining wages, 'frontline' jobs, a collapsing healthcare system (which was already stretched), 'underlying medical conditions', police violence and imprisonment combined in a very deadly way in 2020 and in doing so, laid starkly bare longstanding forms of systemic racism.

Histories of violence and corrupt police in South LA

Police violence in communities like South LA has been relentless for generations, and uprisings have been a critical way of drawing attention to these injustices in an effort to create change. The 1992 Los Angeles Uprisings were a pivotal moment, and particularly impactful for South Los Angeles communities. These began on 29 April 1992 and lasted six days, after a jury acquitted four LAPD officers caught on tape beating Rodney King, a Black Angeleno. As in 2020, the Army National Guard and the Marines were brought in to try to stop the protests. In South Los Angeles, 55 people were killed, over 2,000 people injured and property damage was estimated at one billion dollars.

For many residents, these 1992 uprisings were yet another iteration of the Watts rebellion of 11 August 1965, when the Watts area of South Los Angeles erupted into protests after an incident of police brutality with a Black motorist. On this occasion, there were at least 34 deaths and an estimated $40 million in property damage. Again, the National Guard was brought in to quell the situation.

During these earlier uprisings in response to police violence against Black community members, the damaged property was largely confined to majority Black neighbourhoods. Most buildings were commercial or retail. In the aftermath of the protests, many local businesses closed and never reopened, with consequent job losses and increased unemployment.

The 1992 uprisings drew international attention to Los Angeles. People worldwide were made aware of the stark inequalities between the LA they saw on TV and the LA in which many lived. This attention to disparities yielded some good – organisations and money began to go toward thinking through how to improve conditions. Nearly 30 years on, however, South LA continues to suffer from race-based marginalisation and underdevelopment. An estimated 31 per cent of South LA households are below the poverty line; 39 per cent of residents have not graduated from high school – the highest in the country. Post-1992, there have been ongoing problems associated with job insecurity, declining real wages and police violence. In the context of the rapid spread of COVID-19, a system where access to healthcare is tied to job-based health insurance, job insecurity and low wage insecure labour can brew a public health disaster in areas like South LA.

Nearly 30 years later ...

In early June 2020, as Los Angeles was in the midst of the BLM uprisings, community leader, food justice activist and US Navy Iraq-War Veteran Dr D'Artagnan Scorza posted the following on Facebook:[2]

> The civil unrest across the nation and here in our community is not the product of an isolated incident. These protests are part of a rebellion spurred on by centuries-old racism and oppression manifested in the killing of unarmed black men and women. These men and women, like George Floyd and Breonna Taylor, died at the hands of those who were tasked with protecting and serving them. Their deaths violate the social contract between the community and police.
>
> From the 1964 Watts uprising to the 1992 Los Angeles uprisings (which I lived through) to today, there have always been calls for restraint. But, how can you ask us to restrain ourselves when this country has allowed knees to be pressed upon our collective necks?

Scorza, a widely respected local leader, is not someone I would describe as having very radical politics. However, he has a clear understanding of the role that racism and police violence play in his community and in the everyday lives of those who live in and near South Los Angeles. He continues, connecting the uprisings with his personal story:

> As a Black man who leads an organisation supporting the growth and development of Black male youth, and as a father of a young Black boy, I am anguished and enraged. I'm beyond tired and fed up with these cycles of police violence and the promise of change. I can't remain silent because silence equates to consent and I don't consent to what happened to George Floyd, Breonna Taylor, and the many others who have died at the hands of police who use their power to destroy life.
>
> But, I'm tired of the words that I've used in the past to try and make meaning of what's happening right now. I'm tired of saying 'we need change', 'reform the system', 'we need review boards' and everything else that comes with calls for change. What we really need is to LIVE and do so with the dignity of our lives uninhibited. We not only need to Live, but we are demanding the right to Live. The right to jog in peace. The right to sit in our homes in peace. The right to breathe in peace ...

Here, Scorza openly shifts from a reformist position toward an abolitionist position, underscoring that his previous calls for reform and review have not worked. He fears for his own life and the life of his Black son. He continues:

> It is clear that our policing institutions have utterly failed us and we need to rethink what 'protection', not policing looks like. Much like the military, our police need to be overseen by civilians who make determinations about when force is to be used. The fact that police even have the power to use 'force' is a power in and of itself we have the right to revoke. No individual should be allowed to make that determination on their own.
>
> More so, what we need is solidarity and the complete obliteration of White Supremacy. We need to tear down the ideology that devalues Black life and Black bodies. America must boldly affirm that Black lives matter and in doing so put a knee in the neck of police brutality, systemic and institutionalised racism. This is not a moment to 'protect', we must act swiftly with courageous leadership to ensure that White Supremacy dies, not us.

Scorza highlights that the issues that fuelled the 2020 uprisings are the long-standing, structural problems of South Los Angeles that derive from and build on centuries of racism and anti-Blackness. He notes the lack of response to calls for police reform and the urgent need for a system that actually protects everyone from harm. This system cannot come from a foundation of white supremacy.

From 2000 to early 2020, police had killed 886 people in LA County; the majority were Black or Latinx. While many Black activists had long understood the connections between white supremacy, structural inequality and poverty in Black and Brown communities, the uprisings of 2020 and the COVID-19 pandemic illuminated these connections for many more people. It was clear that at national and local levels, the current political system was not going to eliminate white supremacy or the forms of structural inequality perpetuated by it that deeply impact living conditions in places like South Los Angeles. The problems we were seeing more clearly with the spread of COVID-19, and the poor response to it, also illuminated some of the core problems that Black Lives Matter activists care about: the ways in which our social support systems fail us under contemporary capitalism. The healthcare system, school system, food distribution system and many others that were essential for the wellbeing of all Angelenos, but have been unable to function properly under the conditions of the COVID-19 pandemic, are intricately interwoven with settler colonialism, racial capitalism, white supremacy and the carceral state (Beliso-De Jesús and Pierre 2020; Ralph 2019; Speed 2020).

COVID-19 and health inequality

Whitney N. Laster Pirtle has argued, 'Racial capitalism is a fundamental cause of the racial and socioeconomic inequities within the novel coronavirus pandemic (COVID-19) in the United States' (2020, 504). The epidemiological patterns of COVID-19 have made clear the ways in which racial capitalism results in unequal access to basic services in response to human needs. This is embodied as differential risk for contracting disease, and differential experiences of morbidity and mortality. The problematic disparities along lines of race and socioeconomic status were evident early in the pandemic. In places like South Los Angeles, it was clear that COVID-19 would capitalise on structural violence and vulnerability (Manderson and Levine 2020, 368). By 26 April, LA County (excluding Long Beach and Pasadena) had 19,516 confirmed cases, with data on race and ethnicity for 10,699 cases (LA County 2020): 46.4 per cent were Latino, 23.7 per cent were white, 11.5 per cent were Asian, 8 per cent were African American. Native Hawaiians or other Pacific Islanders had the highest population rate of COVID-19 cases (840 per 100,000), followed by Latinos (114 per 100,000), African Americans (102 per 100,000), then white people (78 per 100,000). When some businesses were allowed to reopen in late July, these disparities widened. Latinos and African Americans are more likely to work in high-risk businesses such as restaurants and grocery stores, and are more likely to rely on public transportation, so increasing their risk of exposure to coronavirus. For these essential workers, 'social distancing and self-isolation are luxuries they cannot afford' (Polonijo 2020). Lower income areas had less testing availability initially, but by early July access to testing in low-income areas improved. On 9 July, Public Health Director Barbara Ferrer reported that 'Latinos are now more than twice as likely as whites to be infected with the novel coronavirus and twice as likely to die. Blacks were 27 per cent more likely to be infected and nearly twice as likely to die from the virus compared to whites' (Rosenfeld 2020).

By 10 September, African Americans and Latinos were over-represented in deaths from COVID-19: African Americans represented 7.7 per cent of COVID-19 deaths, but only 6.0 per cent of the population.

Latino deaths were 48.4 per cent of COVID-19 deaths, but 38.9 per cent of the population (CDPH 2020). Jim Mangia, CEO of St John's Well Child and Family Center, commented: 'When you're in the middle of a pandemic, you really get a sense of where the priorities lie. More people got COVID in South L than in any other part of the county. More people died of COVID here'. The disparities were not only about the types of work and other activities in which residents of South LA might have disproportionately engaged. Long-standing structural problems such as lower rates of health insurance and a general lack of sufficient infrastructure and services in lower-income areas disproportionately characterised the lives of Black and Latino residents (Artiga et al. 2020). As Barbara Ferrer noted, 'the most prominent conditions that lead to death among COVID-19 patients – heart disease, respiratory illness and diabetes – are also more common in communities with higher rates of poverty. They are also less likely to have access to care' (Rosenfeld 2020).

The disparities of COVID-19 and the Black Lives Matter uprisings of 2020 are inextricably linked, and build upon a foundation of racial capitalism and the general devaluation of Black lives in the US. Cedric Robinson (1983) argues that all forms of capitalism are racialised because the historical development of capitalism was based on the forces of racism and hierarchy. Tracing forms of racialised social hierarchy from the formation of Europe, Robinson shows the continued entwining of capitalism and racialised hierarchy. Racial capitalism has a 'fundamental impact on health inequities' (Laster Pirtle 2020, 504). LA area leaders and politicians are increasingly recognising the links between racism, discrimination and health inequities, and are also beginning to see the connection to policing and prisons. In early June, Los Angeles County Supervisor Hilda Solis opened a news briefing on COVID-19 with the statement that COVID was joined by a second public health crisis – 'unabated and unaccountable police violence':

> We've seen another public health crisis highlighted. According to the (American) Public Health Association, addressing law enforcement violence should be a public health priority. The root cause of health inequities, especially during the pandemic, is systemic racism and discrimination (KCET 2020).

In her analysis of the events of 2020 in Los Angeles, Supervisor Solis laid bare the connections between racial capitalism, the carceral state and health inequalities. Just as jobs were eliminated and real wages declined in places like South LA, the state of California significantly expanded its prison system. City budgets were increasingly allocated to policing at the expense of healthcare, mental health, housing programmes, healthcare and food programmes. As people struggled with job loss and declining wages, the social programmes that could have been a safety net were eliminated or reduced, and instead residents faced the threat of police violence and imprisonment (Gilmore 2007; Ralph 2020).

Abolition as a public health measure

On 5 June 2020, National Public Radio aired a report by Ailsa Chang. Chang interviewed three Black men who had lived through multiple uprisings as residents of South Los Angeles. Bruce Patton, one of the interviewees, told her: 'There's no need for a policeman to have a gun. That is what gives them the propensity to kill you. It's their approach to the people in these communities that make police officers fear for their lives'. Chang summarised Patton's understanding that his 'community has been fighting back against a problem that never seems to change – police violence against black people. And for Patton, at least, the solution to that problem is very clear. He says we need to take all guns away from the police' (Chang 2020). Marqueece Harris-Dawson, another native of South LA and city councilman, told Chang that while he thought there was a use for LAPD and other police departments, the police needed to focus on fewer things: 'We ask police departments to solve homelessness. We ask them to solve truancy. We ask them to solve blight, traffic problems, pedestrian safety. We ask them to solve a whole bunch of problems that they oftentimes are not the appropriate set of individuals to do'. Harris-Dawson suggested that instead of (over)funding the police to do this, we should spend more money on schools and healthcare. Chang's third guest, Gilbert Johnson, reflected: 'The community is rising up. Right now, we have opportunity. We have a chance to really organise and galvanise all this momentum and push it in a positive way. We're going to see a lot more change, and a lot more people are out protesting because they want change. So, yes, I see this as a moment of hope amidst all the chaos' (Chang 2020).

Although local residents have varying views on the role of the police, Black Lives Matter LA calls for law enforcement, as it currently exists, to be completely abolished. In general, Black Lives Matter groups carefully craft their messaging so they can maintain abolitionist visions of eradicating the police and prisons, but not be seen as too radical for progressive uptake and media coverage (Shange 2016). The recent calls have been for abolition to happen through defunding police departments, with governments allocating police budgets to reinvest in community needs. The abolition of policing as we know it is tied to the abolition of jails (local city or county level institutions), prisons (state or federal level institutions) and detention centres, which all function together and are central to the state enactment of anti-black violence. As the quote from Supervisor Solis illustrates, police violence is a public health crisis, and addressing this should be a public health priority. One way to do so is to completely abolish the law enforcement system as we currently know it.

The protests of 2020 were peaceful but forceful, and the protestors drew attention on a worldwide scale to the horrors of our carceral state and the relentless murders of Black people by law enforcement officers. At the extreme end of the 2020 uprisings, people set fire to police cars, a few businesses and burned trash to create fires in the streets. The protests themselves did not involve much looting, but after the protesters moved through the streets of Los Angeles, looters moved in. We watched from our living room as dozens of people broke into local stores, taking shoes, clothing and pharmaceuticals from a local drug store. The local news media focused on the looters, insinuating that police force against the protestors was acceptable; the language of 'looting' and 'rioting' was used to delegitimise protests in which all Americans have the right to engage, and to cast protestors as violent and unruly, so justifying even more police violence against them (Bonilla and Rosa 2015). The response from law enforcement was disturbing. An LAPD SUV drove into a crowd, striking protestors. Tear gas was launched at protestors holding the line. And with the nightly curfews, whether peaceful or not, protestors were arrested if they were out after 6 p.m. Like Robin D.G. Kelley (2020), I wondered, 'what kind of society values property over Black lives?'

The initial response from city leadership was chilling. On 1 June, I watched LAPD Chief Michel Moore announce at a live press conference, as Mayor Garcetti looked on, that 'the blood of George Floyd's death is on the hands of protesters'. But this marked a turn, and Moore was forced to recant, claiming that he 'misspoke'. Later, outside LAPD headquarters Mayor Garcetti joined protestors and 'took a knee', an act of kneeling now widely recognised as a silent protest against police brutality and racism in the US. Soon after, he announced that he would take $100 million dollars from the LAPD budget and give it to communities of colour. The city later agreed to reduce the police department budget by $1.8 billion, a step some viewed as moving in the right direction toward abolition and others viewed as insufficient and inadequate. Things seemed to shift at the national level as well. The streets in front of the White House were renamed Black Lives Matter Plaza. The officer who killed Floyd was arrested and charged. Minneapolis banned police use of chokeholds, and (then) presidential candidate Joe Biden asked the US Congress to outlaw chokeholds.

This was just the beginning. More text messages came from the M4BL; we had to keep going; these small concessions were not enough. It is our duty to fight for our freedom. By 4 June, the curfews stopped. On Sunday 7 June, protestors danced and sang at the largest gathering to date at one of LA's famous intersections, Hollywood and Highland, near the Dolby Theater where the Academy Awards or 'Oscars' are usually hosted. The protests continued across the city, with people socially distanced and masked lining major boulevards, holding signs proclaiming Black Lives Matter. It seemed that more white people were turning out to support Black Lives Matter than ever before. Those who took their support beyond symbolic gestures and actually marched and gave monetary support strengthened the power of the uprisings in cities across the US and the world. The City of Dallas announced a 'duty to intervene' rule that requires officers to stop other officers who engage in inappropriate use of force. Statues and monuments celebrating racist figures were officially and unofficially removed in cities across the US. Confederate flags were removed and banned by organisations nationwide, including the US Marine Corps.

State systems, inequality and the Black radical tradition

Using the Black radical tradition to analyse the junctures of the 2020 uprisings and the disparities of COVID-19, it is clear that the liberal capitalist state played a significant role in the state sanctioned killing of Black people, both from a virus and from murderous police (Robinson 1983). The state response to COVID-19 prioritised reopening the economy over public safety. Black and Latino laborers had to return to work in order for the most fundamental elements of the economy – grocery stores, warehouses, public services – to continue functioning, demonstrating some of the ways in which racial capitalism and incessant drive for profit are lethal for Black and Latino communities under COVID-19 (Dawson 2018).

Just before the uprisings of 2020, LA had been reeling from the effects of COVID-19, in terms of morbidity, mortality and economics. In a population of around 10 million, by late May there were over one million unemployment claims filed in Los Angeles County. One article reported that only 45 per cent of LA residents were employed in March 2020 (Wagner 2020). This led to deep concerns about housing and food insecurity. Springing into action, community organisations seemed to come together around mutual aid, and local organisations were quick to pivot their services toward the needs of the COVID-19 era. For instance, to mitigate housing loss, on 4 March LA County invoked an eviction moratorium, banning evictions on residential and commercial tenants. Organisations across the city offered programmes for emergency food distribution. The Los Angeles Regional Food Bank ramped up its distribution programmes. Approximately 405,000 students, or 72.4 per cent of students of Los Angeles Unified School District (LAUSD) qualified for free and reduced-price meals, based on their family's income. These children normally eat free breakfast and lunch at school during the school year and receive free meals during summer programmes through the school district or Los Angeles area Parks and Recreation programmes. On 18 March, a week after closing the schools, LAUSD – the second largest public school system in the US – began distributing food at some of the closed school sites and other central locations across the city. Initially, the food was only intended for students and their families, but, shortly thereafter, it began to be distributed to anyone in need. Smaller organisations, like Community Services Unlimited Ltd. in South Los Angeles, also quickly developed systems for distributing food in their neighbourhoods. These forms of coming together as a community to support one another in times of crisis, as Nancy Burke also illustrates for Cuba (Chapter 2), are precisely the kinds of futures that Black Lives Matter is fighting for.

Under COVID-19, Angelenos started to see the ways in which our systems – education, healthcare, food distribution – were still expected to be supported by the state, but had long been precarious. COVID-19 was the tipping point, causing a complete breakdown of these systems as healthcare systems were overloaded with COVID-19 cases and people seeking preventative healthcare and 'nonessential care' were turned away. Grocery store shelves were empty and store managers did not know when they would be restocked. Schools closed completely leaving hundreds of thousands of kids with nothing but a promise that online learning would come soon. The pandemic led to a devastating loss of life, and a great increase in inequality and precariousness for low-income Angelenos. In realising this, Angelenos came together around fear and devastation, but with a sense of hope and an understanding that only through community organising, and not dependence on that state, could lives be saved (Sojoyner 2017; Vargas 2010). People started to see the connections between school and food, between work and healthcare. They questioned what it meant that school closures could lead to massive food insecurity, and that schools had long been responsible for ensuring that children and their families had enough to eat. Similarly, people started to see that if healthcare was tied to work and people lost their jobs due to business closures, then millions of people would be without access to healthcare. It became increasingly clear how current infrastructure was putting people in increasingly precarious situations.

This understanding of how government systems and state infrastructures fail us also opened many people to the possibility of abolition – abolishing the police and prisons. This did not mean police reform, but the full abolition of policing, of corrupt political systems that protect law enforcement officers that murder Black people, and everyone else who is complicit with this system. The abolition of the prison system dovetails with the abolition of policing. The goal to eliminate both of these racist systems is part of a broader vision to transform education, healthcare and other systems deeply enmeshed in the current economic system. These need to be untethered from racial capitalism so that our communities can survive and thrive. This was what Black Lives Matter LA was fighting for and increasing numbers of Angelenos were joining the fight.

Conclusions

On 9 June, George Floyd was laid to rest in Houston, Texas, and, again, we watched from our living room as crowds gathered outside the cemetery, and stood witness as his casket passed by in a horse-drawn carriage. They gathered to celebrate his life, mourn his loss and to mourn the violent loss of thousands of other Black people at the hands of the police. Some were outraged by the crowds that gathered during a surge in the COVID-19 pandemic in Texas. But the political moment, the need to gather and physically be present in the fight for Black freedom, seemed to outweigh the risk of COVID-19. After all, we may outlive the virus, but we will still face the battle against state-sanctioned anti-Black violence. Whereas we understand the COVID-19 pandemic to be temporary, police violence against Black people is endemic, part of a total climate of anti-Blackness (Sharpe 2016).

Thinking of the COVID-19 pandemic and the violence of the carceral state as parallel plagues that have differential patterns of endangering lives and ending lives across the world, anthropological and social theory can help to illuminate their uneven impacts and consequences in places like South Los Angeles. The forms of police violence and murder that sparked the BLM uprisings of 2020 are distinctly racialised and impact Black Angelenos at significantly higher rates than white Angelenos. And while the virus does not discriminate along racial or socioeconomic lines as it invades and attacks human bodies, how the virus attacks the body, and bodily vulnerability to severe disease, are the outcomes of pre-existing conditions, access to healthcare, workplace conditions and other social and economic factors. The COVID-19 virus is loaded onto a long history of inequality and racialised state violence.

Yet, as we fight against racialised police violence under COVID-19, governments worldwide are enlisting new forms of surveillance and monitoring tied to military and policing, as a number of authors in this volume illustrate. As militarised surveillance is ramped up to fight off the spread of COVID-19, Saiba Varma (2020, 376) reminds us,

> COVID-19 offers us something. It raises profound questions about our reliance on policing as a catchall solution. Even in an unprecedented health crisis, the state's carceral capacities are bolstered – in calls to 'put the military in charge of health care expansion', in surveilling and fining violations of pandemic restrictions, and in everyday descriptions of the pandemic as war.

In our highly connected, unequal world, the focus on investing money and energy into solutions that bolster the capability of military and police to fight disease and kill potential 'threats' is also directly tied to the failures of governments to provide for people's basic needs. As tech developers and companies profit from surveillance technologies, under racial capitalism this likely translates into heightened surveillance and arrests, and potentially moves us towards increasing rates of incarceration and death in Black communities. The 2020 uprisings and COVID-19 have revealed the ways in which the drastic disparities in disease incidence are tied to the overfunding of policing at the expense of community services. But while the COVID-19 pandemic fuelled a political drive to 'flatten the curve' in Los Angeles, little effort has been made to flatten the curve of increasing inequities.

Acknowledgements

I thank Alicia Wright for research assistance, and Saiba Varma for feedback on drafts of this chapter. I thank Nancy J. Burke, Ayo Wahlberg and Lenore Manderson for their editorial feedback, which served to significantly improve this chapter.

Notes

1   https://www.nytimes.com/interactive/2020/07/03/us/george-floyd-protests-crowd-size.html.
2   Used here with permission from Dr Scorza.

References

Artiga, Samantha, Rachel Garfield and Kendal Orgera. 2020. 'Communities of color at higher risk for health and economic challenges due to COVID-19'. KFF.org, 7 April 2020. Accessed 6 September 2020. https://www.kff.org/coronavirus-covid-19/issue-brief/communities-of-color-at-higher-risk-for-health-and-economic-challenges-due-to-covid-19/.
Beliso-De Jesús, Aisha M. and Jemima Pierre. 2020. 'Special section: Anthropology of white supremacy'. *American Anthropologist* 122(1): 65–75.
Bonilla, Yarimar and Jonathan Rosa. 2015. '#Ferguson: Digital protest, hashtag ethnography, and the racial politics of social media in the United States'. *American Ethnologist* 42(1): 4–16.
Burton, Orisanmi. 2015. 'Black Lives Matter: A critique of anthropology'. Hot Spots, *Fieldsights*, 29 June 2015. Accessed 6 September 2020. https://culanth.org/fieldsights/black-lives-matter-a-critique-of-anthropology.
CDPH. 2020. 'COVID-19 race and ethnicity data'. Accessed 9 November 2020. https://www.cdph.ca.gov/Programs/CID/DCDC/Pages/COVID-19/Race-Ethnicity.aspx.
Castillo, Andrea. 2020. 'How two Black women in LA helped build Black Lives Matter from hashtag to global movement'. *Los Angeles Times*, 21 June 2020. Accessed 6 September, 2020. https://www.latimes.com/california/story/2020-06-21/black-lives-matter-los-angeles-patrisse-cullors-melina-abdullah.
Chang, Ailsa. 2020. 'LA's history of racial tensions and police brutality, revisited. National Public Radio all things considered'. *National Public Radio*, 5 June 2020. Accessed 6 September 2020. https://www.npr.org/2020/06/05/871083491/las-history-of-racial-tensions-and-police-brutality-revisited.
Cox, Aimee Meredith. 2020. 'No, I am not OK'. *Transformations*, 3 September 2020. Accessed 6 September 2020. https://www.transformationnarratives.com/blog/2020/09/03/no-i-am-not-ok.
Dawson, Michael. 2018. 'Racial capitalism and democratic crisis'. SSRC Items Essay, 4 December 2020. Accessed 6 September 2020. https://items.ssrc.org/race-capitalism/racial-capitalism-and-democratic-crisis/.
Garth, Hanna. 2020. 'Blackness and "justice" in the Los Angeles Food Justice Movement'. In *Black Food Matters: Racial justice in the wake of food justice*, edited by Hanna Garth and Ashanté Reese, pp. 107–30. Minneapolis, MN: University of Minnesota Press.
Garth, Hanna and Ashanté Reese. 2020. *Black Food Matters: Racial justice in the wake of food justice*. Minneapolis, MN: University of Minnesota Press.
Gilmore, Ruth Wilson. 2007. *Golden Gulag: Prisons, surplus, crisis, and opposition in globalising California*. Berkeley, CA: University of California Press.
KCET. 2020. 'Racial disparities in COVID-19 cases, deaths called "devastating"'. *City News Service*, 5 June 2020. Accessed 6 September 2020. https://www.kcet.org/coronavirus-covid-19/racial-disparities-in-covid-19-cases-deaths-called-devastating.

Kelley, Robin D.G. 2016. 'What does Black Lives Matter want?' *The Boston Review*, 17 August 2016. Accessed 6 September 2020. http://bostonreview.net/books-ideas/robin-d-g-kelley-movement-black-lives-vision.

Kelley, Robin D.G. 2020. 'What kind of society values property over Black lives?' *New York Times*, 18 June 2020. Accessed 6 September 2020. https://www.nytimes.com/2020/06/18/opinion/george-floyd-protests-looting.html.

Kerrigan, Dylan. 2015. 'Transnational anti-Black racism and state violence in Trinidad'. Hot Spots, *Fieldsights*, 29 June 2015. Accessed 5 December 2020. https://culanth.org/fieldsights/transnational-anti-black-racism-and-state-violence-in-trinidad.

LA County. 2020. 'COVID-19 racial, ethnic & socioeconomic data and strategies report'. Report on LA County COVID-19. Data disaggregated by race/ethnicity and socioeconomic status, 28 April 2020. Accessed 6 September 2020. http://publichealth.lacounty.gov/media/coronavirus/data/index.htm.

Laster Pirtle, Whitney N. 2020. 'Racial capitalism: A fundamental cause of novel coronavirus (COVID-19) pandemic inequities in the United States'. *Health Education & Behavior* 47(4): 504–8.

Manderson, Lenore and Susan Levine. 2020. 'COVID-19, risk, fear, and fall-out'. *Medical Anthropology* 39(5): 367–70. https://doi:10.1080/01459740.2020.1746301.

Polonijo, Andrea. 2020. 'How California's COVID-19 surge widens health inequalities for Black, Latino and low-income residents'. *The Conversation*, 30 July 2020. Accessed 6 September 2020. https://theconversation.com/how-californias-covid-19-surge-widens-health-inequalities-for-black-latino-and-low-income-residents-143243.

Ralph, Laurence. 2019. 'The logic of the slave patrol: The fantasy of black predatory violence and the use of force by the police'. *Palgrave Communications* 5: 1–10.

Ralph, Laurence. 2020. *The Torture Letters: Reckoning with police violence*. Chicago, IL: University of Chicago Press.

Robinson, Cedric J. 1983. *Black Marxism: The making of the Black radical tradition*. Chapel Hill, NC: University of North Carolina Press.

Rosenfeld, David. 2020. 'LA County's racial disparities endure, even as coronavirus testing access improves: Latino and Black residents are roughly twice as likely to die from COVID-19 than whites in Los Angeles County'. *The Daily Breeze*, 10 July 2020. Accessed 6 September 2020. https://www.dailynews.com/2020/07/09/la-countys-racial-disparities-endure-even-as-coronavirus-testing-access-improves/.

Shange, Savannah. 2016. 'Unapologetically Black?' *Anthropology News* 57(7): 64–6.

Sharpe, Christina. 2016. *In the Wake: On Blackness and being*. Durham, NC: Duke University Press.

Smith, Christen A. 2015. 'Blackness, citizenship, and the transnational vertigo of violence in the Americas'. *American Anthropologist* 117(2): 384–7.

Smith, Christen A. 2017. 'Battling anti-black genocide in Brazil'. *NACLA Report on the Americas* 49(1): 41–7. https://doi:10.1080/10714839.2017.1298243.

Sojoyner, Damien M. 2017. 'Another life is possible: Black fugitivity and enclosed places'. *Cultural Anthropology* 32(4): 514–36.

Speed, Shannon. 2020. 'The persistence of white supremacy: Indigenous women migrants and the structures of settler capitalism'. *American Anthropologist* 122(1): 76–85.

Wagner, David. 2020. 'LA's latest unemployment numbers are staggering. An estimated 1.3m jobs have already been lost'. Laist.com, 17 April 2020. Accessed 1 September 2020. https://laist.com/2020/04/17/unemployment_numbers_job_loss_california.php.

Vargas, Joao H. Costa. 2010. *Never Meant to Survive: Genocide and utopias in Black diaspora communities*. New York: Rowman & Littlefield Publishers, Inc.

Vargas, Joao H. Costa. 2015. 'Black lives don't matter'. Hot Spots, *Fieldsights*, 29 June 2015. Accessed 5 October 2020. https://culanth.org/fieldsights/black-lives-dont-matter.

Varma, Saiba. 2020. 'A pandemic is not a war: COVID-19 urgent anthropological reflections'. *Social Anthropology*, 19 May. https://doi:10.1111/1469-8676.12879.

6
The biopolitics of COVID-19 in the UK
Racism, nationalism and the afterlife of colonialism
Jennie Gamlin, Sahra Gibbon and Melania Calestani

Historical social inequalities continue to shape the epidemiological profile of COVID-19, visibilising how some bodies are more exposed than others. While there has long been evidence of health disparities among Black, Asian and ethnic minorities in the UK, and growing concern with the role of racism in perpetuating them (Nazroo 2003), the finding that certain communities face a higher risk of contracting and dying from COVID-19 has newly exposed deep-rooted national divisions. The brutal killing of George Floyd in the US in May 2020,[1] and the global protest and activism led by the #BlackLivesMatter movement, reignited discussion around the relationship of racism and life expectancy. By mid-July 2020, as transmission steadied in the first wave of the pandemic, the UK had reached the highest overall and population level COVID-19 mortality in Western Europe, with clear disproportionately high death rates among Black, Asian and Minority Ethnic populations. The stark embodied effects of racism and inequality precipitated growing public calls to consider how colonialism and imperialism continues to have consequences for the health of minority communities (Siddique and Grierson 2020). We refer to these historically defined patterns and processes, along with the presence of colonial structures within the National Health Service itself, as the *afterlife of colonialism*, as they represent the permanence of the past in the present.

In this chapter, by analysing the government's response of putting forth policy decisions by a bullish go-it-alone strategy that initially rejected WHO advice and European Union (EU) collaborative preparations, we draw on anthropological insights to consider the presence of Britain's colonial past in the populations, biopolitics and institutions that defined the handling and impact of COVID-19. The overrepresentation of Black and ethnic minority populations in UK[2] death toll figures for coronavirus tracks the fault lines of social and economic exclusions that give continuity to colonialism and its production and exploitation of racial hierarchies. We examine how the acronym BAME (Black, Asian and Minority Ethnic) has become a proxy for social and economic differences and inequalities, while reinforcing the *othering* of specific groups along lines established by colonialism. Building upon and extending approaches to power and structural inequalities (Farmer 1999; Fassin 2007, 2013) by drawing on Hartman's notion of the 'afterlife of slavery' (2007), we argue that ethno-racial differences in the epidemiological profile of coronavirus are the afterlife of colonialism – the persistence of political domination in the bodies of racialised people.

This afterlife also operates at the level of biopolitics through the lingering sentiments of Empire and we bring in Franklin's discussion of 'nostalgic nationalism' (2019) to unpack the post-Brexit management of this global emergency. The political moment in which COVID emerged coincided with the UK's departure from the EU, which was itself the outcome of a very close referendum result. The Brexit moment on 31 January 2020 was one of a newfound ideational sovereignty, an imagined identity that hinged almost entirely upon a colonially-given political superiority, and the subsequent belief in British exceptionalism that has proven to endure long beyond the UK's political dominance. We examine these complex intersections with the material politics of epidemic response (Lynteris and Poleykett 2018), and the ongoing isolationism arising from the UK's tortured pathway to leaving the EU, particularly in the allocation and resourcing of personal protective equipment (PPE). Populations and biopolitics also collide in the colonial patterning of care provision by Britain's National Health Service (NHS), the centrepiece of the UK's epidemic response, an institution sustained in large part by the combined labour of EU and colonial diaspora communities. Hence the afterlife of colonialism is both lived and delivered as a mentality and a relational dynamic. These same populations, including first, second and later generations of families invited to the UK in the days of dwindling colonial power, are also caring for the ill and dying. In association with mortality rates, we will reflect upon the ethnic patterning of care provision and the coloniality of the NHS.

Epidemiological histories and contemporary revelations

Through its long history of longitudinal cohort studies, the UK has been at the forefront of a global effort to demonstrate the social determinants of health. The Whitehall Studies on the health of British civil servants, and other epidemiological studies, have provided powerful evidence of how social inequalities shape chronic disease morbidity and mortality and pattern the social gradient in health (Marmot 2005). While some have pointed to the failure of a social determinants approach to fully address 'structural inequalities' (Breilh 2013; Yates-Doerr 2020), a succession of UK conservative governments has done little to address the inequalities upon which COVID has played. As a result of the policy of austerity that has characterised the UK's health and social policy since the economic crisis of 2008, inequalities have become more entrenched, increasing alongside unemployment and poverty and affecting healthcare services (Stuckler et al. 2017); in this sense, unequal morbidity and mortality from COVID-19 could have been anticipated and expected. Black men were, during the first wave of the pandemic, at least three times more likely to die than white men, and men and women of Bangladeshi origin were twice as likely to have died. As of 30 June 2020, people of Indian, Chinese, Pakistani, other Asian and Black ethnicity were 10–50 per cent more likely to have died than their white counterparts (PHE 2020).

Racism is causally implicated in health inequalities among minority communities and race is increasingly recognised as a 'social determinant of health' (Williams et al. 2019; Marmot 2020), but there has been little work at a national level to analyse the intersections of race with other social and economic factors (Chouhan and Nazroo 2020). There are significant data gaps on ethnicity and health, with ongoing questions about the quality and accuracy of information collected (Aspinall et al. 2003). Until June 2020, there was no comprehensive disaggregated national data about ethnicity on death certificates. In relation to COVID-19, this has been described as a form of 'state negligence' (Hirsch 2020). There is no epidemiological research on why generations of diasporas with heritage in British colonies still experience excess burdens of morbidity, the 'underlying conditions' now explanatory variables of COVID-19 mortality in the UK. Despite an emerging terrain of epigenetic research (Kuzawa and Sweet 2009), the link between present-day health and inequality and past histories of exploitation, domination and violence has not yet been included in policy-focused research into health inequalities. The fact that epidemiologists and the media alike did not anticipate excess mortality during a pandemic in the most vulnerable populations is a sign of the naturalisation of social inequalities and how entrenched racism has rendered race inequality and health invisible. Perhaps, as Davis (2019) suggests, through the stereotype of the *afterlife of slavery*, we have naturalised the idea that non-white bodies are stronger and more resilient than white bodies.

The emerging narrative of BAME and COVID-19

Black, Asian and Minority Ethnic – in its acronym form as BAME – has become the accepted label to define and sort many different ethnic groups by their shared characteristic of not being of white European descent. It also defines different peoples whose histories largely return to once colonised locations in the Global South. This categorisation of difference serves to define the self as much as the other, making it a relational identity. This must be historicised in the context of colonial hierarchies based on racial and often 'biologised' notions of superiority as culture is transposed onto race. These diaspora populations and subsequent generations who have settled in the UK do not share homogenising biological characteristics that differentiate them from white Europeans, other than not having whiter skin. This category suggests that non-whiteness, where 'whiteness' is a racialised and privileged social category (Echeverría 2016), somehow makes a person more vulnerable to the virus. The lumping together of Black, Asian and ethnic minority groups under 'BAME' is inherently racist as it does not describe who they are, their ancestry or heritage, but who they are not, as we discuss later.

The term BAME, while widely used in the UK including by advocates within and for ethnic minority communities, is problematic when ascribed to social and ethnic groups in relation to health. It suggests that innate biological, genetic or essentialised cultural factors are at play. This disguises the role of social and political history, the afterlife of colonialism. The widespread use of this acronym during the pandemic obscures social causality and demonstrates the coloniality of contemporary social and political dynamics and their embodiment.

With no national requirement to record the ethnicity of hospital patients, the first suggestion that in the UK ethnic minorities were more severely affected by COVID-19 came not from demographic data, but from anecdotal evidence on nightly news reports and reports of deaths and local hospitalisation rates. The first 12 doctors known to have died after contracting coronavirus were 'non-white' (Siddique and Marsh 2020). From mid-March, a distorted picture of disease distribution and death began to emerge. According to the 2011 census in England and Wales, non-white ethnic minority communities constituted 14 per cent of the population, but in April 2020, 35 per cent of almost 2,000 critically ill patients were in this category (Intensive Care National Audit and Research Centre 2020). Local surveys published in *The Guardian* and *Times* newspapers in early April suggested that 19 per cent of recorded hospital deaths to this date were from ethnic minority communities, with higher numbers of ethnic minority residents having higher death rates (Barr et al. 2020). The evidence began to grow across media outlets as the tributes, memorials and daily roll call of faces and names to those who had died from COVID-19 appeared – health professionals, porters, cleaners and other key workers such as bus drivers. Here was visible evidence of the disproportionate effect on communities by COVID-19.

Dr Ayache was one. Syrian-born Fayez Ayache had treated three generations of Jennie Gamlin's family at the local village practice, retiring from full-time employment in 2018. He rejoined the service during the pandemic. On 8 April, six days after being admitted to the same hospital in Ipswich at which he had given a lifetime's service, he died, positive for COVID-19 (BMA 2020). In a statement made after his death, his daughter Layla recalled her father's dedication to his work and to the NHS:

> This is why the NHS was important to dad; because it brought people together, it gave a freedom that some had never experienced before, and it gave hope and light to those who were wandering a darkened path. The NHS is a lifeline for so many that dad felt it his duty to serve within (BMA 2020).

By mid-April, the UK government's rallying call that 'we are in this together' was increasingly hollow as the unequal impact of COVID-19 became clearer. Bowing to public pressure and criticism, the government launched an inquiry into the disproportionate deaths among BAME communities by Public Health England (PHE), led by its National Director for Health and Wellbeing, Professor Kevin Fenton. PHE also recommended that health workers from BAME communities should be 'risk assessed' to consider whether their assigned roles placed them at increased risk of infection (Kanani and Issar 2020). By early May, comprehensive data on ethnicity and hospital deaths began to provide a more robust picture of inequalities. One report suggested that between the end of February and April 2020, 'Black and Asian' people in the UK were 71 and 62 per cent more likely to die from COVID-19 than 'white' people (Williamson et al. 2020). Another report by the Institute for Fiscal Studies suggested that even after adjusting for age, sex and geography, the death rate for 'people of black African descent' was 3.5 times that of 'white British people' (Platt and Warwick 2020). In early June, PHE confirmed that people from Black, Asian and Minority Ethnic communities were twice as likely to die as 'white' communities if they developed COVID-19. However, PHE did not offer explanations or propose any policy interventions to address this disparity, leading to immediate accusations that this final section of the report, purportedly concerning the need to address structural racism, had been censored by the Health Secretary. The report was finally published two weeks later after leaks to the press indicated specific mention of structural racism. The controversy around this report, which coincided with and was informed by widespread activism around the murder of George Floyd in the US and the Black Lives Matter movement, opened up dialogue on the health effects of institutional and historical racism. We return to this later in this chapter.

The specific patterning of care, as the wider context within which the British response to coronavirus played out, is itself an afterlife of colonialism (Fitzgerald et al. 2020), reflecting the permanence of the past in the present through an attitude of nostalgic nationalism. In the following section, we explore this further through the idea of 'heroism' – a description of health and social care workers at the height of the first wave of the epidemic – and how this was belied by the UK's Brexit-fuelled isolationist policy.

Occupational health and Brexit isolationism

From mid-March to July 2020, countrywide, 'Thank you' signs with rainbows for NHS workers appeared in street-facing windows of homes and chalk messages on pavements (Figure 6.1). Thousands of people came outside their houses to 'clap for carers' each Thursday at 8 p.m., thanking mainly NHS healthcare professionals for their outstanding work during these unprecedented times.

Some healthcare professionals were frustrated with this Thursday ritual, arguing that 'the health service is not a charity and it is not staffed by heroes' (*The Guardian* 21 May 2020). On Thursday 28 May, as Prime Minister Boris Johnson was clapping for carers, a silent protest ('Doctors, not Martyrs' – *The Times of India* 29 May 2020) was held outside Downing Street, organised by Indian-origin doctor Meenal Viz, who had raised more than £53,000 towards a legal battle against the UK government over the lack of PPE. Similarly, the previous week, an anonymous NHS doctor

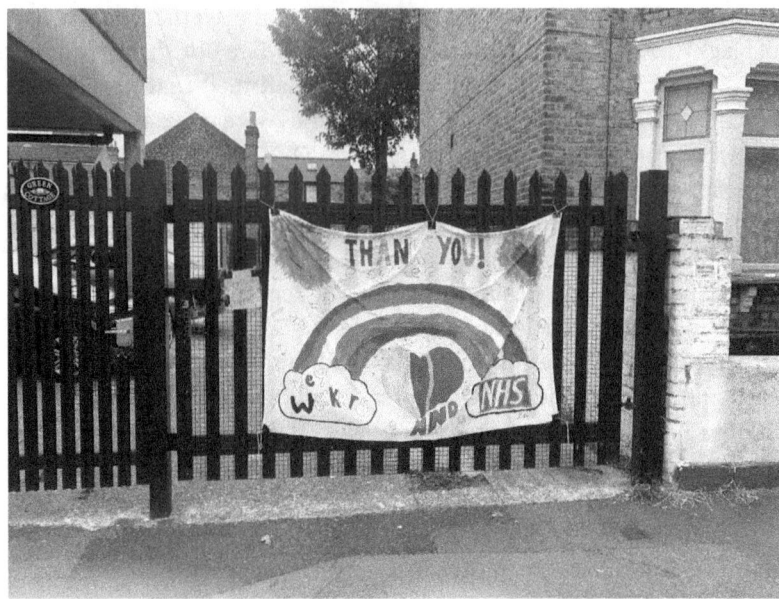

Figure 6.1 Handmade banner supporting the National Health Service (NHS) in south London in response to the COVID-19 pandemic. Photo: Sahra Gibbon

wrote an article in *The Guardian*, emphasising some of the issues at stake when analysing the material politics of the UK epidemic response to COVID-19:

> It would ... be nice to have clarity about many things, from testing to isolation to proper use of personal protective equipment (PPE). It would also be nice to have worked for the past 10 years in an adequately funded NHS, staffed by people listened to by the government. It would be nice to see appropriate remuneration for the low-paid staff holding the service together, to see that the value of immigrants to the NHS is appreciated (Anonymous, *The Guardian* 21 May 2020).

The notion of heroism echoes wartime victories, but the underfunding of the NHS, and the availability of PPE and virus testing, intersects with the politics of the UK COVID-19 response in more complex ways. The WHO has emphasised the need to consider how the social determinants of health and health inequalities are shaped 'by the distribution of money, power and resources at global, national and local levels'

(Gideon 2014, 31). In the UK, recent and more distant historical entanglements, including Brexit and the foundational history of the NHS, must be understood as central in shaping occupational health at the time of COVID-19 and in understanding the disproportionate rate of deaths among ethnic minority NHS employees. Of the initial 119 NHS staff known to have died during the first wave, 64 per cent were from an ethnic minority background (Cook et al. 2020).

Key workers such as NHS staff, and food supply chain and utility workers, continued of necessity to work outside their homes, exposing them more to infection (van Dorn et al. 2020). According to the independent charity The Health Foundation (2020), in London, ethnic minority key workers constitute 54 per cent of the food production, process and sale sector (including all food retail and processing) and 48 per cent of the health and social care sector; 11 and 13 per cent for areas outside London. An NHS Workforce Race Equality Standard Report (2019) emphasised that ethnic minority staff members are underrepresented in senior pay bands and are overrepresented in band 5 – the lowest band, in which salaries start from £22,128 (Royal College of Nursing, 2020).

The majority (44.9 per cent) of ethnic minority health workers are employed in NHS trusts, although their role has been marginalised (Simpson et al. 2010), overrepresented in the lowest band with more difficulties in reaching senior positions. Moreover, a report published in October 2020 by East London Care and London Partnership demonstrated that their experience as ethnic minority employees is mixed, with the COVID-19 pandemic reinforcing health inequalities, racism and discrimination. Their current experiences cannot be disentangled from the foundational history of the NHS.

Fitzgerald and colleagues describe the NHS as 'imperially-resourced' (2020, 1169), with today's NHS an afterlife of colonialism. The first significant wave of overseas-trained doctors, many Jewish and other Central European refugees from fascist states, entered Britain in the thirties (Simpson et al. 2010). In the fifties, migration from the Indian subcontinent became important in recruiting doctors, nurses and other health workers in Britain. In 1948, qualified nurses were recruited for the newly formed NHS, mainly from 16 colonies, particularly the Caribbean (Fitzgerald et al. 2020, 9); in the early 2000s trained nurses migrated for work from various South Asian and African countries (Mackintosh et al. 2006). The London School of Hygiene and Tropical Medicine's continued dominance in global health is another afterlife of colonialism, within which an 'us and them' pervades in their institution's name (MacLeod and Lewis, 1988).

Although nationality is not an indicator of ethnicity, today 37 per cent of doctors employed in the NHS received their primary qualification outside the UK, and the top seven countries of origin of doctors and top five of nurses to the NHS are former British colonies – India, Pakistan, Nigeria, Ghana, Sri Lanka, Zimbabwe and Egypt (Fitzgerald et al. 2020, 9). In addition, some 144,000 EU health and care workers in England and 30,000 doctors, totalling 11 per cent of the 280,000 doctors currently on the register, gained their primary medical qualification in the European Economic Area (EEA) (Simpkin and Mossialos 2017).

A disproportionate number of ethnic minority NHS staff members from various socio-economic backgrounds, including hospital consultants, nurses and healthcare assistants, have died as a result of COVID-19. Five days before admission to hospital with COVID-19, consultant urologist Abdul Mabud Chowdhury appealed for 'appropriate PPE and remedies' to 'protect ourselves and our families' (BBC News, 10 April 2020). Dr Chowdhury died on 8 April, one of 1,431 deaths, still (in December 2020) the highest daily mortality of COVID-19 (Office of National Statistics, 12 June 2020). The lack of availability of PPE was documented closely in the press as a contributing factor in the death of health workers. A shipment of PPE from Turkey did not meet the UK safety standards (Rawlinson 2020), further aggravating the crisis. A survey of 3,500 UK nurses, conducted early April 2020 (Dean 2020), identified that 67 per cent did not have access to sufficient PPE, leaving them terrified. Serena, a nurse in her 40s, elaborated on this with the third author, Melania, during an interview at the end of April 2020, after relocating to her home country in continental Europe.[3] She had been in the UK for 20 years, living in London and working in an NHS high dependency unit (HDU). She described how, in the last month of her employment (March 2020), the health system was 'under a massive strain' and she felt unsafe at work because of unavailable PPE:

> When the first patients came through with 'query COVID', that was probably February, March already. There wasn't actually even testing provided yet for these patients. I remember one of the first patients being tested and it came back as positive. By then I literally was wearing my normal uniform and a pair of gloves. That uniform, I also took [it] home to wash. That was the first positive case.

Serena continued; after that, scrubs were provided by the hospital and staff members were no longer required to wash uniforms at home. However, PPE was allocated regionally on the basis of confirmed

COVID-19 cases, and there was no standardisation of PPE across different units within her hospital or across the NHS:

> Only once there is chest compression, intubation, defibrillation done, or any invasive or non-invasive oxygen therapy then you get the full PPE which is a visor; a facemask; a hair hat; a full gown; and double, triple gloving. This is provided in ITU [Intensive Therapy Unit]. On the HDU [High Dependency Unit] setting I've been working in, this was not provided. We would have literally just had a surgical face mask and a pinny, which is an apron [with] no sleeves and a pair of gloves.

The lack of PPE also has to be understood in light of Brexit. Following a UK-wide referendum in June 2016, in which 52 per cent voted in favour of leaving the EU, the government began to withdraw with the aim of completing this on 31 December 2020. A key message of the Vote Leave campaign during the 2016 Brexit Referendum, which appeared on its campaign bus, was *We send the EU £350m a week – let's fund our NHS instead*, implying that the underfunding of the NHS was due to Britain's obligations to the EU rather than decisions of the Conservative government. The promise to fund the NHS was disowned immediately after the referendum (Simpkin and Mossialos 2017).

COVID-19 presented the UK's Conservative government with its first opportunity post-Brexit to demonstrate national prowess as a 'sovereign' nation. Its 'go it alone' strategy, driven by the idea of a national past characterised by 'multiple nostalgias' (Balthazar 2017; Berliner 2012; Franklin 2019), had profound negative consequences for healthcare professionals' occupational health. By 12 March, the UK dropped the Test and Trace system, claiming that it was no longer feasible due to the level of contagion (Mueller and Bradley 2020), although this had been highly successful in Germany and Vietnam. Instead, the UK assumed a stance of isolationism, reinforcing the government's determination to present itself as independent from the EU.[4] In the coming weeks, it emerged that the UK simply did not have the testing capacity. On 16 March, it was announced that NHS staff could access COVID-19 testing (Moore 2020), although it was unclear how this would be implemented. When Serena developed a cough after her first patient tested positive, she was not offered a COVID-19 test. Neither was another colleague who had attended the same patient. Serena explained, 'it's not the routine that you get swabbed … Unfortunately, staff sickness is very high, so my understanding is that the testing is literally for staff to return to work instead of prevention from spreading it to anyone else'.

A strong sense of obligation to work during epidemics/pandemics coexists with concerns about lack of protection, lack of testing and the welfare of dependents (Shaw et al. 2006). While this affects all health workers and others employed in health facilities, it is widely hypothesised that people from minority groups are less likely to raise concerns about adequate protection (for example PPE) and are at increased risk of infection (Kapilashrami and Bhui 2020). For instance, the death of three ethnic minority cleaners at St George's Hospital in Tooting (London) in May 2020 led their colleagues to discuss strike action amid claims that their own and their families' health was at risk every time they did a shift (Porter 2020) because of the lack of PPE and test provision.

The material politics of epidemiological control, as this concerns PPE and testing in the UK, enact and constitute relations of power (see Lynteris and Poleykett 2018). The availability of PPE and tests intersects in complex ways with the UK epidemic response and the ongoing isolationism arising from UK's withdrawal from EU. The UK government missed out on four rounds of procurement of PPE and ventilators launched by the EU in late February and March (Wintour and Boffey 2020), leaving healthcare professionals, other hospital staff members and their respective families feeling unsafe. While key workers played a huge part of the coronavirus response, there is continued reluctance to acknowledge the historical nature of inequalities, to recognise the UK's dependency on non-British born key workers, or to reward them with good pay and conditions and/or preferential access to citizenship. This essentially discriminates against foreign workers who pay through their taxes into the NHS system, and staff the system, but do not have equal access to it. This is clearly illustrated by the UK's 'immigration health surcharge' (IHS), created in 2015, which resulted in all migrant workers paying twice to use the NHS, both through their taxes and the charge.[5]

The emerging picture of this injustice filtered through the individual voices of migrant health workers using social media. Syrian refugee and NHS hospital cleaner Hassan Akkad, for example, filmed himself sitting in his car after his work shift and called for 'fairer treatment'.[6] This was picked up across national and high-profile social media outlets.[7] Akkad responded, again from his car, that the support expressed to his first post had 'restored his faith in this country' adding that 'Britain is great because of you'. While this sentiment reflected the nostalgic nationalism that characterised discourse around COVID-19 and the NHS, the public profile of social media discourse and the growing pressure from trade unions and campaigners, highlighting the moral injustice of the situation, ultimately forced a humiliating reversal of the government IHS policy in early May.

The IHS, also known as the NHS or 'healthcare' surcharge, is a levy on the majority of UK visa applications, in addition to other Home Office immigration fees. This essentially adds £624 per year per person to the cost of a UK visa, or £470 a year for children, students and Youth Mobility visas. This fee will also apply to EU citizens after Brexit in 2021. Although NHS and care workers are now exempt, critics continue to press for further changes, such as extending the IHS exemption to other categories of essential workers.

National identity and the underlying conditions of racism

The 'afterlife of colonialism' acknowledges the legacy of institutional and historical racism and its role in the biopolitics of COVID-19 in the UK. This was both revealed and compounded by the events that unfolded in June 2020 in response to Black Lives Matter and the findings of PHE's investigation into COVID-19 and Black, Asian and Minority Ethnic groups.

The afterlife of slavery is a 'measure of man (sic) and ranking of life and worth that has yet to be undone ... skewed life chances, limited access to health and education, premature death, incarceration and impoverishment' (Hartman 2007, 6). Adapting this idea to contemporary Britain, we use the afterlife of colonialism as a method of reasoning and knowledge production that 'brings the past and present closer together' by theorising how 'racial hierarchies have been and continue to be replenished' (Davis 2019, 13). This illuminates relationships between the British state and diverse black and ethnic minority groups, whose bodies are entangled with past articulations of empire and white native British superiority, specifically through ideas of race and identity as biologically inherited. These inequalities are related to social deprivation, often with reference to how jobs, work environments and housing make it difficult to 'socially distance' and because complex sociocultural aspects of working and living environments heighten vulnerability, making COVID-19 contagion more likely. 'Underlying health conditions' such as diabetes, heart disease and obesity may also heighten vulnerability to COVID-19 among members of these communities. While these chronic 'underlying' conditions are frequently framed as 'epigenetic'[8] or 'biological' factors, they are the dynamic outcome and product of embodied social inequalities and interactions (Gravlee 2020; Lock 2015).

Afua Hirsch (2020) writes: 'Racism is a system that kills our bodies'. The disproportionate burden of 'underlying health conditions' and generalised social inequalities from systemic or structural racism reflects the embodied afterlife of colonialism. But also, identities such as those of British Black and ethnic minority groups, historically associated with the Global South, have now become social locations or positionalities defined by colonial history. As Kapilashrami and Bhui state, '(e)thnic inequalities in the experience and outcomes of illnesses, especially mental illnesses, have a long research history of contested explanations and evidence [that] fails to capture the complexity of life-course adversity, combined with social structures and interactions with pathophysiologies' (2020, 2). For many people who belong to ethnic minority groups, life course experiences of social location, defined by a colonial past, continue to lead to work stress due to race inequality, racism and discrimination.

Relational identity categories such as BAME are a constant reminder of non-whiteness in a white state, making skin colour an identifier of national belonging and social location. As Appadurai writes in *The Heart of Whiteness* (1993), nations are not natural facts and the linking of state and nation was a tenuous collective project to which a sense of national identity was key. This process implied racial hierarchies. In *Violence and the Body* (2003), Aldama emphasises the role of discursive violence in reinforcing othering, subalternity and the abjection of those positioned at the margins and borders of dominant cultural apparatuses: this social location traumatises the interior psyche formation of subjects. The 'otherisation' of certain bodies, central to the process of identity formation under colonial domination, is 'in some cases more extreme and oblique under the new social orders of the global economy' (Aldama 2003, 5). This otherisation as inferior is the basis of racism as a structural determinant of health and the outcome of intergenerational trauma (Kuzawa and Sweet 2009; Guthman 2014) that was, and continues to be, part of the ongoing process of British national identity.

The idea of a nation-state was aligned to western theories of state and involved the erasure of non-European structures of social organisation through colonialism. As both western economies and epistemologies expanded colonially across the globe, so too, through capitalist expansion, nation-states emerged as the only legitimate geopolitical formations (Mignolo 2002). Race and the idea of biological inheritance were key, defining an imaginary biological origin to attach to the state and national identity. In the UK, Black, Asian and Minority Ethnic share *not belonging* to a biologically inherited identity (white British), so that the BAME category was colonial in origin and is relational in practice. Historians of the colonial period, such as Fisher and O'Hara (2009), have demonstrated how colonisation effectively created the scientific concept of race.

As Laura Briggs suggests (2015, 27), 'science and medicine made race their object', with the dichotomy of modern and pre-modern contingent on racial hierarchies in what Silverblatt (in Fisher and O'Hara 2009, iv) describes as a 'revolution in the possible ways of being human' that attributed different human status depending on skin colour (see also Smith 2003; Wolfe 1999).

This fitting together of race, nation and identity, for Britain, hinged on creating and maintaining an imaginary superiority and imagined inferiority. Yet, as the collective experience of COVID-19 has demonstrated, this ideational sense of superiority is detached from Britain's actual performance as a nation. COVID-19 presented an opportunity to demonstrate post-imperialist exceptionalism. However, the nativist notion of national identity, that plays to a nostalgia for the past, consistently harmed the UK's response. Sarah Franklin (2019) uses the concept of 'nostalgic nationalism' to frame discourse around individual and national belonging. At the heart of this is a sense of loss, derived from a loss of command power over an empire. Injured white nationalism played a very important role in influencing millions to vote to leave the EU in June 2016. The campaign slogans of 'take back control' and 'Let's give 3.5 million to the NHS instead' were hugely influential. Boris Johnson, then campaign leader not yet prime minister, was the personification of the specific brand of nationalist Britishness that he was selling, inviting film crews to cover him eating ice cream cones by the seaside and bringing trays with mugs of tea to journalists.

This aspirational nationalism is reinforced by the NHS. As we have shown, this is an institution served by Black and ethnic minorities for the benefit of a white nation, so mirroring British colonialism and tying Britain's imperialist past to its divided present. The reminder that Britain was once an empire reinforces their otherisation in relation to their social location as 'colonised subjects' (Aldama 2003, 8) or people of empire. Without present-day BAME, there can be no coloniser. The NHS helps Britain retain this status as a coloniser. The irony of this post-empire dynamism is clear in the Brexit–NHS–COVID-19 trilogy. Writing before COVID-19 emerged, Fitzgerald and colleagues (2020) argue that Brexit must be situated in relation to biomedical policy in Britain in order to capture understandings of ancestry and health along with the forms of racial inheritance that structure the state and its welfare system. The Leave campaign's appeal to 'nostalgic nationalism' led to patterns of voting shaped by emotions. The NHS conjures up a similar nationalistic sentiment; the offer of exchanging the EU for the NHS, a centrepiece of the Leave campaign, generated a similarly emotional reaction.

The vital roles of EU citizens and Black, Asian and Minority Ethnic healthcare workers to ensure that the NHS functioned and survived, to save the lives of COVID-19 patients, to clean hospitals and drive buses, has brought inequality in health outcomes to the fore. It has also demonstrated their vital contribution to British society. While the UK appeared to have flattened the initial curve of coronavirus infections, it did not do so in relation to ethnic diversity: Britain did not become a multicultural network of equals, nor a cultural 'melting pot', but rather an uneven nation of whites and non-whites that extends to more recent diasporas of diverse origins. The idea of a category for all non-white people creates discomfort, yet the concept of whiteness makes visible the privileges that have protected some and made others more vulnerable. The COVID-19 pandemic made this starkly visible. Positioning whiteness as a category of experience, analogous with the afterlife of colonialism, Ahmed (2007) describes how groups of white people 'take up space', making this a category of experience not biology. 'Whiteness could be described as an ongoing and unfinished history which orientates bodies in specific directions' (Ahmed 2007, 150), a 'property of persons, cultures and places'. Institutional spaces are shaped by their proximity to certain bodies. The British National Health Services is a rare outlier, a British institution where whiteness does not dominate; the bodies that shape the NHS are Black and ethnic minority staff – healthcare providers, support and managerial staff, cleaners and technicians. However, this diversity has not led to equality – rather, it is evidence of entrenched inequality.

Conclusion

The COVID-19 pandemic has evidenced the inseparability of Britain's imperial past from its divided present, suggesting an afterlife of colonialism that undermines the life chances of many, while reproducing patterns of racial inequalities. The overrepresentation of Black and ethnic minority populations in daily UK death toll figures for coronavirus tracks the fault lines of social and economic exclusions that we argue were defined through colonialism.

In a global pandemic, critical medical anthropology has the task to draw to the surface the social and political origins of illness (Sesia et al. 2020; Pfeiffer and Nichter 2008). Rather, racism, national identity, nationalism and class, and their entanglement, continue to bear down on systemic embodied inequalities in the British healthcare system and have left specific groups particularly vulnerable to COVID-19. Asymmetrical power structures also dominate global health, so that 'the contemporary health crisis can serve as a reminder that the colonisation of medicine, economics and politics remains alive' (Ghilardi et al. 2020). Understanding how social and lived environments shape biological vulnerability without newly homogenising or re-stigmatising already vulnerable communities in an era of COVID-19 is a profound challenge. In post-Brexit UK, the afterlife of colonialism and nostalgic nationalism continues to be relevant. The danger comes from long standing and older risks of biologising inequality and social difference, where poverty, adversity or lived environments permanently mark bodies across lifetime and generations. Negotiating biosocial differences in the time of coronavirus is a fraught terrain. It provides both the opportunity to reveal the profound extent to which structural social inequalities shape health, while risking the ever-present danger that these differences will be subsumed by rendering the biological immutable.

Acknowledgements

We would like to thank the participants of the study 'Healthcare professionals' experiences and challenges at the time of COVID-19' (Kingston University REC reference number LR1545) who generously volunteered their time to be interviewed.

Notes

1 On 25 May 2020, George Floyd, a 46-year-old Black American man, was killed in Minneapolis, Minnesota, during an arrest for allegedly using a counterfeit bill (Hill et al. 2020).
2 The term United Kingdom (UK) refers to the union of all four nations, Northern Ireland, Scotland, Wales and England. However, Britain (which is the same as Great Britain) only includes Scotland, Wales and England. Citizens of the UK all have 'British' nationality as well as their individual nationality – Irish, Welsh, Scottish or English. Southern Ireland or Éire, is a separate country and is not part of the UK or Britain; however, the islands of Ireland and Britain are collectively known as the 'British Isles', although this does not confer political unity.
3 The real name has been changed and continental European nationality has been used to protect the research participant's identity, as requested by the interviewee. This interview was part of the study 'Healthcare professionals' experiences and challenges at the time of COVID-19'. The study received favourable ethical approval by Kingston University Ethics Committee (REC reference number LR1545).
4 This was in contrast to the EU response. The European Commission recommended a common EU approach towards contact-tracing apps (New European Parliament, 6 May 2020).
5 This was linked to a slightly different controversy that had excluded particular NHS migrant workers such as porters and cleaners from the government's 'bereavement scheme'. There was a similar dramatic reversal of this policy in mid-May.
6 https://www.bbc.co.uk/news/av/uk-politics-52761960/hassan-akkad-explains-the-video-which-caused-a-u-turn.

7   See, for instance, Gallagher, Paul. 2020. 'Syrian refugee behind viral NHS video to carry on fight for migrants' rights'. *inews.co.uk*, 21 May 2020. Accessed 2 August 2020. https://inews.co.uk/news/hassan-akkad-syrian-refugee-nhs-viral-video-boris-johnson-430090.
8   See, for instance, https://www.telegraph.co.uk/global-health/science-and-disease/burden-covid-19-falls-poorer-backgrounds-uk/.

References

Ahmed, Sara. 2007. 'A phenomenology of whiteness'. *Feminist Theory* 8(2): 149–68.
Aldama, Arturo J. 2003. *Violence and the Body: Race, gender and the state*. Bloomington, IN: Indiana University Press.
Appadurai, Arun. 1993. 'The heart of whiteness'. *Callaloo* 16(4): 796–807.
Aspinall, Peter, Bobbie Jacobson and Givanna Polato. 2003. 'Missing record: The case for recording ethnicity at birth and death registration'. London Health Observatory. Accessed 2 July 2020. https://www.kent.ac.uk/chss/docs/Births_Deaths_Reg1.pdf.
Balthazar, Ana Carolina. 2017. 'Made in Britain: Brexit, teacups, and the materiality of the nation'. *American Ethnologist* 44(2): 220–24.
BBC News. 2020 'Coronavirus: NHS doctor who pleaded for PPE dies'. 10 April 2020. Accessed 2 July 2020. https://www.bbc.co.uk/news/uk-england-london-52242516.
Berliner, David. 2012. 'Multiple nostalgias: The fabric of heritage in Luang Prabang (Lao PDR)'. *Journal of the Royal Anthropological institute* 18(4): 769–86.
Breilh, Jaime. 2013. 'La determinación social de la salud como herramienta de transformación hacia una nueva salud pública (salud colectiva)'. *La Revista Facultad Nacional de Salud Pública* 31(1): S13–27.
Briggs, Laura. 2015. 'Making race, making sex'. *International Feminist Journal of Politics* 17(1): 20–39.
British Medical Association (BMA). 2020. 'The ultimate price'. BMA. 13 May 2020. Accessed 2 July 2020. https://www.bma.org.uk/news-and-opinion/the-ultimate-price.
Barr, Caelainn, Niko Kommenda, Niamh McIntyre and Antonio Voce. 2020. 'Ethnic minorities dying of Covid-19 at higher rate, analysis shows'. *The Guardian*, 22 April 2020. Accessed 2 July 2020. https://www.theguardian.com/world/2020/apr/22/racial-inequality-in-britain-found-a-risk-factor-for-covid-19.
Chouhan, Karen and James Nazroo. 2020. 'Health inequalities'. In *Ethnicity, Race and Inequality in the UK: State of the nation*, edited by Bridget Byrne, Claire Alexander, Omar Khan, James Nazroo and William Shankley, pp. 73–92. London: Polity Press.
Cook, Tim, Emira Kursumovic and Simon Lennane. 2020. 'Exclusive: Deaths of NHS staff from Covid-19 analysed'. *HSJ*, 22 April 2020. Accessed 26 November 2020. https://www.hsj.co.uk/exclusive-deaths-of-nhs-staff-from-covid-19-analysed/7027471.article.
Davis, Dána-Ain. 2019. *Reproductive Injustice: Racism, pregnancy and premature birth*. New York: New York University Press.
Dean, Erin. 2020. 'COVID-19: Nurses say they are not getting adequate PPE'. *Nursing Standard*, 10 April 2020. Accessed 2 July 2020. https://rcni.com/nursing-standard/newsroom/analysis/covid-19-nurses-say-they-are-not-getting-adequate-ppe-159881.
East London Care and London Partnership. 2020. *Turning the Tide: The experiences of Black, Asian and Minority Ethnic NHS staff working in maternity services in England during and beyond the Covid-19 pandemic*. October 2020. Accessed 26 November 2020. https://www.eastlondonhcp.nhs.uk/downloads/ourplans/Maternity/Turning%20the%20Tide%20Maternity%20Report%20-%202020.pdf .
Echeverría, Bolivar. 2016. *Modernidad y blanquitud*. Mexico City: Era.
Farmer, Paul. 1999. *Infections and Inequalities: The modern plagues*. Berkeley, CA: University of California Press.
Fassin, Didier. 2007. *When Bodies Remember, Experiences and Politics of HIV in South Africa*. Berkeley, CA: University of California Press.
Fassin, Didier. 2013. 'A case for critical ethnography: Rethinking the early years of the AIDS epidemic in South Africa'. *Social Science & Medicine* 99: 119–26.
Fisher, Andrew B. and Matthew O'Hara. 2009. *Imperial Subjects: Race and identity in colonial Latin America*. Durham, NC: Duke University Press.

Fitzgerald, Des, Amy Hinterberger, John Narayan and Ros Williams. 2020. 'Brexit as heredity redux: Imperialism, biomedicine and the NHS in Britain'. *The Sociological Review* 68(6): 1161–78.

Franklin, Sarah. 2019. 'Nostalgic nationalism: How a discourse of sacrificial reproduction helped fuel Brexit Britain'. *Cultural Anthropology* 34(1): 41–52.

Ghilardi, Giampaolo, Laura Leondina Campanozzi, Massimo Ciccozzi, Giovanna Ricci and Vittoradolfo Tambone. 2020. 'The political nature of medicine'. *The Lancet* 395(10233): 1340–41.

Gideon, Jasmine. 2014. *Gender, Globalization, and Health in a Latin American Context*. New York: Palgrave Macmillan.

Gravlee, Lance. 2020. 'Racism, not genetics, explains why Black Americans are dying of COVID-19'. *Scientific American*, 7 June 2020. Accessed 7 June 2020. https://blogs.scientificamerican.com/voices/racism-not-genetics-explains-why-black-americans-are-dying-of-covid-19/.

Guthman, Julie. 2014. 'Doing justice to bodies? Reflections on food justice, race, and biology'. *Antipode* 46(5):1153–71.

Hartman, Saidiya. 2007. *Lose Your Mother: A journey along the Atlantic slave route*. New York: Farrar, Straus and Giroux.

Hill, Evan, Ainara Tiefenthäler, Christiaan Triebert, Drew Jordan, Haley Willis and Robin Stein. 2020. 'How Floyd George was killed in police custody'. *The New York Times*, 31 May 2020. Accessed 31 May 2020. https://www.nytimes.com/2020/05/31/us/george-floyd-investigation.html.

Hirsch, Afua. 2020. 'The racism that killed George Floyd was built in Britain'. *The Guardian*, 2 June. Accessed 3 June 2020. https://www.theguardian.com/commentisfree/2020/jun/03/racism-george-floyd-britain-america-uk-black-people.

Intensive Care National Audit and Research Centre. ICNARC report on COVID-19 in critical care 24 April 2020. Accessed 25 April 2020. https://www.icnarc.org/Our-Audit/Audits/Cmp/Reports.

Kanani, Nikki and Prerana Issar. 2020. 'A note for all BAME colleagues working in the NHS'. 1 May 2020. Accessed 2 July 2020. https://www.england.nhs.uk/blog/note-for-all-bame-colleagues-working-in-the-nhs/.

Kapilashrami, Anuj and Kamaldeep Bhui. 2020. 'Mental health and COVID-19: Is the virus racist?' *The British Journal of Psychiatry* 217(2): 405–7.

Kuzawa, Christopher W. and Elizabeth Sweet. 2009. 'Epigenetics and the embodiment of race: Developmental origins of US racial disparities in cardiovascular health'. *American Journal of Human Biology* 21(1):2–15.

Lock, Margaret. 2015. 'Comprehending the body in the era of the epigenome'. *Current Anthropology* 56(2): 151–77.

Lynteris, Christos and Branwyn Poleykett. 2018. 'The anthropology of epidemic control: Technologies and materialities'. *Medical Anthropology* 37(6): 433–41.

Mackintosh, Maureen, Parvati Raghuram and Leroi Henry. 2006. 'A perverse subsidy: African trained nurses and doctors in the NHS'. *Soundings* 34(34): 103–13.

Macleod, Roy and Milton Lewis. 1988. *Disease, Medicine and Empire: Perspectives on Western medicine and the experience of European expansion*. London: Routledge.

Marmot, Michael. 2005. 'Social determinants of health inequalities'. *The Lancet* 365(9564): 1099–104.

Marmot, Michael, Jessica Allen, Peter Goldblatt, Eleanor Herd and Joana Morrison. 2020. *Build Back Fairer: The COVID-19 Marmot Review*. London: UCL Institute of Health Equity and The Health Foundation.

Mignolo, Waiter. 2002. 'The geopolitics of knowledge and the colonial difference'. *The South Atlantic Quarterly* 101(1): 57–96.

Moore, Alison. 'NHS staff "can access covid-19 testing", government insists'. *HSJ*, 16 March 2020. Accessed 2 July 2020. https://www.hsj.co.uk/workforce/nhs-staff-can-access-covid-19-testing-government-insists/7027133.article.

Mueller, Benjamin and Jane Bradley. 2020. 'England's "world beating" system to track the virus is anything but'. *The New York Times*, 17 June 2020. Accessed 7 September 2020. https://www.nytimes.com/2020/06/17/world/europe/uk-contact-tracing-coronavirus.html.

Nazroo, James Y. 2003. 'The structuring of ethnic inequalities in health: economic position, racial discrimination, and racism'. *American Journal of Public Health* 93(2): 277–84.

News European Parliament. 2020. 'Covid-19 tracing apps: Ensuring privacy and data protection'. News European Parliament, 6 May 2020. Accessed 2 July 2020. https://www.europarl.europa.

eu/news/en/headlines/society/20200429STO78174/covid-19-tracing-apps-ensuring-privacy-and-data-protection/.

NHS, NHS Workforce Race Equality Standard. 2019 Data analysis report for NHS trusts. February 2020. Accessed 2 July 2020. https://www.england.nhs.uk/wp-content/uploads/2020/01/wres-2019-data-report.pdf.

Office of National Statistics. 2020. 'Deaths involving COVID-19, UK: Deaths occurring between 1 March and 30 April 2020'. 12 June 2020. Accessed 2 July 2020. https://www.ons.gov.uk/peoplepopulationandcommunity/birthsdeathsandmarriages/deaths/bulletins/deathsinvolvingcovid19uk/deathsoccurringbetween1marchand30april2020.

Pfeiffer, James and Mark Nichter. 2008. 'What can critical medical anthropology contribute to global health? A health systems perspective'. *Medical Anthropology Quarterly* 22(4): 410–15.

Platt, Lucinda and Ross Warwick. 2020. 'Are some ethnic groups more vulnerable to Covid-19 than others?' *Inequality the IFS Deaton Review*, 1 May 2020. Accessed 2 July 2020. https://www.ifs.org.uk/inequality/chapter/are-some-ethnic-groups-more-vulnerable-to-COVID-19-than-others/.

Porter, Toby. 2020. 'Tooting hospital's cleaning staff discussed walking out before pandemic over risks and poor hygiene'. londonnewsonline.co.uk, 15 May 2020. Accessed 7 September 2020. https://londonnewsonline.co.uk/tooting-hospitals-cleaning-staff-discussed-walking-out-before-pandemic-over-risks-and-poor-hygiene/.

Public Health England. 2020. 'Beyond the data, understanding the impact of COVID-19 on BAME groups'. Accessed 2 July 2020. https://assets.publishing.service.gov.uk/government/uploads/system/uploads/attachment_data/file/892376/COVID_stakeholder_engagement_synthesis_beyond_the_data.pdf.

Rawlinson, Kevin. 2020. 'Coronavirus PPE: All 400,000 gowns flown from Turkey for NHS fail UK standards'. *The Guardian*, 7 May 2020. Accessed 2 July 2020. https://www.theguardian.com/world/2020/may/07/all-400000-gowns-flown-from-turkey-for-nhs-fail-uk-standards.

Royal College of Nursing. 2020. 'NHS pay scales 2017–18'. Accessed 2 July 2020. https://www.rcn.org.uk/employment-and-pay/nhs-pay-scales-2017-18.

Sesia, Paola, Jennie Gamlin, Sahra Gibbon and Lina Berrio. 2020. 'Introduction'. In *Critical Medical Anthropology: Perspectives in and from Latin America*. London: University College London Press.

Shaw, Kelly, Anna Chilcott, Emily Hansen and Tania Winzenberg. 2006. 'The GP's response to pandemic influenza: A qualitative study'. *Family Practice* 23(3): 267–72.

Siddique, Haroon and Jamie Grierson. 2020. 'Historical racism may be behind England's higher BAME Covid-19 rate'. *The Guardian*, 16 June 2020. Accessed 2 July 2020. https://www.theguardian.com/world/2020/jun/16/historical-racism-may-be-behind-englands-higher-bame-covid-19-rate.

Siddique, Haroon and Sarah Marsh. 2020. 'Inquiry announced into disproportionate impact of coronavirus on BAME communities'. *The Guardian*, 16 April 2020. Accessed 20 July 2020. https://www.theguardian.com/world/2020/apr/16/inquiry-disproportionate-impact-coronavirus-bame.

Silverblatt, Irene. 2009. 'Foreword'. In *Imperial Subjects: Race and identity in colonial Latin America*, edited by Andrew B. Fisher and Matthew D. O'Hara, pp. ix–xii. Durham, NC: Duke University Press.

Simpkin, Victoria L. and Elias Mossialos. 2017. 'Brexit and the NHS: challenges, uncertainties and opportunities'. *Health Policy* 121(5): 447–80.

Simpson, Julian M., Aneez Esmail, Virinder S. Kalra and Stephanie J. Snow. 2010. 'Writing migrants back into NHS history: Addressing a "collective amnesia" and its policy implications'. *Journal of the Royal Society of Medicine* 103(10): 392–6.

Smith, Andrea. 2003. 'The sexual colonisation of native peoples'. *Hypatia* 18(2): 70–85.

Stuckler, David, Aaron Reeves, Rachel Loopstra, Marina Karanikolos and Martin McKee. 2017. Austerity and health: The impact in the UK and Europe. *European Journal of Public Health* 27(4): 18–21.

The Guardian. 2020. 'I'm an NHS doctor – and I've had enough of people clapping for me'. 21 May 2020. Accessed 2 July 2020. https://www.theguardian.com/society/2020/may/21/nhs-doctor-enough-people-clapping.

The Health Foundation. 2020. 'Black and minority ethnic workers make up a disproportionately large share of key worker sectors in London'. 7 May 2020. Accessed 2 July 2020. https://www.

health.org.uk/chart/black-and-minority-ethnic-workers-make-up-a-disproportionately-large-share-of-key-worker.

The Times of India. 2020. 'Indian-origin doctor leads Downing Street silent protest'. 29 May 2020. Accessed 2 July 2020. https://timesofindia.indiatimes.com/world/uk/indian-origin-doctor-leads-downing-street-silent-protest/articleshow/76089400.cms.

van Dorn, Aaron, Rebecca E. Cooney and Miriam L. Sabin. 2020. 'COVID-19 exacerbating inequalities in the US'. *The Lancet* 395(10232): 1243.

Williams, David, Jourdyn Lawrence and Brigitte Davis. 2019. 'Racism and health: Evidence and needed research. *Annual Review of Public Health* 40: 105–25.

Williamson, E., A.J. Walker, K. Bhaskaran, S. Bacon, C. Bates, C.E. Morton, H.J. Curtis, A. Mehrkar, D. Evans, P. Inglesby and J. Cockburn. 2020. OpenSAFELY: factors associated with COVID-19-related hospital death in the linked electronic health records of 17 million adult NHS patients. MedRxiv. Accessed 16 April 2021. https://www.medrxiv.org/content/10.1101/2020.05.06.20092999v1.full.

Wintour, Patrick and Daniel Boffey. 2020. 'UK government accused of cover-up over EU scheme to buy PPE'. *The Guardian*, 22 April 2020. Accessed 2 July 2020. https://www.theguardian.com/politics/2020/apr/22/uk-government-accused-of-cover-up-over-eu-scheme-to-buy-ppe.

Wolfe, Patrick. 1999. *Settler Colonialism and the Transformation of Anthropology*. London: Cassell.

Yates-Doerr, E. 2020. 'Reworking the social determinants of health: responding to material-semiotic indeterminacy in public health interventions'. *Medical Anthropology Quarterly* 34(3): 378–97.

7
The shroud stealers
Coronavirus and the viral vagility of prejudice
Aditya Bharadwaj

The emergence of SARS-CoV-2 and the COVID-19 pandemic galvanised global containment, and prophylactic action centred on the strategies of self-isolation and social distancing. These twin procedures of social exclusion quickly became the widely accepted intervention against a viral load currently evading scientific excogitation. This exclusionary approach, undergirding seemingly innocuous global public health measures, is infected with a series of discriminatory assumptions built into the socio-political architecture of democratic states around the globe.

The emergence of SARS-CoV-2 did more than expose the structurally violent and iniquitous stratifications irreversibly scarring lives across the globe. The pandemic sanitised and normalised an inherently violent mode of pandemic governance inaugurated as a benign prophylactic action that rapidly became parasitic on culturally entrenched and socially sanctioned stratifications, including most notably caste, gender, class, race and religion. These social stratifications became unwitting experimental sites for incubating and cultivating alleged herd immunity among those who were already socially isolated, politically excluded and economically marginalised. For example, in some parts of the world the twin prescription of self-isolation and social distancing rapidly exposed existing class (and caste) privilege (see Manderson and Levine 2020), effectively locking out millions for whom the luxury of maintaining and sustaining both distance and isolation turned into an unattainable suicidal feat, as I discuss below. This mode of pandemic governance did not just unleash a vulgar biopolitics of 'make live and let die' (Foucault 2003; Lemke 2011) but rather a form of crass neoliberal fix that allowed a category of subject-citizens to die for the greater good. This inhumane spectacle featuring the untimely demise of an already socially distant and economically isolated citizen was consistently reimagined as prevention, precaution and protection. The vision of the global governing elite – ranging from nation-states to international organisations orchestrating the prophylactic intervention – emerged as inherently blinkered. These governing elites either ignored or elected to remain ignorant of the viral vagility of prejudice already infesting and infecting lives of millions around the globe. This is a tragedy not so much because certain categories of people disproportionately died, such as the 'the footloose' labourers in India, the so-called BAME (Black, Asian and Minority Ethnic) in the United Kingdom, African Americans, 'illegal immigrants' and 'other' minorities in the United States, and vulnerable and frail older people with chronic health problems around the globe. But rather it is an unspeakable tragedy because, to borrow from Foucault, the government of pandemic could not see these subjugated citizens.[1] And when they did finally appear from the ground fog shrouding the stratified polity in which they existed – in most cases broken, isolated, starving or displaced – they were allowed to die for the greater privileged good. A certain vitiation of the biopolitical logic emerged. That is, the purported calculus behind the calculating gaze of the biopolitical state simply missed seeing the many millions assumed to be subjected to its disciplinary logics. For example, while the 'Black Lives Matter' and 'I Can't Breathe' anti-racism protests in the US exposed the state's ruinous complicity in scarring innumerable black lives, the state responded by merely averting its racist gaze. The state saw the protests as just another instance of wanton lawlessness, a predominant attribute it routinely assigns to a figment of its racist imagination: the ungovernable black citizen. This projection also allowed the state to recast the anti-racism movement as nothing more than a breach of its 'pandemic demarche' demanding self-isolation and social distancing from law-abiding citizens. However, the state hypocritically looked away as its 'support base' blatantly violated, often with brazen impunity, the same restrictions in the name of freedom and liberty.

The philosophical commentaries and critiques that followed the emergence of this global emergency were uniquely shaped by the ideological attachments of the commentators. Unmistakeably, as a point of departure, these musings took the lives, rights and liberties of those who could either collaborate with or militate against the disciplinary modality implicit in the proposed distancing and isolating interventions as the norm. Giorgio Agamben (2020) saw the response to be 'disproportionate' and the resultant state of exception as a normal governing paradigm. For Agamben, it was:

> almost as if with terrorism exhausted as a cause for exceptional measures, the invention of an epidemic offered the ideal pretext for scaling them up beyond any limitation. The other no less disturbing factor is the state of fear that in recent years has evidently spread among individual consciences and that translates into an authentic need for situations of collective panic for which the epidemic provides once again the ideal pretext. Therefore, in a perverse vicious circle, the limitations of freedom imposed by governments are accepted in the name of a desire for safety that was created by the same governments that are now intervening to satisfy it.

Povinelli (2016) has already shown that terrorism, exhausted or not, like SARS-CoV-2, is a virus in the late liberal governance modality. For Povinelli, the 'virus is an active antagonistic agent built out of the collective assemblage that is late liberal geontopower' (2016, 19). Geontopower is a 'set of discourse, affects, and tactics used in late liberalism to maintain or shape the coming relationship of the distinction between Life and Nonlife' (Povinelli 2016, 4). While the moving balance between life and non-life – with the figure of the virus as one of its key embodiments (the perennial 'zombie', neither dead nor alive) – somewhat disrupts Agamben's running battle with the biopolitical state, the limits to Povinelli's argument are perhaps reached in cultural contexts such as India. While outside the scope of this chapter, it will probably suffice to say that for millennia *Vedanta* philosophy has mulled over the life and non-life binary as nothing more than alternate states suffusing the Universe: *jad* (matter/unconscious/insentient) and *chaten* (alive/conscious/sentient).

Not to be exceeded in the emerging scene of philosophy gone 'viral', philosophy's self-styled agent provocateur Slavoj Žižek produced extended pamphlets, seeing in the coronavirus epidemic an opportunity to 'give a new boost of life to [reinvented] Communism' (2020). Esposito's blunt organic analogy painstakingly developed in *Immunitas: The Protection and Negation of Life*, equating the human body's immune system to (protective cover of) law, suddenly became timely and prophetic. Similitude between the unfolding pandemic and a search for immunisation against the menacing threat, SARS-CoV-2, looped back to the subliminal thesis of ingesting poison/danger to neutralise poison/danger or, as in the case of COVID-19, vaccine/part virus. Esposito's philosophical sermon was as if proclaiming: immunisation against the other by incorporating the other.

Learning to live with the other. Eliminating incompatibility between (immunitary) self and (communitary) other. In other words, 'to conceptualize the function of immune systems in a different way, making them into relational filters between inside and outside instead of exclusionary barriers … by disabling the apparatuses of negative immunization, and by enabling new spaces of the common' (Esposito in Bird and Short 2013, 6),

However, these philosophical commentaries and others attached to (rightly) critiquing the biopolitical state neglected the rampant re-emergence and re-enactment of brutal old prejudices. These prejudices weren't exactly state generated, but nevertheless they were efficiently mined by the biopolitical state as a governing resource. It was as if the SARS-CoV-2 breathed new life into old discriminations and bequeathed a certain viral vagility to indifference and prejudice. For instance, in the US the pandemic raged like an out-of-control forest fire: on 31 December 2020, in that country alone, nearly 20.5 million people had been reported infected and 355,000 had died from coronavirus. Fatalities were (and are still, at time of writing) disproportionately higher in communities and neighbourhoods with large African American populations (Zephyrin et al. 2020). Additionally, as joblessness and economic precarity deepens, taps are being turned off because of non-payment of bills 'even as the CDC calls for frequent hand washing' (Laxmi 2020). In the UK, a similar story played out as COVID-19 disproportionately impacted Black, Asian and Minority Ethnic people, the so-called BAME. Fatality among doctors and care staff was similarly reported to be higher among 'the BAME'. The virus of prejudice, like SARS-CoV-2, exploited underlying biological weaknesses and socio-political prejudices. The latter is rather well reflected and encapsulated by the use of this offensive acronym, BAME: in one deft move all diversity, complexity and experience was reduced to bureaucratised categories, sutured together as a biopolitical convenience sample. BAME became an alternative to Other. And as I will show later in this chapter, in India the Dalit and other vulnerable groups were singled out to face up to centuries' old persecution, albeit now enjoying a new lease of life in the garb of social distancing and isolation.[2] The word Dalit (dälit) means 'ground down', 'broken to pieces', 'crushed'. It seeks to 'convert a negative description into a confrontational identity and to become a particular sort of political subject' (Rao 2009, 1). Treated as untouchables for millennia, the postcolonial state in India recognised the historic injustice and established the group of Scheduled Castes (SC) within the newly established constitution. The Scheduled Castes are estimated to include around 170 million people. The practice of untouchability was formally banned as the constitution came into force on 26 January 1950.

Key remedial initiatives established constitutionally guaranteed policies of positive discrimination and affirmative action to better support the integration of the SC and ST (Scheduled Tribes, currently numbering 80 million people). However, the cultural force of prejudice continues to vitiate and subvert the constitutionally established principles of equality and non-discrimination. This is notwithstanding the fact that the Dalit community has emerged as a major political force in the Indian democracy (see Rao 2009; Ciotti 2010). It seems the pious utterances enshrined in the constitution continue to be an ineffective vaccine against the virus of culturally entrenched prejudice.

In this chapter, I do no more than grapple with the viral vagility of prejudice in the wake of the COVID-19 pandemic. In so doing, I meditate on the texture of structural violence, exploring how horrific forms of social exclusion and marginalisation exacerbated as the pandemic gained traction. In pointing out this intensification, I take a literary detour to gesture at the 'already there' normalised to euphemised forms of violence that were amplified as states enjoined the citizens to retreat into relative privileged isolation and distancing. Drawing on examples from India, I introduce the notion of 'shroud stealers' to reflect on the unfolding pandemic and to better apportion responsibility, including our own culpability as academic spectators and commentators.

Kafan Chor: 'the shroud stealer' and the pandemic of poverty

The influenza pandemic of 1918 birthed a curious figure in the city of Delhi: *kafan chor*, the shroud thief. Having just lost thousands of Indian soldiers in the First World War, the city was suddenly facing the terrifying spectre of yet more death. From the account provided by writer–poet and scholar Ahmed Ali (1910–94), we learn that 'filled with anger against the inhumanity of man, Nature wanted to demonstrate her own callousness and might' (Ali 1940, 169). Ali vividly captures the unfolding pandemic:

> Men carried dead bodies on their shoulders by the score. There was not a single hour of the day when a few dead bodies were not carried outside the city to be buried. Soon the graveyards became full, and it was difficult to find even three yards of ground to put a person in his final resting-place. In life they had had no peace, and even in death there seemed no hope of rest. A new cemetery was made outside the city where people buried relations by the score.

The Hindus were lucky that way. They just went to the bank of the sacred Jamuna, cremated the dead, and threw away the ashes and unburned bones in the water. Many were thrown away without a shroud or cremation (1940, 169).

At the peak of the pandemic, Ali describes a 'gruesome menace' emerging in Delhi in the form of shroud thieves. Stealing shrouds became a quick way of 'procuring bread' and 'earning a livelihood'. Ali's ghoulish description is written with the anguished authority of an eyewitness. It jolts the reader into sitting up and becoming a spectator – aware but unable to act – given the slow unravelling of the human condition:

> Many went to the graveyards at dead of night with spades and long iron hooks. It was not difficult to dig open the new graves, especially because they had been dug and filled up in a hurry. With the help of their iron hooks they pulled out the winding-sheets and got good money for them. Hyenas and jackals thus found their task made easier for them. They could enter the newly opened graves and fill their bellies to the full (Ali 1940, 170).

According to Ali, the 'grave-diggers' amassed a fortune during the pandemic. The scavenging shroud thieves, for the first time in a long while, did not do too badly either. The cloth merchants, *banias*, raised the price of 'line-cloth' used for 'winding sheets', *kafan*. Those who could not afford a proper *kafan* settled for a cheaper thinner shroud that would barely conceal the dead body, and so 'the person would starve, but spend a little more to give his dear one a decent shroud' (Ali 1940, 171). Similarly, the reader learns that the *ghassals*, whose job it was to wash the dead for their final journey, did 'roaring business' as they 'laved the bodies with water' and pocketed gold and silver rings left on the corpses (Ali 1940, 171).

Ali evokes for the reader a macabre economy that sprang up in the height of the pandemic. His account is not a first-person narrative of unfolding events, nor is it in any straightforward sense rooted in historical evidence. But Ali's pathos laden commentary is a conjuring of collective grief, disbelief transmogrified into memory. It is a traumatic archive of source material which summons pensive reflections on the nature of precarity haunting the human condition. A disparate cast of characters in Ali's account see opportunity in the pandemic, and in their own unique way – digging graves or robbing them, selling shroud or offering *ghassal* – become grotesque iterations of a *kafan chor*, the shroud stealer.

The notion of stealing better typifies the suggested debasement in Ali's account as opposed to mere thievery (thief is the literal English translation for *chor*). The very act of stealing the shroud and its many surrogate enactments in the figure of the *banias* and the *ghassals*, for example, are tantamount to stealing human dignity and losing it altogether. Whether for profit or livelihood, the shroud stealers offer a haunting commentary on human depredation. This theme was elevated in the heart wrenching literary evocations of one of the pioneering figures of modern Hindi and Urdu literature, Munshi Premchand (1880–1936). Premchand wrote over a dozen novels and over 300 short stories describing in vivid detail the tribulations of the middle classes and the crippling poverty of the socially excluded. In his 1936 story *Kafan*, the shroud, Premchand offers a masterful meditation on dehumanising poverty in a stratified social landscape. The story's main protagonists, abjectly poor father (Ghisu) and son (Madho), must face an intractable crisis as Madho's labouring wife, Budhiya, dies in childbirth. The penniless duo neither have the money to buy a shroud nor the means to give the dead woman a decent funeral. While the father and son manage to beg and cobble together enough from the village landlord, merchants and moneylender, they end up spending the money on liquor and a minor feast, even as Budhiya's body languishes in the hut unattended and unshrouded. The decline and descent into this seemingly ugly self-indulgence is gradual:

> 'We need only the shroud now.'
> 'Let's get a cheap one.'
> 'Of course. It will be night when the corpse is carried to the pyre, no one will look at the shroud.'
> 'What an unjust custom! She, who didn't have even tattered rags to cover her body while she was alive, must now have a new shroud.'
> 'And it burns to ashes with the corpse.'
> 'So it does. Now if we had these five rupees earlier, we could've bought her some medicines.' (Premchand 2017, 662)

Premchand suggests that the father and son duo were able to guess the other's weakening resolve. They prolonged their search for the perfect shroud into the evening, only to find themselves at the door of the wine house. It is here their resolve finally crumbles, and with it, the veneer of worldly decorum and appropriacy, the preserve of the well-fed rich.

This surface reading codes a paradigmatic commentary that Premchand rustles into the storyline, straddling multiple narrative devices ranging from darkly comical to manifestly ironic and cathartic. This 'readerly' text, to borrow from Roland Barthes (1974), takes one to the door of a certain 'writerly' complexity. The characters are damned and framed as if embodying prevailing societal judgements and indifference. The potential judgement implicit in a privileged reading is coded into carefully worked up character portraits. Time and again, the author loops the surface reading back to the reader, demanding a deeper incredulous response. Eventually, the reader begins to detect the literary sleight of hand, astutely distilling culturally framed assumptions into the textured but wilfully stereotyped characters. Premchand's characters, in other words, reveal the reader's latent complicity (and by extension society's perfidious culpability) in maintaining structurally violent stratifications that the characters must perennially endure. Premchand hides the cultural context in the narrative fold to expose multiple seething realities haunting the duo. Manifestly, the reader encounters two inherently unsavoury characters: indolent, amoral, insensitive, self-centred, callous, wretched. The reader also learns that the father and son belong to the ostracised Dalit community: in 1936, a Dalit would have been routinely brutalised as an untouchable. However, an array of deeper meanings continually surface to tangle the syntagmatic thread. For example, the protagonists' financial precarity emerges as a feature of their marginal status but equally an element of their everyday resistance practices (torpid laziness) that allowed them to eke out a living under the exploitative and stratified feudal gaze. The fact that the duo end up spending the money for the shroud on feasting and drinking liquor doubles up as an allegory for the caste-based violence scarring their lives. That is, culturally sanctioned upper caste maleficence deprives them both of dignity and of the means to a dignified life. This is also a moment of escape from the guilt and unexpressed trauma of sitting helplessly and watching Budhiya come to a painful end. The story reveals how grovelling, beseeching and snivelling is expediently deployed by Ghisu to extract money from an unjust order that owed him much more than money for a mere shroud. The disgust and condescension with which the landlord obliges, throwing a paltry sum of money at Ghisu, characterises the stratified order in which he has evolved to deploy strategic subservience as a survival strategy. Ghisu knows when to yield and when to wield 'the weapons of the weak' (cf. Scott 1985). At one point in the story, Ghisu sneers at his guilt-ravaged son who is suddenly confronted with the horror of squandering money for the shroud on food and drink: 'The same people who gave us the money [will give the shroud]. They won't hand over the money to us anymore. If they do, we'll have another feast here.

And they'll pay for the shroud again' (Premchand 2017, 664). By about the end of the story, repeatedly punctuated by innovative theodicies justifying their actions, father and son dance and collapse in the throes of inebriate stupor. To the bitter end, Ghisu remains confident of his ability to extract at least a shroud from the unjust society that barely gave him enough to clothe his own existence of bare life.

Premchand paints the unrelenting despoliation of the human condition. These are brought about by practices of ritualised humiliation, built into the architecture of a hierarchically segregated social structure incubating extreme forms of precarity. The feasting and drunken reverie becomes an eerie cipher for near schizophrenic lamenting, a death dance of the living dead, and an outward projection of the internalised societal suggestion that both father and son are at best subhuman. Both Ghisu and his son ventriloquise a culturally sanctioned debasement, electing to become amplified caricatures of an inhumane society personified by the upper caste landlord and moneylender. The need to beg for a shroud by gaming the very people who game into existence the violent stratified order in which one dies, is perhaps the core message in the story. Premchand corrugates into the story the multiple readings of the text; in so doing, he forces the reader to confront the shroud-stealing social order that Ghisu and his son endure on a daily basis.

Stratified proxemics: vitiated life and structural violence

> A baby plays with a shroud covering its dead mother at a station in Bihar, in one of the most tragic visuals to emerge from the daily reports of migrants stranded by the coronavirus lockdown. In a clip widely shared on social media, the toddler tugs at the cloth placed over his mother's body. The cloth comes off but his mother doesn't move; she had died moments before. According to her family, she died of extreme heat, hunger and dehydration (Kumar and Ghosh 2020).[3]

In March 2020, hundreds upon thousands of migrant workers and their families were left stranded as the Indian government ordered a countrywide lockdown in response to the COVID-19 pandemic. The problem was exacerbated by the timeline of the decision: 1.3 billion citizens were given notice of a mere four hours to retreat into self-isolation and to ensure social distance. The lockdown rapidly turned into an extensional threat for India's poor who quickly found themselves out of work and with no safe place to harbour in the city (more on this below; see also Garimella and colleagues, Chapter 11). It seemed that the biopolitical state had no plan. It took, as the norm, the lives and circumstances of those who could isolate and participate in tokenistic display of solidarity with the state. Relatively privileged citizens were summoned to lockdown and called upon to join the state from the comfort of their homes to celebrate the impending end of the pandemic. Mirroring similar public gestures in other settings, the state invited citizens to partake in nightly candle vigils and to beat household utensils, perhaps imagined as a ritual to ward off the evil virus, and to show (middle class) solidarity from the comfort of their balconies, gardens and terraces.[4]

Meanwhile, panic ensued in less salubrious neighbourhoods across the country as people began making contingency arrangements and desperately attempting to stockpile. The suddenness of the lockdown particularly hurt millions of 'footloose' (Breman 1996) daily-wage labourers who, overnight, were without work and money. With infinite foresight, reasoning and desperation, workers decided to retreat to the relative safety of their homes, often thousands of kilometres from megalopolises like Mumbai and Delhi where the majority worked as daily wage labourers (EPW 2020). The ILO noted that 'the lockdown measures in India, which are at the high end of the University of Oxford's COVID-19 Government Response Stringency Index, have impacted these workers significantly, forcing many of them to return to rural areas' (ILO 2020, 6). With no means of other transportation available, workers and their families began converging to walk home along national highways. Thousands continued the trek on foot; a lucky few persuaded interstate haulers to ferry them in the back of their trucks. Hunger, dehydration, heat stroke, exhaustion and vehicle accidents claimed many lives. An exact account of these fatalities, collateral damage of COVID-19, is not yet available.[5] Further, India's surprisingly low death rate linked to COVID-19, with a case fatality rate of 1.8 per cent, is being questioned (Lancet 2020a, b); India lacks the capacity to count and certify deaths due to COVID-19 using the RT-PCR test (Nature 2020). This is hardly surprising given the lopsided nature of India's vast healthcare system – from state-of-the-art hubs for medical tourists to decrepit rural healthcare centres of questionable quality and few resources. Healthcare in India is incorporated under 'the 'State' list of legislation and jurisdiction, different from the 'Union' and 'Concurrent' lists, thus enabling various state governments to assume control and responsibility of health provision for their populations' (Bharadwaj 2016, 110).[6] The Indian healthcare landscape can at best be defined as 'mixed', a vestige of its post-colonial mixed economy developmental planning. In the emerging neoliberal India of the twenty-first century, however, this mixed approach championing public primary health and private curative healthcare provision has further consolidated as a two-tier system skewed in favour of private healthcare delivery. It is this mixed-up model that the state's pandemic response scrambled into action. The true extent of the pandemic and how it impacted the Dalit and other vulnerable groups in India will probably never emerge. This pessimism is only exacerbated by the prevailing state of chronic underinvestment and concomitant limited capacity to test and trace, and to establish a credible and coordinated, nationwide, pandemic surveillance system.

When the state did finally rouse from its candle-lit vigil torpor, it responded to the unfolding tragedy by commandeering special trains and buses to transport people home. However, bureaucratic hurdles and delays, general confusion and lack of information, coupled with rumour and panic, made the task even more arduous. Left wageless and eventually homeless, daily-wage labourers and itinerant workers were rapidly recapitulated and euphemised – both in government and media discourse – as 'migrants' in their own country.[7] The searing heat and unending wait in queues, the overcrowded trains, running often without water or adequate sanitation, added to the fatalities – as in the case of a woman whose partially shrouded anonymity, thanks to gawking smartphone-wielding bystanders, momentarily went 'viral' on social media (see Narasimhan, Chittem and Purang, Chapter 19). The footage was seized by local politicians to expediently criticise the sitting administration in an election year (DNA 2020; Kumar and Ghosh 2020).

As Breman (1996) showed more than two decades ago, the footloose proletariat in India is largely detached from its place of origin, and seldom grows roots in the workplaces to which it temporarily finds employment (also see Sainath 1996). The bulk of such labour is drawn from the Dalit community and other oppressed groups low down on the caste pecking order. Emerging data indicate the deepening economic impact of the entwining of caste and the COVID-19 pandemic. Drawing on nationally representative panel data for 21,799 individuals between May 2018 and April 2020, Deshpande and Ramachandran (2020) show that far from being a 'great leveler', the COVID-19 pandemic disproportionately impacted lowest-ranked castes due to 'lower levels of human capital and over-representation in vulnerable jobs'. The study found that 'the rate of job loss was three times higher for the SCs (Scheduled Castes) and job loss for individuals involved in daily wage jobs, relative to December 2019, was more than nine times higher' (Deshpande and Ramachandran

2020, 1, 10). While the pandemic and resulting lockdown exacerbated pre-existing inequalities, the resulting economic precarity will only increase as the pandemic wears on. This is particularly true in the light of emerging analysis from the World Bank (2020). The World Bank assessment notes that while India has made progress in reducing absolute poverty, declining from 21.6 per cent in 2011 to 13.4 per cent in 2015, thus lifting more than 90 million people out of extreme poverty, India's GDP contracted (year-on-year in quarter 1, financial year 2021) by an astonishing 23.9 per cent because of pre-existing domestic issues and the pandemic-linked national lockdown. The sudden collapse has hit poor people particularly hard. To date, the ILO predicted that 90 per cent of about 400 million workers in the informal economy faced serious risk of falling deeper into poverty during the pandemic (ILO 2020, 6).

The pandemic accentuated the scale of social exclusion, marginalisation and discrimination experienced by the Dalit. For instance, the National Campaign for Dalit Human Rights (NCDHR) in India has actively monitored the impact of the pandemic and the subsequent lockdown on the Dalit, Adivasi (tribal) and other marginalised communities. A press statement released by the National Dalit Movement for Justice (NDMJ-NCDHR) and data collected by NDMJ show how the pandemic has worsened the situation (International Dalit Solidarity Network 2020). One can glean from these emerging data sources a clear rise in instances of caste-based untouchability, physical and sexual assaults, police brutality, reported and unreported murders, inadequate to no PPE for Dalit sanitation workers, and rising levels of hunger and deaths during the lockdown period (International Dalit Solidarity Network 2020). The NCDHR pointed out that the deployment of the term 'social distancing' as a safety measure simply bled into established upper caste prejudice and the practice of 'untouchability' in both subtle and egregious ways. Dalit activist Ramesh Nathan explained:

> But what happened was that the Hindu fundamentalist organisations gradually started using this to justify *Manusmriti* (ancient legal Hindu text dated 100 CE). They did a lot of propaganda in the social media and other media, saying 'this is what we have been saying' and 'we should not let people in our homes, we should not touch other people, we should not shake hands'. They started to reinforce the caste system. For us, the term social distancing has already prevailed in our society due to the caste system. The Dalits have been presented as unseen-able, unapproachable and untouchable. These are the major elements of the caste system. Social distancing

reinforced these ideas. We are hurt that the dominant caste system is taking advantage of the situation to once again push for casteist ideas (*sic*) (TwoCircles.net 2020).

It has become common at mere mention, even in liberal western media, to qualify – often in parentheses – the word Dalit as 'former untouchables'. This is legally accurate. The Untouchability (Offenses) Act, 1955, was amended and renamed in 1976 the Protection of Civil Rights Act, 1955 (PCR Act), in addition to the Scheduled Castes and Scheduled Tribes (Prevention of Atrocities) Act, 1989 (POA Act) (see Thorat 2009). But the notion of 'former untouchable', like the homogenising BAME acronym in the British media and policy discourse, is both offensive and inadequate. As the lived experience of segregation of over 200 million Dalit demonstrates, the practice of 'untouchability' remains a festering legacy of caste-based social distancing. Thus a well-established prejudice further validated 'distancing' while singling out the Dalit body as the primary source of (COVID-19) contagion.

The spatial separation of individuals and classes in India has a long history, marking, maintaining and restricting commensality (Ghurye 1961). The ideologically policed and scripturally sanctioned separation of humans is hierarchically arranged and horizontally divided so as to separate ideals of purity from sources of pollution. This is not just a simplistic opposition of the pure and impure (Dumont 1970; also see Dirks 2001; Jodhka 2018); it is also a feature of a long cultural process of reimagining the impure as perennial contagion stalking and staking the pure. The impure in this respect does not emerge as a site for pollution per se but, more pertinently, as the source of defilement. In classical Brahminical puritanism, defilement assumed a certain mobile and projectile velocity and ferocity. It encompassed an array of bodily organs, discharge and matter, and corporeal contact; even the shadow of impure subjects were menacing sources of contamination and defilement (also see Fuller 2004). The solution against such a spectral menace was reconceived under the modernising impulse of colonial rule (Dirks 2001). As a form of social distancing, literal and metaphoric, this reconceiving disallowed the sources of imagined pollution and abject defilement to infect the pristine sociality fenced off for the untouched pure. The resultant violence – symbolic and graphic, between the untouched and the untouchable – stood for a purity that could not be touched by the untouchable 'super spreaders' of contagious pollution. The dehumanisation that grew out of culturally sanctioned 'concepts of hygiene, purity and contamination' (cf. Savage 2007) became key to both maintaining distance and enforcing isolation between stratified categories of humans. In this respect, the separation of castes was a foundational source of violence between the untouched and the untouchable. The tropes of purity and pollution emerged as a legitimising justification to sustain and contain a violent mode of social control. This structurally violent system of stratification, euphemised as the caste system, institutionalised inequality so as to contain and maintain social distance between humans.

There is a well-documented history of prejudicial barriers and caste-based dogmas in moments of rupture like plagues and pandemics (see Kidambi 2004; Ramanna 2012). For instance, in 1896 the Hindu Plague Hospital in Pune was managed by the priestly caste, Brahmins, and as British colonial officer Charles Rand reported, it was only open to Brahmins and other upper castes (Chamadia 2020). In its inaugural year alone, Brahmins formed 62.2 per cent of the total number of patients (Chamadia 2020), although they were likely around 7 per cent of the population (Plowden 1883, 227). Similarly, Kidambi (2004) described how the draconian measures employed by the colonial administration to control the bubonic plague of the 1890s repeatedly ran into caste-based objections, especially when measures involved coming into contact with lower castes or accepting food cooked by a subordinate caste. The upper caste preoccupation with the inherent contagious impurity of lower castes ironically mirrored not only the iniquitous colonial hierarchy but also its unshakeable belief in 'sanitary disorder' predicated on an 'orthodox contagionist doctrine' (Kidambi 2004, 51).

Dr B.R. Ambedkar, the father of the Indian constitution, a Dalit, scholar and advocate for Dalit rights, powerfully dissected the rabid anatomy of caste and caste prejudice in a paper presented at an anthropology seminar at Columbia University in 1916. Ambedkar located the viral vagility of prejudice in the 'fissiparous character of caste, as a consequence of the virtue of self-duplication that is inherent in it' (Pritchett 1979, 21). In 1948 he further developed the fissiparous character of caste structuring untouchability, explaining how and why 'the Hindu will not live in the quarters of the untouchables and will not allow the untouchables to live inside Hindu quarters' (Ambedkar 1948, 22). For Ambedkar, the caste system cordoned off territory to create permanent spaces of segregation, 'a *cordon sanitaire* putting the impure people inside a barbed wire, into a sort of a cage' (1948, 22). The untouchable ghetto for Ambedkar was an unending and inherently violent form of social distance.

SARS-CoV-2 offers a unique opportunity for reflection, and an opportunity to revisit Ambedkar's life's work. The virus of caste and the *cordon sanitaire* imposed by the caste system reproduce the viral vagility of SARS-CoV-2 in the here and now. And as some of us spectate and protest with anguished horror in privileged quarantine, we must remain attentive to our own culpability.

Addendum

We are all shroud stealers now. As we begin to imagine life beyond the pandemic, some of us will be forced to reimagine the metaphor of *kafan* and *kafan chor* afresh. The shroud, *kafan*, and the thief, *chor*, are ultimate allegories: the former representing peeling away the frayed shards of human dignity and the latter typifying profit-making from structurally violent contexts overseeing unshrouded demise of vulnerable others. This is not mere production of 'bare life' under a 'state of exception' (Agamben 1998), for the excluded, the marginal and the poor are often expediently included in the project of state formation (see Gupta 2012). The notion of *kafan* and *chor* reveals the amorphous indeterminacy of structural violence. As Gupta rightly reminds us, structural violence 'is a crime without a perpetrator', that is, it is hard to identify the perpetrator (2012, 21). Akhil Gupta argues that 'one must keep in mind that certain classes of people have a stake in perpetuating a social order in which such extreme suffering is not only tolerated but also taken as normal' (2012, 21). He further contends that those who disproportionately benefit from the status quo are complicit in the violence directed against the poor. However, he singles out the agents of such violence 'in a country like India', as including not only the (ruling and other) elites, but also the burgeoning middle class. Vocalising this partial truth in different guises is the predominant approach employed by the purveyors of liberal critique, so as to diagnose and locate the mêlées elsewhere. The globally distributed classes of people who circuitously benefit from insidious structural violence (myself and Gupta included) emerge as conscious-stricken diagnosticians and commentators. This faceless crowd of innocent bystanders grows on the margins of a carefully crafted problem space that includes the biopolitical state, its crony elites and the vast swathe of indifferent middle class. The diagnosis remains partial, inherently incomplete and vulnerable to degenerating into sanctimonious politics of outrage and condemnation. Thus we, the faceless liberal crowd, are *kafan chor* in two significant ways. First, we wittingly or unwittingly obfuscate our involvement in the violence against so-called marginalised people: Dalit, 'BAME', Black, Roma, or 'similar others' (cf. other discussions on race, ethnicity and inequality in this volume). In so doing we further feed biopolitical turpitude, forcing inhumane options (disguised as choice) on those who seldom experience choice in choice-obsessed neoliberal formations. Second, we set up home on the margins of structurally violent spaces, sometimes literally but mostly metaphorically, so as to live off the life, labour and death of our entrapped neighbours. Through our vote or support for the biopolitical state or via our schizophrenic relationship to neoliberal citizenship, we remain complicit.

In this sense, Premchand's heart-wrenching literary virtuosity forces a certain ethical recognition. Stratified poverty and social exclusion dehumanises the very humans it ensnares. More importantly, Premchand successfully jolts a reflexive awareness – of the reader's own moral and ethical poverty – into existence. The well-ingrained impulse within us to critique the biopolitical calculus of the modern state aside, one hopes the pandemic will also unleash a moment of critical self-appraisal of our self-centred solipsism. After all, the biopolitical state works for us, and its egregious overreach is almost always justified, sanitised in our name. This is a certain post-pandemic condition in the making: shroud stealers (like me and you) mulling innovative theodicies to better understand how and why the pursuit of an untrammelled life made us complicit in foisting an undignified end on a category of people who, as in life, died without a shard of shroud to their name.

The 'government of pandemic' working to protect both fragility and vulnerability endemic to privilege operates by tapping into vagile prejudices of our times. Perhaps we needed a global pandemic so as to wake up to the subcutaneous biopolitical brutality lurking under the thick skin of the modern state – to reiterate, empowered by us to speak and act in our name. This also means that the logic of *make live and let die* needed to appear that much more clearly and show how an exceptional state of exception further extended and distended state power to allow a certain category of people to perish (as opposed to merely die). But more crucially, the pandemic revealed unsavoury truths about us, a faceless crowd of shroud stealers, content with merely critiquing the biopolitical excesses of the governing elite. And, we are able to do so safe in the knowledge that our ends will be shrouded in a modicum of dignity, even as our picket fenced life will struggle to obfuscate the ugly, poverty-stricken and violent existence of our irreversibly scarred and socially distant neighbours.

Notes

1. According to Foucault, government 'must be allowed the very broad meaning it had in the sixteenth century. "Government" did not refer only to political structures or to the management of states; rather, it designated the way in which the conduct of individuals or of groups might be directed – the government of children, of souls, of communities, of the sick' (2002, 326).
2. At a cursory glance, class in contemporary neoliberal India may appear to be overtaking caste as the primary source of social stratification. In this respect the upper caste poor may now be 'outcaste', to be avoided for fear of contracting COVID-19. However, caste privilege continues to dominate; it allows an upper caste person, even in an economically marginal state, to benefit from caste-ordained prejudices and suffer none of the culturally sanctioned outcomes a Dalit routinely endures (see further below; see also Ciotti 2010). A good comparison is between white working-class poor and African American poor in the US. An outcome rooted in economic precariousness may be unfavourable for both, but the actual consequence is almost always worse if the protagonist is Black. There is little evidence that class privilege fails to guarantee a good health outcome because racist prejudices are built into the biomedical view of the Black body (Davis 2019; see also Maybank et al. 2020).
3. At the time of going to press the horrifying second wave is unfolding in India. The appalling mismanagement and cavalier overconfidence of the state resulted in severe vaccine and oxygen shortages. The daily infection and mortality rates are simply incalculable due to sporadic recordkeeping. As funeral pyres burn day and night and the poor who cannot afford cremations abandon their dead in rivers or bury the dead in river sandbanks, the state's complicitous silence has become deafening. To add to the horror stories about a gang stealing shrouds from crematoriums to sell on the market began circulating in local media (Times of India 2021).
4. It is highly likely that this 'pandemic ritual' was inspired by the impromptu balcony concerts and community singing in Italy, but in India it was an invitation from the sovereign rather than a spontaneous show of solidarity, reducing the ritualised display to mere political theatre.
5. Even when information is available, reports suggest rampant 'undercounting' of COVID-19 linked fatalities (Pulla 2020).
6. According to Balarajan and colleagues, 'India's total expenditure on health was estimated at 4.13% of the Gross Domestic Product (GDP) in 2008–09, with public expenditure on health being 1.10% of the share of GDP. Private expenditures on health have remained high over the last decade, with India having one of the highest proportions of household out-of-pocket expenditures on health in the world, estimated at 71.1% in 2008–09' (2011, 4).
7. In India, mass media, particularly new media, is in a state of crisis. A large section of news media is criticised as having thrown its weight behind the state. Euphemistically referred to as the *godi* media, literally 'lap' or cradling something or someone in one's lap. A vast section of regional and national media is being dismissed by critics in India as compromised or in the 'lap' of the state. These *godi* media outlets routinely peddle fake news, often bordering on shrill jingoism and bigotry. However, a section of independent news media channels and newspapers have asserted journalistic freedom and resisted the '*godi*' news outlets'. A growing number of people are also turning to these sources for more accurate information and editorial assessments.

References

Agamben, Giorgio. 1998. *Homo Sacer: Sovereign power and bare life*. Stanford, CA: Stanford University Press.

Agamben, Giorgio. 2020. 'L'invenzione di un'epidemia'. *Quodlibet*, 26 February 2020. Accessed 22 December 2020. https://www.quodlibet.it/giorgio-agamben-l-invenzione-di-un-epidemia

Ali, Ahmed. 1940. *Twilight in Delhi*. 1994 ed. Delhi, India: New Directions Books.

Ambedkar, B.R. 1948. *The Untouchables: Who were they and why they became untouchables?* New Delhi, India: Amrit Book Co.

Balarajan, Y., S. Selvaraj and S.V. Subramanian. 2011. 'Health care and equity in India'. *Lancet* (London, England) 377(9764): 505–15. https://doi.org/10.1016/S0140-6736(10)61894-6.

Barthes, Roland. 1974. *S/Z*. (Translated by R. Miller). New York: Hill & Wang.
Bharadwaj, Aditya. 2016. *Conceptions: Infertility and procreative technologies in India*. Oxford, UK: Berghahn Books.
Bird, Greg and Jonathan Short. 2013. 'Community, immunity and the proper: An introduction to the political theory of Roberto Esposito'. *Angelaki* 18(3): 1–12.
Breman, Jan. 1996. *Footloose Labour: Working in India's informal economy*. Cambridge, UK: Cambridge University Press.
Chamadia, Anil. 2020. 'Plague and COVID-19: An insight into the role of caste and religion during pandemics in India'. *National Herald*, 7 September 2020. Accessed 20 December 2020. https://www.nationalheraldindia.com/opinion/plague-and-covid-19-an-insight-into-the-role-of-caste-and-religion-during-pandemics-in-india.
Ciotti, Manuela. 2010. *Retro-modern India: Forging the low-caste self*. London: Routledge.
Davis, Dána-Ain. 2019. *Reproductive injustice: Racism, pregnancy, and premature birth*. New York: New York University Press.
Deshpande, Ashwini and Rajesh Ramachandran. 2020. *Is Covid-19 'The Great Leveler'? The critical role of social identity in lockdown-induced job losses*. GLO Discussion Paper, No. 622. Essen, Germany: Global Labor Organization (GLO).
Dirks, Nicholas B. 2001. *Castes of Mind: Colonialism and the making of modern India*. Princeton, NJ: Princeton University Press.
DNA. 2020. 'Toddler tries to wake up dead mother at Bihar's Muzaffarpur railway station, video goes viral'. *DNA*. 28 May 2020. Accessed 26 December 2020. https://www.dnaindia.com/lifestyle/report-toddler-tries-to-wake-up-dead-mother-at-bihar-s-muzaffarpur-railway-station-video-goes-viral-2826180.
Dumont, Louis. 1970. *Homo Hierarchicus*. Chicago, IL: University of Chicago Press.
EPW. 2020. 'Plight of the stranded workers: India's urban economies depend on migrant labour who should not be treated like "problems" during a lockdown'. *Economic & Political Weekly (EPW)* lV(16): 8.
Foucault, Michel. 2002. *Michel Foucault, Power: Essential works of Foucault 1954–1984, Vol. 3*, translated by Robert Hurley, edited by James D. Faubion. London: Penguin.
Foucault, Michel. 2003. *Society Must Be Defended: Lectures at the College De France 1975–1976*, translated by David Macey, edited by Mauro Bertani and Alessandro Fontana. New York: Picador.
Fuller, Chris. 2004. *Camphor Flame: Popular Hinduism and society in India*. Princeton, NJ: Princeton University Press.
Ghurye, Govind Sadashiv. 1961. *Caste, Class, and Occupation*. Bombay, India: Popular Book Depot.
Gupta, Akhil. 2012. *Red Tape: Bureaucracy, structural violence, and poverty in India*. Durham, NC and London: Duke University Press.
ILO. 2020. *ILO Monitor: COVID-19 and the world of work*, 2nd ed., updated estimates and analysis. Accessed 29 December 2020. https://www.ilo.org/wcmsp5/groups/public/---dgreports/---dcomm/documents/briefingnote/wcms_740877.pdf.
International Dalit Solidarity Network. 2020. 'Surge in atrocities against Dalits and Adivasis under COVID-19 lockdown in India reported'. 15 June 2020. Accessed 22 December 2020. https://idsn.org/surge-in-atrocities-against-dalits-and-adivasis-under-covid-19-lockdown-in-india-reported/.
Jodhka, Surinder, S. 2018. *Caste in Contemporary India*. London: Routledge.
Kidambi, Prashant. 2004. '"An infection of locality": Plague, pythogenesis and the poor in Bombay, c. 1896–1905'. *Urban History* 31(2): 249–67.
Kumar, Manish and Deepshikha Ghosh. 2020. 'Baby tries to wake dead mother at Bihar Station in endless migrant crisis'. *NDTV*. 27 May 2020. Accessed 22 December 2020. https://www.ndtv.com/india-news/coronavirus-a-baby-and-its-dead-mother-at-bihar-station-in-continuing-migrant-tragedy-2235852.
Lancet. 2020a. 'Is India missing COVID-19 deaths?' *Lancet* 396(10252): 657. Accessed 26 December 2020. https://www.thelancet.com/journals/lancet/article/PIIS0140-6736(20)31857-2/fulltext.
Lancet. 2020b. 'COVID-19 in India: The dangers of false optimism'. *Lancet* 396(10255): 867. Accessed 26 December 2020. https://www.thelancet.com/journals/lancet/article/PIIS0140-6736(20)32001-8/fulltext.
Laxmi, Nina. 2020. '"It feels like nobody cares": The Americans living without running water amid Covid-19'. *The Guardian*, 1 May 2020. Accessed 22 December 2020. https://www.theguardian.com/environment/2020/may/01/water-shutoffs-us-coronavirus-utilities-economy.

Lemke, Thomas. 2011. *Biopolitics: An advanced introduction. Biopolitics, medicine, technoscience, and health in the 21st century*. New York: New York University Press.

Manderson, Lenore and Susan Levine. 2020. 'COVID-19, risk, fear, and fallout'. *Medical Anthropology* 39(5): 367–70.

Maybank, Aletha, Camara Phyllis Jones, Uché Blackstock and Joia Crear Perry. 2020. 'Say her name: Dr Susan Moore'. *The Washington Post*, 26 December 2020. Accessed 27 December 2020. https://www.washingtonpost.com/opinions/2020/12/26/say-her-name-dr-susan-moore/.

Nature. 2020. '"The epidemic is growing very rapidly": Indian government adviser fears coronavirus crisis will worsen'. 26 June 2020. Accessed 26 December 2020. https://www.nature.com/articles/d41586-020-01865-w.

Plowden, W. Chichele. 1883. *Report on the census of British India taken on the 17th February 1881*. London: Eyre and Spottiswoode.

Povinelli, Elizabeth A. 2016. *Geontologies: A requiem to late liberalism*. Durham, NC: Duke University Press.

Premchand, Munshi. 2017. *The Shroud. Premchand: The complete short stories, Vol. 4*, edited by Mohammad Asaduddin. New Delhi, India: Penguin Random House.

Pritchett, Frances W., ed. 1979. *Dr Babasaheb Ambedkar: Writings and speeches, Vol. 1*. Bombay, India: Education Department, Government of Maharashtra.

Pulla, Priyanka. 2020. 'India is undercounting its COVID-19 deaths. This is how'. *The Wire*, 4 August 2020. Accessed 26 December 2020. https://science.thewire.in/health/india-mccd-comorbidities-covid-19-deaths-undercounting/.

Ramanna, Mridula. 2012. *Health Care in Bombay Presidency, 1896–1930*. Delhi, India: Primus Books.

Rao, Anupama. 2009. *The Caste Question: Dalits and the politics of modern India*. Berkeley, CA: University of California Press.

Sainath, Palagummi. 1996. *Everybody Loves a Good Drought*. New Delhi, India: Penguin Books.

Savage, Rowan. 2007. 'Disease incarnate: Biopolitical discourse and genocidal dehumanisation in the age of modernity'. *Journal of Historical Sociology* 20(3): 404–40.

Scott, James C. 1985. *Weapons of the Weak: Everyday forms of peasant resistance*. New Haven, CT: Yale University Press.

Thorat, Sukhadeo. 2009. *Dalits in India: Search for a common destiny*. Delhi, India: Sage.

Times of India. 2021. Gang which stole shrouds from crematoriums to sell again busted in UP's Baghpat. Accessed 19 May 2021. http://timesofindia.indiatimes.com/articleshow/82505425.cms?utm_source=contentofinterest&utm_medium=text&utm_campaign=cppst

TwoCircles.net. 2020. 'Social distancing being used to reinforce caste bias, justify Manusmriti, says Dalit activist Ramesh Nathan'. Accessed 22 December 2020. http://twocircles.net/2020jul09/437975.html.

World Bank. 2020. 'The World Bank in India: Overview'. Accessed 26 December 2020. https://www.worldbank.org/en/country/india/overview.

Zephyrin, Laurie, David C. Radley, Yaphet Getachew, Jesse C. Baumgartner and Eric C. Schneider. 2020. 'COVID-19 more prevalent, deadlier in US counties with higher Black populations'. *To the Point*. Commonwealth Fund, 23 April 2020. Accessed 22 December 2020. https://www.commonwealthfund.org/blog/2020/covid-19-more-prevalent-deadlier-us-counties-higher-black-populations.

Žižek, Slavoj. 2020. 'Monitor and punish? Yes, please!' *The Philosophical Salon*, 16 March 2020. Accessed 22 December 2020. http://thephilosophicalsalon.com/monitor-and-punish-yes-please/.

8
Unprecedented times? Romanian Roma and discrimination during the COVID-19 pandemic

Cristina A. Pop

Romania has the largest Roma minority in Europe, and here, the COVID-19 pandemic has revealed a pattern of anti-Roma attitudes that have infused the government's attempts to contain the virus. In this essay, I consider two events revolving around the Romanian Roma – the lockdown of Țăndărei, a town with a significant Roma minority, and the public controversy surrounding the publication on social media of a derogatory meme about the Roma stuck in Țăndărei during the lockdown. I examine the ways in which the pandemic has intensified and even institutionalised racist attitudes against Roma, and I show how the Roma have worked around public attempts to confine and ridicule them. While the COVID-19 crisis raises unprecedented challenges for many around the globe, to the Romanian Roma the pandemic may just be the latest in a series of instances in which they have found themselves shamed for their transnational mobility and subjected to containment. I review two such precedents – the swine flu (H1N1) pandemic of 2009–10 and the measles epidemic of 2016–18 – to show that, in contexts of heightened public concern about confinement and contagion, the Roma have been at the same time subjected, and creatively resistant, to biopolitical constraints.

Romanian Roma include several heterogenous groups. While many Roma live in permanent settlements, either as city dwellers or village residents, some are more itinerant, traveling across Romania or back and forth between Romania and other countries in eastern and western Europe. A minority of the Romanian Roma display their wealth by living in opulent mansions whose intricate and pharaonic architectural designs often make headlines in the tabloid press (Dumbara 2016). These contrast with Roma communities of people living in extreme poverty in decrepit neighbourhoods, sometimes in landfill slums. Many Roma have assimilated, to various degrees, with the Romanian majority; fewer continue to practise traditional crafts such as tinsmithing and coppersmithing. Yet notwithstanding their diversity, most Romanian Roma share several potentially unifying ethnic identity markers, such as the high value attached to notions of purity, respect and shame, honour and family (Pons 1995; Tesăr 2012; Berta 2019). Despite their diversity, the majority of Romanians reify the Roma as a monolithic entity, and refer to them in stereotypical terms as unlawful, unclean, underclass and itinerant, but also as talented musicians and dancers, and family-oriented people (Szeman 2018). Fonseca, for example, details various Roma communities in Albania, Poland, Bulgaria, Slovakia and other countries in her ethnography about European gypsies, and describes the Romanian Roma as 'the least obedient people in the world' (1995, 140).

From their first arrival in the fourteenth century into the Carpathian territories situated at the north of the Danube river, the Roma (designated in the past as 'gypsies' [*țigani*]) were enslaved and used as an unpaid labour force, especially in Christian Orthodox monasteries. This continued until the mid-nineteenth century when they were liberated once a new generation of politicians who had been educated in western Europe during the 1848 revolutions came to power in Romania's historical provinces of Moldova and Valachia (Fonseca 1995; Djuvara 2008). Between 1946 and 1989, under the communist regime which prioritised class struggle over ethnic identity, the Roma were not officially recognised as an ethnic group. With notable exceptions, such as the 1977 Plan for the Forced Integration of Nomadic Gypsies (Ștefănescu 2020), the communist state did not try to assimilate the Roma, and communist policies emphasised social emancipation for all classes. Ideas of progress rather than ethnic assimilation informed state programmes to force nomadic Roma into permanent settlements, discontinue their traditional occupations and enrol their children in Romanian schools (Pons 1995; Szeman 2018). Like other Romanian citizens, the Roma benefited from social welfare and free medical care, but given their resistance to assimilationist policies of the communist state, they continued to be discriminated against (Pons 1995; Fonseca 1995). Most Romanian citizens were denied transnational mobility in this Cold War period, yet despite being enclosed behind the Iron Curtain, the Roma managed to engage in international travel, often smuggling coveted western merchandise, from blue jeans to contraceptive pills, back into Romania. They were border-crossers even at a time when the outside world was out of reach of most Romanians. The Roma's transnational mobility reinforced the Romanian majority's stereotypes about their structural nomadism. This established the foundation of their future casting as scapegoats in the time of epidemics. After all, people do not travel alone across borders; viruses travel with them.

After the demise of the communist regime in 1989, the Romanian state formally recognised the Roma as an ethnic group, using the ethnonym 'Roma' [*Rrom*]. While most prefer to be called *Rrom*, some would still favour to be called *țigan* [gypsy], despite the derogatory connotations of this former ethnonym. Their official acknowledgment as an ethnic group subjected Roma to new forms of marginalisation and discrimination (Vincze and Raț 2013), and sometimes to racially motivated violence. For instance, the state has differentially targeted the fertility of various socio-demographic groups, incentivising increased fertility for high-income urban professionals but discouraging it for minorities – especially the Roma (Raț 2009). Universal child allowance, introduced in 1993, was only distributed through schools for children over seven, although in 2007 the law was modified to allow children who did not attend school – the majority Roma – to also receive the allowance. Paid maternity leave is available only for a mother's first three births and only for mothers who were employed and had contributed to the public insurance fund for at least 12 months before giving birth. These elitist family policies have daunted the most fertile categories of population – especially the Roma minority – which is also the poorest. In an eugenicist-sounding comment, political analyst Ionuț Popescu asked the state to decide 'what [type of] natality should be encouraged'. Alluding to Roma parents, Popescu cautioned against the commodification of having children (Benezic 2011).

The Roma were among the first Romanian citizens to take advantage of the post-communist dismantling of previous policies. In the early 1990s, with the removal of the Iron Curtain and European borders gradually opening up to eastern Europeans, many Roma began to migrate to western Europe in search of economic opportunities. Some surrendered Romanian citizenship and became stateless persons in the hope, seldom fulfilled, of being granted refugee status or western country citizenship (Pons 1995). With Romania struggling to attest to its commitment to 'European values' in preparation to joining the European Union, negative stereotypes about the 'uncivilised' Roma became more prevalent in public discourses. The Roma became the designated scapegoats for Romania's geopolitical fiascos (Pons 1995; Fonseca 1995). After Romania was finally admitted to the European Union in 2007, Romanian Roma joined millions of other Romanian citizens in seasonal or, in some cases, permanent economic-driven transnational migration to other European countries, particularly to Italy, Spain, France and the United Kingdom (Berta 2019; Szeman 2018).

For over seven centuries of cohabitation, Romanians have developed stigmatising stereotypes about *țigani*. The dehumanising and marginalising lens through which Roma are viewed is evident in extensive idiomatic expressions, images and stories about gypsies. In general, Roma are represented as delinquent, lazy, untrustworthy and dirty. In its form as a verb, 'to gypsy' (*a se țigăni*) denotes nagging, bartering or excessive negotiating for a minor thing. People speak idiomatically of 'drowning like the gypsy ashore' (*a se îneca ca țiganul la mal*) to denote failing a project or an endeavour in its final stage; '[swallowed food] taking the gypsy's way' (*a se duce pe calea țiganului*) to refer to choking; 'tossing death at the gypsies' (*a arunca moartea în țigani*) to refer to wrongfully blaming someone; 'moving around, like the gypsy and his tent' (*a se muta ca țiganul cu cortul*) to denote instability and untrustworthiness. The most common ethnic slur that non-Roma Romanians use to refer to Roma is 'crow' [*cioară*], a reference to the fact that Roma are believed to have dark complexions, although many 'white gypsies' have very light skin, blond hair and light-coloured eyes, and for this reason, are assumed to be kidnapped Romanians. As a child growing up in Romania, to ensure that I stayed close to my adult family members in a crowded place, I was told that *țiganii* were child abductors. In an ironic twist, it was the ethnic majority of Romanians who feared assimilation by the Roma through human trafficking. As we shall see, these ethnic slurs acquired new meanings during the COVID-19 pandemic.

On 16 March 2020, in response to the emerging coronavirus pandemic, the president of Romania, Klaus Iohannis, issued Decree 195 and declared a state of emergency. The Romanian government periodically updated the stipulations of the decree through 11 military ordinances, issued between 17 March and 11 May. On 4 April 2020, the government issued Military Ordinance 7, which stipulated the lockdown of Țăndărei, a town of 12,000 in southern Romania, about 150 kilometres east of the capital city of Bucharest (Budușan 2020). A significant minority of Roma – 30 per cent of the town's population – live in Țăndărei. As European countries implemented lockdowns and closed borders following coronavirus outbreaks, hundreds of thousands of Romanian citizens, including Romanian Roma, working in Italy, Spain, France and other western European countries, returned to Romania. In a 24-hour period on 25 and 26 March, two Roma men from Țăndărei, aged 60 and 39, died after testing positive for COVID-19. These deaths, along with other cases of people surviving the coronavirus – a total that would rapidly escalate to seven deaths and 37 cases by 6 April – were traced to a funeral that took place in the Roma community of Țăndărei in mid-March (Pocotilă 2020). In response to this outbreak, the Romanian Minister of Internal Affairs, Marcel Vela, declared on 1 April 2020: 'The main issue is that they [the Roma of Țăndărei] are remaining in contact with one another. They don't follow the rules, they move around and are hard to contain' [my translation from Romanian] (Pocotilă 2020; Duminică 2020). In this discourse, Vela points to the irreconcilable otherness of the Roma; he insinuates derogatory connotations to social values otherwise widely recognised as positive, such as closeness, and alludes to the stereotype of the Roma as being obstinate unruly wanderers. Three days later, on 4 April, Țăndărei was placed under lockdown by police and special forces, as specified under Military Ordinance 7. While the lockdown came in response to the increase of COVID-19 cases among the Roma community of Țăndărei, the non-Roma majority of the town was subjected to the same restrictions. The town reopened on 14 May, following the stipulations of Military Ordinance 11.

    Days after the lockdown of the town, several Romanian intellectuals shared on social media an offensive meme that ridiculed the Roma confined in Țăndărei. Vladimir Tismăneanu, professor of politics at the University of Maryland (College Park) in the United States, posted on his Facebook account a meme that he had received from Denisa Comănescu, the general director of Romania's most well-known academic publishing house, *Humanitas*. The meme, posted on 10 April, was the picture of a flock of crows sitting on a wooden fence, with text that read: 'Țăndărei Airport. All flights have been cancelled'. Tismăneanu shared the meme with the comment: 'Super cool, thank you, Denisa Comănescu'. [*Super tare, mulțumesc Denisa Comănescu.*] Tismăneanu, born into a family of communist activists, had defected from Romania in 1981 and has been living in the US since 1982. A prominent intellectual figure of the Romanian diaspora, he is also the director of the Centre for the Study of Post-communist Societies at the University of Maryland (College Park). Although Tismăneanu deleted his Facebook post minutes after publishing it, a public controversy ensued. Sociologist and Roma activist Ciprian Necula publicly denounced Tismăneanu's post as racist. Later the same day, Tismăneanu published 'An error, an explanation' [*O eroare, o precizare*] on his Facebook page, acknowledging his previous posting of the meme, but claiming that he had missed its 'racist implications' because he no longer lived in Romania (Necula 2020). He later deleted this explanation as well. On 11 April, Tismăneanu posted an apology for having circulated the 'racist, inappropriate, and most importantly, hurtful meme', and admitted that not residing in Romania was no excuse for his actions. Romania's National Council Against Discrimination [*Consiliul Național pentru Combaterea Discriminării* CNCD] filed a formal complaint, fined Tismăneanu and notified the University of Maryland. The University's officials acknowledged and firmly condemned the racist character of Tismăneanu's post but did not further sanction their professor, on the grounds that he had not displayed any racist behaviour prior to this incident. Denisa Comănescu, general director of *Humanitas* publishing house and the original source of the meme, also apologised publicly, claiming that she had not realised the racist undertones of the image (Păvălucă 2020). The controversy dragged in other prominent Romanian intellectuals, among them celebrated writer Mircea Cărtărescu, who, in a Facebook post also later deleted, praised Tismăneanu for apologising and denounced those who had shamed him as hypocrites (Mutler 2020; Dobrescu 2020; Tolontan 2020).

In the context of the COVID-19 pandemic, the 'crow' ethnic slur acquired new meanings. 'Crow' had been previously used to refer to the Roma in reference to the stereotype that most Roma have darker complexions than other ethnic groups, just as crows are darker than other birds. But crows also have the ability to fly, and the picture that Comănescu and Tismăneanu circulated showed the birds sitting on a fence. The immobile crow became an ironic allusion to the fact that Roma were deprived of their stereotypical proclivity for mobility by the forced quarantine. The intended humour of the meme depended upon pre-existing derogatory characterisation of Roma as 'unruly wanderers', now forced to stay in place. The wooden fence that stands for 'Țăndărei Airport' can be seen as an intended comic hint to the quasi-rural infrastructure of the town.

On 1 May 2020, in response to the Țăndărei lockdown but unrelated to the racist meme scandal, the former president of Romania, Traian Băsescu, declared on live TV that:

> The gypsies have to understand that their way of life cannot be tolerated. Romania has to be a country where state institutions have control over all territory. No matter how much [the gypsies] protest, they have to understand that, neither police nor constabulary, and, if necessary, not even the armed forces will ever step back' [my translation from Romanian] (Mihai 2020).

Băsescu had been Romania's president for two consecutive terms between 2004 and 2014, and the COVID-19 pandemic was not the first time he had publicly expressed anti-Roma attitudes. Despite being officially recognised as an ethic group in 1989, Romania has never officially acknowledged that, alongside Jews, Roma were subjected to extermination during the Holocaust. In a press release published during Băsescu's first term on the Romanian Presidency website in 2005, the Roma were excluded from the Holocaust commemorations. This omission prompted calls from the Roma community to review the content of the press release.[1] Even if, in 2010, Băsescu declined to sign into law a nationalist proposal to officially replace the ethnonym 'Roma' with the more derogatory 'gypsy', he made repeated racist comments about the Roma, whom he frequently called 'gypsies'. In 2014, he was finally fined by the CNCD for his disparaging statements.

As often happens during social and political crises, xenophobic attitudes are activated by a collective search for a scapegoat. In such circumstances, 'the other' is suddenly more noticeable and potentially culpable. In Romania, the COVID-19 public health crisis granted renewed but unwarranted visibility to the Roma (Matache and Bhabha 2020), in ways that are reminiscent of how they were treated during earlier pandemics and epidemics. Continually socialised into circumstances of discrimination, the Roma have previously been quick to work around forms of biopolitical surveillance. This is why their responses to coronavirus events, including Țăndărei's lockdown and the public controversy surrounding the meme, were neither dramatic nor unprecedented. As anthropologists Veena Das and Erving Goffman (Das and Goffman 2013) remind us, even though 'stigma' and 'contagion' are 'theoretically distinct concepts', they 'tend to slide in each other' especially when 'stigmatized diseases lead to the drawing of boundaries within the domestic and its immediate environment of kinship and village or neighborhood community'. To better understand the Romanian Roma's earlier experiences of being subjected to prejudice in the context of intense public concerns about contagion and confinement, I consider two recent examples: the swine flu (H1N1) pandemic of 2009–10 and the measles epidemic of 2016–18.

Romanian medical care facilities, including maternity hospitals, were placed under quarantine during the 2009 H1N1 pandemic, with strict limitations of access for everyone but medical workers and patients. In December 2009, as a parturient mother in a public maternity clinic in a large city in northern Romania, along with my family members, I had to observe these restrictions to access healthcare. While hospitalised in the quarantined clinic, I noticed the presence of members of extended families of several Roma women who had given birth. A rumour circulated among patients and medical staff that the Roma had bribed the hospital doorman to secure access to their parturient relatives. Despite the rumours and the disparaging comments about breaking the quarantine rules, the medical workers turned a blind eye and the Roma women's family members were not forced to leave the hospital.

As a patient and newly delivered mother myself, I observed ethnic segregation in that maternity hospital on four distinct occasions between 2002 and 2009. Roma women were put together in the room closest to the hospital's entrance, with the least privacy. They were separated from Romanians, Hungarians and members of other ethnic groups in a space closest to hospital hallway traffic. Two Roma women from a town in southern Romania, who I interviewed later as part of a research project (Pop 2016), recalled being segregated in the public maternity hospital in Romania's capital city Bucharest where they had given birth. The practice of segregating people of Roma ethnicity appears to be widespread in Romanian public hospitals, especially in maternity wards, as stated in Open Society Foundation and World Health Organization reports (Refworld 2015, WHO 2013). Similar practices have also been documented in Bulgaria and Hungary, where parturient Roma women are routinely placed together in 'gypsy rooms' (Iszák 2004).

This concern about segregating the Roma from the other patients inside the hospital during the H1N1 pandemic of 2009–10 overlapped with the temporary quarantine provision of separating all hospital patients from the outside world. Ironically, this confinement within confinement created a breaching opportunity for Roma family members. Since the practice of segregating Roma patients was already part of the default racist setting of the hospital space, the family members of the Roma women were prepared to penetrate spatial boundaries and successfully used informal payments for that purpose. The fact that they were only aiming to visit 'the gypsy room' – a quasi-liminal space, already separated from the rest of the hospital – may explain why medical staff seemed unconcerned that Roma family members were being granted access inside the hospital during the flu quarantine. Perhaps Roma's intrusion seemed less real or less important to medical personnel, since they only had access to the actual (and metaphorical) margins of care; for this reason, there was little risk that they might infect other patients. The Roma disregarded the interdiction to enter the quarantined hospital, and successfully worked their way around it. In some sense, like the medical staff, they may have felt that the quarantine did not even apply to them because they only needed access to a marginalised part of the building, which already ensured that they were separated from others in the hospital. Roma family members found ways to break access interdictions precisely because their previous exposure to quotidian forms of structural violence prepared them to expect segregation and discrimination and to develop strategies to overcome these instances. While medical workers and other patients viewed the informal payments to the doorman as bribery – a form of corruption that reinforced the majority's stereotypes of Roma's unlawfulness – the success of informal contributions raises questions about how these perpetuate structural violence and racism against the Roma. 'Bribery' only worked with the complicity of the non-Roma majority (represented in this context by the doorman and hospital medical workers). The non-Roma rewarded transgressive behaviours by granting the Roma family members access to the quarantined hospital only to denounce such behaviours as expressions of Roma's inclination toward illicit action. Roma constantly face segregation and marginalisation (Vincze and Raț 2013; Szeman 2018), and on a daily basis work around formal interdictions. Overcoming barriers to hospital access during the swine flu pandemic provides only one example of many that prepared the grounds for Roma to not take the COVID-19 quarantine seriously.

During the 2016–18 measles outbreak, the Romanian Roma were alleged to have brought the disease from Italy. Measles spread to Romania in January 2016 and peaked in 2018. It has continued to spread; according to statistics released by CNSCBT, by May 2020, 20,107 cases and 64 fatalities had been reported. Data from the European Centre for Disease Prevention and Control identified epidemic spread in several European countries, but Italy and Romania accounted for 34 per cent and 30 per cent respectively of all cases by March 2018. With a notification rate of 226.8 per million population (compared to the European average of 28.7 per million population), Romania was by far the most affected country, with the deadliest outbreak among European nations. According to Romania's National Centre for Surveillance and Control of Communicable Disease [CNSCBT], the epidemic had started in a rural community from north-western Romania, whose members, mostly Roma who traded clothing and household goods, were consistently travelling back and forth between Romania and Italy (Măgrădean and Tobias 2016). Genetic analysis established that the B3 strain of the measles virus had been brought from Italy and was different from the endemic D4 type that had circulated in eastern Europe during past epidemics (CNSCBT 2016).

Measles infection spread rapidly around Romania, and was particularly deadly among Roma infants and children. This influenced claims that the Roma had brought the virus from Italy (Măgrădean and Tobias 2016) despite the fact that, in 2016, over one million Romanians lived and worked in Italy and they too regularly travelled between the two countries. The higher measles incidence and mortality among the Roma was therefore a symptom of a structural rather than contingent problem.

Designed as a one-size-fits-all national scale programme rather than a targeted regional and local project, Romania's measles-mumps-rubella (MMR) vaccination campaign failed in its outreach to many Roma communities and reproduced old discriminations while creating new excluded populations. Community health workers blamed the low vaccination rates on Roma's 'lack [of] identification papers' and 'itinerant lifestyles' (Coman 2017): they argued that many Roma were officially registered neither in Romania nor Italy, and therefore fell between the national immunisation programmes of the two countries. However, investigative journalists who covered the measles outbreak in several, mostly poor and rural, Roma communities in southern and western Romania found that parents had expressed their intention to vaccinate their children, and complained about being forgotten by public health authorities. From the Roma's perspective, the measles outbreak became 'an epidemic of neglect' (Drăgan et al. 2018). Excluded from the healthcare systems of both Romania and Italy, some Roma used traditional healing remedies against measles. Without access to vaccination and allopathic medical care, some Roma community members attempted to prevent measles with imitative magic methods, like dressing babies in red clothes – a reference to the fact that *rujeolă*, the word for measles in Romanian, designates the colour red. Others used traditional folk remedies, such as rubbing the baby's body with brandy or wine (Simina 2017). Journalists highlighted the prejudice held by the Romanian majority against the Roma minority, reporting the manner in which social workers, family doctors and other health providers used ethnic slurs and talked about Roma in a condescending manner (Drăgan et al. 2018). Ignoring some of the structural reasons for low vaccination rates, a few welfare assistants admitted to having used intimidation tactics, such as withholding financial aid to low-income Roma parents on the grounds that they had not vaccinated their children (Ursu 2018). These people, who represented state authority, dismissed the Roma as superstitious and ignorant about the benefits of biomedicine. The use of alternatives to allopathic medicine only reinforced, among the non-Roma majority, clichés about gypsies practising the occult. However, Roma's resort to symbolic magic and traditional prevention can be understood in a more pragmatic manner, as an attempt to use the only available resources at their disposal to prevent illness. The structural violence that shapes the provision of care to many Romanian Roma explains these alternative tactics of prevention and healing.

Even when the MMR vaccination was available, ethnic discrimination prevented Roma children's access to the vaccine. A 2016 study comparing paediatric vaccination in Roma and non-Roma children in countries from central and eastern Europe, including Romania, found that the odds of being vaccinated for a Roma child was 38.6 per cent that of a non-Roma child for MMR for the region. In Romania there is a 31.1 per cent gap in MMR vaccination between Roma and non-Roma, which places Romania, along with Bosnia and Herzegovina, as the country with the highest vaccination gap in the region (Duval et al. 2016). Ethnic origin, lack of access to healthcare, socio-economic status, lack of awareness of the need for immunisation, and perceived and real discrimination have all contributed to this immunisation gap. Overall, the measles epidemic of 2016–18 exposed the existence of entire Roma populations who were omitted from mainstream healthcare because of structural barriers such as poverty, racism and discrimination. The epidemic also highlighted the centrality of stereotypical narratives in official public health discourses that shame the Roma for their transnational mobility.

The systemic forces through which the Roma were singled out during the H1N1 flu pandemic of 2009–10 and the measles epidemic of 2016–18 serve as the background against which we should understand Roma's reactions to confinement in Țăndărei during the early months of the COVID-19 pandemic. Their resistance to the normative powers of biomedicine and the state is more practical than ideological. The Roma have naturalised structural vulnerability to a degree that has prepared them to effectively elude it. While enclosure in their town was enforced by both police and military forces, the Roma live-streamed parties on TikTok, to the despair of authorities. One man from Țăndărei recorded his coronavirus hospitalisation and healing process. In his vlog, posted on YouTube and widely circulated by Romanian mass media, he first speaks through a mask, advising people to stay home and take the virus seriously, and later emerges from his hospital bed, takes off his mask, and invites family and friends to a welcome home party (Literas 2020a, 2020b). Although the non-Roma population of Țăndărei was subject to the same lockdown measures, national TV aired only footage of the streets of the Roma neighbourhoods of the town, with adults and children ignoring social distancing requirements and wandering around. This prompted several other TV channels to feature footage of the police and armed forces patrolling the streets of Țăndărei and enforcing the quarantine under the caption 'game of cat and mouse between the population and the police' (Știrile PROTV 2020).

Structural violence against the Romanian Roma, in the present as in the past, has taken the form of discrimination, segregation, prejudice, marginalisation and poverty. These structural forces expand beyond Romania, impacting the lives of Roma throughout central and eastern Europe. In Bulgaria, Hungary and Slovakia many Roma live in extreme poverty, in crowded dwellings, with no access to running water, under conditions that impede their capacity to adhere to the simplest preventive measures. During the COVID-19 pandemic, similar racialised anxieties about infection and about the Roma spreading the virus were recorded in Bulgaria, Hungary and Slovakia (Neuberger 2020; McLaughlin 2020). While Romania is not the only country to witness pandemic-triggered prejudice against the Roma, the Țăndărei lockdown exposed the full extent of state's and civil society's institutionalised racism.[2]

In the last decade, Țăndărei has been repeatedly featured in the national and even international news. In 2010, several men among the very affluent Roma of Țăndărei were charged with human trafficking, accused of taking children from Romania and forcing them to panhandle in the United Kingdom. The lawsuit dragged on for almost 10 years before the case was dismissed in court in February 2020 due to insufficient evidence. The verdict was controversial and allegations of corruption circulated in the mass media. Wealthy Roma were suspected of having bought the state authorities' complicity to hide incriminating evidence. Though there seems to be no causal link between the accusations of human trafficking against the Roma of Țăndărei and the subsequent lockdown of the town as COVID-19 gained ground, many Romanians connected the two instances (Ștefănescu 2020); they both illustrated a perception about the Roma as situated beyond and above the state's regulations. However, some Roma challenged this perception, arguing instead that both the human trafficking case and Roma's civil disobedience during the lockdown should be understood as examples of the government's inability to punish and discipline the delinquent Roma (Baias 2020; Barberá 2020). Roma activist Duminică (2020) argued for the need to shift the focus from a particular ethnic group to the state and its governance style. In his opinion, the fact that the Roma escaped state control both before and during the COVID-19 pandemic illustrated the state's complicity and corruption. The pandemic, then, exposed and deepened existing mutual mistrust between the Roma minority and Romanian authorities, and reinforced stereotypes on both sides about 'unlawful gypsies' and the 'weak state'. The public health crisis produced by COVID-19 brought into public visibility old and new assumptions about the need to purify the 'social body' from 'corruption', 'superstition' and 'civil disobedience' (see also Matache and Bhabha 2020).

Locking down entire communities because of COVID-19 was unprecedented in Romania. Yet, as suggested by previous instances such as the swine flu pandemic and measles epidemic, the discourses that circulated about the Romanian Roma among ordinary citizens, intellectual and political elites, and authorities during the coronavirus pandemic were not without precedent. By successfully – in a pragmatic rather than ideological manner – working around discrimination by (literally or figuratively) breaking boundaries, the Roma at the same time reinforced stigmatising narratives and attitudes held by the Romanian majority. The COVID-19 pandemic set the ground for future discrimination against Roma.

Notes

1 In fact, Romanian lexicons do not agree with definitions of the Holocaust. In the Romanian academy thesaurus (DEX 1996, 463), the meaning of the 'Holocaust' is the 'killing (through fire) of a very large number of people', while in the Abridged Dictionary of the Romanian Language MDLR (Breban 1997, 281), the Holocaust is defined as 'the massacre of the Jews by the Nazis'. There are no changes in more recent editions of these lexicons.
2 The only other Romanian area to be quarantined was Suceava, a city of 100,000 people from northeast Romania. As stipulated in Military Ordinance 6 from 30 March 2020, Suceava was locked down along with eight other adjacent villages, after the public health authorities recorded 593 cases. To compare the magnitude of the outbreaks, by the time Țăndărei was quarantined on 4 April, there were approximately 30 cases in a town one-tenth the size of Suceava.

References

Baias, Ionut. 2020. 'Cazul Țăndărei, cu 25 de achitări: Nu a existat nicio probă directă din care să rezulte în mod indubitabil vinovăția – instanță'. 11 February 2020. Accessed August 2020. https://www.hotnews.ro/stiri-esential-23655602-cazul-tandarei-25-achitari-nu-existat-nicio-proba-directa-din-care-rezulte-mod-indubitabil-vinovatia-instanta.htm.
Barberá, Marcel Gascón. 2020. 'Romania isolates human trafficking hotspot to limit outbreak'. 5 April 2020. Accessed 31 August 2020. https://balkaninsight.com/2020/04/05/romania-isolates-human-trafficking-hotspot-to-limit-outbreak/.
Benezic, Dollores. 2011. 'Depinde ce fel de natalitate vrem să încurajăm'. 26 January 2011. Accessed 30 August 2020. https://cursdeguvernare.ro/ionut-popescu-depinde-ce-fel-de-natalitate-ne-hotaram-sa-incurajam.html.
Berta, Péter. 2019. *Materializing Difference: Consumer culture, politics, and ethnicity among Romanian Roma*. Toronto, Canada: University of Toronto Press.
Breban, Vasile. 1997. *Mic Dicționar al Limbii Române*. Bucharest, Romania: Editura Enciclopedică.
Budușan, Iulian. 2020. 'Ce prevede Ordonanța Militară cu numărul 7. Orașul Țăndărei se închide, iar zborurile spre zonele roșii sunt anulate'. 4 April 2020. Last modified 31 August 2020. https://www.libertatea.ro/stiri/ordonanta-militara-sapte-text-integral-ce-prevede-2940847.

CNSCBT. 2016. 'Evoluția rujeolei in România, 2016'. Accessed 31 August 2020. https://www.cnscbt.ro/index.php/informari-saptamanale/rujeola-1/560-evolutia-rujeolei-in-romania-2016/file.

Coman, Octavian. 2017. 'Fatal inaction: How measles made a comeback'. 30 November 2017. Accessed 31 August 2020. http://www.balkaninsight.com/en/article/fatal-inaction-how-measles-made-a-comeback-11-30-2017.

Das, Veena and E. Goffman 2013. 'Stigma, contagion, defect: Issues in the anthropology of public health'. Accessed 30 August 2020. https://pdfs.semanticscholar.org/5113/ba09191943a0234e59f5d5ef37b683d502a8.pdf?_ga=2.257549451.1265060091.1598834583-2075407597.1598834583.

DEX. 1996. *Dicționarul Explicativ al Limbii Române*. Bucharest, Romania: Univers Enciclopedic.

Djuvara, Neagu. 2008. *Între Orient și Occident. Țările Române la începutul epocii moderne*. Bucharest, Romania: Editura Humanitas.

Dobrescu, Petre. 2020. 'Mircea Cărtărescu îl apără pe Vladimir Tismăneanu și îi numește "farisei" pe criticii acestuia'. 11 April 2020. Accessed 31 August 2020. https://www.libertatea.ro/stiri/mircea-cartarescu-sare-in-apararea-prietenului-vladimir-tismaneanu-dupa-postarea-rasista-priviti-cum-i-au-sarit-la-gat-toti-fariseii-2950868.

Drăgan, Flavia, Marian Mircea and Ramona Ursu. 2018. 'Epidemia nepăsării'. *Newsweek* 1(4): 13–23.

Dumbara, Ana. 2016. 'The Romanian town built on British benefits: Mansions bigger than the average UK semi and BMWs with British number plates parked in the drives paid for with taxpayer cash'. 5 April 2016. Accessed 24 August 2020. https://www.dailymail.co.uk/news/article-3518736/The-Romanian-town-built-British-benefits-Mansions-bigger-average-UK-semi-BMWs-British-number-plates-parked-drives-paid-taxpayer-cash.html.

Duminică, Gelu. 2020. 'Focarul de coronavirus din Țăndărei n-are legătură cu etnia, ci cu eșecul statului roman'. 6 April 2020. Accessed 31 August 2020. https://www.vice.com/ro/article/dygqwm/focarul-de-coronavirus-din-tandarei-si-statul-roman.

Duval, Laetitia, Francois-Charles Wolff, Martin McKee and Bayard Roberts. 2016. 'The Roma vaccination gap: Evidence from twelve countries in Central and South-East Europe'. *Vaccine* 34: 5524–30.

Fonseca, Isabel. 1995. *Bury Me Standing: The gypsies and their journey*. New York: Vintage Books.

Iszák, Rita. 2004. '"Gypsy rooms" and other discriminatory treatment against Romani women in Hungarian hospitals'. 15 December 2004. Last modified 27 August 2020. http://www.errc.org/roma-rights-journal/gypsy-rooms-and-other-discriminatory-treatment-against-romani-women-in-hungarian-hospitals.

Literas. 2020a. 'Literas eduard bolnav de COVID19 la tandarei live din spital live 1'. 2 April 2020. Accessed 31 August 2020. https://www.youtube.com/watch?v=cPLxxEIe0V4.

Literas. 2020b. 'Literas eduard bolnav de COVID19 la tandarei live din spital live 2 vindecat'. 2 April 2020. Accessed 31 August 2020. https://www.youtube.com/watch?v=MlaIssIb-8Q.

Matache, Margareta and Jacqueline Bhabha. 2020. 'Anti-Roma racism is spiralling during COVID-19 pandemic'. 7 April 2020. Accessed 31 August 2020. https://www.hhrjournal.org/2020/04/anti-roma-racism-is-spiraling-during-covid-19-pandemic/?fbclid=IwAR1z_7ZLp1bfWmRRCuP96tuAbydcaYNVo219U7NayFM-QM5Jt-A_X2p_2mw.

Măgrădean, Vasile and Andreea Tobias. 2016. 'Epidemia de rujeolă. Focarele au apărut în comunități de romi din Bistrița. Copiii nu au fost vaccinați'. 22 September 2016. Accessed 27 August 2020. https://www.mediafax.ro/social/epidemia-de-rujeola-focarele-au-aparut-in-comunitati-de-romi-din-bistrita-copiii-nu-au-fost-vaccinati-15742362.

McLaughlin, Daniel. 2020. 'Coronavirus pandemic deepens despair and danger for Europe's Roma'. 5 April 2020. Accessed 31 August 2020. https://www.irishtimes.com/news/world/europe/coronavirus-pandemic-deepens-despair-and-danger-for-europe-s-roma-1.4221540.

Mihai, Alina. 2020. 'Traian Băsecu reclamat și el la CNCD pentru afirmații incitatoare la ură. Ce a spus fostul președinte despre etnicii romi'. 3 May 2020. Accessed 31 August 2020. https://www.mediafax.ro/politic/traian-basescu-reclamat-si-el-la-cncd-pentru-afirmatii-incitatoare-la-ura-ce-a-spus-fostul-presedinte-despre-etnicii-romi-19112378.

Mutler, Alison. 2020. 'Depiction of Roma as crows exposes deeper racism in Romania'. 16 April 2020. Last modified 31 August 2020. https://www.rferl.org/a/depiction-of-roma-as-crows-exposes-deeper-racism-within-romania/30558933.html.

Necula, Ciprian. 2020. 'Vladimir Tismăneanu, un rasist chiulangiu. Cum a ajuns un professor roman din SUA să posteze fotografii cu "ciorile de la Țăndărei"'. 11 April 2020. Accessed 31 August 2020. https://www.libertatea.ro/opinii/vladimir-tismaneanu-un-rasist-chiulangiu-ciorile-de-la-tandarei-2950585.

Neuberger, Eszter. 2020. 'Europe's marginalised Roma people hit hard by coronavirus'. 11 May 2020. Accessed 31 August 2020. https://www.theguardian.com/world/2020/may/11/europes-marginalised-roma-people-hit-hard-by-coronavirus.

Păvăluca, Luana. 2020. 'Vladimir Tismăneanu își cere scuze pentru meme-ul rasist, dar amintește că atunci când el a fost atacat, CNCD nu a intervenit'. 12 April 2020. Accessed 31 August 2020. https://www.digi24.ro/stiri/actualitate/social/vladimir-tismaneanu-isi-cere-scuze-pentru-meme-ul-rasist-dar-aminteste-ca-atunci-cand-el-a-fost-atacat-cncd-nu-a-intervenit-1290509.

Pocotilă, Andreea. 2020. 'COVID-19. Bomba cu ceas din Țăndărei'. 1 April 2020. Accessed 27 August 2020. https://recorder.ro/covid-19-bomba-cu-ceas-din-tandarei/.

Pons, Emmanuelle. 1995. *Les tsiganes en Roumanie: des citoyens à part entière?* Paris, France: Editions L'Harmattan.

Pop, Cristina. 2016. 'Locating purity with corruption rumours: Narratives of HPV vaccination refusal in aperi-urban community of southern Romania'. *Medical Anthropology Quarterly* 30(4): 563–81.

Raț, Cristina. 2009. 'Disciplining mothers: Fertility threats and family policies in Romania'. In *Family Patterns and Demographic Development*, GESIS Thematic Series on Social Sciences in Eastern Europe, Issue 1: 75–86. Mannheim, Germany: Leibniz Institut für Sozialwissenschaften.

Refworld. 2015. 'Romania: Situation of Roma, including treatment by society and government authorities; state protection and support services available to Roma (2011–2015)'. Accessed 31 August 2020. https://www.refworld.org/docid/563c58104.html.

Simina, Codruța, 2017. 'Pojarul statului. În focar de rujeolă, copiii sunt dați cu răchie și îmbrăcați în roșu'. 14 May 2017. Accessed 31 August 2020. https://pressone.ro/pojarul-statului-in-focar-de-rujeola-copiii-sunt-dati-cu-rachie-si-imbracati-in-rosu/.

Szeman, Ioana. 2018. *Staging Citizenship: Roma, performance and belonging in EU Romania*. Oxford, UK: Berghahn Books.

Ștefănescu, Cristian. 2020. 'Cazul Țăndarei. Sunteți pe o pistă greșită, dragilor'. Accessed 31 August 2020. https://www.dw.com/ro/cazul-%C8%9B%C4%83nd%C4%83rei-sunte%C8%9Bi-pe-o-pist%C4%83-gre%C8%99it%C4%83-dragilor/a-53056793.

Știrile PROTV. 2020. 'Țăndărei a intrat în carantină. Joc de-a șoarecele și pisica între locuitori și polițiști'. 6 April 2020. Accessed 31 August 2020. https://www.youtube.com/watch?v=k58yPWzQn9I.

Tesăr, Cătălina. 2012. 'Becoming Rom (male), becoming Romni (female) among Romanian Cortorari Roma: On body and gender'. *Romani Studies* 22: 113–40.

Tolontan, Cătălin. 2020. 'Tismăneanu, Cărtărescu și "ciorile de la Țăndărei". Toate zborurile și toate responsabilitățile sunt anulate'. 11 April 2020. Accessed 31 August 2020. https://www.tolo.ro/?s=Toate+zborurile+%C8%99i+toate+responsabilit%C4%83%C8%9Bile+sunt+anulate.

Ursu, Ramona. 2018. 'Epidemia nepăsării. "Mica înțelegere", strategia antirujeolă aplicată în Dolj'. *Newsweek* 1(4): 20–21.

Vincze, Enikő and Cristina Raț. 2013. 'Spatialization and racialization of social exclusion: The social and cultural formation of gypsy ghettos in Romania in a European context'. *Studia Universitatis Babeș-Bolyai* 58(2): 5–21.

WHO. 2013. 'Roma health mediation in Romania: Case study'. Accessed 20 October 2020. http://www.euro.who.int/__data/assets/pdf_file/0016/235141/e96931.pdf.

9
Turkey's Diyanet and political Islam during the pandemic

Oğuz Alyanak

On 10 January 2020, two months before the first COVID-19 positive case was announced in Turkey but anticipating its eventuality, a taskforce led by the country's Minister of Health, Fahrettin Koca, was formed to oversee efforts to tackle the pandemic. Like his counterparts in other countries, as cases began to be reported, Koca addressed the nation regularly on measures taken by the government to contain the spread of the virus. Schools were closed on 12 March and a partial flight ban was put in place the next day. Leisure venues such as bars and nightclubs were shut down and the ban was extended to gatherings in mosques on 16 March. All hospitals with infectious disease units were transformed into pandemic hospitals, and from the last week of March, partial curfews were enforced nation-wide. For most Turks used to seeing the Turkish president, Recep Tayyip Erdoğan, addressing them daily through their television screens, Koca's regular appearance was a somewhat welcome change.

Yet the measures mandated by Turkey's Scientific Advisory Board, which to Koca's dismay were not followed literally by government officials, were insufficient to contain the spread of the virus. In the first three weeks of April, Turkey experienced a daily average of 97 deaths and 3,907 cases. Then came a rather abrupt change of discourse. Turks started to see their president and other state representatives, such as the head of the Presidency of Religious Affairs (Türkiye Cumhuriyeti Cumhurbaşkanlığı Diyanet İşleri Başkanlığı, *Diyanet* hereafter), Ali Erbaş, take the stage to comment on the pandemic. Other religious scholars were also invited to participate in televised debates. Although these actors were not public health experts, they weighed in on the discussion and brought to it a new dimension which had less to do with the pandemic's biological tenets, and more with its moral foundations. But why the change of discourse?

In this chapter, I examine how Turkey's ruling Adalet ve Kalkınma Partisi (Justice and Development Party, AKP hereafter) relied on a moralist discourse to retain its legitimacy while facing mounting criticism amid the pandemic. Reflecting on scholarly conversations on moral authority and politics, with a particular emphasis on the notion of political Islam, I show how the use of a moralist discourse enabled new configurations of state power during the first wave of COVID-19 in Turkey. Through the deployment of the Diyanet, which weighed in on conversations on the pandemic during its initial peak in mid-April,[1] the AKP was able to divert attention from any mishandling of the situation, such as not enforcing measures to quarantine Turkish citizens, including those returning from the Islamic holy sites, as I describe in the next section. The Diyanet continued to be an instrumental actor. Rather than providing moral guidance on what it considered catastrophe sent by Allah, it also pursued a moralist discourse by blaming actors and forces that it considered to be behind COVID-19. One such force was the neoliberal world order, which, according to the Diyanet, led individuals to lose their moral compass, so bringing this calamity onto them. Another was one of the AKP's usual targets: individuals who practise non-heteronormative relations, particularly members of the LGBTQI+ community in Turkey, who the Diyanet designated the perpetrators of COVID-19 in late April.

'Searching for someone to blame', Atlani-Dault and colleagues argued in a recent paper on COVID-19, 'is part of the process of making sense of any disaster, akin to the phenomenon of moral panic' (2020, e137). However, the act of blaming does more than contribute to growing anxieties during epidemics and pandemics. It also plays into the hands of public authorities such as politicians who are intent on evading criticism while garnering popular support.

Naming the crisis: public health or political survival?

From the first case of COVID-19 documented in Turkey on 11 March, the AKP was under attack for failing to take the necessary measures to prevent the spread of the virus. First, criticism was levelled at the AKP's handling of pilgrims returning home from Saudi Arabia in mid-March. Rather than enforcing the quarantine of those who had returned back from the holy sites, which by then were considered COVID-19 hotspots, AKP officials initially advocated self-isolation measures. The second criticism came in response to the AKP's delay in enforcing a suspension of religious services such as the *Cumas* (Friday prayers), which required the temporary closure of the country's 82,000 or so mosques. The failure to institute harsh responses in both cases were cited by critics as causing the spike in infections in early April (Tremblay 2020). In subsequent months, scholars and healthcare workers criticised the government for not taking seriously the warnings issued by members of independent scientific councils, such as the Turkish Medical Association (Türk Tabipleri Birliği, TTB hereafter), which advocated a strict lockdown. A report by regional officers of the TTB in late August 2020, for example, indicated that many ICU units in COVID-19 wards were running at near-full capacity, raising concerns for how hospitals might manage increasing numbers of severe cases anticipated in the winter months of 2020–21 (Ahval 2020a).

Critics also questioned the veracity of state-issued COVID-19 statistics (Evin 2020). Even though, in government's accounts, COVID-19 related deaths had not reached numbers comparable to countries like Italy or France, the TTB drew attention to the government's failure to disclose data on cases, counting only symptomatic individuals (Reuters 2020a). In a televised statement on 1 October, Koca acknowledged that this was the case, and that since 29 July the country had only been reporting data on 'patients' with symptoms and had excluded asymptomatic COVID-19 positive 'cases' from the count (bianet English 2020a). In response, the World Health Organization issued a statement inviting Turkey to report data on all positive cases. Koca rejected this, arguing that 'the current stage of the pandemic justifies shifting the emphasis from the number of positive cases to patients' (Ahval 2020b). Backing his Health Minister, Erdoğan went a step further, calling the TTB chair a 'terrorist' and suggesting the medical group be closed (bianet English 2020b).[2]

In Turkey, according to Kirişçi (2020), COVID-19 was not a public health crisis but a crisis of political survival. The AKP had faced numerous crises during nearly 20 years in power but, given the scale and direct impact on the economy and people's livelihoods, COVID-19 was seen by some analysts as the ultimate blow to its rule (Schenkkan 2020). At its first peak in mid-April, the pandemic led to the resignation of Turkey's interior minister, which, although quickly overruled by the Turkish president, was perceived as a sign of tensions building within the administration (Reuters 2020b). There were also rumours that the minister of health was considering resignation (Uğurluoğlu 2020). Globally, however, rather than catalysing a crisis of legitimacy, the pandemic presented an opportunity for most autocrats around the world to strengthen their rule (The Economist 2020). In Turkey as elsewhere, COVID-19 enabled increased authoritarianism, with individuals detained over provocative posts on social media (Reuters 2020c). Doctors and healthcare workers were probed over statements that contradicted official accounts (Human Rights Watch 2020a), and journalists were arrested for reporting on cases of infection (Reporters Without Borders 2020).

One part of AKP's strategy to retain its legitimacy amid the pandemic was to suppress critical voices. Another part was to construct an alternative discourse, which would resonate with large segments of the population and garner popular support. To that end, the AKP shifted public discussion on the pandemic from its scientific roots to its moral tenets, and in this shift, the Diyanet played an instrumental role. This was not the first time that the Diyanet was instrumentalised to overcome a crisis. Mosques in Turkey are governed by the Diyanet, and in July 2016, following a coup attempt, the Diyanet took on a central role in backing the government. By mentioning the failed coup in Friday sermons, which would normally concern practical issues pertaining to religious life, the Diyanet assisted the AKP in constructing a narrative that exculpated its politicians, many of whom were criticised for prior ties to the clique behind the coup, thereby directing attention to the enemies within. The Diyanet also used its mosques to recite prayers, such as the *sela* (salat-al-Janazah) and the *ezan* (the call to prayer) outside regular *namaz* times, reminding people of its support of government's policies and inviting all Muslims to do the same (Gill 2016).

As positive cases of Coronavirus soared across Turkey from late March, the Diyanet used its mosques once again to capture the country's soundscape by reciting prayers outside regular namaz times, and by preaching to the public on television, online and in Friday sermons (Alyanak 2020). It also assisted the government to initiate a funding campaign led by the Ministry of Family, Labor and Social Services to help ease the financial burdens of the pandemic on individuals. On 1 April 2020, the head of the Diyanet, Ali Erbaş, made a televised statement on Turkey's official news channel, *TRTHaber*, declaring his institution's support for the Presidential COVID-19 campaign, *Biz Bize Yeteriz Türkiyem*/We Are All We Need Turkey (Biz Bize Yeteriz Türkiyem 2020). There, Erbaş pointed out religion's historical role in overcoming obstacles, directly referencing to the coup attempt. He drew on verses from the Qur'an to make a case for favourable returns by Allah to those who support this campaign. The *zekats*, or alms, which Muslims are obliged to donate throughout Ramadan, could be sent to this campaign, Erbaş stated. By mid-November 2020, over 41 billion liras (US$5.5 billion) had been paid to households under the campaign budget.

Political Islam as a public health hazard

In early March, *The Washington Post* published a trenchant op-ed on Turkey. Its author, Can Dündar, a prominent Turkish journalist who currently lives in exile, pointing to the Diyanet, argued that political Islam was obstructing rational health policy in Turkey. 'The government's enormously influential Directorate of Religious Affairs, an agency that is supposed to regulate the role of Islam, has become one of the key institutions in the fight against COVID-19 – and not always for the better', wrote Dündar. He continued: 'By obstructing science and misallocating vital resources, political Islam in Turkey has become a direct threat to the health of the nation. Turks now find themselves fighting the virus even as they confront the ignorance that leads to bad policy'. Dündar spoke of an ongoing 'tug of war between reason and belief' in Turkey – a confrontation from which the AKP benefited as the majority of its voters were conservative constituents. Not only did the Diyanet weigh in on debates about the pandemic, but the Turkish president also adopted a discourse akin to it, arguing that the pandemic would be overcome through 'patience and prayers' (Dündar 2020). Critics like Dündar found such statements dangerous as they saw the need for scientific/medical authority to address the pandemic, albeit cognisant of how far the moral discourse could go in convincing millions in the country to retain their support of the AKP.

Why the Diyanet? To address this question, we need to take a moment to clarify the Diyanet's role in Turkey, and its growing influence under AKP's rule. The Diyanet was established in 1924 not as a ministry, but a separate state institution responsible for curbing religion's encroachment in politics by serving as the central authority on Islam. Its purpose was to fill the gap left as a result of the abolition of the Caliphate and Sharia, as well as the dismantlement of religious institutions and foundations (such as *tekkes*, *medreses*, *zaviyes* and *dergahs*) – key institutions of civil society in the Ottoman Empire – following the collapse of the Ottoman Empire,[3] thereby acting as 'a new structure of control and oversight between the state and Islam' (Davison 2003, 338). Representing official Islam, the Diyanet was to take over the role traditionally assumed by religious congregations (Mardin 1977). However, it failed in this role, as many of these top-down reforms did not resonate with the rural population, and different factions within Turkey's Islamic movement continued to operate in covert ways.

Following Turkey's transition into a multiparty system in 1950, Turkish politicians benefited from *de facto* links to these religious congregations for popular support (Çakır 1990) and used the Diyanet as 'an administrative tool to indoctrinate and propagate official ideology regarding Islam' (Gözaydın 2014: 13). Over time, this became known as political Islam. Several political parties have been accused of political Islamic policies, and some have been closed down for their ties to religious congregations. In 2008, the AKP, too, was accused of using Islam for political gain and was charged with violating the constitution's secularism clause. The case was shy by one vote for AKP's closure in Turkey's Constitutional Court. The AKP continued to rely on its allies in Turkey's Islamic movement, most notably, the alleged perpetrator of the 2016 coup attempt, the Gülen movement. Yet, as relations between the Gülen movement and the AKP soured, Erdoğan started to revamp the influence of the Diyanet as the official source of moral authority in order to undermine the influence of 'unofficial' Islamic discourses in Turkey and overseas (Bruce 2019). In the last decade, the Diyanet's budget has increased over five-fold. Today, the institution sits on a budget of 11 billion Turkish lira, exceeding most other ministries in Turkey (T24 2019). It has its own publications and a television channel and runs a fatwa hotline for individuals to consult on practical matters pertaining to Islamic doctrines.[4] Moreover, the Diyanet acts as a key commentator on controversial matters that pertain to public and private life (Mutluer 2018; Kocamaner 2019). Recent examples include Diyanet's comments equating feminism with immorality on International Women's Day in 2008; recommendations extended to single individuals, such as college students, to refrain from cohabitation in 2013, to engaged couples to not flirt or hold hands in 2016, and to married women to submit to their husband even in cases of domestic violence in 2020. A controversial fatwa issued in 2018 legitimised a father's lust for his own daughter; in 2019, a fatwa criticised television series considered to promote nonheteronormative and premarital relations, and deemed un-Islamic and morally corrupting; and, most recently, the Diyanet linked the coronavirus pandemic to non-heteronormative relationships.

The Diyanet's conservative stance on these issues is not surprising. Many religious authorities around the world draw on conservative guidelines to regulate affairs pertaining to the family, public morality and gender. Oftentimes, these guidelines resonate with certain segments of the population while drawing criticism from others. Yet, a legitimate question to ask that is relevant to the pandemic is whether the appeal of such views warrants religious authorities like the Diyanet taking a stance on issues that are tangential to their mission to enlighten the public on religious matters. In Turkey, the Diyanet's intervention in the COVID-19 debate came at the expense of resources allocated to battling the pandemic. Islamic authority was not used to protect human life, which, in Islam, is considered a gift from Allah that should be revered and protected (Daar and al Khitamy 2001; Shomali 2008). Rather, it was used to exculpate a government that had failed to do so. To illustrate this point, I now turn to two critical interventions made by the Diyanet during the peak of the pandemic in April.

Blaming the neoliberal world order: Islam's view on disease outbreaks

In late April 2020, the Diyanet committee, Supreme Council for Matters of Religion, issued a 56-page document entitled *İslam'ın Salgın Hastalıklara Bakışı* (Islam's View on Disease Outbreaks). The document is structured with 13 chapters, each addressing a question posed and accompanied by a lengthy appendix detailing the doctrinal genealogy of practical measures, such as the interruption of communal prayers, funerary services and possible modifications to the imminent Ramadan fasting. Of the 13 chapters, 5 related to questions asking whether outbreaks such as COVID-19 were a test or an opportunity for people to pull themselves together (Chapter 3); if people had brought onto themselves such diseases and catastrophes, and the lessons to be learned from them (Chapter 4); whether outbreaks were a warning sign from the Divine (Chapter 5); if they were a punishment or torment sent by Allah (Chapter 6); and whether they could be read as omens signalling the Day of Judgement (Chapter 7).

The theme underlying these chapters was that the pandemic was not caused by a virus alone, but by humans due to their own moral failures. The virus should therefore be perceived as a lesson from Allah to avoid 'mistakes, denial (of Allah's omnipresence), rebellion, oppression, unruliness, heresy, perversion, and exploitation, which in the past has led Allah to destroy certain nations and tribes' (Din İşleri Yüksek Kurulu 2020b, 17). Science and technology are seen not as an aid in overcoming hardship, but the cause of such hardship. Greater reliance on science and technology, according to the document, has led humans to see themselves as independent of their creator, thereby forgetful of the presence of a higher authority: 'Allah, the Holy, sent a virus barely visible under the microscope to the modern human who has forgotten the presence of his Creator, who has gone astray from his very *raison d'être* of being a *kul* [submitting pupil], and started seeing himself as the owner and conqueror of all things' (Din İşleri Yüksek Kurulu 2020, 20b).

As one of Diyanet's main missions is to enlighten society on matters pertaining to religion, what it can offer best is a religious explanation of a disease outbreak. In Islamic discourse, everything experienced on Earth – good and bad, fortunate and unfortunate – is willed by Allah. COVID-19 is no exception. On this point, the document states the following:

> One of the major trials of humans is diseases. According to Islamic belief, just like goodness and good deeds, diseases and calamities, too, are created by Allah, the Supreme, for various reasons … Without Allah's permission, no calamity reaches its destination. It is Allah the Almighty who also provides the cure and it is Allah who is Almighty (Din İşleri Yüksek Kurulu 2020b, 9).

Facing the inevitability of Allah's will, a person of faith is asked to contemplate the reasons behind Allah's doing in dispatching a calamity that brings life to a halt: 'It is necessary to see these outbreaks and catastrophes as verses sent by Allah for believers and all humans to draw lessons' (Din İşleri Yüksek Kurulu 2020b, 10). Yet, the Diyanet does more than invite believers to (re)turn to religion. The document also claims that the contemporary world order pushes believers to adopt choices which run contrary to Islamic guidelines. For the Diyanet, the underlying cause behind the pandemic needs to be sought in this world order:

> On the one side, there is hunger, starvation, drought, and illnesses which have not been experienced, and on the other, there is exploitation due to brutal capitalism, wars, invasions, migrations, injustices etc. which has disrupted the order of our old world, and has laid bare once again that humans, as our Creator has stated, 'are of a blood-shedding and malice-bringing kind' (Din İşleri Yüksek Kurulu 2020b, 20).

A few pages later, the document again invites humans to comprehend the order created by Allah on the principles of accident and fate, which differs from the order that we abide by today. Those who understand this order, and who abide by divine laws, will succeed in it. The caveat with the

Diyanet's advice, however, is that the world order that leads to tests such as COVID-19 is also one in which the Turkish state is deeply embedded. Not only was Turkey one of the main exporters of personal protective equipment throughout the pandemic,[5] that is, by Diyanet's logic, a profiteer of Allah's wrath, it had also been transformed into a largely privatised economy that relied heavily on the construction and tourism sectors, both threatened by the pandemic. Some critics today view AKP's reluctance to enforce a total lockdown even during the peak of the pandemic as a manoeuvre to save the economy (Erdemir and Lechner 2020). Yet, if the economy matters, then the Diyanet's critique of the neoliberal world order risks harming the very establishment that it relies on both financially and politically. To evade such an outcome, the AKP's neoliberal agenda was not criticised. No decision maker in the political or economic realm was called to task. Moral failures were described as the failure of individuals to break free from exploitative and unjust conditions. No explanation was given regarding the political actors in Turkey who perpetuate these conditions.

One of the risks in making morally charged statements is that they render the agents behind such remarks vulnerable to the criticisms that they extend. In this case, although the Diyanet reprimanded individuals for participating in a neoliberal world order that prioritises consumption over frugality, and worldly temptations over heavenly rewards, over the years, both the Diyanet and the AKP had been criticised for the lavish lifestyles sought of their own members, such as riding in imported luxury cars or living in the newly built Presidential Palace. This left the Diyanet in a discursive conundrum. Yet, as I illustrate below, the Diyanet was able to invent a way out of this conundrum by fabricating a new culprit. Moving beyond its usual judgements pertaining to the moral realm, the Diyanet shifted gears and directly intervened in the realm of public health where COVID-19 became not only the result of perceived moral failures of individuals and neo-liberal structures, but also a disease caused by some of these individuals. These were people following non-heteronormative values.

Reframing the narrative: non-heteronormativity as the cause of COVID-19

LGBTQI+ communities around the world have long faced blame for disease outbreaks. Same-sex couples, and others engaging in non-heteronormative practices, have not only encountered severe discrepancies in accessing healthcare due to being posited as perpetuators of infectious diseases (Lichtenstein 2003), they have also been directly targeted by conservative groups and politicians. Much of the scholarship on the stigmatisation of these groups has focused on the HIV pandemic, but blame for other disease outbreaks including the most recent COVID-19 pandemic continues to be attached to marginalised communities (UNAIDS 2020). A report circulated by the United Nations Office of the High Commissioner of Human Rights in mid-April made this precise point by calling on state authorities and stakeholders 'to speak out against stigmatisation and hate speech directed at LGBTQI+ people in the context of the pandemic' (United Nations Office of the High Commissioner for Human Rights 2020, 8). Despite the call, in several cases LGBTQI+ people were accused of spreading the disease. In South Korea, for example, where the government's intensive tracing of the virus resulted in public disclosure of patient information, the discussion of nightclubs, described in the media as COVID-19 hotspots, quickly turned into gay-bashing because some of these venues were associated with the country's LGBTQI+ community (Kwon and Hollingsworth 2020).

In Turkey, the backlash against the LGBTQI+ community and others living non-heteronormative lifestyles was government sanctioned. While there is no body of law that directly targets members of the LGBTQI+ community or limits their public presence, Turkey is not a signatory to any LGBTQI+ resolutions enacted by the United Nations Human Rights Council and the General Assembly, including the 2008 statement on LGBTQI+ rights (Human Rights Watch 2008). Same-sex marriages and civil unions are considered unconstitutional and remain outlawed. Annual Pride parades have been banned since 2016 to ensure the so-called safety of Turkish citizens and to protect public order. Here the term 'public' continues to be defined through a narrow and moralist definition that excludes relationships that lie outside a heteronormative and conjugal frame. More recently, television channels portraying same-sex couples or promoting promiscuity or homosexuality have been fined for corrupting general morality and the family unit (Muedini 2018, 43–5; bianet English 2019). There have also been several attempts to pass laws to ban 'promiscuous' relations such as *zina* (extramarital sex/adultery) and to regulate cohabitation and unmarried life, as evident in the President's proposal of measures to reinstall the ban on zina that had been retracted by the Turkish Constitutional Court in 1999 (Alyanak and Üstek 2013).

A few days after the circulation of Diyanet's document on disease outbreaks, the head of the Diyanet, Ali Erbaş, made the following statement in his address to the public through the *Cuma hutbesi* [the communal Friday namaz sermon]:

> Islam accepts adultery as one of the biggest sins [*haram*]. It curses homosexuality. What is the reason of that? The reason is that it brings with it illnesses and decay to lineages. Every year, thousands of people are exposed to HIV virus caused by this big sin – committing adultery, living out of wedlock, whose name is 'unchastity' in Islamic literature. Let's take action together to protect people from these evils. (DuvaR.English 2020).

It is no surprise to see the Diyanet take a position that condemns non-heteronormative relations. Like most religious institutions around the world, the Diyanet condemns same-sex and promiscuous relations. Its rationale for this comes from a particular reading of the Qur'an, whereby relations outside of marriage incite Allah's wrath. The oft-cited example here is the plight of Lut (Lot), which is brought up in several *surahs* (chapters) of the Qur'an. According to the story, Lut, the nephew of Prophet Abraham, was sent to the people of Lut (Sodom and Gomorrah in the Book of Genesis) to plead with them to stop their sexual perversions, such as sodomy, prostitution and extramarital affairs. However, the people, including Lut's own wife, dismissed his recommendations. Allah consequently ordered Lut to leave his wife and the tribe, and decimated the tribe.

For Erbaş, the story of the Lut has direct parallels to the plight faced by humans during the COVID-19 pandemic. But this is not the first time that Erbaş had drawn on this story. In 2019, in another *hutbe* that he delivered in a mosque in the Central Anatolian city of Konya, Erbaş reminded the congregation of the dire consequences of dismissing Allah's commands in the Qur'an: 'Our Rabb [Lord] has reminded us that many times in history tribes who faced moral decay and perversions were decimated' (Evrensel 2019).

Similar comments are regularly made by conservative pundits in Turkey, who – unlike those defending LGBTQI+ rights, who are fined for their statements – do not face legal consequences of hate speech. But in this instance, these comments came from a religious institution which acts within the capacity of an official state apparatus responsible for guiding millions of believers in Turkey and overseas. The Diyanet's statement should therefore be read as one that reveals the contours of religion as sanctioned by the Turkish state, which singles out a part of the population, targets those within it as carriers of disease, and sees them as worthy of punishment and decimation.

A few days after Erbaş made this comment, critics targeted him for his hate speech, which is prohibited in the Turkish constitution and criminalised under the penal code. The Ankara branch of the Human Rights Association in Turkey and the Ankara Bar Association both filed cases against Erbaş, asking for his resignation (Human Rights Watch 2020b). However, rather than finding his assertion discriminatory, the Turkish president sided with him. 'An attack against the Diyanet is an attack on the state', argued Erdoğan. Overnight, hundreds of thousands of AKP supporters shared their backing on Twitter by commenting under #AliErbasYalnizDegildir [Ali Erbaş is not alone] (Öztürk 2020). Other trending hashtags in subsequent days included #YallahHollandaya [Go to Holland], suggesting that critics pack their bags and move to the Netherlands, which in Turkey is characterised by its liberal politics on same-sex relations, and #LGBTIstemiyoruz [We don't want LGBT]. Other actors soon joined this debate. Kerem Kınık, the head of the Turkish branch of the Red Crescent, the international non-governmental organisation that provides disaster relief, made a claim similar to Erbaş. Using his Twitter account, Kınık argued on 28 June, a day after the International Pride Day, that his institution would fight anyone who promoted a corrupting mentality, spoke of abnormalities as the new normal, or forced paedophilic dreams on young minds. In response, the International Red Cross Committee, IFRC, issued a declaration disapproving of this comment, which led to the head of Communications for the Turkish Presidency issuing a denunciation of IFRC (Reuters 2020d). Furthermore, an inquiry was opened against the Ankara Bar Association by the Attorney General for insulting religious values, and soon after, the Turkish president once again took centre stage, targeting LGBTQI+ groups as the hub of perversions and spreaders of disease. In his national address on 27 April, the Turkish president attacked the proponents of LGBTQI+ rights directly, arguing that they were complicit in these perversions and asking the Turkish population to take a stance against them.

Seeking blame in LGBTQI+ groups is an easy – and oft utilised – political ploy to manufacture consent among the public – not just in Turkey but in other countries, too. Similarities with Russia and Brazil, run by leaders with authoritarian tendencies, are obvious. So too was the similarity with the US under the presidency of Donald Trump. Same-sex relationships have long provided an easy way out of political blunders in Turkey. Each time governments were accused of corruption or criticised for their lack of competency in navigating Turkish national and international policy, themes such as family values and same-sex relationships have been brought into the conversation. Seen as a danger to moral integrity, non-heteronormative lifestyles were put under the spotlight when bills were proposed by government officials to ban these choices. In the midst of the COVID-19 pandemic, these discussions took a new and poignant turn. Not only were extra-marital relations and homosexuality seen as moral perversions, they were also seen as epicentres of the disease, thereby constituting a public health hazard. As fears among the Turkish public heightened over the spread of the virus, overnight discussion focused on non-heteronormativity as the source of the pandemic.

What the Diyanet, and the Turkish president, did was more than blame a marginalised community for moral decay. Blaming moral ills on what these actors consider to be sexual perversions, with the focus most notably on same-sex couples, is an unfortunate norm in Turkey that many LGBTQI+ institutions are trying to debunk. In a recent Pew Research survey, 57 per cent of the population in Turkey still views homosexuality unfavourably, and only 25 per cent of those surveyed indicated that homosexuality should be accepted by society (Poushter and Kent 2020). The Turkish president speaks directly to this 57 per cent, assuring them that he shares a similar sentiment by making statements that affirm his belief that same-sex relations are a sexual perversion with no place in Turkish culture and morals. In the COVID-19 moment, he further spoke of those associated with this 'perversion' as the main culprit of the disease outbreak, emphasising the presumption that sexual 'perversions' are more than a moral threat. Members of the LGBTQI+ groups in Turkey already face many obstacles in the country, and having the Diyanet and the Turkish president view them as morally perverse, though terrifying, is nothing new. What is different during the COVID-19 pandemic, however, is that the Diyanet, and Erdoğan, hold these groups responsible for a disease outbreak that continues to agitate the public on a daily basis, and that generates uncertainties and fear for people's very lives and livelihoods.

What really does COVID-19 have to do with non-heteronormative relations? Epidemiologically, there are no links between promiscuity, or homosexuality, and the coronavirus. From a political perspective, however, there is much at stake in creating a link between the virus and what is seen as sexual perversity, as it helps to divert attention away from the actions and accountability of state actors.

Conclusion

I opened this chapter with the Turkish Minister of Health, Fahrettin Koca, and his Scientific Advisory Board, heralding Turkey's initial response to the pandemic. As the cases and deaths related to COVID-19 began to soar from late March, however, we witnessed in Turkey a rather abrupt change of discourse propagated by a new set of actors, including the Turkish president and the head of the Diyanet. I asked why that was the case. My intention in asking this question was not to downplay the social or cultural tenets of the disease outbreak. I do not advocate a scientific approach that dismisses the contributions of moral authorities to the debate on COVID-19. However, in Turkey, the contribution of religious authorities to understanding and responding to COVID-19 had less to do with devising culturally sensitive modes of healing, and more with seeking blame in actors who have long been subject to the government's disciplinary measures. Rather than seek morally and biomedically attuned solutions to the pandemic, what we saw in Turkey during the first wave of the pandemic was religious authorities such as the Diyanet engaging in a blatant attack on AKP's ideological opponents. This explains how political Islam hindered the makings of what critics such as Dündar called a rational public health policy in Turkey.

The Diyanet's controversial intervention into the debate also played into the hands of the AKP – not only by furthering a repressive political agenda that it has adopted over the years, but also by helping change the narrative on the pandemic. The Diyanet's statement was so controversial that it alone sufficed to turn public attention to LGBTQI+ groups overnight, leading to the tabling of discussions on measures taken by the AKP government to tackle the pandemic. Criticism over the government's handling of the pandemic, as evident in its delayed response to returning pilgrims and its hesitation to close down mosques, swiftly transformed into criticism of homosexuality.

Scholars working on stigma and disease outbreaks have shown how certain groups, who are readily marginalised in their specific societies, are targeted in the midst of public health crises (Songwathana and Manderson 2001; Castro and Farmer 2005; Singer 2009; Gregg 2011). While much of this conversation draws on evidence provided by studies on HIV, COVID-19 follows this trend. In Turkey, marginalised groups were targeted specifically to divert attention from the practical responses, or their lack, of the government. Other critics who have pointed out the shortcomings of the AKP's strategy to tackle the pandemic were also criticised by Erdoğan as well as by other figures close to the AKP government, such as the Turkish chief of the International Red Crescent. Can Dündar, a journalist in exile, was one such critic whom Erdoğan considers a member of a terrorist organisation (International Press Institute 2015). The TTB chair, Şebnem Korur Fidancı, is another figure whom Erdoğan publicly called a terrorist for having previously signed a petition in support of a peaceful negotiation of the country's Kurdish conflict. Yet, this kind of targeting also had a practical impact on the livelihood of marginalised communities. By falsely identifying them as responsible for COVID-19, the government exposed them to further stigma, with the potential to quickly turn into other kinds of violence (Yuzgun 1993; Biçmen and Bekiroğulları 2014; Başaran 2014; Özbay 2015; Yenilmez 2017).

In Turkey, political Islam jeopardises public health, and helps the AKP deflect criticism for its mishandling of the pandemic. This strategy comes at the cost of the lives of the very people whom the Turkish state is meant to protect – not just those who agree with the government's vision of a proper mode of sexual relations and romance, but also those who choose to disagree with it. The preamble of the Turkish constitution considers the right for all Turkish citizens to lead an honourable life as a birth right. This law should apply to all.

Acknowledgements

I would like to thank Funda Üstek-Spilda for commenting on earlier drafts, and the editors of this volume for extending an invitation to contribute.

Notes

1. According to the Turkish health minister, Turkey had experienced its second peak in the first wave of the pandemic after the Eid-al-Adha holiday (30 July–3 August 2020), with hospitals and intensive care units reaching 47 and 60 per cent occupancy rates respectively (Hurriyet Daily News 2020). The first peak here corresponds to the initial spike in the number of cases in mid-April, when the cases more than doubled (from 2,148 to 5,138) within the first ten days of the month.
2. A month later, Fahrettin Koca reverted from his initial stance, and decided to disclose the total number of cases in Turkey. On 25 November, 28,351 cases were announced – the fourth highest number of daily cases in the world following the US, India and Brazil. The numbers continued to climb in the following days (bianet English 2020c).
3. After the Republic of Turkey was founded in 1923, a string of reforms – known today as the Kemalist reforms – was passed by the Turkish Grand National Assembly, which led to the abolishment of the Islamic state known as the Caliphate (1924), the sharia courts which relied on Islamic law (1924) and numerous religious institutions (1925). The Diyanet was established in 1924 to undertake the tasks previously undertaken by these institutions, but due to the country's secular (*laik*) outlook, its role was limited to the regulation of texts for *hutbes*, or religious sermons (Mutluer 2018, 4).
4. Fatwa (*fetva* in Turkish) – religious advice and rulings – are issued by muftis, or Islamic jurists, in response to questions pertaining to religious conduct. For example, a Muslim with diabetes may ask a mufti whether it is acceptable to take medication while fasting. In response, the mufti

would refer to Islamic texts, including the Qur'an, and a collection of Prophet Muhammed's sayings and deeds, known as the hadiths, to pass a judgement on the issue (Alobalan and Al-Moujahed 2017). Fatwas can be issued via telephone or email or consulted by going to the Diyanet's Supreme Council for Matters of Religion (Din İşleri Yüksek Kurulu) website (Bruinessen 2018; Din İşleri Yüksek Kurulu Başkanlığı 2020a).

5 During the first week of May, with Turkish authorities calling the pandemic in Turkey under control, a decree was passed to lift restrictions on the export of personal protective equipment to Western European countries. The shipment of PPE had previously led to rising diplomatic tensions between Turkey and countries in Western Europe, which were hit hard during the first wave, such as Spain, Italy and the UK (Ant 2020; Sabbagh and McKernan 2020).

References

Ahval. 2020a. 'Turkey's intensive care units full, doctors forced to choose between patients – TTB chairman'. 30 August 2020. Accessed 16 April 2021. https://ahvalnews.com/covid-19/turkeys-intensive-care-units-full-doctors-forced-choose-between-patients-ttb-chairman.

Ahval. 2020b. 'Turkey defends decision to stop counting asymptomatic patients as COVID-19 numbers increase'. 2 October 2020. Accessed 16 April 2021. https://ahvalnews.com/fahrettin-koca/turkey-defends-decision-stop-counting-asymptomatic-patients-covid-19-numbers.

Alobalan, Heba and Ahmad Al-Moujahed. 2017. 'Muslim patients in Ramadan: A review for primary care physicians'. *Avicenna Journal of Medicine* 7(3): 81–7. https://doi.org/10.4103/ajm.ajm_76_17.

Alyanak, Oğuz. 2020. 'Faith, politics and the COVID-19 pandemic: The Turkish response'. *Medical Anthropology* 39(5): 374–5. https://doi.org/10.1080/01459740.2020.1745482.

Alyanak, Oğuz and Funda Üstek. 2013. 'Extreme measures: Invoking moral order in Turkey'. openDemocracy. Accessed 16 April 2021. https://www.opendemocracy.net/en/north-africa-west-asia/extreme-measures-invoking-moral-order-in-turkey/.

Ant, Onur. 2020. 'Turkey rolls back curbs on medical exports as outbreak subsides'. *Bloomberg*, 2 May 2020. Accessed 16 April 2021. https://www.bloomberg.com/news/articles/2020-05-02/turkey-rolls-back-curbs-on-medical-exports-as-outbreak-subsides.

Atlani-Dault, Laetitia, Jeremy K. Ward, Melissa Roy, Celine Morin and Andrew Wilson. 2020. 'Tracking online heroisation and blame in epidemics'. *The Lancet* 5(3): e137–8. https://doi.org/10.1016/S2468-2667(20)30033-5.

Başaran, Oyman. 2014. '"You are like a virus": Dangerous bodies and military medical authority in Turkey'. *Gender & Society* 28(4): 562–82. https://doi.org/10.1177/0891243214526467.

bianet English. 2019. '"Homophobic fine" against Fox Life by RTÜK'. 12 April 2020. Accessed 16 April 2021. https://m.bianet.org/english/media/207420-homophobic-fine-against-fox-life-by-rtuk.

bianet English. 2020a. 'Turkey admits not announcing numbers of all COVID-19 cases'. 1 October 2020. Accessed 16 April 2021. https://bianet.org/english/health/231876-turkey-admits-not-announcing-number-of-all-covid-19-cases.

bianet English. 2020b. 'Erdoğan calls Turkish Medical Association chair "a terrorist", hints at new law'. 14 October 2020. Accessed 16 April 2021. https://bianet.org/english/politics/232726-erdogan-calls-turkish-medical-association-chair-a-terrorist-hints-at-new-law.

bianet English. 2020c. 'Turkey starts including asymptomatic cases in its daily count, reports 28,351 cases'. 25 November 2020. Accessed 16 April 2021. https://bianet.org/english/health/235027-turkey-starts-including-asymptomatic-cases-in-its-daily-count-reports-third-highest-number-in-world?bia_source=rss.

Biçmen, Zümrüt and Zafer Bekiroğulları. 2014. 'Social problems of LGBT people in Turkey'. *Procedia-Social and Behavioral Sciences* 113: 224–33. https://doi.org/10.1016/j.sbspro.2014.01.029

Biz Bize Yeteriz Türkiyem. 2020. Ministry of Family, Labor and Social Services. Accessed 16 April 2021. https://bizbizeyeteriz.gov.tr/.

Bruce, Benjamin. 2019. 'The many faces of official Islam in Turkey'. In *Governing Islam Abroad*, edited by Benjamin Bruce, pp. 15–43. Cham, Switzerland: Springer. https://doi.org/10.1007/978-3-319-78664-3_2.

Bruinessen, Martin. 2018. 'The governance of Islam in two secular polities: Turkey's Diyanet and Indonesia's Ministry of Religious Affairs'. *European Journal of Turkish Studies* 27: 1–26.

Castro, Arachu and Paul Farmer. 2005. 'Understanding and addressing AIDS-related stigma: From anthropological theory to clinical practice in Haiti'. *American Journal of Public Health* 95(1): 53–9. https://doi.org/10.2105/AJPH.2003.028563.

Çakır, Ruşen. 1990. *Ayet ve Slogan: Türkiye'de İslami Oluşumlar*. İstanbul: Metis Yayınları.

Daar, Abdallah S. and A. Binsumeit al Khitamy. 2001. 'Bioethics for clinicians: 21. Islamic bioethics'. *CMAJ* 164(1): 60–3.

Davison, Andrew. 2003. 'Turkey, a "secular" state? The challenge of description'. *South Atlantic Quarterly* 102(2–3): 333–50. https://doi.org/10.1215/00382876-102-2-3-333.

Din İşleri Yüksek Kurulu. 2020a. *Fetva Yöntemimiz*. Accessed 16 April 2021. https://kurul.diyanet.gov.tr/FetvaYontem.

Din İşleri Yüksek Kurulu. 2020b. *İslam'ın Salgın Hastalıklara Bakışı*. Ankara: Dini Yayınlar Genel Müdürlüğü Basılı Yayınlar Daire Başkanlığı.

duvaR.English. 2020. 'Turkey's top religious official once again targets LGBT individuals' 25 April 2020. Accessed 16 April 2021. https://www.duvarenglish.com/domestic/2020/04/25/turkeys-top-religious-official-once-again-targets-lgbt-individuals/.

Dündar, Can. 2020. 'In Turkey, political Islam is getting in the way of rational health policy'. *Washington Post*, 26 March 2020. Accessed 16 April 2021. https://www.washingtonpost.com/opinions/2020/03/26/turkey-political-islam-is-getting-way-rational-health-policy/.

Erdemir, Aykan and John A. Lechner. 2020. 'The coronavirus will destroy Turkey's economy'. 8 April 2020. Accessed 16 April 2021. https://foreignpolicy.com/2020/04/08/the-coronavirus-will-destroy-turkeys-economy/.

Evin, Mehveş. 2020. 'Is this struggle against the virus, or against Turkey's doctors?' 9 July 2020. Accessed 16 April 2021. https://www.duvarenglish.com/columns/2020/07/09/is-this-struggle-against-the-virus-or-against-turkeys-doctors/.

Evrensel. 2019. 'Diyanet İşleri Başkanı Ali Erbaş, Cuma Hutbesinde LGBT+ları HEdef Aldı'. 5 July 2019. Accessed 16 April 2021. https://www.evrensel.net/haber/382508/diyanet-isleri-baskani-ali-erbas-cuma-hutbesinde-lgbti-lari-hedef-aldi.

Gill, Denise. 2016. 'Turkey's coup and the call to prayer: Sounds of violence meet Islamic devotionals'. *The Conversation*, 10 August 2016. Accessed 16 April 2021. https://theconversation.com/turkeys-coup-and-the-call-to-prayer-sounds-of-violence-meet-islamic-devotionals-63746.

Gözaydın, İştar. 2014. 'Management of religion in Turkey: The Diyanet and beyond'. In *Freedom of Religion and Belief in Turkey*, edited by Özgür Heval Çınar and Mine Yıldırım, pp. 10–35. Cambridge, UK: Cambridge Scholars Publishing.

Gregg, Jessica L. 2011. 'An unanticipated source of hope: Stigma and cervical cancer in Brazil'. *Medical Anthropology Quarterly* 25(1): 70–84. http://doi.org/10.1111/j.1548-1387.2010.01137.x.

Human Rights Watch. 2008. 'UN: General Assembly statement affirms rights for all'. 18 December 2008. Accessed 16 April 2021. https://www.hrw.org/news/2008/12/18/un-general-assembly-statement-affirms-rights-all.

Human Rights Watch. 2020a. 'Turkey: Probes over doctors' Covid-19 comments'. 10 June 2020. Accessed 16 April 2021. https://www.hrw.org/news/2020/06/10/turkey-probes-over-doctors-covid-19-comments.

Human Rights Watch. 2020b. 'Turkey: Criminal case for opposing homophobic speech'. 1 May 2020. Accessed 16 April 2021. https://www.hrw.org/news/2020/05/01/turkey-criminal-case-opposing-homophobic-speech.

Hurriyet Daily News. 2020. 'Turkey in Second Peak of First Wave of Outbreak, Says Health Minister'. 1 September 2020. Accessed 16 April 2021. https://www.hurriyetdailynews.com/turkey-in-second-peak-of-first-wave-of-outbreak-says-health-minister-157881.

International Press Institute. 2015. 'Erdogan threatens journalist in latest attack on media'. 2 June 2015. Accessed 16 April 2021. https://ipi.media/erdogan-threatens-journalist-in-latest-attack-on-media/.

Kirişci, Kemal. 2020. 'The coronavirus has led to more authoritarianism for Turkey'. *The Brookings Institute*, 8 May 2020. Accessed 16 April 2021. https://www.brookings.edu/blog/order-from-chaos/2020/05/08/the-coronavirus-has-led-to-more-authoritarianism-for-turkey/.

Kocamaner, Hikmet. 2019. 'Regulating family through religion: Secularism, Islam, and the politics of the family in contemporary Turkey'. *American Ethnologist* 46(4): 495–508. https://doi.org/10.1111/amet.12836.

Kwon, Jake and Julia Hollingsworth. 2020. 'Virus outbreak linked to Seoul clubs popular with LGBT community stokes homophobia/' *CNN*, 13 May 2020. Accessed 16 April 2021. https://edition.cnn.com/2020/05/12/asia/south-korea-club-outbreak-intl-hnk/index.html.

Lichtenstein, Bronwen. 2003. 'Stigma as a barrier to treatment of sexually transmitted infection in the American deep south: Issues of race, gender and poverty'. *Social Science & Medicine* 57(12): 2435–45. https://doi.org/10.1016/j.socscimed.2003.08.002.

Mardin, Şerif. 1977. 'Religion in modern Turkey'. *International Social Science Journal* 29(2): 279–97.

Muedini, Fait. 2018. *LGBTI Rights in Turkey: Sexuality and state in the Middle East*. Cambridge, UK: Cambridge University Press.

Mutluer, Nil. 2018. 'Diyanet's role in building the '*Yeni* (new) *Milli*' in the AKP era'. *European Journal of Turkish Studies* 27: 1–24. https://doi.org/10.4000/ejts.5953.

Özbay, Cenk. 2015. 'Same-sex sexualities in Turkey'. In *International Encyclopedia of the Social & Behavioral Sciences*, edited by James D. Wright, pp. 870–74. Exeter, UK: Elsevier Ltd. https://doi.org/10.1016/B978-0-08-097086-8.10219-3.

Öztürk, Fundanur. 2020. 'Diyanet İşleri Başkanı neden eleştirildi, Cumhurbaşkanı Erdoğan Ali Erbaş'ı nasıl savundu?' *BBC News Türkçe*, 27 April 2020. Accessed 16 April 2021. https://www.bbc.com/turkce/haberler-turkiye-52447722.

Poushter, Jacob and Nicholas Kent. 2020. 'The global divide on homosexuality persists'. *Pew Research Center*, 25 June 2020. Accessed 16 April 2021. https://www.pewresearch.org/global/2020/06/25/global-divide-on-homosexuality-persists/.

Reuters. 2020a. 'Doctors group says Turkey "hid the truth" by reporting only those with COVID-19 symptoms'. 1 October 2020. https://www.reuters.com/article/us-health-coronavirus-turkey-idUSKBN26M71J.

Reuters. 2020b. 'Turkish minister's resignation exposes tensions in Erdogan's AKP'. 14 April 2020. Accessed 16 April 2021. https://www.reuters.com/article/us-turkey-politics-erdogan/turkish-ministers-resignation-exposes-tensions-in-erdogans-akp-idUSKCN21W2M1.

Reuters. 2020c. 'Turkey rounds up hundreds for social media posts about coronavirus'. 25 March 2020. Accessed 16 April 2021. https://www.reuters.com/article/us-health-coronavirus-turkey/turkey-rounds-up-hundreds-for-social-media-posts-about-coronavirus-idUSKBN21C1SG.

Reuters. 2020d. 'Turkey defends anti-gay tweet by head of Turkish Red Crescent'. 29 June 2020. Accessed 16 April 2021. https://www.reuters.com/article/us-turkey-rights-lgbt-idUSKBN24023P.

Reporters Without Borders. 2020. 'Turkish journalist arrested for reporting Covid-19 cases'. 11 May 2020. Accessed 16 April 2021. https://rsf.org/en/news/turkish-journalists-arrested-reporting-covid-19-cases.

Sabbagh, Dan and Bethan McKernan. 2020. 'RAF plane sent to pressure Turkey to release gowns for NHS'. *The Guardian*, 20 April 2020. Accessed 16 April 2021. https://www.theguardian.com/society/2020/apr/20/raf-planes-await-order-to-set-off-to-collect-ppe-from-turkey.

Schenkkan, Nate. 2020. 'As COVID-19 threatens Turkey, Erdoğan's authoritarian playbook may undermine his own rule'. *Freedom House*, 27 April 2020. Accessed 16 April 2021. https://freedomhouse.org/article/covid-19-threatens-turkey-erdogans-authoritarian-playbook-may-undermine-his-own-rule.

Shomali, Mohammad Ali. 2008. 'Islamic bioethics: a general scheme'. *Journal of Medical Ethics and History of Medicine* 1(1): 1–8.

Singer, Merrill. 2009. 'Pathogens gone wild? Medical anthropology and the 'swine flu' pandemic'. *Medical Anthropology* 28 (3): 199–206. https://doi.org/10.1080/01459740903070451.

Songwathana, Praneed and Lenore Manderson. 2001. 'Stigma and rejection: Living with AIDS in villages in Southern Thailand'. *Medical Anthropology* 20 (1): 1–23. https://doi.org/10.1080/01459740.2001.9966185.

T24. 2019. 'Diyanet'in 2020 Bütçesi Sekiz Bakanlığı Geride Bıraktı, Bütçenin 125 Milyon Lirası Derneklere Aktarılacak'. 24 October 2020. Accessed 16 April 2021. https://t24.com.tr/haber/diyanet-in-2020-butcesi-sekiz-bakanligi-geride-birakti-butcenin-125-milyon-lirasi-derneklere-aktarilacak,845137.

The Economist. 2020. 'The coronavirus pandemic has exposed fissures within religions'. 11 April 2020. Accessed 16 April 2021. https://www.economist.com/international/2020/04/11/the-coronavirus-pandemic-has-exposed-fissures-within-religions.

Tremblay, Pınar. 2020. 'Turkey's state religious body undermines anti-coronavirus efforts'. *Al-Monitor*, 7 April 2020. Accessed 16 April 2021. https://www.al-monitor.com/pulse/originals/2020/04/turkey-religious-body-diyanet-mired-coronavirus-controversy.html.

Uğurluoğlu, Orhan. 2020. 'Orhan Uğuroğlu, Bakan Soylu'nun İstifasının Perde Arkasını Açıkladı'. YeniÇağ Gazetesi, 12 April 2020. Accessed 16 April 2021. https://www.yenicaggazetesi.com.tr/orhan-uguroglu-suleyman-soylunun-istifasinin-perde-arkasini-aciklayacak-274968h.htm.

UNAIDS. 2020. 'UNAIDS and MPact are extremely concerned about reports that LGBTI people are being blamed and abused during the COVID-19 outbreak'. 27 April 2020. Accessed 16 April 2021. https://www.unaids.org/en/resources/presscentre/pressreleaseandstatementarchive/2020/april/20200427_lgbti-covid.

United Nations Office of the High Commissioner for Human Rights. 2020. 'COVID-19 guidance'. 13 May 2020. Accessed 16 April 2021. https://www.ohchr.org/Documents/Events/COVID-19_Guidance.pdf.

Yenilmez, Meltem Ince. 2017. 'Socio-political attitude towards lesbians in Turkey'. *Sexuality & Culture* 21(1): 287–99. https://doi.org/10.1007/s12119-016-9394-6.

Yuzgun, Arslan. 1993. 'Homosexuality and police terror in Turkey'. *Journal of Homosexuality* 24(3–4): 159–70. https://doi:10.1300/J082v24n03_12.

10
Citizen vector

Scapegoating within communal boundaries in Senegal during the COVID-19 pandemic

Ato Kwamena Onoma

The Ministry of Health and Social Action of Senegal reported the first positive test for COVID-19 in the country on 2 March 2020. Thereafter, there was a slow but steady growth in the numbers of confirmed cases and fatalities, with the Ministry's Communique No. 198 of 15 September 2020 listing a total of 14,529 cases, 10,692 recoveries and 298 deaths.[1] Initial cases were all people who were infected abroad and had travelled to the country; the first case of community transmission was reported on 12 March 2020 in the Ministerial Communique No. 11. While the metropolitan area of Dakar, the capital of the country, recorded the highest number of cases, by September 2020, cases had been reported in all 14 regions of the country.

The state adopted an approach which focused on slowing the spread of the disease. Early on, it had emphasised an aggressive process of contact tracing, hospitalisation of positive cases, and testing and isolating the contacts of those who tested positive in specific locations (Faye 2020b). Measures adopted in mid-March 2020 included the closure of the country's airspace and land borders, suspension of commercial passenger flights and interregional travel within the country, and the closure of schools, places of worship, bars, night clubs, restaurants and beaches. All forms of assembly were banned in public and private spaces, a night-time curfew was imposed, and markets were closed on certain days of the week to facilitate their disinfection (Faye 2020a). Senegalese social anthropologist Sylvain Faye (2020a) has written on people's resistance to some of these measures, many of which were progressively eased from

11 May 2020 as the president, Macky Sall, sought to reduce the economic impact of the pandemic by encouraging Senegalese to 'learn how to live in the presence of the virus' (BIG 2020).

The first four cases of disease involved European citizens who had travelled to the country. On 11 March 2020, the Ministry of Health and Social Action reported COVID-19 case No. 5 to be a male Senegalese emigrant based in Italy and visiting relatives in the country. In the days that followed, both the Ministry and the media reported more cases of Senegalese emigrants returning from Southern European countries like Spain and Italy who tested positive for COVID-19. These emigrants, based in Southern Europe, are predominantly from the central west and major urban areas across the country, and so they include a mix of ethnic groups. They started migrating to Italy and Spain in the 1980s, marking a turn from earlier migration that originated in the Senegal River Valley and tended to flow towards France and other African countries (Fall 2017; Mbaye 2005; Riccio 2008; Tall 2008a; Mboup 2000). Popular views on these migrants have swayed over time and space, from adulation and glorification to vilification and derision (Mbodji 2008; Uberti 2014; Riccio and Uberti 2013). They are commonly referred to in Senegal as 'Modou'; 'Modou' is a shortened form of the name 'Momodou', a variant of the name of the Prophet Mohammed and a common given name among these migrants. The repetition follows similar patterns of double iteration in the Wolof language, the lingua franca in Senegal. In this chapter, I use the term 'Senegalese emigrants' because some regard 'Modou' as pejorative (Thiam 2020). I note otherwise when I refer to other migrant populations.

While a number of these emigrants travelled legally to their destination countries and then overstayed visas, many more migrated illegally, using routes that involved dangerous crossings over the Atlantic Ocean, Mediterranean Sea and Sahara Desert (Willems 2008; Tall 2008b; Riccio 2008; Tall 2008b; Uberti 2014). Most earlier migrants were farmers from rural areas who lacked formal education; those who migrated more recently were from urban areas and were informal sector workers, unemployed youth, small business owners, and in some cases, employed professionals (Uberti 2014; Tandian 2008; Tall 2008a). In their host countries they took up diverse employment opportunities, with many working as hawkers, farm labourers, and unskilled and semi-skilled capacity in manufacturing industry and the construction and hospitality sectors (Riccio 2008, 85–7; Tall 2008b). The vast majority of these migrants are male. They often leave their wives and children in Senegal, partly to maximise the savings they can repatriate back home (Tall 2008a, 53–4; Uberti 2014).

The announcement of COVID-19 case No. 5 and media coverage of other Senegalese emigrants returning to the country from areas with high numbers of COVID-19 cases raised concerns about returning citizens, as evident in many other countries across the world (Zeidan 2020; Boda 2020; Online Reporters 2020). In Senegal, these concerns degenerated into scapegoating these emigrants (Faye 2020a). On radio, various social media platforms including WhatsApp and Facebook, and in comments on news stories, people widely blamed these emigrants for spreading the disease in the country. In comments in response to online news stories, some Senegalese portrayed these emigrants as negligent or thoughtless, unwittingly spreading the disease by refusing to respect the lockdown rules in Europe and by not getting tested or self-isolating before interacting with people upon their return to Senegal (Gueye 2020a, 2020b, 2020c; Seneweb News 2020a, 2020b, 2020c). Other commentators of online news stories cast them as unpatriotic and wilful, returning to Senegal knowing they carried the virus and intent on spreading the disease and ruining the country (Gueye 2020a, 2020b, 2020c; Seneweb News 2020a, 2020b, 2020c).

In online comments on news stories, people called on these emigrants to stay away from Senegal and put pressure on the government to suspend commercial flights, close the country's land borders and refuse entry at border posts, thus forcing emigrants to return to their points of departure or languish in the desert (Seneweb News 2020b, 2020c; Gueye 2020c). These online comments mirrored thoughts expressed on radio and on social media platforms like Facebook and WhatsApp. Across the country, people reported returning emigrant neighbours to the authorities who proceeded to round up, question, test and quarantine them (Dakaractu 2020; Sakhanokho 2020). The Observatory of the Senegalese of the Diaspora, a non-governmental organisation created in 2013 with the stated goal of 'promoting the interests of Senegalese Diasporas around the world by all legal means', condemned this scapegoating in a communique on 13 April 2020 (Thiam 2020). These attacks were so pervasive even earlier that on 17 March 2020, the Ministry of Health and Social Action decided to reduce the amount of detail it provided in its daily communiques to curb the scapegoating of 'foreigners and emigrants' (Willane 2020).

The scapegoating of migrants during the COVID-19 pandemic in many ways mirrored the ways Peul migrants from Guinea to Senegal were cast as vectors during the 2013–16 outbreak of Ebola Virus Disease (EVD) that centred on the Mano River Basin countries of Sierra Leone, Liberia and Guinea. The difficult days under the first president of Guinea, Sekou

Touré, saw large-scale migration of Peul – known as Fulani in other areas of West and Central Africa – to Senegal; this flow of migrants has continued in a less intense manner since then (Diallo 2009). As the EVD epidemic of 2013–16 threatened to spread beyond the borders of the Mano River Basin countries, Peul migrants were described as spreading EVD in Senegal. Some Senegalese began to call for the country's borders with Guinea to be closed to curb what was portrayed as an uncontrolled 'horde' of Peul migrants entering the country. Others called for Peul migrants to be counted and secluded, and for others to avoid physical contact with them by boycotting their shops and sitting apart from them on public transportation (Onoma 2020a). The diagnosis of the only case of EVD in Senegal in August 2014 – a young Peul student who was in Senegal to visit relatives – only heightened the scapegoating of this community (Onoma 2017).

The treatment of Senegalese emigrants as vectors of COVID-19 in Senegal differs from that of Peul migrants during the EVD epidemic in important ways. Unlike Peul migrants who were scapegoated in Senegal where they were considered as foreigners, Senegalese emigrants were scapegoated in their country of origin, a place where they are not only recognised as citizens but are also usually celebrated as national heroes toiling abroad for the benefit of their families, communities and country (Diop 2008, 28; Riccio 2005; 2008; Tall 2002; Fouquet 2008; Mbodji 2008).

The scapegoating of certain populations during disease outbreaks is very common and has been widely studied across public health outbreaks including the plague, cholera, yellow fever, HIV, MERS, SARS and EVD (Benton and Dionne 2015; M'Bokolo 1982; White 2010; Mason 2012; Echenberg 2002; Eichelberger 2007; Markel and Stern 2002; Ngalamulume 2012; Ginzburg 1990; Eamon 1998). These outbursts usually target non-citizens, foreigners and those generally cast as 'other'. People blame these outsiders for the origin and spread of diseases, subject them to verbal and physical attacks, and advocate their exclusion from the national territory or mass seclusion (Onoma 2020a; Benton and Dionne 2015; Monson 2017; Eichelberger 2007; Markel and Stern 2002). Motivations for these outbursts include concern over their spreading of germs from their places of origin, and broader anxieties over what is portrayed as their resistance of public health measures (White 2010; Gussow 1989; Echenberg 2002; Onoma 2017; Mason 2012; Trauner 1978; Onoma 2018). The process of constructing these others as public health dangers is often embedded in long-standing processes of identity formation that fashion the civilised and hygienic self by distinguishing it from the other cast as uncivilised and insalubrious (Onoma 2017), and anxieties over the potential propagation of diseases are enmeshed in concerns over the spread of what are portrayed as the less than desirable behaviours and values of these others.

In this chapter, I explore the scapegoating of Senegalese emigrants in their country of origin by their fellow citizens to reflect on the extent to which communal boundaries shape scapegoating during public health crises. I elaborate on the lively debate between Senegalese based in the country and emigrants over citizenship and its value, during the troubling times of the COVID-19 pandemic. I examine the gap between discourses that portray communal boundaries as critical in social interactions, and the lived experiences of people who regularly work around these boundaries in their quotidian interactions. Pointing out that scapegoating during public health crises is not reserved for those portrayed as 'foreigners' adds to the literature on social relations in Africa and beyond. This raises questions of the extent to which a focus on these boundaries affords an understanding of the intricacies of social interactions during times of crisis when such boundaries are most vociferously invoked.

I base this chapter on my analysis of online comments on news stories concerning the evolution of the COVID-19 pandemic and its unfolding in Senegal. These online comments only constitute one facet of popular discourses that occurred over radio, social media platforms like WhatsApp and Facebook, and in face-to-face interactions. There are clear challenges with the use of online comments in social analysis (Henrich and Holmes 2013; Taylor et al. 2016), including knowing whether people are who they claim to be. Also, the propensity for anonymity to encourage people to express their views without censure or restraint makes it difficult (for social analysts) to claim that comments online represent wider social views. The use of spam bots to comment on online content further undermines our capacity to gauge popular views (Schneier 2020). At the same time, these comments are readily accessible and perceived anonymity may encourage people to share their 'true' views (Henrich and Holmes 2013; Taylor et al. 2016).

Communal boundaries and social relations

During public health crises, those outside of communal boundaries, identified as strangers and foreigners, can become the targets of scapegoating and abuse, while those within these lines, defined as citizens and autochthones, are spared maltreatment and cast as unfortunate victims (Benton and Dionne 2015; M'Bokolo 1982; White 2010; Mason

2012; Eichelberger 2007; Markel and Stern 2002; Ngalamulume 2012; Ginzburg 1990; Eamon 1998; Onoma 2020a). In exclusionary discourses that proliferate worldwide, citizens and autochthones are said to properly belong to the territory in which they reside, where they are imbued with a plenitude of rights, including to residence, land ownership, participation in economic activities and politics, and standing before judicial systems. Strangers across the intercommunal line, in contrast, are cast as interlopers who have left their own homes to appropriate and settle in the territories of others. Their rights to own land, participate in economic activities, contest elections, vote and enjoy a peaceful life are challenged in discourses that urge them to go back to where they properly belong. Such invective is often accompanied by physical attacks and this has sometimes led to xenophobic terror, mass expulsion and genocide (Mamdani 2002; Onoma 2013; Jackson 2006; Geschiere 2009).

While exclusionary discourses often portray boundaries between communities as thick walls that prevent links and interactions across groups, the specification of these boundaries is characterised by great ambiguity. The idea of origins as deployed in these discourses is nebulous and the subject of both manipulation and contestation. Autochthones are described alternately as those who have sprung out of their territory, as opposed to those who moved there from elsewhere, those who arrived first in the territory, those who arrived there before other populations against whom they are involved in contestations, and so on (Jackson 2006; Konings 2008; Nyamnjoh 2015; Geschiere and Nyamnjoh 2000). As noted in the literature, the determination of precedence in these discourses and disputes is a highly political process to which various resources, including force, are regularly deployed (Berry 2000; Murphy and Bledsoe 1987).

The specification of territory to which groups belong invokes deeply contested geopolitical questions. Actors involved in disputes over where communal markers lie and who lives on either side of these boundaries regularly switch between geopolitical scales (village, town, district, region, nation-state), making these contestations complex and leaving very few safe from potential accusations of being strangers (Jackson 2006; Onoma 2018). While judico-legal citizens of a country may band together to expel migrants from another country, citizens belonging to an ethnic group may expel their fellow citizens from what is cast as an ethnic homeland, demanding that they go back to their own area of the country (Eyoh 1999; Geschiere and Nyamnjoh 2000; Geschiere 2009).

In conjuring neatly bounded communities demarcated by thick boundaries, these discourses underestimate the flux and fluidity of (inter) communal markers, the politics of borderlines, and the tendency of people to cross boundaries and go where they are thought to not belong (Nyamnjoh 2016; Jackson 2006; Bauman 1997; Douglas 1984). They underestimate the extent to which borders between communities constitute zones of encounters and interactions rather than barriers that are immutable and able to guarantee absolute separation (Nyamnjoh 2015a, 2015b; Hay 2014, 2016). Given this, we need to critically examine the ability of these boundaries to protect those within their confines from indignities and violence, while exposing those outside of their ambit to scapegoating and social exclusion during public health crises.

The situation of migrants troubles assumptions about the extent to which communal lines serve to protect those within them – citizens – from exclusion in their homelands, while exposing 'strangers' who have wandered away from their homelands to scapegoating. Those who discriminate against immigrants and ask them to 'go back home' imply that these travellers and their offspring only properly belong in the 'places of origin' that they have left behind (Eyoh 1999; Geschiere and Nyamnjoh 2000; Onoma 2013). The ties of emigrants to and their standing in their places of origin are far more precarious than these exclusionary discourses suggest. These ties are the subject of constant negotiation and contestation (Onoma 2018; Nyamnjoh 2005; 2011). Scholars recognise that the extent to which those at home see generations of emigrants as still possessing the full plethora of rights that accrue to 'sons and daughters of the soil' depends on factors that go beyond their ability to prove deep family ties to 'home' areas. Scholars have cited visits to these home areas, financial support of family and friends there, restraint in the face of exploitative and abusive behaviour by relatives at home, accessibility at all times to those at home, support of community members who also happen to be abroad, and participation in local development projects and investment in their home country, as determinants of the status of these ties (Ferguson 1999; Englund 2004; Tabappsi 1999; Nyamnjoh 2001; 2005; de Sardan 1999; Lindley 2007; Geschiere and Nyamnjoh 2000; Onoma 2018; Tazanu 2012). Emigrants who neglect these 'duties' potentially face sanctions that include insults and name-calling, threats of and reported mystical attacks, including through witchcraft and marabouts, and ostracism by their families and communities at large (Tabappsi 1999; Nyamnjoh 2001; 2005; Lindley 2007; Onoma 2018; Tazanu 2012).

Remittances have come to assume a central position in interactions between migrants and people left in their home communities, and the perceived refusal of some migrants to remit is a central cause of problems with their relatives in home communities (Nyamnjoh 2006; Onoma 2018; Lindley 2007). But the attitude of home communities to remittances is ambivalent, mixing covetousness with concern (Nyamnjoh 2011). Remittances, like other forms of external interventions, reshape landscapes and reorder hierarchies by favouring and empowering some while disempowering and marginalising others. Concern over financial remittances also coincides with trepidation over 'foreign' values, norms and practices that are brought back by migrants from their travels abroad (Riccio 2005, 2008; Uberti 2014; Nyamnjoh 2011). Anxiety over emigrants bringing COVID-19 to Senegal plays into the tensions between gratitude for remittances and apprehension about the invasion of Senegal by not only of remittances, norms and practices, but also disease. Fears of the spread of COVID-19 by returning migrants capture broader preoccupations with the transgression of boundaries and upending of social orders by movements and flows, which people at once embrace, agonise over and even resist.

COVID-19 and the lightness of citizenship in Senegal

Senegalese emigrants in Southern European countries are widely recognised as investing significantly to maintain healthy relations with their home communities (Daffe 2008; Tall 2008b; Riccio 2005; 2008; Mboup 2000; Tall 1994; Barro 2008; Gueye 2002). Like the Cameroonian 'bushfallers' described by Nyamnjoh (2011), they approach migration as going abroad to work, where they amass and repatriate wealth, returning back home at the earliest possibility (Tall 2008b). Once they acquire residential and work permits, many regularly visit Senegal to spend time with wives and children left behind, to see other members of the family, to attend religious events, and to establish and monitor businesses that many of them create in the retail and wholesale, real estate, transportation, agriculture and fisheries sectors. Many are uninterested in integrating into the communities abroad where they find themselves, often seeing themselves strictly as sojourners (Riccio 2002, 2008; Fouquet 2008).

These emigrants contribute to the livelihoods of their families by paying utility bills, covering the costs of schooling, hospitalisations, funerals and baptisms, and covering daily expenses on food. They contribute to community development projects in their areas of origin, including the construction of mosques, schools and clinics, the acquisition of ambulances, sinking of boreholes and so on. In addition, they invest heavily in many sectors of the Senegalese economy (Daffe 2008; Tall

2008b; Riccio 2005; 2008; Mboup 2000; Daffe 2008; Tall 1994; Barro 2008; Gueye 2002). Senegal is one of the highest recipients of migrant remittances in Africa (Diop 2008), and these transfers were estimated at US$2.5 billion in 2019 (World Bank n.d.). In a 2001 study, in some villages in the Louga Region of Senegal, 90 per cent of household revenue was identified as coming from migrant remittances (Tall 2008b, 54).

In this context, the question of citizenship assumed a central position in conversations on scapegoating; it was one of the principal grounds on which some emigrants and some Senegalese residents questioned the legitimacy of scapegoating, because people who were targeted were within the ambit of their own communities. One version of this argument focused on the space where scapegoating was taking place, contending that emigrants could not be scapegoated in Senegal because they were Senegalese, were born in the country and had sacrificed themselves through travel for the wellbeing of their families, communities and country (Seneweb News 2020a). This argument partakes in the fetishisation of citizenship that was a feature of early responses to the COVID-19 pandemic. Border closures that ostensibly sought to curb the spread of the virus through international travel were often carefully crafted to allow citizens to return 'home', including when they were infected by COVID-19. This move ignored the fact that many people do not call their countries of citizenship 'home', and had no interest in going to these places to shelter from the pandemic. Further, it elides the fact that many people call territories where they do not have citizenship home, and that they needed, for various reasons, to return to these places during the pandemic (Onoma 2020c). These moves are grounded in the territorialisation of identity that ties people to specific geographical terrains (Mamdani 2002; Malkki 2009), ignoring the ability and tendency of people to fashion temporary and situational ties to multiple homes.

A second argument focused on the perpetrators of scapegoating. The contention was that Senegalese could not scapegoat these emigrants since they were of the same nationality. One can understand from this argument that scapegoating should only occur between people on opposing sides of intercommunal boundaries. One commentator, on an online news story, exclaimed: 'Unbelievable! Brothers who are racist toward their fellow citizens!' (Seneweb News 2020a). There were overt efforts by some to shift attention to the 'proper' targets of scapegoating, 'foreigners'. People repeatedly brought up the fact that the first four cases of coronavirus infection in Senegal were European citizens, and that while news stories proliferated about the threat posed by Senegalese emigrants, Europeans infected with the disease continued to enter the country. These Europeans, instead of the emigrants, some commentators implied, should be held responsible for the spread of disease. One commentator on an online news story could not hide his or her incredulity at the 'misplaced' targeting of the Senegalese: 'You people like to lynch your own compatriots, but as for strangers, they are just great!' (Seneweb News 2020d). Other online commentators blamed conspiracies that shifted blame away from 'strangers' and onto Senegalese emigrants as perpetrated by European embassies, the Senegalese state and even sections of the media (Seneweb News 2020a).

Underlying this incredulity over the scapegoating of 'fellow citizens' and 'compatriots' was a primordialist vision of identity and ties imbued with notions of blood and origins. This perspective posits interactions as posterior to and almost entirely shaped by ties of blood and common origins (Mbembe 2001; Diagne 2002). It strays from the view that context-laden interactions are what define ties, which are always tentative and evolving.

The urge to respect the law of communal boundaries, by showing solidarity towards fellow Senegalese emigrants and scapegoating Europeans instead, reflected a global pandemic of xenophobia that accompanied the public health crisis of COVID-19 (Zhu 2020; Human Rights Watch 2020; Eric 2020), as also occurred in other disease outbreaks (Benton and Dionne 2015; White 2010; Mason 2012; Eichelberger 2007; Markel and Stern 2002). In Senegal, these calls did not always fall on receptive ears. Being a citizen, including one who had contributed to the development of the country, their community, and the wellbeing of their kin, it was asserted, did not give a person the right to endanger the country and those who live in it (Gueye 2020d). A commentator on one online story pointed out that '(t)he fact that you send Western Union or Ria to your family in need does not give you the right to contaminate Senegalese' (Seneweb News 2020b).

People argued that what was important was not which community people belonged to, but what threat they posed to other Senegalese and to the country. Some argued that Senegalese emigrants from Southern European countries posed a greater danger than foreigners on account of their numbers, their membership of wider networks in Senegal, and the difficulties they faced in self-isolating and practising social distancing relative to foreigners (Seneweb News 2020a, 2020e). Sylvain Faye (2020a) has written on the challenges with social distancing, self-isolation and confinement in Senegal. In addition to these challenges, people invoked the supposedly 'uneducated', 'undisciplined' and 'stubborn' character of these emigrants. Faye has also discussed the 'authoritarian' visions and measures that undergird the tendency to denounce, as evidence of stubbornness and indiscipline, people's efforts to balance the imperative of pandemic control and prevention with the needs of precarious lives lived in a context where propitiousness for these measures are far from certain (Faye 2020a, 2020b). For Senegalese emigrants, these characterisations also suggest frustrations over the new-found celebrity status of formerly unemployed youth, who after high-risk voyages abroad, occasionally return with fortunes that better educated and formally employed relatives and neighbours in Senegal could only dream of.

The focus on xenophobia during epidemics accords with the broader view that posits communal lines as overwhelmingly influential on social interactions (Ekeh 1975; Jackson 2006; de Sardan 1999; Geschiere 2009; Geschiere and Nyamnjoh 2000). While the literature emphasises 'others' as the targets of scapegoating during epidemics and pandemics (Onoma 2017; Benton and Dionne 2015; M'Bokolo 1982; White 2010; Mason 2012; Echenberg 2002; Eichelberger 2007; Markel and Stern 2002; Ngalamulume 2012; Ginzburg 1990; Eamon 1998), the scapegoating of fellow citizens in Senegal shows that communal boundaries do not always exert determinate influences on social interactions. This insight ties in with a wealth of work that questions the extent to which communal lines shape quotidian interactions. Nyamnjoh (2015a, 2015b), in his work on conviviality, has emphasised the ways in which people and communities, including those who emphasise these lines as primordial to social interactions, routinely work around these boundaries. The literature on the incorporation of strangers in African communities (Guyer 1993; Bledsoe 1980; Colson 1970) has emphasised the capacity of people to rope those considered as assets into their families and clans regardless of which side of the communal line they fell. This same literature underlined the limited extent to which belonging on the same side of the communal line, including having jural ties, influenced the tendency toward conviviality in African society (Murphy and Bledsoe 1987). In my previous work on refugee-host relations (Onoma 2013), I have shown how belonging to different ethnic groups did not discourage Guineans from incorporating refugees from Sierra Leone and Liberia during recent civil wars in those countries.

In social research on medicine and diseases, Cohn's reflections (2018) on solidarity across communal lines during communicable disease outbreaks question the tendency to see periods of epidemics as always coinciding with xenophobia. My previous reflections (Onoma 2020b) on how acts of xenophilia and conviviality persist even during outbreaks of xenophobia further illustrate the tendency to work around communal lines, even when people invoke these boundaries most vociferously. This work of destabilising the influence of communal boundaries on social relations is also evident in Napier's reflections on the implications of advances in the fields of theoretical immunology and stem cells, regenerative medicine and epigenetics, for our understanding of social relations (2012, 2017). He points at our frequent and almost compulsive search for and outreach to the other over lines that bound the self, and argues that such outreach is beneficial to the self. Of particular importance in the work of Napier is the way in which he casts this outreach and its consequences as fundamental to the constitution of the self. This raises the spectre that there may not be a well bounded and stable self that is anterior to these interactions across lines (2012, 2017).

Conclusion

This account of Senegalese emigrants who are scapegoated by their 'compatriots' in 'their own country' suggests that communal lines do not necessarily help us make sense of the social dynamics that are characteristic of epidemics. Consistent with other literature on relations between migrants and home communities, and the exploitation, contestations and tensions that bedevil these relations, I suggest that citizenship and being on the 'right side' of communal boundaries does not necessarily protect emigrants from the indignity of scapegoating during crises such as that of pandemics.

In scapegoating Senegalese emigrants based in Southern Europe during the COVID-19 pandemic, no effort was made to question their Senegalese citizenship, and participants in debates over these emigrants displayed their capacity to scapegoat even those who they recognise as legitimate members of the Senegalese body politic. People did not claim that these emigrants were 'no longer part of us'. Instead, the argument was that 'they are dangerous so we should keep them at arm's length even if they happen to be part of us'. People did not cast them as other in order to scapegoat them. The understanding instead was that certain members of the body politic can be dangerous, and the community has a right to protect itself by ensuring their distance. Communal boundaries did not have a determinate effect on how people pursued what they saw as the goal of securing their health, no matter how problematic their actions were.

Note

1 The communiques of the Ministry of Health and Social Action are on the website of the Ministry at http://www.sante.gouv.sn/taxonomy/term/14 (accessed 16 September 2020).

References

Barro, Issa. 2008. 'Emigration, transferts financiers et creation de PME dans l'habitat'. In *Le Senegal des Migrations: Mobilites, Identities et Societies*, edited by Momar-Coumba Diop, pp. 133–52. Paris, France: Karthala.
Bauman, Zygmunt. 1997. *Postmodernity and its Discontents*. New York: New York University Press.
Benton, Adia and Kim Yi Dionne. 2015. 'International political economy and the 2014 West African Ebola outbreak'. *African Studies Review* 58(1): 223–36.
Berry, Sara. 2000. *Chiefs Know Their Boundaries: Essays on property, power, and the past in Asante, 1896–1996*. Portsmouth, UK: Heinemann.
BIG (Bureau d'Information Gouvernmentale). 2020. '"Nous devons apprendre a vivre en presence du virus" SEM Macky Sall, President de la Republique du Senegal'. Accessed 16 September 2020. http://www.big.gouv.sn/index.php/2020/05/12/nous-devons-apprendre-a-vivre-en-presence-du-virus-sem-macky-sall-president-de-la-republique-du-senegal/.
Bledsoe, Caroline. 1980. 'The manipulation of Kpelle social fatherhood'. *Ethnology* 19: 29–45.
Boda, Tharun, 2020. 'Returnees contribute to rise in COVID-19 infections'. *The Hindu Times*, 30 May 2020. Accessed 5 June 2020. https://www.thehindu.com/news/national/andhra-pradesh/returnees-contribute-to-rise-in-covid-19-infections/article31712804.ece.
Cohn, S. 2018. *Epidemics: Hate and compassion from the plague of Athens to AIDS*. New York: Oxford University Press.
Colson, Elisabeth. 1970. 'The assimilation of aliens among Zambian Tonga'. In *From Tribe to Nation in Africa: Studies in incorporation processes*, edited by Ronald Cohen and John Middleton, pp. 35–54. Scranton, PA: Chandler Publishing Company.
Dakaractu. 2020. 'Coronavirus à Touba /Modou-Modou rentrés à Touba en catimini: Les voisins versent dans la dénonciation pour se tirer d'affaire'. 19 March 2020. Accessed 5 June 2020. https://www.dakaractu.com/CORONAVIRUS-A-TOUBA-Modou-Modou-rentres-a-Touba-en-catimini-Les-voisins-versent-dans-la-denonciation-pour-se-tirer-d_a185606.html.
Daffe, Gaye. 2008. 'Les transferts d'argent des migrants senegalais entre espoir et risqies de dependence'. In *Le Senegal des Migrations: Mobilites, identities et societies*, edited by Momar-Coumba Diop, pp. 105–31. Paris, France: Karthala.
de Sardan, Jean-Paul Olivier. 1999. 'A moral economy of corruption in Africa?' *The Journal of Modern African Studies* 37(1): 25–52.
Diagne, Souleymane Bachir. 2002. 'Keeping Africanity open'. *Public Culture* 14(3): 621–23. https://muse.jhu.edu/article/26293.
Diallo, Papa Ibrahima. 2009. *Les Guinéens de Dakar: Migration et intégration en Afrique de l'Ouest*. Paris: L'Harmattan.
Diop, Momar-Coumba. 2008. 'Presentation. Mobilites, etat et societe'. In *Le Senegal des Migrations: Mobilites, identities et societies*, edited by Momar-Coumba Diop, pp. 13–36. Paris, France: Karthala.
Douglas, Mary. 1984. *Purity and Danger: An analysis of the concepts of pollution and taboo*. London: Routledge.
Eamon, William. 1998. 'Cannibalism and contagion: Framing syphilis in counter-reformation Italy'. *Early Science and Medicine* 3(1):1–31.
Echenberg, Myron. 2002. *Black Death, White Medicine: Bubonic plague and the politics of public health in colonial Senegal, 1914–1945*. Portsmouth, NH: Heinemann.
Eichelberger, Laura. 2007. 'SARS and New York's Chinatown: The politics of risk and blame during an epidemic of fear'. *Social Science & Medicine* 65(6): 1284–95.
Ekeh, Peter. 1975. 'Colonialism and the two publics in Africa'. *Comparative Studies in Society and History* 17(1): 91–112.
Englund, Harri. 2004. 'Cosmopolitanism and the devil in Malawi'. *Ethnos* 69(3): 293–316.

Eric. 2020. 'An unprecedented rupture in China-Africa relations'. 13 April 2020. Accessed 5 June 2020. https://mailchi.mp/chinaafricaproject/a-rupture-in-china-africa-relations-1182057?e=ea9eb5ea5e.

Eyoh, Dickson. 1999. 'Community, citizenship and the politics of ethnicity in postcolonial Africa'. In *Sacred Places and Public Quarrels: African cultural and economic landscapes*, edited by Ezikiel Kalipeni and Paul Tiyambe Zeleza, pp. 271–300. Trenton, NJ: Africa World Press.

Fall, Papa Demba. 2017. *Des Francenabe aux Modou-Modou: L'émigration sénégalaise contemporaine*. Dhaka, Senegal: L'Harmattan.

Faye, Sylvain. 2020a. 'La distanciation sociale au Sénégal, un remède au Covid-19 qui a du mal à passer'. *The Conversation*, 29 May 29. Accessed 16 September 2020. https://theconversation.com/la-distanciation-sociale-au-senegal-un-remede-au-covid-19-qui-a-du-mal-a-passer-134810.

Faye, Sylvain. 2020b. 'La peur, la stigmatisation et la culpabilisation expliquent le refus de certains malades de révéler les cas contacts'. *Le Soleil*, 11 May 2020. Accessed 16 September 2020. https://4bee979e-9181-4f06-b0c4c163999ccbbf.filesusr.com/ugd/4f395b_27944c5272a94271927ee6bd6cdf389c.pdf.

Ferguson, James. 1999. *Expectations of Modernity: Myths and meanings of urban life on the Zambian copper belt*. Berkeley, CA: University of California Press.

Fouquet, Thomas. 2008. 'Migrations et "glocalisation" dakaroises'. In *Le Senegal des Migrations: Mobilites, identities et societies*, edited by Momar-Coumba Diop, pp. 241–76. Paris: Karthala.

Geschiere, Peter. 2009. *The Perils of Belonging: Autochthony, citizenship and exclusion in Africa*. Chicago, IL: University of Chicago Press.

Geschiere, Peter and Francis Nyamnjoh. 2000. 'Capitalism and autochthony: The seesaw of mobility and belonging'. *Public Culture* 12(2): 423–52.

Ginzburg, Carlo. 1990. 'Deciphering the sabbath'. In *Early Modern European Witchcraft: Centres and peripheries*, edited by Bengt Ankarloo and Gustav Henningsen, pp. 121–38. New York: Oxford University Press.

Gueye, Cheikh. 2002. *Touba: La capital des Mourides*. Paris: Karthala.

Gueye, Salla. 2020a. 'Coronavirus "Une vingtaine de 'Modou-Modou' suivis à Louga" (Médecin-chef)'. 20 March 2020. Accessed 4 June 2020. https://www.seneweb.com/news/Societe/coronavirus-laquo-une-vingtaine-de-lsquo_n_312153.html.

Gueye, Salla. 2020b. 'Coronavirus: Le "Modou-Modou" vavait regagné Touba à bord d'un "Allo taxi"'. 12 March 2020. Accessed 4 June 2020. https://www.seneweb.com/news/Societe/coronavirus-le-laquo-modou-modou-rsquo-r_n_311400.html.

Gueye, Salla. 2020c. '[Photos-Vidéo] Coronavirus: 13 "Modou-Modou" bloqués à la frontière entre le Maroc et la Mauritanie'. 19 March 2020. Accessed 4 June 2020. https://www.seneweb.com/news/International/coronavirus-13-quot-modou-modou-quot-sen_n_312017.html.

Gueye, Salla. 2020d. 'Covid-19: Le Modou-Modou de Touba craque et demande pardon aux Sénégalais'. 14 April 2020. Accessed 4 June 2020. https://www.seneweb.com/news/Sante/covid-19-le-modou-modou-de-touba-craque-_n_314647.html.

Gussow, Zachary. 1989. *Leprosy, Racism, and Public Health: Social policy in chronic disease control*. Boulder, CO: Westview Press.

Guyer, Jane. 1993. 'Wealth in people and self-realisation in Equatorial Africa'. *Man* 28(1): 243–65.

Hay, Paula. 2014. *Negotiating Conviviality: The use of information and communication technologies by migrant members of the Bay Community Church in Cape Town*. Bamenda, Cameroon: Langaa RPCIG.

Hay, Paula. 2016. 'Negotiating intimacy, distance and marginality: Migration, religion and the use of ICTs at the Bay Community Church in Cape Town'. In *Mobilities, ICTs and Marginality in Africa: Comparative perspectives*, edited by Francis Nyamnjoh and Ingrid Brudvig, pp. 71–84. Cape Town, South Africa: HSRC Press.

Henrich, Nathalie and Bev Holmes. 2013. 'Web news readers' comments: Towards developing a methodology for using on-line comments in social inquiry'. *Journal of Media and Communication Studies* 5(1): 1–4.

Human Rights Watch. 2020. 'Covid-19 fueling anti-Asian racism and xenophobia worldwide: National action plans needed to counter intolerance'. 12 May 2020. Accessed 5 June 2020. https://www.hrw.org/news/2020/05/12/covid-19-fueling-anti-asian-racism-and-xenophobia-worldwide.

Jackson, Stephen. 2006. 'Sons of which soil? The language and politics of autochthony in Eastern D.R. Congo'. *African Studies Review* 49(2): 95–123.

Konings, Piet. 2008. 'Autochthony and ethnic cleansing in the post-colony: The 1966 Tombel disturbances in Cameroon'. *The International Journal of African Historical Studies* 41(2): 203–22.
Lindley, Anna. 2007. 'Remittances in fragile settings: A Somali case study'. HiCN Working Papers 27. Households in Conflict Network. https://ideas.repec.org/p/hic/wpaper/27.html.
Malkki, Liisa. 2009. 'National Geographic: The rooting of peoples and the territorialisation of national identity among scholars and refugees'. *Cultural Anthropology* 7(1): 24–44. https://doi.org/10.1525/can.1992.7.1.02a00030.
Mamdani, Mahmood. 2002. *When Victims Become Killers: Colonialism, nativism and genocide in Rwanda*. Princeton, NJ: Princeton University Press.
Markel, Howard and Alexandra Stern. 2002. 'The foreignness of germs: The persistent association of immigrants and disease in American society'. *The Milband Quarterly* 80(4): 757–88.
Mason, Katherine. 2012. 'Mobile migrants, mobile germs: Migration, contagion, and boundary-building in Shenzhen, China after SARS'. *Medical Anthropology* 31(2): 113–31. https://doi.org/10.1080/01459740.2011.610845.
Mbaye, S.A. 2005. *Modou*. Las Palmas, Spain: Antoart Ediciones.
Mbembe, Achille. 2001. 'African modes of self-writing'. *Identity, Culture and Politics* 2(1): 1–39.
Mbodji, Mamadou. 2008. 'Imaginaires et migrations: Le cas du Senegal'. In *Le Senegal des Migrations: Mobilites, Identities et Societies*, edited by Momar-Coumba Diop, pp. 305–19. Paris, France: Karthala.
M'Bokolo. Elikia. 1982. 'Peste et société urbaine à Dakar: L'épidémie de 1914'. *Cahiers d'Études Africaines* 22 (85/86): 13–46.
Mboup, Mourtala. 2000. *Les senegalais d'Italie. Emigres, agents du changement social*. Paris, France: l'Harmattan.
Monson, Sarah. 2017. 'Ebola as African: American media discourses of panic and otherization'. *Africa Today* 63(3): 2–27.
Murphy, William and Caroline Bledsoe. 1987. 'Kinship and territory in the history of a Kpelle Chiefdom (Liberia)'. In *The African Frontier: The Reproduction of Traditional African Societies*, edited by Igor Kopytoff, 121–47. Bloomington, IN: Indiana University Press.
Napier, A. David. 2012. 'Nonself help: How immunology might reframe the Enlightenment'. *Cultural Anthropology* 27(1): 122–37.
Napier, A. David. 2017. 'Epidemics and xenophobia, or, why xenophilia matters'. *Social Research* 84(1): 59–81.
Ngalamulume, Kalala. 2012. *Colonial Pathologies, Environment, and western medicine in Saint-Louis-du-Senegal, 1867–1920*. New York: Peter Lang.
Nyamnjoh, Francis. 2001. 'Delusions of development and the enrichment of witchcraft discourses in Cameroon'. In *Magical Interpretations, Material Realities: Modernity, witchcraft and the occult in postcolonial Africa*, edited by Henrietta L. Moore and Todd Sanders, pp. 28–49. London: Routledge.
Nyamnjoh, Francis. 2005. 'Images of Nyongo amongst Bamenda grassfielders in whiteman kontri'. *Citizenship Studies* 9(3): 241–69.
Nyamnjoh, Francis. 2011. 'Cameroonian bushfalling: Negotiation of identity and belonging in fiction and ethnography'. *American Ethnologist* 38(4): 701–713. https://doi.org/10.1111/j.1548-1425.2011.01331.x.
Nyamnjoh, Francis. 2015a. 'Incompleteness: Frontier Africa and the currency of conviviality'. *Journal of Asian and African Studies* 52(3): 253–70. https://doi.org/10.1177/0021909615580867.
Nyamnjoh, Francis. 2015b. 'Amos Tutuola and the elusiveness of completeness'. *Stichproben Wiener Zeitschrift für kritische Afrikastudien* 15(29): 1–47
Nyamnjoh, Francis. 2016. *#Rhodes Must Fall: Nibbling at resilient colonialism in South Africa*. Mankon, Cameroon: Langaa RPCIG.
Onoma, Ato. 2013. *Anti-Refugee Violence and African Politics*. New York: Cambridge University Press
Onoma, Ato. 2017. 'The making of dangerous communities: The "Peul-Fouta" in Ebola weary Senegal'. *Africa Spectrum* 52(2): 29–51.
Onoma, Ato. 2018. 'Epidemics and intra-communal contestations: "Les Guinéens" and Ebola in West Africa'. *Journal of Modern African Studies* 56(4): 595–617.
Onoma, Ato. 2020a. 'Xenophobia's contours during an Ebola epidemic: Proximity and the targeting of Peul migrants in Senegal'. *African Studies Review* 63(2): 353–74. https://doi.org/10.1017/asr.2019.38.

Onoma, Ato. 2020b. 'Epidemics, xenophobia and narratives of propitiousness'. *Medical Anthropology: Cross-Cultural Studies in Health and Illness* 39(5): 382–97. https://doi.org/10.1080/01459740.2020.1753047.

Onoma, Ato. 2020c. 'COVID-19, liberalism and the (non)citizen'. SCRIPTS Cluster of Excellence. 22 July 2020. Accessed 16 September 2020. https://www.scripts-berlin.eu/blog/Covid-19_-liberalism-and-the-_non_citizen/index.html.

Online Reporters. 2020. '17 new Covid-19 cases among returnees from Mideast'. *The Bangkok Post*. 4 June 2020. Accessed 5 June 2020. https://www.bangkokpost.com/thailand/general/1929328/17-new-covid-19-cases-among-returnees-from-mideast.

Riccio, Bruno. 2002. 'Senegal is our home: The anchored nature of Senegalese transnational networks'. In *New Approaches To Migration? Transnational communities and the meaning of home*, edited by Nadge Al-Ali and Khalid Koser, pp. 68–83. London: Routledge.

Riccio, Bruno. 2005. 'Talkin' about migration. Some ethnographic notes on the ambivalent representation of migrants in contemporary Senegal'. *Vienna Journal of African Studies* 8: 99–118.

Riccio, Bruno. 2008. 'Les migrants senegalais en Italy. Reseaux, insertion et potential de co-developpement'. In *Le Senegal des Migrations: Mobilites, identities et societies*, edited by Momar-Coumba Diop, pp. 69–104. Paris, France: Karthala.

Riccio, Bruno and Stefano degli Uberti. 2013. 'Senegalese migrants In Italy: Beyond the assimilation/transnationalism divide'. *Urban Anthropology and Studies of Cultural Systems and World Economic Development* 42(3/4): 207–54.

Sakhanokho, Salif. 2020. 'Sénégal: Le statut des "modou-modou" a été sali par le coronavirus'. 26 March 2020. Accessed 5 June 2020. https://www.pressafrik.com/Senegal-le-statut-des-modou-modou-a-ete-sali-par-le-coronavirus_a213668.html.

Schneier, Bruce. 2020. 'Bots are destroying discourse as we know it'. 7 January 2020. Accessed 1 December 2020. https://www.theatlantic.com/technology/archive/2020/01/future-politics-bots-drowning-out-humans/604489/.

Seneweb News. 2020a. 'Covid-19: 3 des 4 nouveaux cas sont des "Modou-Modou"'. 18 March 2020. Accessed 4 June 2020. https://www.seneweb.com/news/Societe/covid-19-3-des-4-nouveaux-cas-sont-des-q_n_311892.html.

Seneweb News. 2020b. 'Coronavirus: Le "Modou-Modou" d'Espagne testé positif savait qu'il était malade'. 16 March 2020. Accessed 4 June 2020. https://www.seneweb.com/news/Sante/covid-19-le-quot-modou-modou-quot-d-espa_n_311653.html.

Seneweb News. 2020c. 'Coronavirus: 25 Sénégalais venus d'Espagne en quarantaine'. 20 March 2020. Accessed 4 June 2020. https://www.seneweb.com/news/Sante/coronavirus-25-senegalais-venus-d-espagn_n_312121.html.

Seneweb News, 2020d. 'Coronavirus: Les premiers mots du "Modou-Modou" d'Italie qui a contaminé 16 personnes'. Accessed 4 June 2020. https://www.seneweb.com/news/Sante/coronavirus-les-premiers-mots-du-quot-mo_n_311664.html.

Seneweb News. 2020e. 'Coronavirus: Onze nouveaux cas au Sénégal'. 13 March 2020. Accessed 4 June 2020. https://www.seneweb.com/news/Sante/coronavirus-onze-nouveaux-cas-au-senegal_n_311474.html.

Tabappsi, Timothee. 1999. *Le modèle migratoire bamiléké (Cameroun) et sa crise actuelle: perspectives économique et culturelle*. Leiden, Netherlands: CNWS.

Tall, Serigne Mansour. 1994. Les investissements immobiliers a Dakar des emigrants senegalais. *Revue Europeenne des migrations internationals* 3(10): 137–51.

Tall, Serigne Mansour. 2002. 'L'emigration international senegalaise d'hier a demain'. In *La societe senegalaise entre le local et global*, edited by Momar-Coumba Diop, pp. 549–78. Paris, France: Karthala.

Tall, Serigne Mansour. 2008a. 'Les Senegalais en Italie: Transferts financiers et potential de development de l'habitat au Senegal'. In *Le Senegal des Migrations: Mobilites, identities et societies*, edited by Momar-Coumba Diop, pp. 153–77. Paris, France: Karthala.

Tall, Serigne Mansour. 2008b 'La migration international senegalaise: Des recrutements de main-d'oeuvre aux pirogues'. In *Le Senegal des Migrations: Mobilites, identities et societies*, edited by Momar-Coumba Diop, pp. 37–67. Paris, France: Karthala.

Tandian, Aly. 2008. 'Des migrants senegalais qualifies en Italie: Entre regrets et resignation'. In *Le Senegal des Migrations: Mobilites, identities et societies*, edited by Momar-Coumba Diop, pp. 365–87. Paris, France: Karthala.

Taylor, Catherine A., R. Al-Hiyari, Shawna J. Lee, A. Priebe, L.W. Guerrero and Ana Bales. 2016. 'Beliefs and ideologies linked with approval of corporal punishment: A content analysis of online comments'. *Health Education Research* 31(4): 563–75.

Tazanu, Primus. 2012. *Being Available and Reachable: New media and Cameroonian transnational sociality*. Bamenda, Cameroon: Langaa RPCIG.

Thiam, Jamil. 2020. 'Covid-19: Les Sénégalais de la Diaspora dénoncent la stigmatisation et les statistiques erronées'. 13 April 2020. Accessed 5 June 2020. https://www.socialnetlink.org/2020/04/13/covid-19-les-senegalais-de-la-diaspora-denoncent-la-stigmatisation-et-les-statistiques-erronees/.

Trauner, Joan. 1978. 'The Chinese as medical scapegoats in San Francisco, 1870–1905'. *California History* 57(1): 70–87.

Uberti, Stefano Degli. 2014. 'Victims of their fantasies or heroes for a day?' *Cahiers d'études africaines* 213–14. https://doi.org/10.4000/etudesafricaines.17599.

White, Cassandra. 2010. 'Déjà vu: Leprosy and immigration discourse in the twenty-first century United States'. *Leprosy Review* 81(1): 17–26.

Willane, Babacar. 2020. 'Absence de détails dans le communiqué: Le ministère de la Santé s'explique'. Seneweb. 18 March 2020. Accessed 4 June 2020. https://www.seneweb.com/news/Sante/absence-de-details-dans-le-communique-le_n_311922.html.

Willems, Roos. 2008. 'Les 'fous de la mer': Les migrants clandestins du Senegal aux iles Canaries en 2006'. In *Le Senegal des Migrations: Mobilites, identities et societies*, edited by Momar-Coumba Diop, pp. 277–303. Paris, France: Karthala.

World Bank. n.d. 'Personal remittances, received (current US$)- Senegal'. Accessed 17 December 2020. https://data.worldbank.org/indicator/BX.TRF.PWKR.CD.DT?end=2019&locations=SN&start=1974&view=chart.

Zeidan, Karim. 2020. 'Vidéo: Algérie: Le Diaspora priée de rester dans le pays d'accueil'. 3 March Accessed 5 June 2020. https://afrique.le360.ma/algerie/politique/2020/03/13/29799-video-algerie-la-diaspora-priee-de-rester-dans-les-pays-daccueil-29799.

Zhu, April. 2020. 'Sinophobia spreads faster than the coronavirus'. February 28. Accessed 5 June 2020. https://www.theelephant.info/culture/2020/02/28/sinophobia-spreads-faster-than-the-coronavirus/.

Part III
Unequal burdens

11
Pandemic policy responses and embodied realities among 'waste-pickers' in India

Surekha Garimella, Shrutika Murthy, Lana Whittaker and Rachel Tolhurst

Accounts of hardship among waste-picking communities and sanitation workers have appeared intermittently in the print and social media since March 2020, as the COVID-19 pandemic took hold in India. These accounts brought to public consciousness the lack of personal protective equipment (mainly gloves and masks) among sanitation workers, and the risks they faced in relation to exposure to the virus, in the context of increased medical waste, including masks, that were being seen in public spaces and landfill areas. There were also accounts of loss of livelihoods because of the nation-wide lockdown for three weeks from 25 March to 14 April 2020. During this time waste pickers were unable to go out and collect and recycle dry waste, and this severely impacted their ability to feed themselves. Emerging accounts highlighted the negative impact of measures taken to contain COVID-19, while they also laid bare the troubling reality of waste-picking communities, of lives lived on the margins of societies, with little to no recognition and protection (social, income, health and safety protections) despite the crucial work they do to keep cities and commons clean. For these communities, COVID-19 has intensified the uncertainty hardwired into their work, their living spaces and their everyday lives. Public health practices around masking, washing hands and physical distancing, while necessary to reduce the risk of contracting the virus, have little resonance with the living and working conditions of waste-picking communities; for these community members, protecting and taking care of themselves is extremely difficult (Figure 11.1).

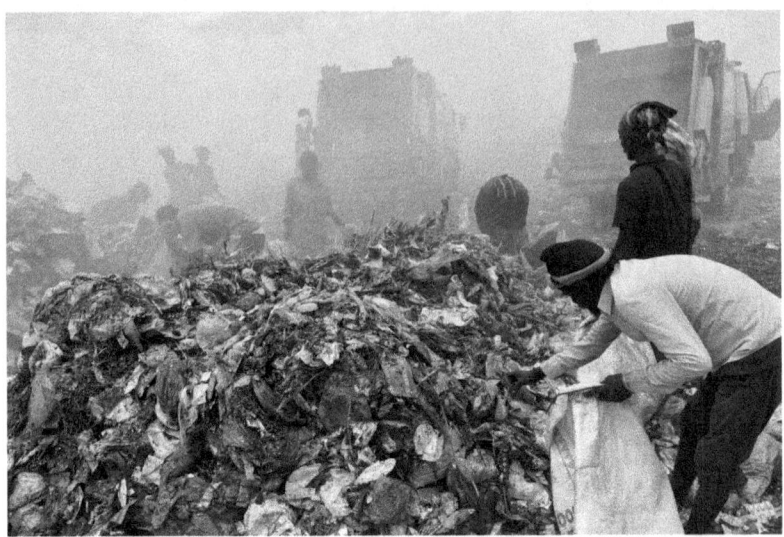

Figure 11.1 Sifting and collection of recyclables at Naidupeta dump yard at Guntur, Andhra Pradesh, India. Photo: Arise Hub, The George Institute for Global Health India

The word 'waste' can be traced back to the Latin word, *vastus*, which means 'unoccupied, uncultivated' (Gidwani and Reddy 2011). Gidwani and Reddy trace the entry of waste as a political-juridical concept to late-thirteenth century England, where it was used in the context of usufructuary[1] rights of tenants. The tenant could not allow the land to go to waste if he (never she) were to continue to hold such right. Waste therefore originated in the context of property and land. In India, in some local contexts, this still remains the case. For instance, in Tamil the word *poramboke nilam* means land which is outside the revenue accounts of the government, but literally the term means waste land. Barbara Harriss-White (2020), among others, has noted that along with the proliferation of waste, research on waste and waste work is also rapidly expanding although still fragmented. Rarely is the waste economy looked at as a whole.

Waste pickers are among the poorest, most marginalised and stigmatised in India (Harriss-White 2020; Doron 2018; Kornberg 2019; Shankar and Sahni 2017). Waste makes us uneasy, it reminds us of our 'all-too-mortal bodies'; and this discomfort is, as Martha Nussbaum notes, 'projected outward onto groups who can serve as, so to speak, the surrogate dirt of a community, enabling the dominant group to feel clean and heavenly' (Morrison 2015, 37). Waste pickers mainly come from the most marginalised castes and communities in India. In his essay, 'Untouchability and Lawlessness', B.R. Ambedkar (Maharashtra 1989) writes that under the caste order, 'the scavenger's work is beneath the dignity of the Hindus'.[2] Even today in India, the occupation of handling waste, both formally and informally, remains a function of caste (Singh 2014; Doron 2018). Other sites of inequity operate along with caste (Gidwani and Maringanti 2016; Gidwani 1992; Gidwani and Baviskar 2011). For instance, poor working-class people who migrate to cities in search of other work are often absorbed into waste-picking work (Kornberg 2019; Shankar and Sahni 2017).

In India, in The Solid Waste Management Rules (SWM), waste pickers were for the first time explicitly recognised and defined by the government (GOI 2016b).[3] A waste picker was defined as:

> A person or groups of persons informally engaged in collection and recovery of reusable and recyclable solid waste from the source of waste generation, the streets, bins, material recovery facilities, processing and waste disposal facilities for sale to recyclers directly or through intermediaries to earn their livelihood.

Urban India generates around 42 million tonnes of municipal waste and the Twelfth Schedule[4] mandates local urban administrative bodies to maintain the streets and keep cities clean. The formal structures of urban municipalities are able to recycle only 30 per cent of the waste and rely on waste pickers and existing informal waste collection and recycling networks to meet the larger tasks of keeping cities clean. Waste picking is informal work, but it plays a key role in waste management. Waste-picking communities save resources for the municipality by collecting over 80 per cent of total recyclable waste and contributing to a substantial portion of the waste economy (Harriss-White 2020). The current system of waste management in India is built on this informality, and relies on the coercive and unequal power relations that arise out of these informal arrangements as well as caste-derived ideas of purity and pollution. According to the Constitution of India, public health and sanitation are state[5] matters. However, solid waste management is the responsibility of local urban administration. Article 243W of the Constitution refers to 'public health, sanitation conservancy and solid waste management' as a direct responsibility of municipalities. Though waste management is a municipal responsibility, it is fast moving away from public sector control, bringing 'private players into confrontations with informal waste pickers' (Shankar and Sahni 2017: 55). No official data are available on the number of people engaged in waste picking, but up to one and a half million people are estimated to be involved in this work, accounting for up to 10 per cent of waste pickers globally (GOI 2016a; Bose and Bhattacharya 2017).

Waste pickers face constant harassment from state institutions and are often suspected as 'thieves masquerading as waste collectors' (Shankar and Sahni 2017: 61) by residents and police.[6] Women enter the workforce on an unequal footing with men (Sankaran 2013) due to the sexual division of labour, and this affects their standing in the public sphere as much as in private life.[7] Wages for the kinds of work performed 'typically by women' are classified as 'light work', thus attracting lesser wages than those paid to men (Sankaran 2013). In waste picking, women occupy the bottom of the wage ladder, their working conditions differing from men even when they pursue similar activities. Shankar and Sahni (2017) argue that in the informal waste sector, men occupy the 'transactional' segment of the 'waste ladder', while women and children are usually at the bottom of the hierarchy and 'handle waste in its raw form' (Shankar and Sahni 2017: 251). Caste-patriarchy[8] shapes the lives of both men and women waste pickers.[9]

The informal waste economy comprises socially, occupationally and economically differentiated categories of 'waste people' – waste pickers/collectors, ragpickers, manual scavengers and sanitation workers among other categories. This line of work is characterised by the symbolic and practical manifestations of caste, religion and gender. Most waste pickers/collectors are poor Scheduled Castes (Dalits) and Muslims who have been systematically forced into this profession because of their status as lower caste and low status. Exiting from this occupation remains difficult. It is often argued that the labour in waste economies is deliberately informalised to contain costs (by paying low wages) and to express contempt for Dalits (by subjugating them and suppressing particular communities). Increasingly, informal activity has become hard-wired into the business model of municipal contracting wherein acute revenue stress and practices of new public management have forced the municipality to subcontract services, including that of sanitation. Informal labour contractors often bring in labourers and their families from adjoining states and pay them to work as waste pickers in cities. These migrant labourers are often heavily disadvantaged: they are paid abysmal wages without any perks, housed on common land in tent-like shacks without proper access to water and electricity; they are unable to communicate and integrate with the local population; are constantly regarded as 'outsiders'; and are further discriminated against because of the nature of their work. Recent governance shifts toward reforming the waste management sector through increased privatisation and mechanisation threaten to dispossess waste pickers from their livelihoods (Gidwani and Corwin 2017). These precarious conditions are manifestations of intersectional linkages of hierarchies of gender, caste, class and religion interlocking with processes of economic liberalisation, urbanisation and migration among others (Butt 2019). Waste pickers' marginalisation, enmeshed in the gender, caste and class axis, is simultaneously associated with both the materiality of waste and the ritual and symbolic pollution of untouchability, further entrenching their exclusion (Gill 2009; Reddy 2018).

Despite the social, economic, public health and ecological importance of their work, waste pickers are not given due recognition for their role, and they continue to struggle under the pressures of poverty, stigma and compromised citizenship. In contrast, '(w)ithin the waste economy, the municipal sanitation workers are considered to be the 'aristocracy' of waste labour' (Harriss-White 2017, 421); they benefit from higher salaries, better living conditions, job security and health insurance, in comparison to informal waste pickers/collectors. But, even for this aristocracy: 'Sanitation for sanitation workers is conspicuously absent; the dirtier and more dangerous the work, the lower the pay and the more physically taxing the work conditions' (Harriss-White 2020, 8).

We share preliminary insights from our ongoing work with waste pickers in India in the ARISE (Accountability for Urban Informal Equity) project in this chapter. We analysed selective policies that were in place pre-COVID-19 and additional policies that were introduced during the pandemic. In addition, we share what we are learning from ongoing work with waste-picking communities.

Policies and what they reveal

In the wake of the COVID-19 outbreak, the Indian government announced a nation-wide lockdown to start on 25 March, thereby severely restricting the movement of individuals across the country. The lockdown was initially imposed for 21 days, and it was extended to a period of three months. This large-scale restriction on movement was particularly disruptive for poor, marginalised and vulnerable sections of population. Waste-picking communities found themselves in a situation where they could no longer go out and collect waste. The immediate fall out of this was the fear of going hungry. Waste needs to be collected and sold on a daily basis to ensure a cash flow in people's homes and sufficient money to buy food to eat.

At the same time as initiating the lockdown, the federal and state governments and the courts announced various social security measures, some of which specifically focused on the most vulnerable. The scale and frequency of these announcements was unprecedented, with many orders amended then revoked within hours of their release, and often not updated on the official government websites, making it increasingly difficult to track these updates. In this light, a group of activists, researchers, lawyers and students came together collectively to set up a crowdfunded COVID-19 India policy tracker called 'COVIDIndiaTrack'.[10] The main objectives of this tracker were to make information easily accessible on a real-time basis, monitor the implementation of policies, and demand some basic accountability. For sourcing policies pertaining to COVID-19, we relied on this tool extensively. In addition, we frequently checked the official government handles used on social media platforms, especially Twitter, in order to keep abreast with the latest announcements.

The policy analysis we attempted involved three stages. First, we searched for policies pertaining to waste-picking communities before and after COVID-19. Second, we scrutinised these for fit and relevance, based on a dynamic and evolving criteria of inclusion and exclusion (see Table 11.1, below). Finally we analysed a subset of these policies based on Carol Bacchi's 'What's the problem represented to be?' approach (2014). The search strategy was split into two streams: pre-COVID-19 and post-COVID-19. The post-COVID stream was further split into federal and state governments (Andhra Pradesh, Himachal Pradesh and Karnataka), where the cities in which we work are located. An evolving inclusion and exclusion criteria also aided the policy screening process.

The main objective of the policy screening was to identify policies of direct relevance to waste-picking communities. However, most of the post COVID-19 policies made no explicit mention of 'waste-picking communities' or 'waste pickers'. Instead, they used overarching categories like vulnerable sections of society, poor persons, homeless and street children, to name a few. As a result, we included these policies for analysis because these spaces are where the waste-picking communities are located. Based on the first round of searches, we shortlisted 150 policies announced by the union government and 30, 13 and 6 policies announced by the state governments of Karnataka, Himachal Pradesh and Andhra Pradesh, respectively.

In the first round of screening, we read through the summaries that had been drafted by COVIDIndiaTrack and made a quick note of the

Table 11.1 Inclusion and exclusion criteria

Inclusion criteria	Exclusion criteria
Social protection/relief: Provision of food, relief kits, cash, insurance – all the central/state	Test kits
Employment – including government officials as contrast	Hospital management
Orders relating to restriction of movements	Corporate social responsibility (CSR)
Harassment and discrimination	Car insurance
Waste disposal including medical waste	Violence against healthcare workers
Management of dead bodies	Transportation of goods during lockdown (our focus is on movement of people)
Education	Migrant workers and labourers
Continuation of existing health services: immunisation, tuberculosis (TB)	
Access to healthcare	Fake news
Homeless, street/pavement dwellers	Containment – travellers coming into India
	Pharmaceutical interventions
	Personal protective equipment (PPE) – only if sanitation workers employed in hospitals
	Testing – only if experienced
	Agriculture/rural areas focus
	Documents detailing safety measures/employment within specific government departments
	Child protection

central topics that were the focus of the policy and relevant to our analysis. Based on this screening, we identified 22 policies pre-COVID and 97 policies post-COVID: 75 policies released by the union government and 11, 7 and 4 policies released by the state governments of Himachal Pradesh, Karnataka and Andhra Pradesh respectively

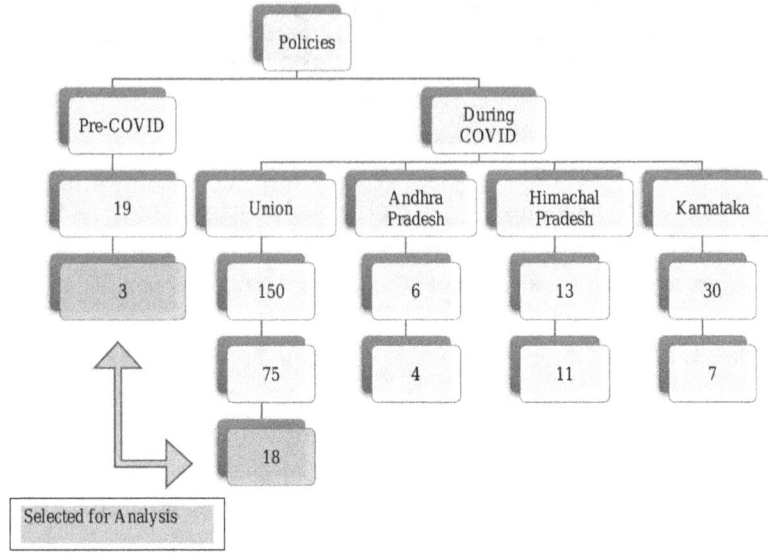

Figure 11.2 Policy screening flow. Source: authors

(see Figure 11.2). In the second round of screening, we read through the shortlisted policies in greater detail and made a note of those that would classify for Carol Bacchi's 'What's the problem represented to be?' approach and those that would be good for providing background information. Finally, 18 policies were selected for analysis. We chose to use Bacchi's framework because it looks at problem definitions and solutions as inextricably linked together.

Pre-COVID-19

Representation and visibility

The policies that apply to waste picking are located in a sociocultural and economic context within which people handle waste to earn their livelihoods. Policies are not merely spaces to search for gaps but provide insight into how waste pickers and their problems are represented. A common thread in pre-COVID-19 policies[11] was emphasis on the importance of the role of the informal sector as the 'backbone of municipal solid waste management (MSWM) value chain in India' (GOI 2016b), which includes the *kabaadi* system and waste pickers, and the relevance of legal recognition to strengthen the informal systems of collection that are integral to MSWM. In India, the *kabaadi* system consists a network of *kabaadiwalas* (junk or scrap dealers), itinerant waste collectors and buyers. The latter collect recyclables from households (such as cardboard, newspapers, glass bottles and plastic) and sell these to scrap dealers at a fixed rate per kilogram, depending upon the composition and valuation of items collected. The Solid Waste Management Rules (GOI 2016b) recognise the role of the informal sector in waste management and emphasise the establishment of a system for the integration of authorised waste pickers and waste collectors (by issuing identity cards and formation of self-help groups) to facilitate their participation in the solid waste management system, including door-to-door collection of waste. But silence on the issue of caste and its centrality in waste picking remains, and to a great extent there are efforts to gloss over the intertwining of caste and waste and render it as a managerial issue (Gatade 2015). Treating caste and waste as a bureaucratic issue is not new, and Butt (2019) has shown in his work on colonial Punjab how the colonial regime cemented links between waste work, governance and caste.

For unspecified reasons, different typologies are used to classify waste-picking communities in different policy documents. The First National Commission on Labour of 1969 (GOI 1969) used the terms 'sweepers' and 'scavengers', while The Second National Commission on Labour of 2002 (GOI 2002) used all terminologies – ragpickers, waste pickers, scrap collectors and waste collectors – interchangeably. 'Waste workers' as a term was used to refer to all workers who earned their livelihoods by dealing with waste, including the municipal sanitation workers and 'manual scavengers'. The National Commission for Enterprises in the Unorganised Sector, 2007 (NCEUS) (GOI 2007) identified 'ragpickers' as self-employed workers; however, the document made a distinction between 'ragpickers' and self-employed persons owning businesses that recycle scrap and junk. The report also positioned the 'ragpicker' as economically better off than a 'casual worker'. Until late 2016, the National Urban Livelihood Mission (NULM) document and Municipal Solid Waste (management and handling) Rules refer to them as ragpickers, and only in later policy documents was the terminology of 'waste pickers' used more consistently. The impact of these ambiguities on the recognition of the work that waste pickers do, on the dignity of their profession, and whether a lack of definition impinges on access to social security schemes of the government, remains poorly understood.

In the policies, there is some recognition of the vulnerabilities of and problems faced by urban poor in general and particular sections of the urban population, including 'Scheduled castes, Scheduled tribes, minorities, female-headed households, persons with disabilities, the destitute, migrant labourers, and especially vulnerable occupational groups such as street vendors, ragpickers, domestic workers, beggars, construction workers, etc.' (Ministry of Housing and Urban Affairs 2016, 11). These include a lack of social security and lack of access to healthcare, and are considered to belong to vulnerable occupational groups. Solutions proffered include the initiation of special projects to address livelihood issues of the most vulnerable sections of this population, including those with physical disabilities, people categorised as ragpickers, domestic workers, rickshaw pullers and sanitation workers (GOI 2018).

Recognition/identity cards

The SWM and PWM rules specifically mandate that waste pickers must be provided with identification documents. Because waste picking is an informal activity and waste pickers mainly live in informal settlements and on pavements, they do not possess identification cards. Not having a card means a lack of access to government welfare schemes. In addition, waste pickers are subject to harassment by the police and the general public. They are commonly assumed to be thieves and tend to be the first people to get picked up by the police in the event of theft. Many organisations that work with waste pickers advocate that they be issued with official identity cards. Reddy and Kumar (2018), for example, make the case that ensuring the welfare of waste pickers lies in issuing them with identity cards that acknowledge their occupation and their right to access, collect and sell waste across their respective states. Waste pickers in turn argue that identity cards will benefit them in multiple ways, including by increasing their access to waste in both private and public areas, and, by giving their occupation legitimacy in the eyes of the police and the citizenry, reducing the harassment they routinely face. In Karnataka, a project for providing identity cards to waste pickers was initiated in 2011 by Bruhat Bengaluru Mahanagara Palike (BBMP), making it the first urban local body to register waste pickers in India. Through this project, over 6,000 waste pickers in the city were identified and issued identification cards, with another 7,000 approved and waiting for cards to be issued (Reddy and Kumar 2018). However, waste pickers noted that the identity cards also had negative impact, since those who were unable to gain these cards, for reasons such as being identified as migrants, faced even greater exclusion and marginalisation.

Access to government health schemes

The Unorganised Workers Social Security Act UWSSA (2008) (GOI 2008) extends to 'ragpickers' and provides for the formulation of welfare schemes related to, inter alia, life and disability cover, and health and maternity benefits. Under Schedule I of the Act, several schemes have been listed to which workers can have access. Among these are the Janani Suraksha Yojana (JSY) of the Ministry of Health and Family Welfare, which is a safe motherhood intervention to reduce maternal and neonatal mortality through promotion of institutional deliveries among poor pregnant women. This federal scheme integrates cash assistance with delivery and post-delivery care. There is also the Rashtriya Swasthya Bima Yojana (RSBY) of the Labour Ministry, a national health insurance scheme for people living below the poverty line which provides protection from financial liabilities that arise out of hospitalisation. This scheme has now moved under the aegis of the Ministry of Health and Family Welfare, and in 2018 it was subsumed by the federal government scheme Ayushman Bharat-Pradhan Mantri Jan Aarogya Yojana (PMJAY), which is implemented by states on a cost-sharing basis. This is meant to avoid duplication of multiple schemes for the same population group, and to reduce the burden of furnishing multiple cards for services by families (because coverage is for families). Earlier, poor people found it very difficult to decipher and understand which scheme covered what services. Changes to schemes aimed to prevent them from having to access multiple service providers as well as being denied services due to non-applicability of specific schemes in specific facilities. While the intent is commendable, in actual practice, the autonomy of states to shape the policies with relevance to their context has been curtailed due to the centralised nature of this scheme (Krishnakumar 2019;[12] The Week 2018[13]). The standing committee report on Urban Development[14] in 2008, among other things, acknowledged the occupational health issues involved with 'rag picking' and recommended that those involved in such work be provided with 'personal protective equipment like gloves and spectacles and things like that so that they do not contract diseases' (55). But the lack of identity cards remains a gatekeeping issue which prevents access to these schemes. In 2013, RSBY was extended to 'ragpickers' and 'sanitation workers'.[15] The RSBY website claims that registration under the scheme is easy. The 2013 notification requires that the state government identify 'ragpickers' provided that they are at least 18 years of age; and 'ragpickers' must provide a self-declaration confirming that they are a 'ragpicker', and a document of proof of occupation. Acquiring proof of occupation is not easy for waste pickers, however.

During COVID times

As indicated earlier, a flurry of orders, guidelines and rules were issued by federal and state governments to deal with COVID-19 and its impact; this remained dynamic to the end of December 2020. Insurance schemes for health workers have been announced; these include sanitation workers but not waste pickers or waste workers. Sanitation workers are formally employed by the city's administration to clean public spaces including sewers and manholes, empty toilet pits and septic tanks, segregate different kinds of waste, and operate pumping stations and treatment plants. They are tenured or 'regular' employees and are given employee benefits such as a pension and health insurance. In times of COVID-19, the government heralded them as 'frontline workers' or 'frontline warriors'. Schemes to provide additional food for the poor were also introduced, but these were limited to a three-month period at the beginning of the lockdown. While these schemes were welcome initiatives, they built onto existing schemes and did not directly address the exclusionary nature of existing schemes. This appears to be based on the assumption that problems in accessing these schemes are only due to COVID-related disruptions, but they do not address the impact of loss of work, hunger and inability to access healthcare, nor do they take into account the problems faced by waste-picking communities in accessing these schemes, even in regular times.

In addition to reviewing policies as part of our ongoing research, we conducted interviews with nine waste pickers and sanitation workers from Bengaluru, Vijayawada and Shimla. We also interviewed five key informants from these cities. Across these sites, we are working with a cross-section of waste workers: in Bengaluru, we are working with waste pickers who engage in door-to-door collection of segregated dry waste. In Vijayawada, we are working with waste pickers in the informal sector who are own account workers (Murthy 2020; Saligram 2020). In Shimla, we are working with tenured sanitation workers and contractual door-to-door garbage collectors.

Tapestries of wellbeing and ill-health

The interviews revealed a preoccupation with food insecurity and hunger, inability to access health services, and the waste-picking community's dependence on non-governmental organisations (NGOs) and other community-based organisations. Some of the interviewees[16] spoke about complete dependence on NGOs to feed themselves and their families, and the difficulties faced by these organisations in delivering medicines to the communities where waste pickers live. Sujatha, one of our interviewees, told us that if her family and others 'had not received any support from the NGO, it would have been very, very tough. They gave us one month's provisions and then we got some from the public distribution system ('ration shop') which helped us "maintain" our lives'. She also went on to say that the organisation had offered to supply the medicines. But this did not happen, and she does not know why; 'they had to go to a nearby medical store and buy it. But mostly people go to the nearby public facility and pick-up medicines'.

Waste pickers depend on the regular flow of cash which they generate through picking, sorting and selling on a daily basis to feed themselves and their families. Because of the lockdown, their only source of income was cut off. People consistently spoke about lack of food, lack of money to seek care if needed and the immense stress/distress in such situations. Kamal, for example, spoke to us about how food relief was necessary and helpful, but it did not resolve other stresses related to cash flow. Being unable to access health services was a major source of stress:

> Each rupee matters now for a person. Just lentils and rice alone won't run the house, right? But the lockdown … honestly has troubled us, no one even has a rupee. We are managing somehow but if someone falls ill at home or if some problems arise then meeting these costs would be a huge issue. We don't have money to go to doctor, so we go to the government hospital here but for the people who work here (indicating migrant workers), their homes run because they send money.

Suresh conveyed the stress due to the lockdown slightly differently, referring to the inability to work, the role of the police, and her perception that the government did not seem to understand their situation:

> We are also struggling more now, we are not allowed to go outside, the police are not allowing anyone to leave their homes. Two to three people are physically challenged; they are not able to do any work. Mainly many are depending on begging at door to door in the near places. They are completely helpless; this needs to be recognised by the government.

People also spoke about feeling distressed at what they were seeing around them, but also solidarity in troubled times and looking out for each other, as Annie put it:

> most of the people are facing problems in this pandemic, they need some food. Some people are in critical position, kids are crying for food. Due to social stigma parents are not ready to ask help. I am also facing problems but two times I have prepared food for the hungry people. They are not my relatives; I don't know who they are when I helped them.

While some of the issues had an urgency shaped by the challenges of managing their lives during the pandemic, the key informants who had worked with waste pickers for many years now shared that many issues that waste pickers were facing were not unique to the pandemic, but were ones that they faced at any time. Indhu, one of our key informants, told us:

> The fear is also there, and they also fear that sometimes they are diagnosed with something that requires 10 days rest or 15 days rest or something like that ... they can't afford that. It sounds like help should not be taken for granted but this is the bitter realities that these people ... there was this one woman ... I can give you a lot of community examples because this is what we encounter on a day-to-day basis. She had elephantiasis on her left leg and she just refuses to go to doctor because she has seven children to take care of and if she loses a day of work what will happen? They won't have anything to eat. So, if there is a community health camp where they can go for one hour come back that is all fine, but not where it takes days for them and regular follow ups for them. Frankly speaking, those who work in the godowns [warehouses] and scrap shops, their owners also exploit them in many ways. I won't say like very good and nice things about them because it is true, this exploitation still happens even if we associate with them it happens back of the hand. So, it's like a daily wage kind of a thing, you lose one day's work if you go to the hospitals, then there is bill and all that.

Most waste pickers constantly struggle to eat and survive, and seek care. While the government has provided welfare and health insurance schemes that are expected to meet the needs of poor people including waste pickers, to what extent these actually meet their needs remains moot. Even when there is a possibility of seeking care, stigma, fear and the experience of being treated poorly by health workers means that they avoid accessing these services. As another key informant elaborated, a lot of hard work and convincing building of trust has to be done before many very poor people will agree to access health services, and they are dependent on NGOs and citizen groups to help them. Previously waste pickers were reluctant to present for care because of fear of stigma. This is particularly so because many belong to Scheduled tribes, and from the perspective of key informants, their persistent experience of stigma and social exclusion impacts their willingness to access health services. Aman, for instance, emphasised the work involved in talking to women about institutional deliveries and antenatal care, and allaying their fears about going to hospitals. Slowly, he remarked, 'we are seeing an increasing willingness to access government services including medical services'. Aman continued:

> There are no medical shops, for example, in dumping yards … they will have to come to the city. They will have to travel around 12 km. And I want to tell you one more thing … with regards to the dumping yard, there's one pregnant woman and they don't follow institutional deliveries … they don't do that. So, they'd rather … they deliver at their houses itself. We spent a lot of time talking to the woman and assured her that we will take her to the government hospital where she can get good care. When she started to experience labour pain she called us and we spoke to her and arranged for an auto to take her to the government hospital, we spoke to the doctor and paid for her medicines too. So, she, her family and the community were very happy that we could help them during this time. And they said … this is the first time … in our community … this is the first time … this much service and care has been provided to us (Aman).

From these narratives, it is clear that while experiences shared find their immediacy in the fallout of COVID-19, these are not unique to the pandemic, but rather are issues that waste-picking communities grapple with on an everyday basis. Living with and through a pandemic adds to their vulnerability; as Bennett and Dewi (this volume) show, the pandemic amplifies their marginality and the health consequences of this.

Accountabilities

The slew of policies released by the federal and state governments during the COVID-19 pandemic allocated responsibilities for implementation to different arms of the bureaucracy. For example, advice on the provision of safe and potable water to those residing in urban slums and belonging to the poorest strata of society simply reinforced what needs to happen with or without the pandemic. Access to safe and potable water for the poor is a longstanding unmet need. The initiation of the lockdown to reduce the spread of the disease ended up further stigmatising waste-picking communities, at a stroke taking away their chances of earning a living and feeding themselves. The efforts to provide food to these communities were not based on their realities as detailed in policy statements, and the exclusions built into public distribution systems remained. The interviewees we spoke with elaborated on the negative impacts of the lockdown:

> Lockdown is a problem. It is tough for people, the labourers like waste pickers … we have no salary … it is not that monthly we get money then we sleep and that's it. For us the money depends on how much work we do. So, government should have thought about us, the sanitation workers on the road who do cleanliness work … they do the work of sanitation workers also so government should have also thought that the one who uses his cycle to pick up materials and sell … whose lives revolve around this … they should have thought about people like us. If they have told us 'okay, you do your work don't create issues' … if we or someone had said this or allowed us to do so, we could have lived better. In such a state how will one feel? You tell me. It was not necessary to do this, people can maintain distance and work. Doing so it would have been better for us, but with lockdown it is like … stay at home like how one has to stay in jail. What is the use of it? Instead … People live their lives to eat food so if we can't get food then what will we do? Better than this is … we do our work but we maintain distance. People have to work, if they cannot work then what will they do? People with money can sit at home, what problems do they have? (Kamal)

Others spoke of the inability to gain access to rations supposed to be provided by the government. From our own interviews and observations, we found that civil society organisations and concerned citizens tried hard to fill this gap and supply food and medicines to the waste-picking communities in the cities where we work. As one of them told us:

> Nothing from either the government or the corporation. The councillor from the ward provided support. He gave us two kilos of rice each and that is not even enough to last one day (Shalini).

> I know this information from the community people, TV news and newspapers. And village volunteers also told. They said to us who

are having ration card, they are only eligible for receiving Rs. 1000. In this community, only two or three families are having ration cards (Suresh).

Affirming what the waste pickers have shared with us, civil society organisations, well-meaning citizen groups, and individuals were the ones supplying food and care. Aman, a key informant, narrated how he reached out to the municipal commissioner and shared a note about the guidelines for sanitation workers during COVID-19. Aman was pleasantly surprised when the commissioner responded by asking Aman if he needed any help to support the waste-picking community with whom he works. Aman immediately brought to the notice of the commissioner that many waste pickers did not have ration cards, and although the government was supplying food aid without these cards, they were unable to access other aid. For example, each family was to get a thousand rupees, but not possessing the card meant that they could not get this small financial relief being offered. He provided a list of names of waste pickers who did not have these cards with the local administration. The following day, Aman found that rice and lentils were being distributed to waste pickers who did not have ration cards. However, the people who were doing this were not local officials, but the wife of the commissioner and her friends who were part of Indian Administrative Service (IAS) Wives Association. Essentially, the administration lacked the mechanisms to give relief to those without ration cards. The inability to access identity cards has remained a problem for many of the waste pickers, although some have fared better than others:

> In my caste, there is no differentiating. But others are facing problems. Those who belong to the Yerukula and Pamula communities are facing problems. But we are not getting any help from the government. I have applied many times for Ration card, Aadhar card and housing, and only after a long struggle I got them (Annie).

Discrimination against and stigmatisation of waste pickers practised in everyday social encounters and in policy spaces remains a huge barrier. Aman spoke of the commonplace discrimination against waste pickers, which he has struggled to counter for over a decade working with them. Discrimination takes many forms, including in governance spaces like municipal corporations. Waste pickers are integrated into waste management systems, but are systematically discriminated against through entrenched hiring practices, which remain contractual and intensify informality and precarity among waste pickers. This is a direct reflection of how little authorities value the work that waste pickers do. Although sympathy was expressed and relief provided by individuals and groups during the lockdown, Aman remains circumspect about whether the realisation of the particular vulnerability of waste pickers will translate into lasting positive or less discriminatory change.

Discussion

Drawing on policy discourse analysis and experiences shared by waste pickers and key informants working with waste-picking communities, we suggest that while the COVID-19 pandemic is in many ways exceptional, the policy responses and their impacts in specific contexts are an acute manifestation of what is already built into the worlds and everyday lives of waste-picking communities. Policy making by design creates and defines different masses of bodies for their government, and defines the contours of embodiment among individuals and groups. To make sense of this, we feel that the concept of 'debility', as articulated by Puar (2017), can allow us to interrogate the experiences of waste pickers in India. Puar articulates debility as a 'durational death', a way in which bodies are allowed neither to live nor to die. By 'creating injury' and maintaining this population as perpetually debilitated, and yet alive, this population can be controlled and used. Debility differs from disability; it foregrounds the 'slow wearing down of populations' (2017, xiv) rather than focusing on the before-and-after of an event that produces disability.

Puar argues that the 'precarity of certain bodies and populations' is maintained by making them available for maiming. As researchers, we are grappling with whether precarity and debility as concepts can be used to understand how waste workers are treated to generate a more holistic and intersectional understanding of waste picking, its markers and the lived realities of those engaged in this work, their families and communities. It helps us to understand how waste workers are deliberately held in a socially and economically constrained position. Their marginalisation is sedimented in both everyday social and national and local policy spaces in order to maintain the status quo, because India cannot function as a clean (pure and modern) state without the marginality of those charged with the work of cleaning. To extrapolate from Deleuze and Guattari, 'the state apparatus needs, at its summit, pre-disabled people' (see Puar 2017, 63) and, we suggest, needs this precarity to continue its claims to cleanliness and purity.

Puar (2017) argues that the social acceptance of disability relies on the obfuscation and deep proliferation of debility. The acceptance of certain kinds of understandings of waste work valorise the fact that waste pickers contribute around 20 per cent of the work involved in recycling waste. This blurs other more obscene aspects of waste work, and articulates waste pickers as hard-working citizens who contribute to society and therefore need to be rewarded.

The experiences of waste pickers highlight an urgent need to rethink overarching governance and accountability structures and systems that define 'waste picking', and those who make their living from this, to provide an accommodative frame of policy making centred on their rights. Such re-thinking demands that we develop an emic understanding of embodiment with those who are marginalised and oppressed. We need to integrate this understanding with discourses of intersectionality to move towards a framing capable of transforming power relations and redressing the inequalities in the health and wellbeing of waste-picking communities.

Acknowledgements

This chapter is written on the basis of our ongoing work with sanitation workers and waste-picking communities in Bengaluru (Karnataka), Guntur, Vijayawada (Andhra Pradesh) and Shimla (Himachal Pradesh), in India through the Accountability for Informal Urban Equity Hub (ARISE). ARISE is funded by the United Kingdom Research and Innovation (UKRI) Global Challenges Research Fund (GCRF). We would like to thank Barathi Nakkeeran and Prasanna Saligram from our team at the George Institute for Global Health, India, for their help and insights on all policy-related issues. Ethical clearance was obtained from the George Institute Ethics Committee and the Liverpool School of Tropical Medicine Research Governance and Ethics Office.

Notes

1. An usufructuary right allows the tenant to use and enjoy a property over a certain period, as long as he or she is able to maintain the property, pay taxes, and whatever else may be required as per applicable laws of the land. It is not ownership.
2. Page 47, https://www.mea.gov.in/Images/attach/amb/Volume_05.pdf .
3. Solid Waste Management Rules. 2016. Government of India, Ministry of Environment, Forest and Climate Change. Rule 3(1)(58).
4. Twelfth Schedule of the Indian Constitution: the Powers, Authority and Responsibilities of Municipalities. This schedule has 18 items. The Twelfth Schedule was added by the 74th

Amendment Act of 1992. In this chapter we refer to items within the purview of the municipalities.
5   Item 6, Seventh Schedule of the Constitution.
6   'It wasn't uncommon for the police to round up waste pickers for investigation in cases of theft in a locality' (Shankar and Sahni 2017, 255).
7   Sankaran (2013) also points out that one of the reasons for the disparity between the wage rates of men and women in India is the interplay between the Minimum Wages Act, 1948 and the Equal Remuneration Act, 1976.
8   Women are 'embraced by multiple patriarchies' that produce different effects on women in different castes and communities (Rao 2003). While there are similarities between the oppression(s) women face across castes and communities, Dalit Bahujan scholarship in this regard suggests that it is crucial to delineate the differences in order to avoid possible erasures.
9   It is crucial, when thinking of structures of power, to think of not only the 'victims' (Andersen and Collins 2015). Relying too heavily on the experiences of Black women can erase our ability to see race, class and gender as an integral part of everyone's experiences: 'What intersectionality does rather than what intersectionality is lies at the heart of intersectionality' (Collins and Bilge 2020, 3).
10 https://covid-india.in.
11 Deendayal Antyodaya Yojana – National Urban Livelihoods Mission, Empowering Marginalized Groups – Convergence Between SBM and DAY-NULM March 2018, National Urban Policy Framework 2018. (GOI 2018). Other policies have been used to support our argument as appropriate.
12 https://frontline.thehindu.com/cover-story/article26641511.ece.
13 https://www.theweek.in/news/india/2018/09/24/modis-ayushman-bharat-scheme-rejected-by-five-states.html.
14 https://eparlib.nic.in/bitstream/123456789/63614/1/14_Urban_Development_38.pdf#.
15 http://www.nrhmhp.gov.in/sites/default/files/files/Extension%20of%20RSBY%20to%205%20new%20Categories%20.pdf.
16 We have used pseudonyms for the interviewees to protect their identities.

References

Andersen, Margaret and Patricia Hill Collins. 2015. *Race, Class, & Gender: An anthology*. Boston, MA: Cengage.
Bacchi, Carol. 2014. *Analysing Policy: What's the problem represented to be?* 1st ed. Melbourne, Australia: Pearson Australia.
Bose, Rajanya and Anirban Bhattacharya. 2017. 'Why ragpickers, unrecognized and unpaid, are critical for waste management in India'. *IndiaSpend*, 12 May 2020. Accessed 4 January 2021. https://www.indiaspend.com/why-ragpickers-unrecognised-and-unpaid-are-critical-for-waste-management-in-india-43164/.
Butt, Waqas H. 2019. 'Beyond the abject: Caste and the organization of work in Pakistan's waste economy'. *International Labor and Working-Class History* 95: 18–33. https://doi.org/10.1017/s0147547919000061.
Collins, Patricia Hill and Sirma Bilge. 2020. *Intersectionality*. Cambridge, UK: Polity Press.
Doron, Assa. 2018. *Waste of a Nation: Garbage and growth in India*. Cambridge, MA: Harvard University Press.
Gatade, Subhash. 2015. 'Silencing caste, sanitising oppression'. *Economic & Political Weekly* 50(44): 29–35.
Gidwani, Vinay. 1992. '"Waste" and the permanent settlement in Bengal'. *Economic and Political Weekly* 27(4): 39–46. http://www.jstor.org/stable/4397526.
Gidwani, Vinay and Amita Baviskar. 2011. 'Urban commons'. *Economic and Political Weekly* 46(50): 42–3.
Gidwani, Vinay and Julia Eleanor Corwin. 2017. 'Governance of waste'. *Economic & Political Weekly* 52(31): 44–54.
Gidwani, Vinay and Rajyashree N. Reddy. 2011. 'The afterlives of "waste": Notes from India for a minor history of capitalist surplus'. *Antipode* 43(5): 1625–58.

Gidwani, Vinay and Anant Maringanti. 2016. 'The waste-value dialectic: Lumpen urbanization in contemporary India'. *Comparative Studies of South Asia, Africa and the Middle East* 36(1): 112–33. https://doi.org/10.1215/1089201x-3482159.
Gill, Kaveri. 2009. *Of Poverty and Plastic: Scavenging and scrap trading entrepreneurs in India's urban informal economy*. New Delhi, India: Oxford University Press.
GOI. 1969. *Report of the National Commission on Labour*. New Delhi, India: Ministry of Labour and Employment and Rehabilitation
GOI. 2002. *Report of the Second National Commission on Labour*. New Delhi, India: Ministry of Labour.
GOI. 2007. *The Challenge of Employment in India: An informal economy perspective*. New Delhi, India: National Commission for Enterprises in the Unorganised Sector.
GOI. 2008. *The Unorganised Workers' Social Security Act*. New Delhi, India: Ministry of Labour and Employment.
GOI. 2016a. *An Inclusive Swachh Bharat through the Integration of the Informal Recycling Sector: A step by step guide*. New Delhi, India: Ministry of Urban Development.
GOI. 2016b. *Solid Waste Management Rules*. New Delhi, India: Ministry of Environment and Forests.
GOI. 2018. *National Urban Policy Framework*. New Delhi, India: Ministry of Housing and Urban Affairs.
Harriss-White, Barbara. 2017. 'Formality and informality in an Indian urban waste economy'. *International Journal of Sociology and Social Policy* 37(7/8): 417–34. https://doi.org/10.1108/IJSSP-07-2016-0084.
Harriss-White, Barbara. 2020. 'Waste, social order, and physical disorder in small-town India'. *The Journal of Development Studies* 56(2): 239–58. https://doi.org/10.1080/00220388.2019.1577386.
Kornberg, Dana. 2019. 'From Balmikis to Bengalis: The "casteification" of Muslims in Delhi's informal garbage economy'. *Economic & Political Weekly* 54(47): 48–54.
Krishnakumar, R. 2019. 'A better option in Kerala'. *Frontline Magazine*, 12 April 2020. Accessed 4 January 2021. https://frontline.thehindu.com/cover-story/article26641511.ece.
Maharashtra, Government of. 1989. *Dr Babasaheb Ambedkar: Writings and speeches, Vol. 5*. Mumbai, India: Government of Maharashtra.
Ministry of Housing and Urban Affairs. 2016. *Deendayal Antyodaya Yojana-National Urban Livelihoods Mission*. Accessed 4 January 2021. https://nulm.gov.in/PDF/NULM_Mission/NULM_mission_document.pdf.
Morrison, Susan Signe. 2015. *The Literature of Waste: Material ecopoetics and ethical matter*. New York: Palgrave Macmillan.
Murthy, Shrutika. 2020. 'Shadowing Suvartha on her waste-picking route in Vijayawada'. Accessed 4 January 2021. http://www.ariseconsortium.org/learn-more/multimedia/shadowing-suvartha/.
Puar, Jasbir K. 2017. *The Right to Maim: Debility, capacity, disability*. Durham. NC: Duke University Press.
Rao, Anupama. 2003. *Gender and Caste*, edited by Rajeshwari Sunder Rajan. *Issues in Contemporary Indian Feminism, Vol. 1*. New Delhi: Kali for Women (in association with the Book Review Literary Trust).
Reddy, Akhileshwari and Alok Prasanna Kumar. 2018. *Wastepicker Welfare Law in Karnataka*. New Dehli, India: The Vidhi Centre For Legal Policy.
Reddy, Rajyashree N. 2018. 'The urban under erasure: Towards a postcolonial critique of planetary urbanization'. *Environment and Planning D: Society and Space* 36(3): 529–39.
Saligram, Prasanna. 2020. 'Shadowing Kishore on his waste-picking route in Vijayawada'. Accessed 4 January 2021. http://www.ariseconsortium.org/shadowing-kishore/.
Sankaran, Kamala. 2013. 'Domestic work, unpaid work and wage rates'. *Economic and Political Weekly* 48(43): 85–9.
Shankar, V Kalyan and Rohini Sahni. 2017. 'The inheritance of precarious labor: Three generations in waste picking in an Indian city'. *Women's Studies Quarterly* 45(3/4): 245–62.
Singh, Bhasha. 2014. *Unseen: The truth about India's manual scavengers*. Translated by Reenu Talwar. London: Penguin.
The Week. 2018. 'Modi's Ayushman Bharat scheme rejected by five states'. 24 September 2018. Accessed 24 December 2020. https://www.theweek.in/news/india/2018/09/24/modis-ayushman-bharat-scheme-rejected-by-five-states.html.

12
The amplification effect

Impacts of COVID-19 on sexual and reproductive health and rights in Indonesia

Linda Rae Bennett and Setiyani Marta Dewi

Indonesia's President Joko Widodo declared the spread of COVID-19 a national disaster on 13 April 2020. Since this declaration, people living in the cities of Jakarta and Yogyakarta have endured extreme flooding, multiple dengue outbreaks, a notable earthquake and a full-scale volcanic eruption within their provincial boundaries. They have lived daily with appalling air, water and waste pollution, abysmal overcrowding in informal urban settlements, and, in the case of Jakarta residents, knowledge that their home is literally sinking. These circumstances typify the ongoing precarity that Indonesians face in their everyday lives, and form critical context for understanding the impacts of additional threats such as the COVID-19 pandemic.

In this chapter, we offer a contextualised analysis of the ways in which COVID-19, and responses to it, have impacted on the sexual and reproductive health and rights (SRHR) of vulnerable Indonesian communities living in Jakarta and Yogyakarta. The communities we focus on are youth, particularly street-dwelling youth, people living with HIV, transwomen and female sex workers. We share the recent experiences of these communities via the observations of frontline workers engaged in the promotion of SRHR both before and during the COVID-19 pandemic. Frontline workers are thus positioned as experts on their experiences of how COVID-19 has impacted their work, as well as mediators seeking to reduce the impacts of the pandemic on the communities they support. Half of the frontline workers we have spoken with are also members of the communities with whom they work.

Through our analysis of frontline worker narratives, we trace how the pandemic has amplified pre-existing inequalities. The concept of amplification has received most attention in the field of risk analysis (Kasperson et al. 1988), with a focus on exploring how media reporting and public communications about epidemics and other threats shape the social construction of risk perception (Masuda and Garvin 2006; Wirz et al. 2018). In this chapter, we are not concerned with risk perception. Rather we use the term amplification to describe how the concrete and often overlapping conditions of deprivation have been intensified within the pandemic. We adapt the notion of deprivation amplification as we identify how everyday lives that are routinely marked by deprivation of income and resources, access to healthcare, and the denial of human rights, respect and citizenship, have been rendered disproportionally vulnerable to the impacts of COVID-19. By focusing on SRHR, we place the larger health footprint of the COVID-19 pandemic at the centre of analysis. We track how COVID-19 has amplified the vulnerability of marginalised communities to poorer health outcomes more widely.

Frontline worker informants paint a vivid picture of Indonesia's brittle, patchy and under-resourced health system. This image is verified by data on health expenditure and sexual and reproductive health (SRH) outcomes, which we outline briefly to contextualise recent declines in the provision of SRH services. Indonesia's expenditure on health as a percentage of GDP is low, remaining below average in comparison with other middle-income countries; last verified in 2017, it was 3.1 per cent of gross domestic product (WHO 2021).[1] Despite the introduction of the national health insurance programme in 2014, the Government of Indonesia's (GoI) contribution to the cost of healthcare remained at 39 per cent in 2017, while out-of-pocket health expenditure was estimated at around 61 per cent (WHO 2021). Additionally, the health worker to population ratio in Indonesia remains lower than recommended by the World Health Organization (WHO) (Anderson et al. 2014; Agustina et al. 2019), with a particular shortage of nurses and midwives who are crucial for the provision of SRH services.

Indonesia's performance against key SRH indicators is highly deficient, with underinvestment in health and failure to address poverty both contributing to poor SRH outcomes. Indonesia's maternal mortality rate was the highest of all ASEAN nations in 2017, with 177 deaths per 100,000 live births (World Bank 2020a), and considerable variation between regions, impacting especially remote, poor and adolescent women (Nababan et al. 2018). Unmet need for contraception is estimated to be approximately 15 per cent among married couples and much higher among unmarried people who have no legal access to contraception (World Bank 2020b).

Legal access to safe abortion in Indonesia is highly constrained, unless a woman's life is deemed to be at risk. Approximately two million induced abortions occur annually, and deaths from unsafe abortion contribute to at least 15 per cent of the country's maternal mortality (Landiyanto 2010). Early marriage and adolescent child bearing are still prevalent, particularly in remote and low-income communities, where up to 40 per cent of women become mothers before the age of 18 (Bennett 2014).

Another indicator of Indonesia's lack of investment in SRHR is the consistent increase in HIV infections since 2012. Heterosexual transmission is now the primary mode of new infections, and a gradual feminisation of the epidemic is occurring, with younger women most vulnerable (Bennett and Spagnoletti 2019). Out of an estimated population of 640,000 HIV positive Indonesians in 2018, only 17 per cent were receiving antiretroviral (ARV) treatment (HIV and AIDS Data Hub for Asia Pacific 2020) and only 15 per cent of HIV-positive pregnant Indonesian women received the WHO-recommended regimen for prevention of mother-to-child transmission (HIV and AIDS Data Hub for Asia Pacific 2020). The under-investment in SRHR and the neglect of vulnerable populations forms the backdrop for understanding the additional SRH burden experienced by these communities since the onset of the pandemic.

Below we address how COVID-19 has necessitated a shift in research praxis, and the importance of resisting closing ethnographic fields in times of crisis. We discuss our inclusive definition of frontline workers and their holistic approach to supporting marginalised Indonesian communities. We establish how access to SRH services for vulnerable communities has been impacted during the pandemic, and how these impacts have been shaped by long-term inequalities. The concept of invisible citizens is then deployed to analyse the systematic exclusion of specific individuals from state-sponsored healthcare and emergency financial assistance. This brings us to our core argument – that COVID-19 has amplified inequalities, making it all the more important to ethno-graphically engage with vulnerable communities and highlight how recent detrimental impacts on their SRHR are embedded in the persistent politics of discrimination and deprivation.

Reshaping research praxis and engaging frontline workers

International border closures, neighbourhood lockdowns and social distancing measures, introduced to slow the spread of COVID-19, inhibit our capacity to enter the ethnographic field, and we do not know when these will be removed. However, rather than accepting a forced closing-off of the field, we chose to adapt, and propelled by the wish to maintain ongoing dialogue with valued Indonesian colleagues at a time when their voices clearly need to be heard, we extended our research praxis. Through online stakeholder consultations we identified several groups particularly vulnerable to the impacts of COVID-19 in Indonesia. These groups are people living with HIV, youth – including street-dwelling youth – transwomen and female sex workers. We then put aside former anxieties over how virtual/digital ethnography could potentially lead to the loss of intimacy, rapport and trust with research participants, although we are mindful (and grateful) that our foray into virtual data collection and collaboration is underpinned by decades of ethnographic research and practice in the SRH field in Indonesia.

Significant attention has been accorded to the crucial roles of frontline health workers, and their vulnerability in the context of COVID-19 (Amnesty International 2020; Nguyen et al. 2020). In Indonesia, very high infection and mortality rates among frontline healthcare workers have been verified, resulting in pressure on the GoI to better protect them (Amnesty International 2020). In this study, we extend the definition of frontline workers from such qualified healthcare workers to others also actively engaged in the promotion of SRHR. We interviewed a total of 20 frontline workers who support vulnerable communities in various ways: providing counselling and clinical SRH services; facilitating access to services and running outreach programmes; providing peer support and distributing condoms; providing information about SRH and available services; managing or implementing targeted programmes; and providing emergency financial assistance.

An eclectic group of frontline workers was purposively sampled to provide access to the first-hand experiences of people whose work focuses on supporting communities with poor access to SRH services under normative (pre-COVID-19) circumstances. Our broad definition of frontline workers recognised the complex needs of and complexity of working with vulnerable communities to address intersecting axes of disadvantage. Our informants viewed biomedical solutions to health problems as 'only one part of the problem' facing their friends and clients. They emphasised that efforts to improve SRH among vulnerable communities should also include: facilitating access to health services; education and advocacy; creating belonging and countering the impacts of stigma; and facilitating poverty alleviation. This holistic conceptualisation of their roles resonates with the observations of Sarradon-Eck et al. (2014) in their research with frontline social workers and urban homeless populations in France. They describe a logic of care (Mol 2008) and support among French frontline workers that propelled them to engage with clients in a more holistic way than hospital-based health workers (Sarradon-Eck et al. 2014, 260). In drawing on narratives from our research, we show how frontline workers reveal a consistent logic of care driven by a commitment to provide broad support to vulnerable community members. The breadth of their work and perspectives enabled us to explore how poorer SRH outcomes for vulnerable communities during the pandemic have been produced by and through pre-existing and intensified patterns of inequality, not merely due to an interruption of routine services.

Our sample of frontline workers included four transwomen, 11 women, four men and one person identifying as queer, reflecting the gender imbalance in the field of SRHR in Indonesia. This gender asymmetry also reflects that many SRH programmes in Indonesia focus on women as recipients, and tend to employ women as programme managers, outreach workers and peer educators/leaders with the exception of programmes dedicated to men who have sex with men. We acknowledge the limits of our inclusion of voices from vulnerable community members (except for the ten frontline workers who were also community members) and hope to remedy this when collaborative community-based research becomes safe. To protect anonymity, pseudonyms are used for direct quotes from frontline workers, and we refer to the gender and professional role of informants only as identifying features.

Data were collected in June and July 2020 via WhatsApp (for recruitment and follow up), email (used for stakeholder consultations, sharing plain language statements and clarifying points of interest from interviews) and Zoom (to conduct and record virtual interviews). While we relied on digital technology to be co-present with our participants, the interviews focused on people's concrete experiences in the physical world. Children, pets and partners drifted in and out of focus during interviews due to the shared 'work from home if you can' situation. We were struck by the parallels in atmosphere between the virtual interviews and experiences of face-to-face ethnography conducted in people's physical homes. An unforeseen but welcome aspect stemming from the infusion of domesticity was an enhanced sense of informality and intimacy in our dialogue, and a willingness of people to share their time generously. Virtual interviews were conducted with relative ease, as most informants were using the chosen communication mediums in their professional lives, and had reliable internet access. While these conditions facilitated dialogue with frontline workers, we note that the vulnerable community members that our informants support are not all in the same position, and many could not be expected to participate in virtual research without significant financial and technological assistance. Thus, the field in this instance could stretch no further than the boundaries of a reliable internet connection and a smartphone with credit enough to run the Zoom application for an hour or more. Most interviews took around one and a half hours and up to two and a half hours.

Impacts of COVID-19 on sexual and reproductive health and rights

While the full extent of COVID-19 impacts on SRH cannot be precisely measured during the crisis, Riley and colleagues (2020) have estimated that a 10 per cent decline in women's access to SRH services and contraception in low- and middle-income countries during the COVID-19 pandemic will have vast impacts, including a rapid escalation in maternal mortality. In Indonesia, where frontline workers have described widespread reductions in the availability of SRH services and the number of women accessing those services, shortages of hormonal contraceptives and condoms, reduced access to voluntary testing and counselling (VCT) and to antiretroviral drugs (ARV), we can expect dramatic increases in negative SRH outcomes. With this knowledge, frontline workers are legitimately arguing for the GoI to recognise SRH services as an essential area of healthcare both during the COVID-19 pandemic and under ordinary circumstances.

Maternal health, family planning and safe abortion services

Frontline workers reported a wide range of interruptions to routine SRH services in Yogyakarta and Jakarta, stemming from the GoI response to COVID-19 and the low capacity of the health system prior to the pandemic. Clinical health workers described recent changes in their roles, such as being seconded to COVID-19 testing and tracing, and to emergency rooms to replace colleagues who were unable to work after contracting COVID-19. This redeployment of staff led to decreased opening hours in both public and private SRH clinics. Our informants reported that early in the pandemic, many clinics were only managing to open one or two days a week, when they had previously been open five or six days a week. In some districts primary health clinics contracted and offered emergency services only, such as responding to birth complications, but offered no other SRH services.

Reduced uptake of SRH services also resulted from communities receiving inadequate information regarding which services were considered essential according to the GoI response plan. Many frontline workers reported that vulnerable community members were confused over which clinics were open, during what hours and what services were available. The GoI health communication efforts during the pandemic firmly focused on messaging related to managing COVID-19 (Hort et al. 2020) and neglected to provide adequate information about how other services have been reorganised.

Melati, who coordinates SRH programmes for youth, explained the increased risks women faced without clear definitions of emergency or essential SRH services:

> For instance, in [location deleted] area ... only pregnant women having a medical situation [emergency] can come to the health service. Well, actually the definition of emergency could be different between the providers and also the clients. And it could be very dangerous because like when the women experiencing the complications and stuff it can lead them to stay away. I mean like, they don't give the parameters on what is considered as an emergency or not.

Others reported that primary health clinics where they worked had attempted to continue offering a range of basic services. However, the definition of essential services by the Ministry of Health did not include programmes for hard-to-reach groups, such as youth-friendly services and dedicated programmes for sex workers, which were part of routine services in highly resourced clinics prior to the pandemic (MOH 2020). As a response to the pandemic, primary healthcare clinics shifted to offering services only by appointment, and increasingly clinics are dictating that appointments must be made online not in person. The length of standard appointments shortened as infection spread, and whenever possible tele-health appointments were (and are) encouraged. These changes represent barriers to participation for vulnerable groups without access to the internet or smartphones, or cash to buy phone credit.

Our participants confirmed that some primary health clinics could not provide women with long-acting reversible contraceptives (LARC) such as inter-uterine devices (IUDs) and implants, because these methods must be administered by clinical health workers, many of whom were seconded to the COVID-19 response. Participants were also concerned about the depletion of LARC supplies at the national level, as Melati explained:

> In April, BKKBN [the National Family Planning Board] said that there will be a stock-out of IUD in the country. And also, we are afraid that it will happen to other contraceptive methods like pills and injectables. Because like, we import them from India, and since India is on lockdown … there is a … shortage in many provinces.

Health workers also expressed concern over their clients' preferences for short-acting contraceptives such as the pill or monthly injectables because free access to these types of contraceptives requires regular visits to health clinics. Clients were less willing to attend clinics due to fear of COVID-19 infection, and delayed access to the contraceptive method of their choice was assumed to be related to the increasing number of women presenting at clinics with unintended pregnancies.

Another consequence of reduced access to free SRH services has been higher demand for services in the private sector, because private SRH clinics are not obliged to offer COVID-related services as are primary health clinics, and thus attending them is perceived as having lower COVID-19 risk. However, there has also been a reported reduction in the availability of safe abortion services, which many people seek to access in the private sector because of the restricted legality of abortion in Indonesia. Hati, a SRH phone counsellor, described the ongoing barriers to accessing safe abortion during the COVID-19 pandemic:

> It's more difficult [to access safe abortion] for people in a less privileged group of course, so … promoting medical abortion [in Indonesia] … may be the only choice that we have now [during the pandemic]. Because if women go to the surgical clinic it will take like … a million rupiah, and then if you want a safe service on abortion, if you want to have … a good service on abortion, you have to pay … multiple times to a doctor. Ya, because it can only happen in a private hospital.

Rising costs of care in the private sector made SRH services increasingly accessible only to middle class and elite Indonesians. Rose, who directs a CBO supporting street-dwelling youth, described how reduced access to free healthcare at primary health clinics at the beginning of the COVID-19 pandemic led to higher costs for pregnant women seeking care from private midwives:

> What we know at that time [at the beginning of the pandemic] the primary health care clinic reached full capacity in offering services, these clinics quickly went over capacity. So pregnant women were not going to the *puskesmas* for service. Many decided to visit private midwives for their check-ups. But the cost for just one visit is very expensive and so they only went once.

Low-income street-dwelling youth who become pregnant are already at higher risk of pregnancy and birth-related complications due to age and poverty, and their ability to access their four pre-natal visits (recommended by the GoI and known as the K4) has been compromised by reduced access to free services.

STI and HIV prevention and related services

Routine STI and HIV testing, and mobile testing, stalled in many of the urban neighbourhoods of Jakarta and Yogyakarta. Free mobile clinics and outreach services offering SRH services to hard-to-reach communities are the most accessible services for vulnerable groups, particularly street-dwelling youth, transwomen and sex workers (Hegarty et al. 2020). The cessation of mobile outreach services that offer VCT and free condoms to hard-to-reach groups amplified the vulnerability of those groups to poor SRH outcomes. Many primary healthcare clinics offering SRH services are poorly equipped to offer non-judgemental and non-discriminatory services (Waluyo et al. 2015), as Niko explains: 'In health facilities [primary healthcare clinics], young people who are vulnerable are often told by a health worker to "stop being sex workers, to stop being gay, and to pray more often"'.

With the suspension of mobile clinics and outreach programmes specialised in the provision of SRH services, highly vulnerable groups lost access to their routine avenues for accessing SRH care. Ari, a peer educator with female sex workers, explains the situation for low-income sex workers unable to access free condoms due to constrained outreach services:

> Many people from the [sex worker] community … complain about this. Sex worker friends who only make 50 thousand rupiah or 30 thousand rupiah per customer cannot also provide condoms …

> So, they [sex workers] really need a free condom, they really need it. I have met a lot of sex worker friends whose fees are cheap, 50 thousand rupiah, yes, some even say that they only get paid 15 thousand rupiah. Well, just imagine if they have to set aside money again for a condom, in one day they will need to increase their customers for example from 10 customers to 15 customers just to cover the condom cost. It should not be like that huh?

Access to free condoms for sex workers also declined as social distancing requirements and funding cuts diminished the capacity of community outreach programmes. Madu, an outreach worker in a HIV prevention and treatment programme, also noted the shortage of condoms among female sex workers: 'We are still [in June 2020] meeting sex workers who have to buy their condoms themselves, they are not receiving them free, first because the supply [of free condoms] is depleted, and second because peer distribution is interrupted because of COVID'. For most sex workers, purchasing condoms is not an option because they are expensive, especially when people experience a dramatic loss of income.

Reduced outreach services for people living with HIV also occurred, particularly affecting the availability of voluntary testing and counselling. Our participants working to support people living with HIV observed that the number of people seeking routine VTC in Jakarta and Yogyakarta dropped by 75 per cent or more between April and August (when we completed our virtual field work), and there is growing concern within the HIV positive community and frontline workers about rising HIV infections. Utama, a programme coordinator and outreach worker with HIV positive Indonesians and LGBTQI+ communities, expressed his concerns as follows:

> Yeah maybe people can go to the private service, go that way [to access VTC], but for the clinic situation, all I hear is that COVID is the primary issue, and for now, other issues are getting less attention. So I'm worried, yes I'm worried about it [the lack of access to VCT] ... if VCT access is low now ... later we can see many new cases, and new cases without a diagnosis. I'm worried ... very worried about this.

While ARV is a necessary treatment for HIV as a chronic condition, it is also an important component to ensure the SRH and wellbeing of people living with HIV, to maintain a low risk of maternal-to-child transmission, and to lower the risk of transmission to sexual partners. At the beginning of the pandemic, there was expressed concern about constrained access to antiretroviral drugs for HIV positive Indonesians (Luis et al. 2020; Pangestika 2020). The Ministry of Health technical guidelines for service provision at primary health clinics during the COVID-19 pandemic state that access to ARV for registered HIV positive individuals should be maintained. However, this guideline is accompanied by an explicit caveat that ARV should be provided only where 'stocks are adequate' (MOH 2020, 15), which the GoI has been unable to guarantee.

Shortages in the supply of ARV were initially reported in Java, Bali and in Ambon and other outer islands of the archipelago between March and May 2020 (Ibnu Aqil 2020). Later in the pandemic, supplies of ARV stock were (in August 2020) reportedly secure on the island of Java, but other locations across Indonesia were still vulnerable to stock-outs, partly due to the interruption of domestic and international transport systems. This resulted in innovative responses among people living with HIV, including sharing limited ARV supplies, making do with out-of-date ARV drugs and visiting hospitals more regularly to access ARV – as often as every four days (UNAIDS 2020). HIV positive and queer communities, international non-governmental organisations and HIV organisations across and beyond Indonesia used crowd sourcing to raise funds and hired special couriers to deliver ARV to remote areas, put highly visible pressure via social media on international suppliers of ARV to increase the pace of shipments to Indonesia, and advocated to the Ministry of Health. Bunga, a programme director who works with HIV positive Indonesians and female sex workers, described lobbying the GoI to prevent future stock-outs of ARV drugs:

> Another work in progress is to ensure this is not happening again in the future [ARV shortages] … The Ministry of Health is only able to procure drugs which are included in the e-catalogue. So, we advocated to influence a faster process for some essential [ARV] drugs to be included in the e-catalogue. Two of them have been included in the last month [May 2020].

The health-seeking behaviour of vulnerable groups has also been shaped by their responses to COVID-19, which frontline workers associate with loss of income stemming from the pandemic. A survey conducted by the UNAIDS Indonesia branch in April 2020, measuring the impact of COVID-19 on the wellbeing of young HIV positive Indonesians, confirmed that 56 per cent of survey participants had lost their jobs since the beginning of the pandemic (UNAIDS 2020). Melati, who coordinates SRH programmes for youth, describes the impact of this on the young people with whom she works:

> Like for young people ... when they lose their job, it makes them become vulnerable because it limits their ability to fulfil their daily basics. So, I mean like if the daily basics are not fulfilled yet, they won't think that their sexual and reproductive health is an important thing.

Reduced mobility, particularly for people who have no independent means of transport, has also constrained access to services. Community-level responses to COVID-19 across Indonesia have varied, with some neighbourhoods imposing strict lockdowns and travel bans, further inhibiting people's ability to access SRH care beyond their immediate neighbourhoods. Low-income communities have fewer transport options, and if they want to access healthcare they must risk exposure on public transport. Ira works for an organisation supporting children living with HIV and their caregivers, and conveys the pressure this has put on families seeking continuity of care for their children:

> According to the policy [regarding HIV care for children] they should be taken to a doctor first if they are ill, not directly to the hospital. So they must take two trips. For them to reach the hospital they only have the option of public transport, they can't use the online motorcycle taxi, as this kind of service has declined due to social distancing. If they don't have a motor bike, the other option is to rent a car and that is much more expensive.

Reproductive cancer prevention and screening programmes

Mobile outreach mammogram services, targeting poor and homeless women in Jakarta, were also reportedly paused due to the perceived COVID-19 risk related to outreach work and the unavailability of healthcare workers to run the mobile units. Again, the same pattern emerges: the most vulnerable members of society are the first to lose access to essential SRH services, as a result of the GoI's priorities in relation to its COVID-19 response. Community-based outreach screening services for cervical and breast cancer also stalled, and are likely to be suspended for at least 12 months. This is due to significant government funding cuts to community-based organisations providing SRH health services for the financial year beginning July 2020 (Spagnoletti et al.

2020). Below, Hannah, a researcher in the area of cervical cancer, describes the likely impact of funding cuts on cervical cancer prevention:

> I just got the news from my colleagues [at a cancer prevention service] that their operating budget for the next 12 months is cut. They will go from 30 staff down to 15, and even those 15 will just be part time. They will only be open three days a week. And they won't be able to offer mass pap smear screenings in the community. There will be a significant reduction in free pap smear tests offered [over the next 12 months], down from 4000 to 1000. This is because the Government decided to focus on COVID-19.

Free human papilloma virus (HPV) vaccination of teenage girls has also been deferred, and it is estimated that around 120,000 girls in 2020 may not receive their second dose of the HPV vaccine, and thus will not be protected against HPV infection (Ramdan 2020). Despite significant lobbying for the HPV vaccination to be added to the national immunisation programme, there is no commitment from the Ministry of Health to do so.

Home-based schooling in response to COVID-19 also means Indonesian adolescents are missing crucial opportunities for SRH education that only occur for most in school. Government funding for adolescent-friendly outreach programmes, run by primary health clinics, has been reduced by up to 70 per cent for the remainder of 2020 due to the redirection of operating funds to the COVID-19 response. Ina, a senior official in charge of adolescent health programmes at district level, describes these funding cuts and their impact:

> The original budget for [youth outreach] this year was about 800 million rupiah ... but it turns out we have received only about 200 million ... This changed in the month of March, when COVID happened ... since April we have received nothing at all, so going out for outreach was only possible from January to March this year.

Invisible citizens

In Indonesia, identity cards confer rights, and without these cards vulnerable communities and individuals are structurally excluded from full citizenship. Currently (and prior to COVID-19), people from within these communities who have no legal identity are, in effect, invisible. In theory, Indonesian citizens are entitled to free healthcare and financial assistance to alleviate extreme poverty, both of which are crucial in the context of catastrophic income loss. The financial assistance schemes introduced in response to COVID-19 are supposed to operate at district and village levels, and provide cash payments of 600,000 rupiah per family, per month.[2] This equates to less than 50 per cent of the minimum wage in Yogyakarta and less than 25 per cent of the minimum wage in Jakarta (Yumna et al. 2020). At the time of writing (October 2020) 600,000 rupiah was equivalent to US$40; the cost of a standard appointment with a private midwife in an urban area around 50,000 rupiah or US$5.

However, a key criticism of the GoI's COVID-19 response has been its failure to ensure that emergency financial assistance reaches the most vulnerable communities – those already living below the poverty line prior to COVID-19. The increased cost of SRH care has been felt acutely within marginalised communities with limited access to financial support from the GoI, and dramatic loss of income for those who cannot work due to social distancing and lockdown measures. Frontline workers identified that a key barrier to those most in need receiving support is their ineligibility for financial assistance and free healthcare. The GoI's COVID-19 social assistance payments are available only to citizens who can produce a current identity card, either the NIK (national identity card) or KTP (residents' card), and are registered as residing in the same locale as they seek benefits. Highly mobile populations, including street-dwelling youth and families, and sex workers, are frequently unable to produce this requisite proof of residence. Because they have no fixed address, or proof of residence, they are rendered invisible. Vin, a director of a transwomen's CBO, explained:

> The help [financial assistance from GoI] so far is not given just by name, right … If you don't have an identity card in the place where you live now, for example, you can't access it [financial assistance] like that. So you do have to have a residence. Not everyone has a regular residence and not everyone has an ID card for where they live, for example some only have one from where they originally come from. Maybe there is a way to access the help via a local community leader, who knows who we are, but until now my friends don't know if this is possible.

Loss of income, lack of a secure residence and the absence of a legal identity therefore converge to result in deprivation amplification, rendering people disproportionally vulnerable to the impacts of COVID-19 compared to those with legal citizenship and relative economic security. Vulnerable community members also reported discriminatory treatment when seeking to access support designed to protect Indonesians during the pandemic, as Anggi, a transwoman activist, described:

> Since the COVID-19 pandemic hit the whole of Indonesia and especially in [location removed], the impact has been very large on the transwoman community and marginal communities in general. This impact is due to limited access to what's it called? … [financial assistance], due to considerable levels of pre-existing stigma and discrimination. The attention given to minority groups has been so drastically reduced it is now almost non-existent. Even those who clearly have ID cards in their area are finding they are not registered to receive the payment. They are missing from the government assistance data base.

Motivated by the introduction of Indonesia's universal healthcare system in 2014, Berenschot and colleagues (2014) documented how Javanese of low-income, rural and remote backgrounds might access the new system, and identified multiple barriers to accessing free healthcare. They observed that 'social marginalization and bureaucratic unresponsiveness – often in vicious combination – generate a gap between rights-on-paper and rights-as-realized' (Berenschot et al. 2018). Six years after the establishment of the national health insurance scheme, the situation has changed little, but now with the amplifying effect of COVID-19 in play. Without a current identity card, it is still impossible to apply for coverage under the national health insurance scheme, and so even nominally free health services must be paid for out-of-pocket. Moreover, low-income communities who experience intergenerational cycles of poverty have low rates of registration of births, marriages and deaths in many parts of Indonesia (Platt 2017). The absence of birth and marriage certificates make obtaining an identity card difficult because this requires an application to a civil court, letters from a village or neighbourhood leader, and witnesses (with their own identity cards) to verify the identity of the person. These processes were described as unnecessarily complicated, arduous and time consuming by our informants.

Currently, the health and welfare needs of people under the age of 18 are assumed by the state to be protected within the family unit. Their ability to access services, hormonal contraceptives, condoms and essential medicines is understood as contingent on their parents' approval and support. Niko works with vulnerable youth including those who are HIV positive, who sell sex and who identify as LGBTQI+. He explains how state regulations are highly problematic for young people without family support:

> According to the law people under 18 need consent from their parents [or guardians] before they can have a test [HIV or other STI test]. But in reality these teenagers are not open to their families about their behaviour outside the house or their sexual orientation. To get access to health services some people under 18 steal their family KTP. There is also some confusion around who is eligible to be a guardian. Some health [youth friendly] services will allow a community worker to act as a guardian, but many of them do not.

Failure to recognise the independence of youth before the age of 18 (or, for many, prior to marriage) prevents them from acquiring individual identity cards, and this in turn prevents them from accessing free SRH healthcare. Moreover, widespread denial and condemnation of youth sexuality in Indonesia mean that youth below age 18 are not considered sexual citizens and subsequently young people have no legal status as consumers of SRH services.

Another vulnerable group with constrained access to identity cards is women living in abusive relationships, whose male partners control their access to the family identity card and subsequently to healthcare, including access to free contraception. Bunga, who works in a HIV prevention and treatment programme, noted that others, too, lacked proof of identity:

> Transwomen and younger sex workers … are most likely not to have the ID card … Without the ID card they are then not linked to the safety net that is provided by the government. It is common [to not have an ID card] among sex workers who are mobile, or living within an abusive relationship. So, I have, I observed many cases of this … their husbands, their boyfriends keep their ID cards.

Bunga also described that identity cards were increasingly being held as collateral by money lenders until such time that debts can be cleared: 'It is now common in Indonesia to have female sex workers who are … trapped in a loan, we now have what we call, like online loans, and also traditional loans. So, you're able to borrow money easily, but you need to give the ID card [as security]'. Low-income women are more likely to be forced into these kinds of debt arrangements than men, because they typically lack other forms of capital that can be used to guarantee repayment. Loss of income due to COVID-19, compounded by debt, and the loss of access to healthcare and financial support, can create a vicious dynamic of deprivation amplification for women.

Conclusion: The amplification effect

Multiple overlapping conditions of exclusion and deprivation, shaping the everyday lives of marginalised urban Indonesian communities, have been amplified during the pandemic. We have used amplification conceptually to capture frontline workers' assertions that COVID-19 is not the root cause of the challenges they are now facing, but rather, that it has revealed and rapidly intensified pre-existing inequalities. In Melati's words, 'We can't blame it all on COVID'. She further explains, 'previously, the access [to SRH services for vulnerable groups] is not really there and because of COVID, like, it's become more visible'. The pre-existing dynamics of under-investment in SRH, the othering of vulnerable communities, and the exclusion of individuals from full citizenship, all contribute to the amplification of poor access to SRH services and other forms of deprivation during the COVID-19 pandemic.

In theory, Indonesia's comprehensive policy should promote the SRHR reproductive rights of citizens, but the implementation of this policy has been limited and variable. Underpinning the GoI's failure to implement this policy is the highly selective allocation of resources, the neglect of many SRH issues and the exclusion of non-conforming groups. Prior to COVID-19, budget allocation and human resources for SRH were overwhelmingly directed towards population control via the vigorous promotion of family planning (for married couples) and maternal health (once a woman is pregnant) (Bennett 2014), perpetuating a narrow focus on SRH concerns for married women who are already pregnant or who are seeking to limit family size. The consequence is that the core operational funds for primary health clinics are delegated to the provision of family planning and maternal health services, while other SRH services must be met by discretionary funds, which are not guaranteed. Frontline workers confirmed that SRH services for groups defined as hard-to-reach or most-at-risk in terms of SRH have not been designated as core services in the context of COVID-19, and were the first to be cut when the pandemic hit Indonesia. The observations of frontline workers are confirmed by the priorities in the Ministry of Health's operational guidelines for primary healthcare centres during the pandemic, issued in May 2020 (MOH 2020).

Critical SRH issues that the government excludes from its health budget include: access to safe abortion including medical abortion (both of which are illegal unless a woman's life is deemed at risk); access to contraception for unmarried people (which is illegal); affordable fertility treatment (excluded from the national health insurance scheme); and screening and treatment for intimate partner violence including sexual violence (guidelines exist but have not been operationalised beyond pilots) (Bennett and Spagnoletti 2019). The government continues to neglect or underinvest in: access to free HIV and other STI testing, counselling and treatment; prevention of HIV[3] and other STI transmission via condom promotion; comprehensive programmes for PMTC; the provision of comprehensive SRH education; access to youth-friendly SRH services; access to non-judgemental SRH services; and the prevention and treatment of reproductive cancers (Bennett and Spagnoletti 2019).

In mainstream GoI health discourses, the latter group of neglected SRH issues is closely associated with practices labelled as deviant, affecting only individuals who engage in deviant behaviour. An entrenched culture of othering, based on the dominant sexual morality of Indonesian society, exists at all levels of the health system from policy and budget allocation to the level of service provision (Bennett 2015). Most of our informants expressed deep concern over the stigmatisation and othering of vulnerable groups, and a small number exhibited discriminatory attitudes towards clients themselves. Jupe is a health worker in a primary health clinic and she shared the following concern: 'Mostly, what I regret, is that they [clients] have no shame when coming to the health service, they are young, unmarried, often having unprotected sex, and they just casually come to us for service … this is what I regret'. Jupe's negative judgement of unmarried youth seeking free SRH care at her clinic is not uncommon. In contrast, when asked what was required to improve the access of vulnerable groups to SRH care, Hati suggested: 'We need to address stigma and discrimination in the system … health workers should be the first group to achieve zero per cent stigma and discrimination in their behaviour'.

We have exposed the invisibility of poor, young (under 18) and marginalised community members as citizens, and illustrated how the lack of a legal identity prevents people from accessing free healthcare or financial assistance. The lack of citizenship is a profound driver of deprivation, and will continue to amplify the vulnerability of marginalised groups over the longer term, cementing pre-existing class inequalities. We have demonstrated that it is crucial to explore the intersections between economic hardship and health impacts to unpick the experiences and patterns of deprivation flowing from COVID-19.

Indonesia's failure to include comprehensive SRH services as essential services within its COVID-19 response (UNFPA 2020) will result in a dramatically larger long-term health footprint stemming from the pandemic, in which women, youth, poor and vulnerable groups will be disproportionally affected. The increasing visibility of Indonesia's failure to protect the SRHR of its citizens due to global media coverage of the pandemic could lead to greater international pressure on the GoI to increase its investment in SRH. However, achieving a more inclusive health system also requires recognition of full citizenship for marginalised and vulnerable groups, including the sexual citizenship of young people. Recognition of the prevalence and impact of stigma among health workers is also essential to improve the uptake of SRH services by vulnerable groups. The government's failure to adequately invest in SRH services as essential, during a state of emergency, is consistent with historical trends of under investment in health and a dangerously narrow definition of what constitutes legitimate SRH concerns. Longstanding politics of neglect and exclusion have been amplified through COVID-19 responses, reinforcing multiple intersecting barriers to peoples' ability to exercise their rights to health and livelihoods.

Acknowledgements

We wish to thank the frontline health workers who generously volunteered their time and energy to participate in this research while also managing an extraordinarily high burden of care in responding to the ongoing COVID-19 pandemic in Indonesia. We also acknowledge the financial support for this project received from the Indonesia Democracy Hallmark Research Initiative administered through the University of Melbourne.

Notes

1   The most recent population-based demographic health survey in Indonesia was conducted in 2017; the next is due to be conducted in 2022.
2   These schemes are called *bantuan sosial tunai* (cash social assistance) and *bantuan langsung tunai* (direct cash assistance).
3   Another structural factor shaping access to SRH services for vulnerable groups is the outsourcing of this work to international non-governmental organisations and CBOs. For instance, in 2016, the GoI dissolved the National AIDS Commission and contracted out this role to UNFPA. The strategy of outsourcing does have some benefits for vulnerable communities, but also reinforces the notion that these communities are, and should remain, other in relation to their SRHR. The outsourcing also gives a clear message that the government does not support the promotion of condoms for HIV prevention.

References

Agustina, Rina, Teguh Dartanto, Ratna Sitompul, Kun A. Susiloretni, Suparmi, Endang L. Achadi, Akmal Taher, Fadila Wirawan, Saleha Sungkar, Pratiwi Sudarmono, Anuraj H. Shankar and Hasbullah Thabrany. 2019. 'Universal health coverage in Indonesia: Concept, progress, and challenges'. *The Lancet* 393 (10166): 75–102. https://doi:10.1016/S0140-6736(18) 31647-7.

Amnesty International. 2020. *Global: Amnesty analysis reveals over 7,000 health workers have died from COVID-19*. Accessed 14 October 2020. https://www.amnesty.org/en/latest/news/ 2020/09/amnesty-analysis-7000-health-workers-have-died-from-covid19/.

Anderson, Ian, Andreasta Meliala, Puti Marzoeki and Eko Pambudi. 2014. 'The production, distribution, and performance of physicians, nurses, and midwives in Indonesia: An update'. Accessed 13 August 2020. https://ideas.repec.org/p/wbk/hnpdps/91324.html.

Bennett, Linda R. 2014. 'Early marriage, adolescent motherhood and reproductive rights for young Sasak mothers in Lombok'. *Wacana: Journal of the Humanities of Indonesia* 15 (1): 66–86. https://doi:10.17510/24076899-01501005.

Bennett, Linda R. 2015. 'Sexual morality and the silencing of sexual health within Indonesian infertility care'. In *Sex and Sexualities in Contemporary Indonesia: Sexual politics, diversity, representations and health*, edited by Linda R. Bennett and Sharyn G. Davies, pp. 148–66. London and New York: Routledge.

Bennett, Linda R. and Belinda Spagnoletti. 2019. 'Reproduction: Health: Indonesia'. In *Encyclopaedia of Women & Islamic Cultures*, edited by Suad Joseph. Accessed 12 April 2021. http://dx.doi. org/10.1163/1872-5309_ewic_COM_002172.

Berenschot, Ward, Retna Hanani and Prio Sambodho. 2018. 'Brokers and citizenship: Access to health care in Indonesia'. *Citizenship Studies* 22(2): 129–44. https://doi.org/10.1080/13621 025.2018.1445493.

Hegarty, Benjamin, Sandeep Nanwan and Ignatius Praptoraharjo. 2020. 'Understanding the challenges faced in community-based outreach programs aimed at men who have sex with men (MSM) in urban Indonesia'. *Sexual Health*. https://doi:10.1071/SH20065.

HIV and AIDS Data Hub for Asia Pacific. 2020. 'Indonesia: Epidemic snapshot'. *HIV AIDS Asia Pacific Research Statistical Data Information Resources AIDS Data Hub* website. Accessed 24 July 2020. https://www.aidsdatahub.org/country-profiles/indonesia.

Hort, Krishna, Angus Campbell and Tiara Marthias. 2020. 'Who to believe: Social media or government? The challenge of coronavirus in Indonesia'. *Indonesia at Melbourne* (blog). 28 February 2020. Accessed 13 August 2020. https://indonesiaatmelbourne.unimelb.edu.au/ who-to-believe-social-media-or-government-the-challenge-of-coronavirus-in-indonesia/.

Ibnu Aqil, A. Muh. 2020. 'HIV drug shortage hits nation as ministry procures supply'. *The Jakarta Post* website, 10 March 2020. Accessed 13 August 2020. https://www.thejakartapost.com/ news/2020/03/10/hiv-drug-shortage-hits-nation-ministry-procures-supply.html .

Kasperson, Roger E., Ortwin Renn, Paul Slovic, Halina S. Brown, Jacque Emel, Robert Goble, Jeanne X. Kasperson and Samuel Ratick. 1988. 'The social amplification of risk: A conceptual framework'. *Risk Analysis* 8(2): 177–87. https://doi.org/10.1111/j.1539-6924.1988.tb01168.x.

Landiyanto, Erlangga Agustino. 2010. 'Abortion policy in Indonesia: Rights, law and religious perspectives'. *SSRN Electronic Journal*. https://doi.org.10.2139/ssrn.1583403.

Luis, Hendry, Wayan Dede Fridayantara, Pande Agung Mahariski, Frank Stephen Wignall, Irwanto and Keerti Gedela. 2020. 'Evolving ART crisis for people living with HIV in Indonesia'. *The Lancet* 7: e384–5. https://doi.org.10.1016/S2352-3018(20)30138-7.

Masuda, Jeffrey R. and Theresa Garvin. 2006. 'Place, culture, and the social amplification of risk'. *Risk Analysis* 26(2): 437–54. https://doi.org/10.1111/j.1539-6924.2006.00749.x.

Ministry of Health Republic of Indonesia (MOH). 2020. *Petunjuk teknis pelayanan puskesmas pada masa pandemi covid-19 (Technical instructions for primary health care centre services during the COVID-19 pandemic)*. Jakarta, Indonesia: MOH.

Mol, Annemarie. 2008. *The Logic of Care. Health and the problem of patient choice*. New York: Routledge.

Nababan, Herfina Y., Md Hasan, Tiara Marthias, Rolina Dhital, Aminur Rahman and Anwar Iqbal. 2018. 'Trends and inequities in use of maternal health care services in Indonesia, 1986–2012'. *International Journal of Women's Health* 10: 11–24. Accessed 14 April 2021. https://doi.org/ 10.2147/IJWH.S144828.

Nguyen, Long H., David A. Drew, Graham S. Mark, Amit D. Joshi, Chuan-Guo Guo et al. 2020. 'Risk of COVID-19 among front-line health-care workers and the general community: A prospective cohort study'. *The Lancet* 5(9): E475–83. https://doi.org/10.1016/S2468-2667(20)30164-X.

Pangestika, Dyaning. 2020. 'Activists urge govt to resolve HIV drugs shortage amid COVID-19 pandemic'. *The Jakarta Post*, 20 March 2020. Accessed 13 August 2020. https://www.thejakartapost.com/news/2020/03/20/activists-urge-govt-to-resolve-hiv-drugs-shortage-amid-covid-19-pandemic.html.

Platt, Maria. 2017. *Marriage, Gender and Islam in Indonesia: Women negotiating informal marriage, divorce and desire*. New York: Routledge.

Ramdan, Dadan. 2020. Komitmen pemerintah dalam vaksinasi HPV disoal (Government commitment to HPV vaccination questioned), *Kontan.Co.ID*, 21 January 2020. Accessed 13 August 2020. https://nasional.kontan.co.id/news/komitmen-pemerintah-dalam-vaksinasi-hpv-disoal.

Riley, Taylor, Elizabeth Sully, Zara Ahmed and Ann Biddlecom. 2020. 'Estimates of the potential impact of the COVID-19 pandemic on sexual and reproductive health in low- and middle-income countries'. *International Perspectives on Sexual and Reproductive Health* 46: 73–6. Accessed 13 August 2020. https://www.guttmacher.org/journals/ipsrh/2020/04/estimates-potential-impact-covid-19-pandemic-sexual-and-reproductive-health.

Sarradon-Eck, Aline, Cyril Farnarier and Takeo David Hymans. 2014. 'Caring on the margins of the healthcare system'. *Anthropology & Medicine* 21(2): 251–63. https://doi.org/10.1080/13648470.2014.924299.

Spagnoletti, Belinda, Hanum Atikasari, Linda Bennett, Henny Putri, Miranda Rachellina and Ardhina Ramania. 2020. 'Hitting the pause button: The impact of COVID-19 on cervical cancer prevention, screening and treatment access in Indonesia'. *Asian Pacific Journal of Cancer Care* 5(1): 255–7. https://doi.org/10.31557/APJCC.2020.5.S1.255-257.

UNAIDS. 2020. 'Report: Rapid survey on the impact of COVID-19 to young key populations and young people living with HIV in Indonesia'. Accessed 13 August 2020. https://unaids-ap.org/2020/05/13/report-rapid-survey-on-the-impact-of-covid-19-to-young-key-populations-and-young-people-living-with-hiv-in-indonesia/.

UNFPA. 2020. 'Coronavirus diseases (COVID-19) preparedness and response UNFPA interim technical brief: Sexual and reproductive health and rights, maternal and newborn health & COVID-19'. Accessed 9 July 2020. https://www.unfpa.org/sites/default/files/resource-pdf/COVID-19_Preparedness_and_Response_-_UNFPA_Interim_Technical_Briefs_Maternal_and_Newborn_Health_-23_March_2020_.pdf.

Waluyo, Agung, Gabriel J. Culbert, Judith Levy and Kathleen F. Norr. 2015. 'Understanding HIV-related stigma among Indonesian nurses'. *Journal of the Association of Nurses in AIDS Care* 26(1): 69–80. https://doi.org/10.1016/j.jana.2014.03.001.

Wirz, Christopher D., Michael A. Xenos, Dominique Brossard, Dietram Scheufele, Jennifer H. Chung and Luisa Massarani. 2018. Rethinking social amplification of risk: Social media and Zika in three languages. *Risk Analysis* 38(12): 2599–624. Accessed 12 April 2021. https://doi.org/10.1111/risa.13228.

World Bank. 2020a. 'Maternal mortality ratio (modelled estimate, per 100,000 live births) – Indonesia'. *The World Bank Group* website. Accessed 24 July 2020. https://data.worldbank.org/indicator/SH.STA.MMRT?locations=ID.

World Bank. 2020b. 'Unmet need for contraception (% of married women ages 15–49) Indonesia'. The World Bank Group website. Accessed 24 July 2020. https://data.worldbank.org/indicator/SP.UWT.TFRT?view=chart&locations=ID.

World Health Organization. 2021. 'Current health expenditure (% of GDP) – Indonesia'. Accessed 14 April 2021. https://data.worldbank.org/indicator/SH.XPD.CHEX.GD.ZS?locations=ID.

Yumna, Athia, Hafiz Arfyanto, Luhur Bima and Palmira Permata Bachtiar. 2020. 'Social safety nets amid the COVID-19 crisis: What should the government do now?' *The SMERU Research Institute* website. Accessed 13 August 2020. http://www.smeru.or.id/en/content/social-safety-nets-amid-covid-19-crisis-what-should-government-do-now.

13
Vulnerabilities within and beyond the pandemic

Disability in COVID-19 Brazil

Claudia Fonseca and Soraya Fleischer

Epidemics affect poor people in disproportional numbers, as illustrated for different eras, regions and pathologies. It is no surprise, therefore, that the coronavirus pandemic, held to be the greatest global health disaster since the 1918 Spanish flu, has not materialised everywhere in the same way. The unpredictable meanders of an 'emerging' and little-known disease such as COVID-19 are compounded by the complex political, economic and social circumstances of each of its concrete manifestations. This complexity is what brings Herring and Swedlund to endorse a 'syndemic approach' to the study of epidemics – one that requires researchers to look:

> beyond individual infections to consider how they may be capacitated by the presence of other diseases and conditions and sustained by social inequity and the unjust exercise of power, which channels and sustains damaging disease clusters in disadvantaged populations (2010, 5).

At the same time, each new pathogen has its own specific properties that, in interaction with the health authorities' leanings of the moment, elicit a certain response. Lakoff (2017), in his analysis of the World Health Organization's reaction to health threats in recent history, reflects on how many of the organisation's authorised experts had come to the conclusion that an alarmist reaction to the outbreak of infectious disease could, in the long run, be counter-productive. Particularly in the case of countries in urgent need of improved sanitation and more efficient health systems, money channelled toward combatting a momentary epidemic might be better spent on infrastructure aimed at attenuating less spectacular (although more epidemiologically significant) contagious diseases and non-communicable chronic conditions (malaria, diarrhoeal infections, diabetes, heart disease, etc.). Specialists had become understandably wary lest the declaration of a 'global health threat', incurring drastic measures, cause more harm than good.

Nonetheless, recognising WHO's failure to apprehend the seriousness of the Ebola outbreak in 2014, its experts revised their stance, once again attending to the very real possibility of a global catastrophe. Thus, with the explosion of COVID-19 globally in early 2020, and in the absence of vaccines or effective medicines to combat the highly contagious and often lethal air-borne virus, the organisation was quick to advocate a radical measure – generalised home confinement – even knowing it might spell out temporary deprivation for a good part of the world's population.

In our syndemic approach to COVID-19 in Brazil, we thus propose, first, to consider how dubious political leadership dovetails with the past decade's neoliberal austerity programmes and budget cuts to produce a national calamity in which deaths by COVID-19 are surpassed only by those in the US. The disadvantaged population that interests us here is people with disabilities, rendered particularly vulnerable by this virus. Whereas epidemics of the past are remembered as having affected younger, able-bodied members of the workforce, COVID-19 is reputed to strike down primarily older people, those with disabilities and people suffering from debilitating chronic conditions. Given this context, we argue that Brazilian president Bolsonaro's negationist stand – his refusal to heed WHO orientations to contain the pandemic, his tireless combat against any change in routine activities, whether school attendance, commerce, travelling, tourism and even the use of face masks – could be seen as the logical offshoot of his radical neoliberalism (Neiburg and Thomasz 2020; Ortega and Orsini 2020). Predicated on the survival of those regarded as physically and morally fit, Bolsonaro's philosophy would tacitly condone a sort of culling of unproductive elements of the population.

Second, by comparing the present situation with the previous epidemic of the Zika virus, which also especially impacted Brazil, we underline how a distinct political mood produced a vastly different *mise-en-scène* of expert knowledge, bringing medical researchers and health specialists to work in concert with public authorities. Furthermore, during the Zika epidemic, those who suffered most from the infection – children born with congenital Zika syndrome – were cast not as lamentably expendable, but as victims worthy of special attention.[1] During COVID-19 however, Zika 'survivors', most classified as severely disabled, live with the spectre of eugenicist discrimination as they vie for medical services grown scarce due to the impact of emergency cases of COVID-19 on health resources and services.

We then focus on a novel feature of the pandemic's recommended preventive measures. To contain the spread of infectious diseases, in the past authorities would typically place only the sick and ailing in quarantine – a policy of variable efficacy. With COVID-19, however, when infection is for many asymptomatic, global health specialists have strongly recommended social distancing for the entire population, raising questions of how such a measure is organised and morally framed by people living in radically unequal conditions. If, in Brazil, Bolsonaro's most rabid supporters viewed these recommendations as the senseless infringement of basic rights that would devastate the economy, other observers tended to depict strict adherence as a life-saving civic virtue to reduce cases of infection and alleviate the load on overburdened hospitals. Here, ethnographic observations[2] defy simplistic conclusions that might link specific political loyalties to one or other course of prevention. They also cast light on community-based strengths as well as structural vulnerabilities, exploring contextually conditioned understandings of how best – morally and pragmatically – to confront the pandemic.

Politics and negationism in Brazil under Bolsonaro

At the end of the 1980s, Brazil emerged from over 20 years of a harsh military dictatorship to a new era of democratic nation-building. The next 30 years witnessed the expansion of public services, as well as varying efforts to diminish the vast gap between rich and poor, the result of the country's long legacy of colonial exploitation and an economy historically dependent on slave labour. The election in 2002 of President Luis Ignácio (Lula) Silva – heralding into national power the left-leaning Workers' Party government with its avowed platform of minority rights, development and social justice for all – appeared to crown these efforts.

Just how Brazil came to plunge in so short a time from Lula's term in office into the elected presidency of Bolsonaro – an obscure, far-right politician with no particular party base – has been the subject of myriad analyses (see, for example, Neiburg and Thomaz, 2020). What interests us here is how, in the wake of economic recession, relentless media scandals on corruption at every level of government, and the impeachment of Lula's anointed successor (the country's first female president, Dilma Rousseff) for minor infringements of budget laws, the country's electorate was polarised between two radically opposed blocks. Voters who saw a more egalitarian income distribution, the expansion of quality public services and the promotion of human rights as priority issues, continued to support the Workers' Party. On the other hand, those most concerned by violent crime, the erosion of 'traditional' family values and political corruption, opted for what they saw as a strong-arm candidate with military sympathies: Jair Bolsonaro.

During Bolsonaro's first year in government, 2019, under the firm hand of a minister of economy trained at the University of Chicago, his administration passed through Congress major institutional reforms that diminished job stability and downsized pension benefits, while it quietly worked toward the privatisation of banks, utilities, universities and other government-run institutions. The Public Health System (*Sistema Único de Saúde*, better known as SUS), that attends over 80 per cent of the country's population, was particularly hard hit by austerity measures. Although guaranteed by the 1988 Constitution, and inaugurated in 1994, the free and universal system of healthcare was slow to gain momentum. High-complexity services are to this day concentrated in the state capitals where ailing patients could be routinely seen forming enormous lines in front of the major public hospitals. The lack of basic equipment, technology, medications and medical specialists has been steadily denounced in newspaper headlines for decades. Never completely satisfactory, in recent years SUS has suffered more than ever from successive financial cuts, structural downsizing and political attacks dictated by the government's openly neoliberal and capital-oriented policies. As a result, patients desperate for treatment have increasingly resorted to juridical procedures to guarantee their constitutional right to health (Biehl, 2016). The system, already ill-equipped to deal with routine sickness and disability, would be pushed to the verge of collapse by the disaster of COVID-19.

The first official death by coronavirus – that of a domestic worker who had caught the virus from her employer recently returned from a trip abroad – was registered on 16 March. Within days, the Minister of Health (Luis Henrique Mandetta, a medical doctor) had confirmed community transmission throughout Brazil. Although after taking office in early 2019 he had done little to reverse the decline of the deteriorated public health system, his prompt reaction to the threat of COVID-19 earned him the respect of most Brazilians. While Bolsonaro followed the example of his idol, US President Donald Trump, referring to COVID-19 as a 'paltry flu' that did not warrant sacrificing economic routine, Mandetta vigorously promoted policies of social distancing that would curb transit across international borders, limit inter-city transportation, suspend school attendance and rein in the activities of most 'non-essential' public and commercial services. While the president adamantly resisted wearing face masks (even after 22 members of his entourage tested positive for COVID-19), his Minister of Health consistently recommended their use. And, countering Bolsonaro's claim that (hydroxy)chloroquine was a miracle treatment for the disease, Mandetta (in keeping with the position of WHO and mainstream medical research) firmly resisted endorsing a protocol to encourage the drug's use.

Regardless of their political leanings, a growing number of state and municipal executives appeared to side with the Minister of Health over the president. Overriding presidential objections, the Supreme Court itself condoned the right of local governments to impose emergency restrictions – closing schools, shutting down non-essential businesses and imposing individual fines on people who refused to use face masks in public. In response, the president and most his cabinet resisted acknowledging the seriousness of the threat. Bolsonaro continued to decry physical distancing, attending rallies throughout the nation where, maskless, he would shake hands and embrace supporters in the crowd. After the president joined protesters calling for military intervention to combat the 'anti-democratic' policies of social distancing imposed by state and municipal authorities, 20 state governors released an 'Open letter to Brazilian society in Defence of Democracy'. Their call for national union against a common enemy, coronavirus, under the guidance of science-based medicine, failed to convince the president.

Given such tensions, it was no surprise when on 16 April – with an explosion of COVID-19 casualties welling on the horizon – Bolsonaro fired his health minister. Mandetta's low-profile successor (also an MD) fell from grace barely a month later. The new minister (the third in five weeks), a military general who openly admitted he had no experience whatsoever in the field of health, began work in mid-May, promptly issuing a protocol to promote the use of chloroquine for all stages of COVID-19 and intensifying the use of army infrastructure for the medicine's frenetic production.[3] As to other demands posed by the pandemic – such as expanding the availability of diagnostic tests and rationalising the distribution of much-needed basic hospital supplies – the new commander of national health exhibited relatively modest interest.

Already at the end of April, it was evident that, in many regions, the precarious conditions afforded by the country's run-down public health system fell far short of the challenges posed by the pandemic. Especially in poorer areas, decentralised and sporadically funded health administrations encountered untold obstacles in their attempts to find and stock test kits for adequate diagnosis, build and equip quality field hospitals, purchase functioning ventilators or even procure routine protective equipment for health workers. Manaus, capital of the State of Amazonas and an important crossroad for a good number of indigenous groups, proved to be one of the first hard-hit capitals. By the second half of May, the town was crawling with national and international reporters anxious to broadcast this worst-case scenario of ill-equipped hospitals, overrun ICUs and a sky-rocketing death toll that required mass burials. The deaths by COVID-19 of indigenous leaders and the pandemic's devastation of their tribes, alongside the government's blind eye to illegal miners and religious missionaries (major vectors of the virus) within their traditional territories, would all come to reinforce the accusation of genocide which, at time of writing (December 2020), is pending against Bolsonaro in the Hague's International Criminal Court.

With the number of cases of infection rising throughout the country, Bolsonaro flailed about for new ways to justify his negationist stance. Among other tactics, he intensified his attacks against news reports and statistics on the disease's high lethality. While observers noted a considerable rise in pulmonary-related deaths compared to previous years and argued that COVID-19 deaths were being underreported, Bolsonaro insisted that their number had been blown completely out of proportion by a conspiracy of journalists, global health specialists and leftist intellectuals out for 'political gain'. Right up to one of the worst moments of the pandemic, with deaths at over a thousand a day, the president insisted that *misinformation* about the pandemic had caused much panic and promised that the 'true' facts would soon be known.

Aside from his disregard for mainstream science, what most disturbed journalists and a good part of the general public was Bolsonaro's apparent lack of empathy for victims of the pandemic. When pressed by journalists to comment on the country's rising death toll, he displayed an indifference bordering on cynicism: 'I'm not a gravedigger, OK?'; 'It's a shame, but what am I supposed to do about it? I may be Messias [his middle name, meaning "Messiah"], but I don't perform miracles'. Citing the opinion of specialists, that eventually 70 per cent of the population would inevitably be infected, he insisted there was 'no running from truth, everyone has to die sometime'.

Bolsonaro's pronouncements echoed that of a small contingent of authorities around the globe who, at the start of the pandemic, had predicted that COVID-19 would prove fatal for only a small percentage of the population – principally the elderly, the disabled and people suffering from debilitating chronic illness. The prognostic supported those decision makers who favoured letting the virus run its course, with economic and other activities in full steam, until the population reached 'herd immunity'. Loss of the population's more fragile members could be minimised by 'vertical segregation', that is, by having those categorised as vulnerable remain homebound, while the younger, hale and hearty masses would go about business as usual. Some deaths would be inevitable, but, from this typically 'ableist' point of view, individuals who deviated from the corporeal standard of the perfect specimen could be considered not fully human (Ortega and Orsini, 2020). Shocking though it may appear, this view has the merit of elucidating a philosophy of government that tolerates the idea of 'letting die' a certain portion of a country's population which, even in normal times, could be seen as a burden on the economy. As a British financial journalist suggested, 'from an entirely disinterested economic perspective, COVID-19 might even prove mildly beneficial in the long-term by disproportionately culling elderly dependants' (Warner, 2020).

The social Darwinist undertones of this discourse have understandably received colossal criticism (Ecks 2020; Butler 2020; Queiroz 2020). We would add that, in the Brazilian context, with the country still coming to grips with the previous epidemic of Zika – and the tide of neurologically disabled children left in its wake – they take on particularly problematic connotations.

Living with disability during successive epidemics

Coronavirus is, of course, far from the first epidemic to cause alarm among Brazilian authorities. From leprosy and syphilis arriving with the first Europeans to epidemics of smallpox, plague and cholera that would periodically erupt in the country's major ports, doctors have worked for centuries alongside government authorities in an attempt to contain damage. Toward the end of the nineteenth century, with European and North American attention turned toward yellow fever and other tropical diseases that threatened colonial endeavours, Brazil became an international centre of medical research. By the early twentieth century, in close collaboration with their overseas counterparts – including specialists from the Pasteur Institute and the Rockefeller Foundation – Brazilian medical researchers were going beyond treatment, applying their research and translation efforts to the systematic prevention of disease (Castro et al. 2010; Lowy 2017).

Over the next decades, a new philosophy of public health, developed in institutions such as Fundação Oswaldo Cruz (with flourishing centres in Rio de Janeiro and Salvador), played a fundamental role in the promotion of not only vaccines, but also – especially after the Spanish flu – sanitary reforms designed to clean up the vectors of infectious diseases (rats, mosquitoes, bacteria-ridden waste products) that plagued urban areas. Aside from developing and deploying a vaccine against yellow fever, national authorities organised effective campaigns against the *Aedes aegypti* mosquito, which was and is responsible for three other less lethal infections: dengue, chikungunya and Zika (Segata 2017). But although these diseases were considered of lesser significance, worries appeared in 2015 as medical observers began to suspect links between a perplexing spate of children born with the severely debilitating condition of microcephaly and the Zika virus (Diniz 2017).

The way President Dilma's administration confronted the Zika epidemic, in comparison with the present national government's treatment of COVID-19, yields insights not only into the ways political leadership can shape the alliance between public health and science but also into the experience of the most vulnerable potential victims rising to the challenges of care and prevention. Zika, like COVID-19, was a relatively unknown entity when it first caught the attention of authorities. A first generation 'Zika mother', living in one of the country's poorer northeastern states, commonly went through her entire pregnancy with no inkling of any serious health threat to herself or to the baby in her womb (Diniz 2017). Primary care centres where most women had prenatal check-ups were generally not equipped with ultrasound technology, and the sonogram was not part of routine protocol. Only those women willing to pay for the exam (motivated, for example, by the desire to know the baby's sex) would have discovered signs of foetal anomaly. For the most part, mothers and their medical attendants were taken by surprise at the arrival of an infant with severe disabilities, and often ill-prepared to deal with the particular risks (for both mother and child) involved in such a birth.

Even during the following year's 'second generation' of victims, including those in Brazil's more prosperous southeast, the imprecision of diagnosis[4] and delay in test results did little to assuage the anxiety of women who had experienced Zika-like symptoms during pregnancy.

Foetal prognosis, plagued with uncertainty, was of little help in a woman's reproductive decisions – whether she should think about a legally questionable abortion (more common in the upper classes) or prepare home and family for the care of a disabled child. In other words, although they were eventually able to tie the significant number of newborns with neurological anomalies to congenital Zika,[5] researchers acknowledged they knew little about the disease – whether concerning its vertical and sexual modes of transmission or its long-term consequences.

In the case of both COVID-19 and Zika, there was an urgent demand for medical research to provide answers. Articulations around the idea of science, however, were of an entirely different order. When Zika first became an issue, President Dilma Rousseff of the Workers' Party was under heavy political siege that would soon bring about her impeachment. Nonetheless, under the slogan 'A mosquito is not stronger than our entire country', her government embraced the combat against Zika, organising campaigns to eradicate vectors, publicly expressing solidarity with its victims, and using financial and administrative incentives to promote university-based research on the disease's various facets. Aside from local scientists, researchers from abroad flocked to the epidemic's geographic epicentre in hopes of mapping the as yet uncharted social and medical territories of the disease. Mothers allowed their bodies (and those of their babies) to be repeatedly scrutinised, their blood samples gathered and stocked, in the hope of accelerating medical discoveries that could eventually help their children lead better lives (Fleischer 2019).

Some women may have been frustrated by the lack of feedback and the discontinuity of interest in their cases; many would lament the inadequacy of available health services. However, neither they nor medical staff, nor even the general media, ever expressed doubt about the validity of the scientific endeavour. The contrast with the present government's reaction to COVID-19 could not be starker. By the time the coronavirus pandemic struck, Bolsonaro and his Minister of Education were systematically denigrating the country's major public universities, cutting funds and downplaying the science produced at mainstream research centres. In the case of COVID-19, the president and his Minister of Health further confounded onlookers by apparently denying the results of any study (on chloroquine, for example) that did not confirm their own preconceived ideas.

During the worst moments of both epidemics, people looked to government for measures that would help minimise suffering and death. In the case of COVID-19, this care was designed to keep affected patients from dying – hence, the rush to multiply intensive care units and to procure respirators. In the case of Zika – not in itself a particularly lethal disease – the 'victims' that demanded the most energies and investments were the babies born to women infected during pregnancy. Even though medical care had guaranteed survival, these young children inevitably suffered sequelae from the disease that left them particularly vulnerable to complications from COVID-19. Yet, to the desperation of their caregivers, at no time were these children included in the pandemic's 'populations at risk', much less singled out to receive priority at hospitals and ICUs.

With general immunodeficiency caused by Congenital Zika Syndrome, these young children lack resistance to colds, and are at heightened risk of eye and ear infections, bronchitis, pulmonary allergies and other childhood diseases. Because of neurological complications, they have difficulty in swallowing. With food and saliva leaking into their lungs, they require frequent hospitalisation for pneumonia and other forms of respiratory intercurrences. Constantly bombarded with analgesics, antibiotics and other medicines, they are also in danger of developing problems linked to overmedication: resistance to certain drugs, liver intoxication and other iatrogenic syndromes. To access high-cost medicines, the children need new prescriptions from doctors every month. And, as they grow, periodic interventions are required to refit feeding tubes, adjust prosthetic devices and perform reparative surgeries (Lima and Fleischer 2020). Yet, faced with hospital services completely flooded with victims of COVID-19, these children find it increasingly difficult to get the routine treatment they need.

During the pandemic, the mothers' fragile hopes – that their children not only survive but lead meaningful lives – have grown dim. Without a regular supply of pharmaceuticals, there is no way to assuage their children's chronic pain, nor regulate their sleep (so as to allow other members of the family some rest). The children are at constant risk of convulsions that may set them back months in terms of cognitive and motor skills. As hospital services have been cut to a bare minimum, suspended altogether, or, at best, gone shakily online, some sectors have posted short videos on social media so that women themselves can give the necessary neuro- and physiotherapy to their toddlers at home. However, many women do not feel competent to replicate rehabilitation exercises on their own. Some may not have access to digital resources; and, even when they do, results may be frustrating, either because older children, now involved in online schooling, monopolise the computer or because, given the mother's already heavy load of domestic chores, she simply cannot find the necessary time to learn and practise new therapeutic techniques.

Today, even for critical situations, these 'micro mothers'[6] ask themselves if it's worth braving public transportation, waiting long hours in hospital corridors and exposing their children to the risk of infection by coronavirus – especially when they are unsure of the reception they will get. During the first years of the Zika epidemic, the babies' need for intensive professional care was recognised as a legitimate cause, thanks largely to collective political action, including street marches and demonstrations in front of government offices. In the present situation of generalised quarantine caused by COVID-19, traditional forms of political organisation are restricted, and the efficacy of online activism (webinars, interviews and podcasts) remains doubtful. The mothers have thus joined a growing number of 'vulnerable' categories of people in Brazil who, following the example of similar groups around the globe, elaborate online manifestos to reiterate the right of all patients – no matter what physical or mental health condition – as equally worthy of attention in any medical emergency. Nonetheless, under the shadow of Bolsonaro's *macho* style of government, patients are left wondering if, in their case, the financial trimming of public services does not spell out the moral withdrawal of state concern.

Social distancing in a setting of inequality

As with Zika and other health emergencies, the pandemic exposed glaring inequalities Brazil's citizens have lived with for decades. The disease wreaked havoc particularly in urban peripheries and rural townships – those regions peopled largely by poor, Afro-Brazilian and indigenous groups (Gragnani 2020). In these areas, with lack of basic infrastructure (piped-in water, city-supervised sewers, routine garbage collection), the vectors of infectious disease proliferate. In this context of 'environmental racism' (Carvalho, 2017), even the simplest measures recommended to avoid COVID-19 (for example frequent handwashing) appear of doubtful application. As to treatment of those infected, most well-off Brazilians have private health insurance which – at least in the past – has guaranteed them adequate hospital care. The rest of the population (i.e. the vast majority) is used to facing crowded public health facilities, praying they will find professionals and equipment available to cure their ills. Acknowledging not only regional differences but also these class- and race-based disparities, one medical specialist after the other, when interviewed about coronavirus, repeats the evidently consensual verdict: in Brazil, there exist many different pandemics.

The apparently democratic preventive measure of social distancing also plays out differently in the various socio-economic groups. On the one hand, individuals from the moneyed sectors may barricade themselves in their relatively comfortable homes. Those lucky enough to have a guaranteed end-of-the-month pay check are able to stock food, construct their home gym and enjoy reliable internet services to make their confinement slightly less trying. The other half of the economically active population – those who are precariously employed and autonomous workers of the informal labour market – is aware that if they do not keep working, they will be unable to maintain even the most modest mode of existence.[7] The few months of emergency aid (just over US$100 dollars) provided by the federal government allowed for some relief, but as the pandemic progressed and lockdowns were extended (or renewed), it became clear that the respite afforded by stop-gap solutions would be short-lived. In such conditions, staying home does not necessarily spell out staying healthy (Yates-Doerr 2020).

The sensitive ethical dilemma between survival and contagion is further complicated in homes including a person with a disability, where the coordination of multiple caregivers must occur while striving to avoid the danger of contamination. Such is the case of Taina's family, an Afro-Brazilian household on the outskirts of Porto Alegre (southern Brazil) that revolves around a spritely pre-teen who, since early infancy, has suffered from an acute form of fibromyalgia. Despite seizures of unbearable pain often accompanied by epileptic-type convulsions that have caused her to miss months of class, when the 2020 school year began (in March), Taina was a well-appreciated eighth-grader at the nearby public school. To some extent, her family is luckier than those of most of her friends whose parents – many of them cleaning ladies and janitors – were laid off with no financial compensation. To complement his minuscule retiree's pension, her father does odd jobs and at the time was being paid to renovate a neighbour's house. Her mother, Aline, works with a nearby NGO, where she supervises extra-curricular activities for around 50 local children. During this period of confinement, however, Aline pays a heavy toll to keep her job, attending simultaneously to household chores and professional obligations (now conducted entirely on WhatsApp) for which she remains on call literally for 12 hours a day.

Given her daughter's needs, Aline now also stands in as physiotherapist, providing twice-daily massages to diminish the frequency of Taina's seizures. The public hospital service attending Taina since her birth suspended activities in mid-March, announcing shortly afterwards it would not reopen, and Aline is still searching for a new facility willing to care for Taina in the event of a life-endangering crisis such as those she has suffered in the past. Lacking the support of a specialised service, mother and daughter have fallen back on their neighbourhood's vastly overburdened primary care unit. Another problem the family must confront is how to guarantee the costly medicine needed to assuage Taina's bouts of intense pain. Public services designed to facilitate the endless bureaucracy required to access government-subsidised medications are all downtown, a good distance away, and many have operated only sporadically during the pandemic. Meanwhile, Aline takes on piecemeal work as a seamstress to cover the higher price she pays for medicines at the local pharmacy.

Perhaps the greatest challenge the family must face during the pandemic is to coordinate the care network that surrounds Taina. At any moment she might have a life-threatening convulsion, and her parents have long since decided she must never be left alone. However, the network they normally rely on, composed of different members of their extended family, has grown tenuous. Taina's grandparents live in their own home at the far end of the back patio, but they are no longer available as before. The grandmother, being treated for diabetes and heart disease, is so worried about contagion that she will not share dinnerware with her near 80-year-old husband because he refuses to give up his job as a doorman at an apartment complex downtown. Aline's sister, owner of a small food store where she attends customers from morning to night, has stopped coming by for fear of contaminating her relatives. Another brother – a delivery boy, now completely swamped with work that constantly exposes him to risk of infection – has reduced contact with his family to an occasional phone call. To keep Taina company, her mother has to rely on the girl's two older siblings – young adults who have not given up their sociable routines.

A closer look suggests that none of the girl's hands-on caregivers follow the rules of social distancing to the letter. Aside from chores (bill payments, health check-ups) that regularly take her outside the home, Aline is frequently involved in volunteer work. In these times of exceptional hardship, she spends Saturdays at the community centre distributing parcels of food and clothes to her students' families and, twice a week, she helps a neighbour ladle out soup (made with food donations) to members of the area's neediest families. The fact that few of their 'clients' wear masks does not appear to deter the volunteers' enthusiasm. Asked if she isn't worried about contamination, Aline answers with an unequivocal 'of course', but it would seem the moral injunction of neighbourhood solidarity overrides even such a fear.

As the pedagogical slogans urging people to stay home gain impetus, debates on the public scene often seem to frame adherence to quarantine as a question not only of personal health and civic morality, but also of party politics. Circumstances conspire to paint a person's free transit in public byways as a proclamation of pro-Bolsonaro political leanings (Canzian 2020). Yet, the alacrity with which observers tend to see those who fail to adhere to total confinement as scientifically illiterate and politically conservative may be ill-advised. True, those shopkeepers constantly lobbying to open commerce apparently adhere to Bolsonaro's cost-benefit evaluations that put the country's economic health above people's lives. The same might be said of the crowds of beautiful people at tourist sites, teenagers herding through the shopping malls and bohemians out for a pick-me-up at their favourite bar. But for the majority of people passing through the streets of working class neighbourhoods where it would appear business carries on almost as usual, our experience suggests that attitudes are characterised more by ambivalence than firm conviction. Observation of the various strategies deployed by working-class families such as Taina's to get through this period of crisis leads us to believe that the class-based parameters of many of our instruments of evaluation do not begin to describe the complex package of acute perception, conditions of possibility and imperatives of social solidarity that permit people to forge meaningful existences during the pandemic.

Conclusion: Coronavirus and culling in the neo-neoliberal age

Our syndemic approach to COVID-19 in present-day Brazil is meant to underline the highly variable ways that the disease plays out in different contexts. Political circumstances that conspired to put a 'negationist' president in power, together with the chief executive's consistent undermining of public trust in science, have no doubt been responsible for a percentage of the country's high death toll (at 31 December 2020). The survival-of-the-fittest philosophy openly avowed by Bolsonaro has also had consequences. On the one hand, it explains the federal government's refusal to elaborate a coordinated plan to contain the pandemic. On the other hand, it has caused many people who are vulnerable – the chronically ill and disabled – to doubt their entitlement to basic constitutional rights. Finally, the colossal number of under- and irregularly employed workers obliged to eke out a daily living renders the major prevention measure against COVID-19 – social distancing – awkward if not entirely unfeasible for a good part of the population. Threading its way through all these contextual particularities, we find the overriding issue of structural inequality.

The neoliberal cut-backs taking place in Brazil, as well as many other countries throughout the world, have been branded by certain scholars as a form of necropolitics (Ortega and Orsini 2020; Yancy 2020). The term is meant to highlight the usually implicit tenets of regimes whose social policies appear to separate 'grievable' from 'ungrievable' lives, that is, those people 'who should be protected against death at all costs and those whose lives are considered not worth safeguarding against illness and death' (Butler 2020, 3). COVID-19 may have exacerbated this trend, but tacit forms of 'culling' the population are not particularly new. As Manderson and Wahlberg (2020) point out, in many parts of the world – especially where resources are scarce – health workers have long been sorting out which patients should receive priority attention.

In Brazil, black, indigenous and poor people – those most likely to be found in the public health facilities – are suffering a mortality rate from COVID-19 many times that of middle-class whites. But how can one forget that in 'normal' times the average life expectancy of an individual from these disadvantaged groups is years shorter than that of their white, middle-class counterparts? Between chronic unemployment, structural racism, police violence, miserable work wages and inadequate and poorly resourced health facilities, one might conclude that the mechanisms that lead to a *de facto* hierarchy of more and less worthy humanities were operational long before COVID-19.

Recognition that Brazilians have learned to live with chronically precarious institutional support expands our focus beyond the present pandemic to the informal means through which most people routinely manage to hold home and hearth together despite adverse conditions. Our observations in this chapter on the care-giving networks of young children with disabilities point to the importance of local forms of social organisation in facing new, acute ordeals within a context of economic and institutional precarity. We would suggest that the strategies mounted by extended families and neighbourhood associations appear to work, at times, even better than many of the state and humanitarian interventions, exactly because they are based on established relations of cooperation and interdependence ensconced in day-to-day tasks (Bersani 2020, 13; see also Ennis-McMillan and Hedges 2020). This sort of spontaneous mutual aid, found in the lower-income urban periphery and isolated rural areas throughout Brazil (as well as in many other regions of the world), may be of limited scope and patchy duration. But so are many of the social programmes organised by public authorities. Any sort of coordinated effort to contain the pandemic and minimise suffering must take into account these community resources as well as local modes of existence. However, if concern with the present catastrophe does not extend to the reformulation of policies for 'normal' times, and the development of long-lasting infrastructures that guarantee wellbeing for the population as a whole, further tragedy is bound to ensue.

Notes

1. These reflections are the result of an ethnographic study under the coordination of Soraya Fleischer, conducted from 2016 to the present in Recife, with parents and family members of children born with congenital Zika syndrome (Fleischer and Lima 2020). In early 2020, the research team branched out from an interest in the everyday challenges faced by these families to contemplate the influence of COVID-19 in this scenario. Funding for this research comes from CNPq and the University of Brasília.
2. Claudia Fonseca has carried out fieldwork on the outskirts of Porto Alegre over the past two decades. Material for the present article was collected through telephone interviews in May and June of 2020 with members of the community organisation *Coletivo Autônomo do Morro* within the framework of 'Living with Disabilities', a research project funded by the Newton Foundation (British Council) and CNPq.
3. Notwithstanding the existence of an abundant national supply, the country received not long afterward a colossal shipment of the product supposedly sent by US President Donald Trump himself.
4. Until 2016, the only existing laboratory tests were for dengue.
5. To date, authorities have tabulated approximately 4,000 children born with what they label Congenital Zika Virus Syndrome (CZVS). Since 2016, numbers have tapered off, leading WHO to pull the disease off the list of immediate epidemiological concerns (Lakoff 2017), but – especially with the detection of a new strain of virus in June 2020 – the disease is still very much on the map of Brazil's public health concerns.
6. 'Micro family', a term coined by the mothers themselves, refers to the major visible symptom of microcephalic babies who suffer from the foetal syndrome.
7. While the officially unemployed fluctuated at somewhere between 11 and 13 million, by late June, surveyors were talking of some 75,000,000 Brazilians outside the job market.

References

Bersani, Ana Elisa de Figueiredo. 2020. '(Extra)ordinary *help*: Untold stories on disaster and generosity in Grand'Anse, Haiti'. *Vibrant* 17: 1–20.

Biehl, João. 2016. 'Patient-citizen-consumers: Judicialization of health and metamorphosis of biopolitics'. *Lua Nova* 98: 77–105.

Butler, Judith. 2020. 'Capitalism has its limits'. 30 March 2020. Accessed 10 April 2020. https://www.versobooks.com/blogs/4603-capitalism-has-its-limits?fbclid=IwAR29tPvGaYcQNgzSvLO99OfWQCRHD4cGJ7ushuTo74D99RKJo5ZiQzn0P4A.

Canzian, Fernando. 2020. 'Falas de Bolsonaro contra isolamento podem ter matado mais seus eleitores, aponta estudo'. *Folha de São Paulo*, 30 June 2020. Accessed 8 December 2020. https://www1.folha.uol.com.br/equilibrioesaude/2020/06/falas-de-bolsonaro-contra-isolamento-podem-ter-matado-mais-seus-eleitores-aponta-estudo.shtml.

Carvalho, Layla Pedreira. 2017. 'Vírus Zika e direitos reprodutivos: Entre as políticas transnacionais, as nacionais e as ações locais'. *Cadernos Gênero e Diversidade* 3(2): 134–57. https://doaj.org/article/4fd5316dcfbe4c809508839500863ad8.

Castro, Arachu, Yasmin Khawja and James Johnston. 2010. 'Social inequalities and dengue transmission in Latin America'. In *Plagues and Epidemics: Infected spaces past and present*, edited by D. Ann Herring and Alan C. Swedlund, pp. 1–21. New York: Berg.

Diniz, Debora. 2017. *Zika: From the Brazilian backlands to global threat*. London: Zed Books.

Ecks, Stefan. 2020. 'Coronashock capitalism: The unintended consequences of radical biopolitics'. *COVID-19 Perspectives*, blog from University of Edinburgh. Accessed 10 April 2020. https://blogs.ed.ac.uk/covid19perspectives/2020/04/10/coronashock-capitalism-the-unintended-consequences-of-radical-biopolitics-writes-stefan-ecks/.

Ennis-Mcmillan, Michael C. and Kristin Hedges. 2020. 'Pandemic perspectives: Responding to COVID-19'. *Open Anthropology* 8(1), April. https://www.americananthro.org/StayInformed/OAArticleDetail.aspx?ItemNumber=25631.

Fleischer, Soraya. 2019. 'But will this research produce any results? Zika, moms and science in Brazil'. *CORTH Blog*, 28 February 2020. Accessed 28 February 2020. http://www.sussex.ac.uk/corth/publications/blog/2019-02-28.

Fleischer, Soraya and Flávia Lima. 2020. *Micro: Contribuições da antropologia*. Brazil: Athalaia. http://www.dan.unb.br/images/E-Books/2020_FLEISCHER_LIMA_Micro.pdf.

Gragnani, Juliana. 2020. 'Por que o coronavírus mata mais as pessoas negras e pobres no Brasil e no mundo'. *BBC News Brasil*. Accessed 8 December 2020. https://www.bbc.com/portuguese/brasil-53338421.

Herring, D. Ann and Alan C. Swedlund, eds. 2010. *Plagues and Epidemics: Infected spaces, past and present*. Oxford/New York: Berg.

Lakoff, Andrew. 2017. *Unprepared: Global health in a time of emergency*. Berkeley, CA: University of California Press.

Lima, Flávia and Soraya Fleischer. 2020. 'Nourishment dilemmas: The complex science of caring for children with CZVS'. Somatosphere, 24 February 2020. Accessed 24 February 2020. http://somatosphere.net/author/flavialima/.

Lowy, Ilana. 2017. 'Leaking containers: Success and failure in controlling the mosquito *Aedes aegypti* in Brazil'. *American Journal of Public Health* 107(4): 517–24.

Neiburg, Federico and Omar Ribeiro Thomaz, eds. 2020. 'Currents: The rise of Brazilian fascism'. *HAU: Journal of Ethnographic Theory* 40(1): 7–53.

Manderson, Lenore and Ayo Wahlberg. 2020. 'Chronic living in a communicable world'. *Medical Anthropology* 39(5): 428–39. https://doi.org/10.1080/01459740.2020.1761352

Ortega, Francisco and Orsini, Michael. 2020. 'Governing COVID in Brazil: Dissecting the ableist and reluctant authoritarian'. *Somatosphere*. Accessed 8 December 2020. http://somatosphere.net/2020/governing-covid-in-brazil-dissecting-the-ableist-and-reluctant-authoritarian.html/.

Queiroz, Aline. 2020. '*Quo Vadis* European Union?' *Social Epistemology Review and Reply Collective* 9(4): 59–64. https://wp.me/P1Bfg0-4Wa.

Segata, Jean. 2017. 'O *Aedes aegypti* e o digital'. *Horizontes Antropológicos* 48(23): 19–48.

Yancy, George. 2020. 'Judith Butler: Mourning is a political act amid the pandemic and its disparities'. *Truthout*. Accessed 8 December 2020. https://truthout.org/articles/judith-butler-mourning-is-a-political-act-amid-the-pandemic-and-its-disparities/.

Yates-Doerr, Emily. 2020. 'Stay home, stay healthy' is dangerous language'. *Ms.* 4 March 2020. https://msmagazine.com/2020/04/03/stay-home-stay-healthy-is-dangerous-language/.

Warner, Jeremy. 2020. 'Does the Fed know something the rest of us do not with its panicked interest rate cut?' *The Telegraph*, 3 March 2020. Accessed 8 December 2020. https://www.telegraph.co.uk/business/2020/03/03/does-fed-know-something-rest-us-do-not-panicked-interest-rate/.

14
'You are putting my health at risk'
Genes, diets and bioethics under COVID-19 in Mexico

Abril Saldaña-Tejeda

On 27 March 2020, as rates of infection were rapidly escalating worldwide, the Mexican government reported 717 confirmed cases of COVID-19 and 12 deaths. For some at least, this suggested that the country would avoid the worst outcome of economic collapse and devastating numbers of fatalities. But due to undertesting and underreporting, many saw these figures as underestimating the problem (Gobierno de Mexico 2020a). From the beginning of the pandemic, Mexico had one of the lowest testing rates in the Americas, with only 2,350 per 1 million residents examined. Some argued that the government's strategy of testing only serious cases made it difficult to develop appropriate interventions (Agren 2020). Others suggested that public health officials followed the only strategy possible in a country within which 41.9 per cent of its 126.2 million population lived in poverty (Coneval 2018), where 56 per cent of the working population were in informal employment (INEGI 2020).

From late February, the government offered daily televised briefings on the pandemic; to the time of writing in mid-September, these were continuous. The briefings were held and hosted by the Undersecretary of Health, Hugo López-Gatell Ramírez, an epidemiologist with an impressive academic record and robust experience in health crises, an engaged public speaker able to captivate the public in a way no previous health authority had before. During the first months of the 'stay at home' campaign, in daily briefings, Gatell and his team covered important issues related to lockdown, including domestic violence and mental health. Gatell also dedicated special briefings to answer questions from children and mothers on their respective national days, taking advantage of the state's presence to promote awareness of self-care practices under COVID-19 and 'healthy lifestyles'. In some ways, these briefings were key to promote an image of Gatell as caring representative of the state. Children and mothers were asked to send their questions through home-made videos; questions were carefully selected and some widely commented in social media. Gatell also aligned with many other social justice agendas; he started to use green ties and later, green facemasks to promote the decriminalisation of abortion in the country.

Soon after the briefings started, Gatell began to be presented as a sex symbol. WhatsApp stickers circulated with Gatell's image, and he was reported to be trending in Twitter, ranked the third most popular epidemiologist in the world (Ojeda de la Torre 2020). By mid-April, piñatas of him were on sale in the streets. In Mexico, being made into a piñata is proof of iconic status, reflecting political and social views of approval, mockery or national indignation.

Gatell made the most of his popularity and high rates of approval to address another public health challenge that, before COVID-19, had ignited heated legislative debate. Gatell had been spearheading the national campaign to legislate the use of warning labels on processed foods and sugar sweetened beverages. The new law, passed just before the country entered into lockdown, required processed food companies to provide easy to understand, correct, direct, simple and visible nutritional information on their products, especially those high in sugar, sodium and saturated fats. This small but significant victory of public health over profit was celebrated by many activists and non-governmental organisations. The COVID-19 crisis seemed the perfect setting to publicly sustain the need to continue to successfully address excessive weight gain and obesity, something that the country had attempted, with little success, since the early 2000s.

In early April, the media drew attention to comorbidities among COVID-19 patients: up to 85 per cent of deaths caused by COVID-19 were associated with cardiometabolic disease, including obesity (Torres 2020). The risk of death due to COVID-19 among those living with obesity increased by 78 per cent, 73 per cent with diabetes and 38 per cent with hypertension (Solís and Carreño 2020). By late July, there were 370,712 confirmed cases and 41,908 fatalities by COVID-19. Some 67 per cent of fatalities had suffered from at least one comorbidity of diabetes, hypertension, obesity and cardiovascular disease. Up to 17 per cent of confirmed cases and 43 per cent of deaths were among people who suffered from hypertension; 17 per cent of confirmed cases and 38 per cent of deaths among those living with diabetes. Finally, up to 18 per cent of confirmed cases and 25 per cent of fatalities were reported as obese (Gobierno de México 2020b).

In this chapter, I explore Mexico's public health campaign against obesity prior to and after the onset of the COVID-19 pandemic, and document the increasing stigmatisation of fatness as a result of contemporary discourses of vulnerability and risk. I first look at genetic and epigenetic approaches to obesity rates among Mexican mestizos before COVID-19. I briefly expose concerns regarding the potential racialising impact of the new life science, and question the tendency among epigenetic studies to place women's reproductive bodies and their consumption choices at the centre of social interventions designed to improve the health of future generations. Through a review of Mexico's long obsession with diets and foodways from colonisation to the eugenic movement of the twentieth century, I argue that a new focus on diets and 'healthy choices' is highly problematic under COVID-19. A renewed focus on individual responsibility continues to occlude major structural problems that would better explain Mexico's food landscape and why people eat what they do.

Second, I look at public and medical discourses that identify a genetic advantage among Mexican mestizos. I argue that the continuous use of genetic profiles as substitutes for national representation converges and supports the resurgence of old eugenic tropes of foodways and diets as ways of enhancing the nation's population. Such obsession with the 'truths' invested in the body – its genetic makeup and its power to 'heal' the nation through social intervention and self-care – silence the (evident) social factors behind the heath disaster that we are witnessing today due to the pandemic. I expose the stigmatising effects of the state's war against obesity and how such effects have materialised in misinformation and discrimination. Finally, I look at the bioethical guide of extreme triage in Mexico and the heated debate around it. I show how the impact of the war against obesity goes beyond fat stigmatisation to directly affect individual possibilities of survival. I argue that notions of vulnerability and risk associated with COVID-19 are materialised in public health policy, and public health debates and policies seem to fuel fatphobic messages and practices that might have a direct impact on people's notions of risk under COVID-19 and on patients' willingness to seek help when needed.

Obesity in Mexico: genetic vulnerabilities and strengths

In Mexico, according to the National Health and Nutrition Survey 2018 (NHNS), seven out of ten adults (aged 20 and older) suffered from overweight and/or obesity (75.2 per cent), along with three out of ten children between the ages of 5 and 11 years old (35.6 per cent) and almost four out of ten adolescents between the ages of 12 and 19 years of age (38.4 per cent) (INSP 2018). During the last decades, these rates have caused great concern for the government, and public health officials have consistently warned against the 'anti-evolutionary essence' of obesity and the threat it represents to the 'viability of the nation' (Secretaría de Salud 2013, 7). These concerns have underpinned substantial private and governmental funding to research the genetic basis of obesity.

From its foundation in 2005, backed by substantial private and governmental funding, the National Institute for Genomic Medicine (INMEGEN) engaged with a series of international collaborations to explore the genetic basis of diabetes and obesity. Mexican mestizos were found to be especially susceptible to obesity due to their Amerindian origin (INMEGEN 2014; SIGMA Type 2 Diabetes Consortium 2014). Official and media outlets were swift to interpret and circulate these findings, strengthening the idea that Mexicans were predisposed to obesity and 'carried it in their genes' (Olivares 2012; Forbes 2013; Ruiz Jaimes 2013), with obesity predisposition often linked to the Thrifty Gene Hypothesis (TGH) (see Saldaña-Tejeda and Wade 2018). In simple terms, this hypothesis supports the idea that where ancestral populations lived in a harsh environment, the natural selection of a thrifty gene allowed them to store energy for times of famine (Neel 1962). In a modern environment of food abundance and sedentary lifestyles, the continued storing of energy explains obesity population clusters. These genetic hypotheses were soon accompanied by epigenetic explanations of obesity that stressed the role of environmental factors to regulate gene function and modification. Epigenetics offered the opportunity to escape the criticism of genetic determinism, while accommodating well to public health agendas by focusing on state interventions that might modify the genetic makeup of the nation. An epigenetic approach backed up the idea that genes could be 'switched' off and on through environmental (often dietary) interventions and foetal developmental programming, often targeting intrauterine environments and therefore women's reproductive bodies (Sharp et al. 2018; Warin et al. 2015). In the last decades, the state has consistently recommended further investment in genetic and epigenetic research and the development of a *genoteca del obeso*, that is, a biobank of samples from obese patients from public clinics and hospitals (Secretaría de Salud 2013). Critics of genomic medicine based on ancestry highlight its potential as a 'racialised science' or a 'backdoor to eugenics' (Duster 2003; Smedley and Smedley 2005; Koenig et al. 2008). Epigenetic approaches do not escape such criticism, given their tendency to focus on the actions of self-disciplining citizens (often poor and/or negatively racialised mothers) and their power to somehow reverse problematic global health rates in future generations (Saldaña-Tejeda and Wade 2019). Epigenetic studies of foetal exposures often centre around the 'abnormal' dietary 'choices' of mothers, positioning women as the main vehicles of poor intergenerational health (Manderson 2016; Pentecost 2018; Yates-Doerr 2015; Saldaña-Tejeda 2018).

Mexico has long seen diets and foodways as pathways to enhance the racial makeup of the population and convert souls to Christianity. From early Spanish colonisation, European foods were presented as morally and nutritionally superior (Earle 2010). Indians were advised to eat 'that which the Castilian people ate' to become 'strong and pure and wise' (Burkhart 1989, 166). After independence, political elites continued to blame indigenous diets for the 'underdevelopment' of the population and favoured the consumption of processed, industrialised foods that signalled a modern, Mexican nation (Pilcher 1998; Aguilar-Rodríguez 2007). Ideas on health and heredity eventually materialised in the eugenic environmentalist measures of the twentieth century. Diets, food practices and hygiene – along with moral values – were believed to be the root of all national problems and were the basis of interventions that targeted Mexican families, particularly indigenous and other poor mothers (Aguilar-Rodríguez 2007; Vargas Domínguez 2017).

Under COVID-19 and its known comorbidities, diets and 'healthy' food choices became again the focus of public interventions. As with genetic and epigenetic approaches to chronic diseases, the focus on individual responsibility worked to silence major structural problems that would better explain Mexico's food landscape and why people eat what they do. As Galvez (2018) shows, the North American Free Trade Agreement (NAFTA) signed in 1994 by Canada, the US and Mexico changed Mexico's food systems and resulted in a deep transformation of the welfare state. Market-based ideas about how to solve society's problems (i.e. chronic diseases) began to frame citizens as consumers able to make rightful choices in the marketplace. In this frame, the medical gaze centred on the need to educate consumers, overlooking the social determinants of health and the effects of neoliberalism on the country's food systems (Galvez 2018). The transformation of Mexico's peasant cooperatives into urban communities is only one example of such effects.

Created after the 1910 Mexican Revolution, peasant cooperatives known as *ejidos* were the centre of an agrarian reform that lasted 60 years. Designed to allocate and redistribute land in order to provide a subsistence base for millions of peasants, ejidos historically entailed a set of obligations for beneficiaries such as working the land and living in villages. However, from the 1980s, socioeconomic processes that led to NAFTA resulted in the commodification of communal land that, in 2017, amounted to 51 per cent of Mexican territory. The use of land for agricultural activities was gradually replaced by mining industry, activities linked to 'flex crops' (for example, corn and soybeans, able to be used for food, feed, fuel or industrial material) and logging. As Torres (2019, 73) states, 'all around Mexico, *ejidatarios* (ejido holders) are selling, renting, or leasing their lands; they have become a new kind of individual owner, with many rights over the ejido plots but without the obligations towards families or communities that they used to have'.

These systemic changes altering the food landscape converged with years of governmental failure to address extreme poverty and food insecurity. For instance, in 2013, when the National Strategy to Prevent Obesity and Diabetes was launched, the administration of Enrique Peña Nieto (2012–18) announced its signature policy, the Crusade Against Hunger. This programme aimed to alleviate extreme poverty by giving a basic allotment of staple food consisting, ironically, largely of processed foods, so increasing the exposure of low-income families to a commoditised food economy (Galvez 2018). Mothers also received cash transfers from the government that, like previous social assistance programmes, were conditional on them attending multiple 'training' sessions to 'learn' how to make healthy choices for their families. The programme failed. In the end, it reached only 0.1 per cent of its initial intended beneficiaries and the population living under extreme poverty increased by up to 13 per cent from 2014 to 2018 (Cruz Vargas 2020). In August 2019, a media investigation revealed that the Crusade Against Hunger was involved in one of the most notorious corruption scandals in the country's recent history. Rosario Robles Berlanga, the head of the programme, was prosecuted for participating in a large corruption network that diverted some US$263 million dollars of public resources from the Crusade (Nájar 2019).

With a renewed focus on genes and/or diets to address COVID-19 and its major comorbidities, the body was, again, placed at the centre of the discussion. Diets, genes and prescriptions of 'self-care' converge to leave the state's failures unaccountable for the devastating effects of COVID-19 so far. As Mendenhall (2012) shows for diabetes, a syndemic framework on chronic diseases helps to unveil the ways that adverse social conditions (for example, poverty, stress, lack of healthcare) weaken a population's defences, exposing it to a cluster of health disasters such as those in Mexico today. In the case of obesity, diabetes and COVID-19, disease clustering is deeply linked to adverse syndemic interactions (Singer 2020). However, an incessant focus on genes, diets and individual choices obscures the social and historically situated dimensions of COVID-19 and creates new barriers and challenges for those defined as the source of the problem.

Mestizaje under COVID-19: from strong national genes to sinful bodies

When the first cases of coronavirus were identified in Mexico, the narrative of genetic health risks associated with mestizaje gave way to a hopeful idea of national genetic strength. At the beginning of the lockdown, a widely-read national newspaper, *El Universal,* published a column by García Soto (2020) in which he described a special meeting between President Manuel López Obrador and the health team coordinating the national COVID-19 strategy. According to García Soto, the president was informed that the country could expect up to 2,000 deaths by COVID-19, but:

> due to genetics, the Mexican race was more resistant to this type of virus than other races, such as the European. It was argued that [resistance] was linked to the Mexican genome and with mestizaje, it was expected that [race] was going to positively affect the impact of the new coronavirus among the Mexican population.

A few days later, Julio Granados Arriola a renowned Mexican immuno-geneticist, spoke out in support of this supposed advantage, stating that 'genetic admixture and not the purity of our populations (was) providing strength in this global crisis' (Gilet 2020). He challenged the idea that we are all exposed to coronavirus in equal ways, and dismissed the idea that a genetic strength among racially mixed populations in Latin America was 'a colonial mechanism' that denied the situated experiences of Mexican mestizos.

Under the COVID-19 Host Genetics Initiative, phenotypes around the world are being investigated to determine major genetic risk factors for the virus across populations (2020). Brazil, Paraguay, Argentina and

Chile have collaborated with the initiative to study the effects of national genetic profiles in the severity of the virus in Latin America. As in Mexico, Chile's media circles and scientists have stressed the need to have their own genetic component represented in the initiative, as clinical outcomes could be unique due to indigenous ancestry (Valenzuela 2020). The increasing use of genetic profiles as substitutes for national representations seems to have prompted the resurgence of old eugenic tropes of foodways and diets believed to be associated with the racial 'betterment' of populations.[1] For instance, in a column supporting Mexican's genetic advantage to navigate the virus, Gil Gamés (2020) explained that ancestral food practices were behind what he called 'gene modification' among Mexican mestizos and that food was the basis of Mexicans' genetic strength; he echoed eugenic ideas of heredity and evolution, and the power of foodways and other environmental factors to 'improve' the racial profile of the nation (Weismantel 1989; Stepan 1991).

The idea of genetic strength linked to mestizaje as protecting against coronavirus was shattered by the rapid increase in confirmed cases and fatalities in Latin America, as naïve ideas in genetic capital were confronted by the social and biological reality of viral encounters. By the first week of July 2020, Latin America, with only eight per cent of the world's population, had accounted for half of COVID-19 global deaths (Tharoor 2020). By 18 May, around 20,000 cases of COVID-19 had been confirmed among indigenous peoples from the Amazonia region and its 2,400 territories across eight countries (Martin 2020). Black Brazilians were said to be 62 per cent more likely to die from the virus than whites (Genot 2020) and migrants, refugees and displaced people were left without basic needs to navigate the virus as borders shut down (Segnana 2020). In Mexico, people treated at a private hospital were reported 60 per cent less likely to die by COVID-19 than those in public health units (Solís and Carreño 2020). Up to 71 per cent of COVID-19 fatalities were among people with an educational attainment of primary school or less (i.e. incomplete primary school or no formal education); up to 46 per cent were retired, unemployed or part of the informal economy (Hernández Bringas 2020). As this suggests, race, class and other social factors are tightly tied to the devastating effects of COVID-19. Nonetheless, public attention focused on what Foucault would call 'truths' invested in the body, the strength of the national genetic makeup to resist the virus, and the strength of character of its citizens to assume responsibility for their individual and collective survival.

The current obsession with the body, which because of shape and weight has been publicly deemed as 'at risk' and 'a risk' of COVID-19, draws

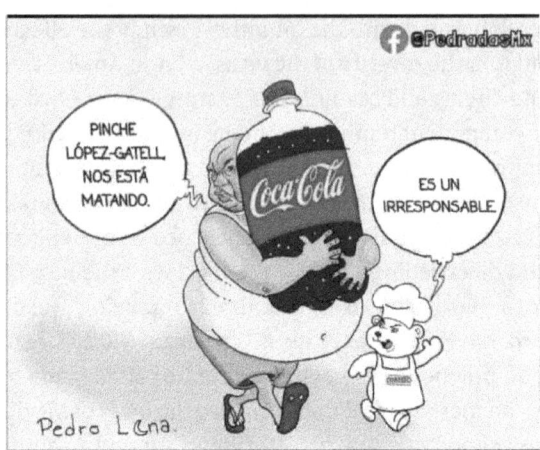

Figure 14.1 Caricature about obesity circulating in social media, source unknown

on and produces misinformation and stigma. Messages and caricatures began to circulate about the virus and people living with excessive weight gain and obesity. In its Twitter account, the national newspaper, *La Jornada*, published the image of a fat man sitting on a couch, watching TV, gorging on junk food, transmogrifying into the virus and dying (*La Jornada* online 2020). In another image, a morbidly obese man carries an oversize bottle of Coca-Cola and angrily states 'Gatell is killing us'. The man is accompanied by the iconic little white bear that represents Mexico's number one high-caloric and processed food label: Bimbo (Figure 14.1). The bear responds to the man: Gatell is irresponsible. In another cartoon, a morbidly obese woman wearing a facemask angrily decries a 'normal weight' young woman for not doing so. 'You must wear a mask' she says. 'You are putting my health in danger' (Figure 14.2). People living with obesity are caricatured as angry, lazy and irresponsible, bad citizens, and embodied obstacles to the government's strategy to address the pandemic and save the nation. The idea is promoted that people living with obesity are the only ones at risk, the only ones expected to wear facemasks.

On 5 November 2020, President Manuel López Obrador announced a government strategy to address obesity and stated that the majority of deaths by COVID-19 was linked to this condition. The president stated that obesity was caused by bad eating habits and presented a cartoon (Figure 14.3) to be distributed among 30 million households in Mexico. In the cartoon, a young thin girl educates an overweight boy about the dangers of junk food. 'You have a junk body' says the girl, as the boy shows

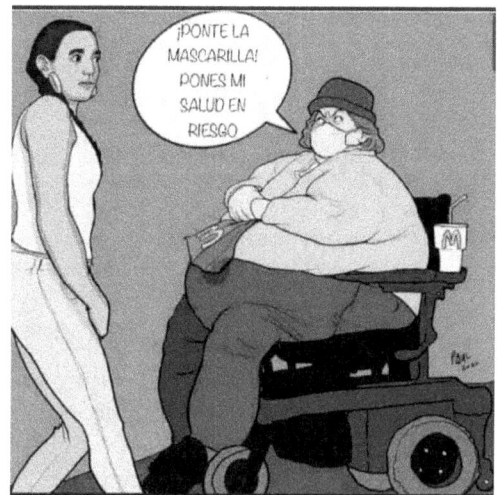

Figure 14.2 Caricature about obesity circulating in social media, source unknown

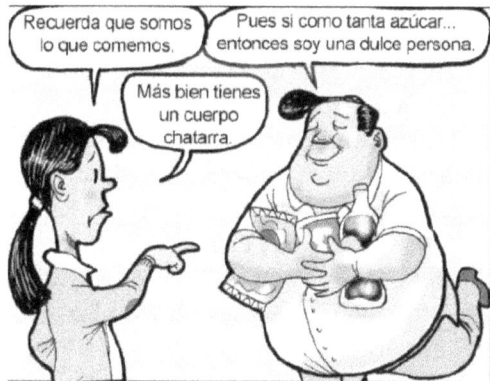

Figure 14.3 Caricature designed to educate children on the dangers of obesity and junk food. Commissioned by Mexican Secretariat of Health and authored by Rafael Barajas (El Fisgón) Source: Gobierno de México: https://www.gob.mx/cms/uploads/attachment/file/590444/CPM_Campan_a_nutricio_n_folleto__05nov20.pdf

her the food items he has brought for school lunch. The cartoon depicts fat children as obsessed with junk food, ignorant and unable to control themselves. It shows the boy eating from a trash can to suggest that junk food is trash, it accuses people diagnosed as overweight or obese as a burden to the state and to taxpayers, and finally (Figure 14.4) it warns against COVID-19's comorbidities and explains other countries' better

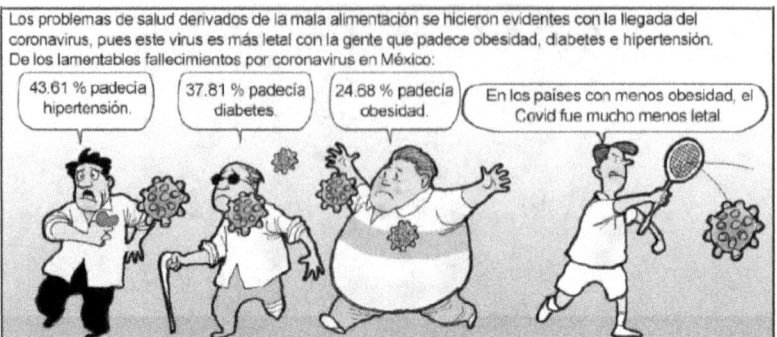

Figure 14.4 Caricature designed to educate children on the dangers of obesity and junk food. Commissioned by Mexican Secretariat of Health and authored by Rafael Barajas (El Fisgón) Source: Gobierno de México: https://www.gob.mx/cms/uploads/attachment/file/590444/CPM_Campan_a_nutricio_n_folleto__05nov20.pdf

outcomes through lower rates of obesity among their population. 'COVID is less lethal' in countries where people eat better and exercise. The cartoon has been widely criticised for stigmatising fatness, promoting fatphobia and strengthening the idea that people's health is the outcome of individual choices and responsibility.

In April 2020, a joint international consensus statement, written by a multidisciplinary group of experts, criticised the gap between stigmatising narratives around obesity and current scientific knowledge (Rubino et al. 2020). At stake were long-lasting effects of stigmatisation on the mental health of people living with obesity and their right to medical care. Le Brocq and colleagues (2020) also pointed to the all-consuming fear, anxiety and uncertainty that COVID-19 had caused among people diagnosed with obesity in the UK. Respondents worried about not getting medical support if they were admitted to hospital, either because of lack of proper equipment or because of stigma or extreme triage guidelines. The authors warned against such stigma leading to people's reluctance to seek healthcare, with the potential of worsening COVID-19 outcomes. This was especially relevant as many identified as particularly vulnerable to COVID-19 were already being denied regular care as hospitals were overwhelmed by emergency admissions of people with COVID-19 (Manderson and Wahlberg 2020).

As always in the normalisation of privilege for certain kinds of bodies (i.e. by race, gender or ability), stigmatisation is often materialised in practices and policies that directly affect people's possible survival. As I illustrate below, the war against obesity as a public health and political strategy extends beyond fat stigmatisation. COVID-19 has forced many countries to swiftly develop bioethical guides to allocate limited medical resources. These guidelines illustrate how notions of vulnerability and risk manifest in public health policy, and how a focus on obesity as risk may extend beyond stigmatisation by conditioning people's possibilities of receiving the care that they deserve and to which they have a right.

Bioethical guidelines of extreme triage under COVID-19

Assuming a shortage of medical resources, many countries in Latin America have discussed or already established bioethical guidelines, referred to as extreme triage, for resource allocation in cases of public health emergency such as COVID-19. Under the principle of social justice, these guidelines propose to allocate resources to save as many lives as possible. Chile, México, Argentina, Colombia, Brazil and Uruguay have developed triage guidelines to administer scarce resources (Carvajal 2020; Woites 2020; Moreno Molina 2020; Giordano 2020). Although these guidelines were drafted independently and not through a regional initiative, they coincided on the main criteria for critical medical care allocation: evaluating the possibility that a patient will improve and survive, with or without comorbidities, and in light of their age, in other words, 'years of life to be saved'. In a brief on ethics guidance on the use of scarce resources for critical healthcare during the COVID-19 pandemic, the Pan American Health Organization stressed the need to treat all people equitably. However, the document also highlights the need to save the greatest number of lives and to prioritise those most likely to survive treatment (PAHO 2020).

An emergency resource allocation strategy involves abandoning the Hippocratic Oath, the idea of equality between people, and the sacredness of life. In a crisis as presently experienced with COVID-19, health professionals require direction to proceed in the face of limited resources. In April 2020, Helen Ouyang (2020), a New York emergency department doctor, vividly described her experience during the first outbreak of the pandemic, as hospitals were flooded by patients, dead and alive. She argued the need for bioethical guidelines of extreme triage for those at the front line, physically and emotionally exhausted by attending to the flow of COVID-19's patients and potentially risking their own health and lives to save others. However, it is possible to support the need for triage guidelines while also questioning the criteria used to evaluate and decide how to allocate critical medical care.

Triage guidelines sparked a heated debate across the globe (Del Missier 2020). Bioethicists were accused of 'playing God' by deciding who deserves the chance to live and who not. In many countries, public opinion forced bioethicists to rewrite and retract recommendations for limited medical resource allocation. In some Latin American countries, the most prominent voices pointed at age discrimination. In Mexico, critics compared the guidelines with Nazi atrocities against people perceived as old or ill (Miranda 2020); in Argentina, bioethicists questioned age as a criterion to determine outcome, given that a young individual could suffer from more severe pathologies than an older one (Woites 2020). Others pointed to increasing evidence that structural factors and comorbidities were more sensitive than age at predicting the lethality and severity of COVID-19 (Bello-Chavolla et al. 2020).

The guidelines also recommended limited resources be allocated in light of patients' 'past situation', that is, 'the presence of pre-existing comorbidities that might impact on the patients' expectation to benefit from treatment' (Consejo de Salubridad 2020, 11). Pre-existing diseases were therefore used to evaluate a patient's eligibility to receive medical care. Vulnerable populations were mentioned throughout the guidelines, but these were narrowed to ethnic minority groups, people who are unemployed, pregnant women, other women and people working in the health sector. The label 'vulnerability' was avoided, so referring to patients' comorbidities suggests that vulnerability implies protection. In contrast, the term 'situation' allows the guidelines to recommend exclusion from medical care without appearing contradictory.

However, as Barnes and colleagues suggest, 'care always has a past and how we respond to past injustices is one of the largest ethical questions we need to face' (2015, 11). In the area of research ethics and public health ethics, vulnerability first appeared in the 1979 Belmont Report, in which populations in need of special protection are described. Some populations – ethnic minorities, people economically disadvantaged, the very sick and those without capacity for free consent (i.e. persons confined to institutions) – were entitled to protection. Other landmark documents in research ethics, including the International Guidelines for Biomedical Research Involving Human Subjects (1982) and the Declaration of Helsinki (2000), also address questions of vulnerability and vulnerable populations (Luna 2019). The former identifies three groups of vulnerable populations that, linked to their social or physical conditions, were 'relatively (or absolutely) incapable of protecting their own interests' (CIOMS 2002, 69). Lack of power was therefore the main criterion defining certain subpopulations as vulnerable and in need of protection.

This lack of power has been at the centre of debates regarding the notion of vulnerability. For many, the notion of vulnerability contains the risk of reducing politics to care, complicating the possibility of a vulnerable political subject (Ferrarese 2016, 157). Such risks derived from the tendency to reflect on vulnerability as embodied and historically are seen as unworthy of the political sphere. Embodied vulnerability, tied to capability/capacity, strengthens the perceived incompatibility between politics and the expression of suffering and needs. The long negligence of the body, as opposed to mind and reason, as a subject of investigation in philosophical thought and sociology, maintains the idea of the body as located in the private realm (Malacrida and Low 2008). Thus, the current focus on the body operates as a mechanism to leave the state unaccountable for the political and social roots of health inequalities, and keeps the individual body in its place through notions of self-care and individual/private responsibility. The body as private or apolitical could also be behind the stigmatisation and condescending practices that often occur when labelling whole groups as vulnerable (Luna 2019). For instance, a private amusement park in the city of Monterrey, northeast Mexico, announced that older adults, children and people with obesity were forbidden entrance for their own protection from coronavirus (Zuñiga 2020). The park did not specify how staff would 'diagnose' someone as obese nor clarify if measures would be implemented to avoid discrimination. People have been reported being denied entrance into casinos if perceived as obese for 'their own protection'. People with other comorbidities, less easy to diagnose by sight, such as diabetes or hypertension, are allowed to occupy these spaces freely. A national newspaper, *Animal Político*, reported that since June 2020, companies started to refuse hiring people with chronic diseases, over 55 years of age, or with other 'risks' linked to COVID-19 (2020). According to an unemployed man interviewed for this chapter, COVID-19 had resulted in discrimination against those suffering from known comorbidities (Casasola 2020). This leads us to ask who or what are these businesses 'protecting'? What forms and meanings does the notion of 'vulnerability' take in these cases? Although, as Ferrarese (2016) argues, the discourse of vulnerability is already fully political through the polemics to which it gives rise, we must be attentive of the ways that both 'vulnerability' and 'risk' are used, as these terms are heavily charged with complex and, sometimes, contradictory meanings.

During their daily briefings, public health officials never referred to obesity as a vulnerability to COVID-19, and instead, spoke of risk when referring to chronic diseases. While vulnerability invokes the need for special protection, risk demands accountability and personal responsibility. This idea of risk works to justify labour and other forms of discrimination. As Kippax and Stephenson (2016) show in the case of HIV prevention, a turn to 'vulnerable populations' rather than 'risky individuals' focused attention on the social and cultural 'drivers' of vulnerability; vulnerability could work to deny the power of collective action and agency over social and cultural structures. Social practices instead of individual behaviours might better account for how peoples' actions contribute to change.

COVID-19 raises how and when languages of vulnerability and risk are deployed, and how these narratives impact people living with obesity. Such narratives have political implications, with potential impact on the health of individuals and possibilities for collective action. We must also acknowledge the agency of those whose bodies are insistently labelled as 'at risk' of infection or 'a risk' (to others) of transmitting infection. The perceptions and experiences of people living with known conditions must be taken into account in any action and public health strategy (Le Brocq et al. 2020). Garland-Thomson et al. (2020), disability bioethicists, remind us of the need to transform medical subjects into political ones. They denounce as unethical and illegal the way in which extreme triage guides under COVID-19 allocate resources unequally on the basis of ability. Eugenics, they remind us, was also a scientific gaze to categorise human variation in order to create 'a better future' with the 'best' kind of people.

Conclusions

Bioethics must go beyond procedures such as informed consent and ethical committees to account for the political nature of health policies and scientific endeavours (Hernández 2019). We must explore the political implications of new public health discourses and policies on peoples' situated experiences. In this chapter, I have illustrated that narratives around obesity increase stigmatisation of fatness, as the government's war against obesity has become a war against people with excessive weight gain and/or obesity. Through an analysis of the guide, I argue that avoiding the notion of vulnerability in relation to COVID-19, and instead using the term 'past situation' to justify the denial of critical medical care to some people, neglects social factors linked to health inequalities and social injustice. This implies that people with serious cardiometabolic disease – obesity, diabetes and heart disease – are at risk of being denied care since they are at risk either of not responding to care and dying anyway, or surviving COVID-19 with compounded comorbidities and reduced life expectancy.

Attention must be given to other forms of vulnerability to COVID-19 beyond known comorbidities. This is urgent as democratic action gives way to the imposition of state emergency measures in order to care, surveil or discipline those deemed 'at risk' and 'a risk' (see Manderson and Levine, Chapter 3). For instance, in Mexico, Giovanni López, a 30-year-old bricklayer, was beaten to death by police officers for not wearing a face mask in public. Police brutality is a pre-existing condition, but it complicates the implementation of state measures to care for the wider population. Similarly, domestic violence has taken a toll on women during lockdown. In Mexico in March 2020 alone, when the 'stay at home' campaign started, 115,614 emergency calls linked to sexual and physical violence against woman were reported (SESNSP 2020). Violence is also a pre-existing condition that impacts women's possibility to survive the pandemic. Similarly, as elsewhere in the world, people working in Mexico's food system have been severely affected by COVID-19 (Gross and Yates-Doerr 2020). By early June, more than 1,000 workers in the country's largest food market, the *Mercado de Abastos*, had tested positive for the virus (Gómez 2020a). Farmers' organisations warned of an unprecedented social crisis due to the lack of social protection and sanitation standards in agriculture (Gómez 2020b). In addition, there is a risk that people may avoid food markets and revert to the processed food that the government is so fiercely fighting to eliminate from people's diets.

What these 'past situations' show is the importance of acknowledging the complex and intricate shapes that vulnerability and risk assume under COVID-19. Language is never neutral, and narratives around COVID-19's comorbidities must be revised with caution to avoid concrete and long-lasting effects upon the people living with these conditions. The current language of risk strengthens fat phobia in a country that has recently started to study the extent of weight discrimination (Soto et al. 2014). The focus on obesity might also produce misleading information (for example, the relative risk to infection of people with obesity) while justifying a public health strategy to tackle COVID-19 that many perceive as disastrous. People living with obesity have been easy targets to blame for the states' pre-existing negligence and failures, including the appalling condition of its healthcare system. COVID-19's comorbidities could be understood as embodied palimpsests not of past situations but past injustices. In the case of obesity, these exist in the colonial erasure of traditional diets in favour of western food practices and in reproducing racial and gendered ideas of heredity and care. This past must be revised to make reparations and allow us to imagine a more just and ethical future for all.

Note

1 To read more about the creation of Mexican national genome see Vasquez and Deister (2019).

References

Aguilar-Rodríguez, Sandra. 2007. 'Cooking modernity: Nutrition policies, class, and gender in 1940s and 1950s Mexico City'. *The Americas* 6: 177–205. https://doi.org/10.1353/tam.2007.0128.
Agren, David. 2020. 'Mexico "Flying blind as lack of Covid-19 testing mystifies experts"'. *The Guardian*, 24 July 2020. Accessed 18 November 2020. https://www.theguardian.com/global-development/2020/jul/24/mexico-covid-19-testing-coronavirus.
Animal Político. 2020. '9 gobernadores de oposición piden renuncia de López-Gatell; ustedes también son responsables, les responde'. *Animal Político*, 31 July 2020. https://www.animalpolitico.com/2020/07/10-gobernadores-de-oposicion-piden-la-renuncia-de-lopez-gatell/.
Barnes, Marian, Tula Brannelly, Lizzie Ward and Nicki Ward. 2015. 'Introduction: The critical significance of care'. In *Ethics of Care: Critical advances in international perspective*, edited by Marian Barnes Tula Brannelly, Lizzie Ward and Nicki Ward, pp. 3–19. Bristol, UK: Policy Press.
Bello-Chavolla, Omar, Jessica Paola Bahena-Lopez, Neftali Eduardo Antonio-Villa, Arsenio Vargas-Vázquez, Armando González-Díaz, et al. 2020. 'Predicting mortality due to SARS-CoV-2: A mechanistic score relating obesity and diabetes to COVID-19 outcomes in Mexico'. *The Journal of Clinical Endocrinology & Metabolism* 105(8): 2752–61. https://doi.org/10.1210/clinem/dgaa346.
Burkhart, Louise M. 1989. *The Slippery Earth: Nahua-Christian moral dialogue in sixteenth-century Mexico*. Tucson, AZ: University of Arizona Press.
Carvajal, Claudia. 2020. '¿A quién conectar y a quién desconectar?: El debate ético que pasa de la teoría a la práctica médica'. *Diario Uchile*, 26 May 2020. Accessed 19 November 2020. https://radio.uchile.cl/2020/05/26/a-quien-conectar-y-a-quien-desconectar-el-debate-etico-que-pasa-de-la-teoria-a-la-practica-medica/.
Casasola, Tania. 2020. 'El COVID nos trajo discriminación: Niegan empleo por tener diabetes, hipertensión y obesidad'. *Animal Político*, 17 September 2020. Accessed 23 November 2020. https://www.animalpolitico.com/2020/09/covid-niegan-empleo-enfermos-diabetes-hipertension-obesidad-discriminacion/.
Coneval (Consejo Nacional de Evaluación de la Política de Desarrollo Social). 2018. 'Pobreza en México. Resultados de pobreza en México 2018 a nivel nacional y por entidades federativas'. Accessed 19 November 2020. https://www.coneval.org.mx/Medicion/Paginas/PobrezaInicio.aspx.
Consejo de Salubridad de México. 2020. 'Guía bioética para asignación de recursos limitados de medicina crítica en situación de emergencia'. http://www.csg.gob.mx/descargas/pdf/index/informacion_relevante/GuiaBioeticaTriaje_30_Abril_2020_7pm.pdf.
Council for International Organizations for Medical Sciences (CIOMS) and World Health Organization (WHO). 2002. *International Ethical Guidelines for Biomedical Research Involving Human Subjects*, 2nd ed. Geneva, Switzerland: CIOMS.
Cruz Vargas, Juan. 2020. 'Cruzada contra el hambre fracasó: ASF; la pobreza extrema alimentaria aumentó 13%'. *Proceso*, February 2020. Accessed 23 November 2020. https://www.proceso.com.mx/nacional/2020/2/21/cruzada-contra-el-hambre-fracaso-asf-la-pobreza-extrema-alimentaria-aumento-13-238873.html.

Del Missier, Giovanni. 2020. 'Overwhelmed by the virus: The issue of extreme triage'. *Alphonsian Academy Blog*. 27 March 2020. Accessed 19 November 2020. https://www.cssr.news/2020/03/overwhelmed-by-the-virus-the-issue-of-extreme-triage/.

Duster, Troy. 2003. *Backdoor to Eugenics*, 2nd ed. London: Routledge.

Earle, Rebecca. 2010. 'If you eat their food: Diets and bodies in early colonial Spanish America,' *American Historical Review* 115(3): 688–713.

Ferrarese, Estelle. 2016. 'Vulnerability: A concept with which to undo the world as it is?' *Critical Horizons* 17(2): 149–59.

Forbes Staff. 2013. 'Descubren gen que provoca la diabetes tipo 2 en los mexicanos.' *Forbes*. 26 December. Accessed 6 June 2021. https://www.forbes.com.mx/descubren-gen-que-contribuye-la-diabetes-tipo-2-en-los-mexicanos/.

Galvez, Alyshia. 2018. *Eating NAFTA: Trade, Food policies, and the destruction of Mexico*. Oakland, CA: University of California Press.

Gamés, Gil. 2020. 'El poder de la genética'. *Milenio*, 24 March 2020. Accessed 19 November 2020. https://www.milenio.com/opinion/gil-games/uno-hasta-el-fondo/el-poder-de-la-genetica.

García Soto, Salvador. 2020. 'Esperan hasta 2 mil muertes por Covid-19 en México,' *El Universal*, 23 March 2020. Accessed 19 November 2020. https://www.eluniversal.com.mx/opinion/salvador-garcia-soto/esperan-hasta-2-mil-muertes-por-covid-19-en-mexico.

Garland-Thomson, Rosemarie, George Daley and Bartha Knoppers. 2020. 'CRISPR and human identity: Governing germline gene editing'. *30 Years of the Genome Integrating and Applying ELSI Research. Columbia University*. Accessed 19 November 2020. https://www.mhe.cuimc.columbia.edu/our-divisions/division-ethics/elsi-virtual-forum/elsi-virtual-forum-video-recordings.

Genot, Louis. 2020. 'In Brazil, Coronavirus hits blacks harder than whites'. *Barrons*, 7 May 2020. Accessed 19 November 2020. https://www.barrons.com/news/in-brazil-coronavirus-hits-blacks-harder-than-whites-01588886404.

Gilet, Eliana. 2020. 'El mestizaje de América Latina como "barrera" ante el COVID-19'. *Sputnik*, 22 May 2020. Accessed 19 November 2020. https://mundo.sputniknews.com/ciencia/202005221091514037-el-mestizaje-de-america-latina-como-barrera-ante-el-covid-19/.

Giordano, Álvaro. 2020. 'El problema ético en la pandemia ¿Cómo podremos trabajar en medio de una demanda extraordinaria de recursos?' *La Diaria Opinión*, 2 April 2020. Accessed 19 November 2020. https://ladiaria.com.uy/opinion/articulo/2020/4/el-problema-etico-en-la-pandemia-como-podremos-trabajar-en-medio-de-una-demanda-extraordinaria-de-recursos/.

Gobierno de México. 2020a. 'Informe diario sobre coronavirus COVID-19. Viernes 27 de marzo 2020'. Accessed 19 November 2020. https://www.gob.mx/insabi/es/videos/informe-diario-sobre-coronavirus-covid-19-viernes-27-de-marzo-2020.

Gobierno de México. 2020b. 'Informe diario sobre coronavirus COVID-19. Jueves 23 de julio 2020'. Accessed 19 November 2020. https://www.gob.mx/insabi/es/videos/informe-diario-sobre-coronavirus-covid-19-jueves-23-de-julio-2020.

Gómez, Carolina. 2020a. 'Movimientos campesinos prevén catástrofe social por Covid-19 en México,' *La Jornada*, 17 July 2020. Accessed 19 November 2020. https://www.jornada.com.mx/ultimas/sociedad/2020/07/17/movimientos-campesinos-preven-catastrofe-social-por-covid-19-en-mexico-1451.html.

Gómez, Carolina. 2020b. 'Mercados de abasto son indispensables y no pueden cerrar frente a Covid-19: expertos'. *La Jornada*, 3 July 2020. Accessed 19 November 2020. https://www.jornada.com.mx/ultimas/sociedad/2020/07/03/mercados-son-indispensables-y-no-pueden-cerrar-frente-a-covid-19-expertos-8190.html.

Gross, Joan and Emily Yates-Doerr. 2020 'Racialized inequalities. Society for Anthropology of Food and Nutrition'. *Food Anthropology*, 23 July 2020. Accessed 19 November 2020. https://foodanthro.com/2020/07/23/op-eds/.

Hernández Bringas, Héctor Hiram. 2020. 'Mortalidad por COVID-19 en México. Notas preliminares para un perfil sociodemográfico'. *Notas de Coyuntura del CRIM* 36: 1–7.

Hernández, Cuauhtémoc. 2019. 'De Van R. Potter a Michel Foucault o de la bioética a la biopolítica como estrategia de análisis en el debate en torno a las biotecnologías'. In *Poder y subjetividad. Emplazamientos para una reflexión sobre el presente*, edited by Javier Corona Fernández, pp. 95–119. México: Itaca/Universidad de Guanajuato.

INEGI (Instituto Nacional de Estadística, Geografía e Informática). 2020. 'ENOE. Primer trimestre de 2020'. *Encuesta Nacional de Ocupación y Empleo*. Accessed 19 November 2020. https://www.inegi.org.mx/programas/enoe/15ymas/.

Instituto Nacional de Medicina Genómica (INMEGEN). 2014. 'Diabetes'. *Boletín Expresión Inmegen*, 4(19). Accessed 19 November 2020. https://boletin.inmegen.gob.mx/boletin19/.

Instituto Nacional de Salud Pública (INSP). 2018. 'Informe de Resultados de La Encuesta Nacional de Salud y Nutrición – 2018'. *ENSANUT 2018*. Accessed 19 November 2020. https://ensanut.insp.mx/encuestas/ensanut2018/informes.php.

Kippax, Susan and Niamh Stephenson. 2016. *Socialising the Biomedical Turn in HIV Prevention*. London: Anthem Press.

Koenig, Barbara, Sandra Lee and Sarah Richardson. 2008. *Revisiting Race in Genomic Age*. New Brunswick, NJ and London: Rutgers University Press.

La Jornada online. 2020. 'Chatarravirus por @monerohernández'. Twitter post by *La Jornada Online*, 24 July 2020. Accessed 23 November 2020 https://twitter.com/lajornadaonline/status/1286849903696650240.

Le Brocq, S., K. Clare, M. Bryant, K. Roberts and A.A. Tahrani. 2020. 'Obesity and COVID-19: A call for action from people living with obesity'. *The Lancet Diabetes & Endocrinology* 8(8): 652–4.

Malacrida, Claudia and Jaqueline Low, eds. 2008. *Sociology of the Body: A reader*. London: Oxford University Press.

Luna, Florencia. 2019. 'Revisiting Vulnerability: Its Development and Impact'. In *Controversies in Latin American Bioethics*, edited by Eduardo Rivera and Martín Hevia, pp. 67–81. Cham, Switzerland: Springer.

Manderson, Lenore. 2016. 'Foetal politics and the prevention of chronic disease'. *Australian Feminist Studies* 31(88): 154–71. https://doi.org/10.1080/08164649.2016.1224056.

Manderson, Lenore and Ayo Wahlberg. 2020. 'Chronic living in a communicable world'. *Medical Anthropology* 39(5): 428–39. https://doi.org/10.1080/01459740.2020.1761352.

Martin, Jamie. 2020. 'Los casos de coronavirus entre los indígenas del Amazonas ascienden ya a 20,000'. *Noticias ONU*, 19 May 2020. Accessed 19 November 2020. https://news.un.org/es/story/2020/05/1474662.

Mendenhall, Emily. 2012. *Syndemic Suffering: Social Distress, Depression, and Diabetes Among Mexican Immigrant Women*. New York: Routledge.

Miranda, Perla. 2020. 'Expertos critican guía que prioriza a jóvenes sobre ancianos con Covid-19'. *El Universal*, 15 May 2020. Accessed 19 November 2020. https://www.eluniversal.com.mx/nacion/expertos-critican-guia-que-prioriza-jovenes-sobre-ancianos-con-covid-19.

Moreno Molina, Julieta. 2020. Recomendaciones generales para la toma de decisiones éticas en los servicios de salud durante la pandemia Covid-19. *Ministerio de Salud, Colombia*, 23 March 2020. Accessed 19 November 2020. https://www.minsalud.gov.co/Ministerio/Institucional/Procesos%20y%20procedimientos/GIPS13.pdf.

Nájar, Alberto. 2019. 'La estafa maestra: de qué acusan a Rosario Robles, la exministra de Peña Nieto arrestada en México, BBC News, 13 August 2020. Accessed 19 November 2020. https://www.bbc.com/mundo/noticias-america-latina-49338467.

Neel, James. 1962. 'Diabetes mellitus: A "thrifty" genotype rendered detrimental by "progress"?' *American Journal of Human Genetics* 14(4): 353–62.

Ojeda de la Torre, Ivonne. 2020. 'López-Gatell ha sido 115 veces TT en Twitter, y como epidemiólogo es el 3 con más fans en el mundo'. *Sin Embargo*, 30 May 2020. Accessed 19 November 2020. https://www.sinembargo.mx/30-05-2020/3795209.

Olivares, Alonso Emir. 2012. 'Los mexicanos tienen predisposición genética a la obesidad, según estudio.' *La Jornada*. 2 August 2012. Accessed 6 June 2021. http://www.jornada.unam.mx/2012/08/02/ciencias/a15n1cie.

Ouyang, Helen. 2020. 'I'm an ER doctor in New York. None of us will ever be the same,' *The New York Times*, 14 April 2020. Accessed 19 November 2020. https://www.nytimes.com/2020/04/14/magazine/coronavirus-er-doctor-diary-new-york-city.html.

Pentecost, Michelle. 2018. 'The first thousand days: Epigenetics in the age of global health'. In *The Palgrave Handbook of Biology and Society*, edited by Maurizio Meloni, John Cromby, Des Fitzgerald and Stephanie Lloyd, pp. 269–94. London: Palgrave Macmillan.

PAHO (Pan American Health Organization). 2020. 'Ethics guidance for the use of scarce resources in the delivery of critical health care during the COVID-19 pandemic,' *PAHO*, 8 May 2020. Accessed 23 November 2020. https://iris.paho.org/handle/10665.2/52096.

Pilcher, Jeffrey M., 1998. *¡Que vivan los tamales! Food and the making of Mexican identity*. Albuquerque, NM: University of New Mexico Press.

Rubino, Francesco, Rebecca Puhl, David Cummings, Robert Eckel, Donna Ryan, et al. 2020. 'Joint international consensus statement for ending stigma of obesity'. *Nature Medicine* 26: 485–97.

Ruiz Jaimes, Elizabeth. 2013. 'Mexicanos Globalmente Gordos.' *El Economista*. 8 September 2013. Accessed 24 November 2020. https://www.eleconomista.com.mx/arteseideas/Mexicanos-globalmente-gordos-20130908-0082.html.

Saldaña-Tejeda, Abril. 2018. 'Mothers' experiences of masculinity in the context of child obesity in Mexico'. *Women's Studies International Forum* 70: 39–45. https://doi.org/10.1016/j.wsif.2018.07.013.

Saldaña-Tejeda, Abril and Peter Wade. 2018. 'Obesity, race and the indigenous origins of health risks among Mexican mestizos'. *Ethnic and Racial Studies* 41(15): 2731–49. https://doi.org/10.1080/01419870.2017.1407810.

Saldaña-Tejeda, Abril and Peter Wade. 2019. Eugenics, epigenetics, and obesity predisposition among Mexican Mestizos. *Medical Anthropology* 38(8): 664–79. https://doi.org/10.1080/01459740.2019.1589466.

Secretaría de Salud. 2013. *Estrategia Nacional Para la Prevención y el Control del Sobrepeso, la Obesidad y la Diabetes*. Mexico City: Secretaría de Salud. Accessed 23 November 2020. https://www.medigraphic.com/pdfs/enfermeriaimss/eim-2014/eim142i.pdf.

Segnana, Juan. 2020. 'La situación de los migrantes en América Latina en el contexto del COVID-19'. *PNUD América Latina y El Caribe*, 19 May 2020. Accessed 19 November 2020. https://www.latinamerica.undp.org/content/rblac/es/home/blog/2020/la-situacion-de-los-migrantes-en-america-latina-en-el-contexto-d.html.

SESNSP (Secretariado Ejecutivo del Sistema Nacional de Seguridad Pública). 2020. 'Información sobre violencia contra las mujeres (Incidencia delictiva y llamadas de emergencia 9-1-1, September 2020'. Accessed 23 November 2020. https://drive.google.com/file/d/1p9M_mt-4jmn3CE8lB9qEu0sYlLAO67fp/view.

Sharp, Gemma C., Deborah A. Lawlor and Sarah. S. Richardson. 2018. 'It's the mother! How assumptions about the causal primacy of maternal effects influence research on the developmental origins of health and disease'. *Social Science & Medicine* 213: 20–27. https://doi.org/10.1016/j.socscimed.2018.07.035.

SIGMA Type 2 Diabetes Consortium. 2014. 'Sequence Variants in SLC16A11 Are a Common Risk Factor for Type 2 Diabetes in Mexico'. *Nature* 506: 97–101. https://doi.org/10.1038/nature12828.

Singer, Merrill. 2020. 'Deadly companions: COVID-19 and diabetes in Mexico,' *Medical Anthropology* 39(8): 660–65. https://doi.org/10.1080/01459740.2020.1805742.

Smedley, Audrey and Brian Smedley. 2005. 'Race as biology is fiction, racism as a social problem is real: Anthropological and historical perspectives on the social construction of race'. *American Psychologist* 60(1): 16–26. https://doi.org/10.1037/0003-066X.60.1.16.

Solís, Patricio and Hiram Carreño. 2020. 'COVID-19 fatality and comorbidity risk factors among confirmed patients in Mexico'. *MedRxiv*, 25 April 2020: 1–8. Accessed 19 November 2020. https://www.medrxiv.org/content/10.1101/2020.04.21.20074591v1.

Soto, Lucero, Ana Lilia Armendáriz-Anguiano, Monserrat Bacardí-Gascón and A. Jiménez Cruz. 2014. 'Beliefs, attitudes and phobias among Mexican medical and psychology students towards people with obesity'. *Nutrición Hospitalaria* 30(1): 37–41. https://doi.org/10.3305/nh.2014.30.1.7512.

Stepan, Nancy. 1991. *'The Hour of Eugenics': Race, Gender, and Nation in Latin America*. Ithaca, NY and London: Cornell University Press.

Tharoor, Ishaan. 2020. 'Latin America's coronavirus crisis is only getting worse'. *The Washington Post*, 25 June 2020. Accessed 19 November 2020. https://www.washingtonpost.com/world/2020/06/26/latin-america-coronavirus-crisis/.

The Covid-19 Host Genetics Initiative. 2020. 'Home'. Accessed 23 November 2020. https://www.covid19hg.org.

Torres, Gabriela. 2019. 'Ejidos/Comunidades'. *Journal for the Anthropology of North America* 22(2): 72–4.

Torres, Yuvenil. 2020. 'El 85% de decesos por el coronavirus en Hidalgo, con comorbilidad'. *Criterio*, 21 April 2020. Accessed 19 November 2020. https://criteriohidalgo.com/noticias/el-85-de-decesos-por-el-coronavirus-en-hidalgo-con-comorbilidad.

Valenzuela, Cecilia. 2020. 'Coronavirus: ¿afecta a los chilenos de igual manera que al resto del mundo?' Noticias Facultad de Medicina de la Universidad de Chile, 20 August 2020. Accessed 23 November 2020. http://www.medicina.uchile.cl/noticias/166641/el-coronavirus-afecta-a-los-chilenos-igual-que-al-resto-del-mundo.

Vargas Domínguez, Joel. 2017. 'Metabolismo y nutrición en el México posrevolucionario: eugenesia y clasificación de la población mexicana entre 1927 y 1943'. PhD thesis, Philosophy of Science, Universidad Nacional Autónoma de México.

Vasquez, Emily Elizabeth and Vivette García Deister. 2019. 'Mexican samples, Latino DNA: The trajectory of a national genome in transnational science'. *Engaging Science, Technology, and Society* 5: 107–34.

Warin, Megan, Vivienne Moore, Michael Davies and Stanley Ulijaszek. 2015. 'Epigenetics and obesity: The reproduction of habitus through intracellular and social environments'. *Body & Society* 22 (4): 53–78. https://doi.org/10.1177%2F1357034X15590485.

Weismantel, Mary. 1989. *Food, Gender and Poverty in the Ecuadorian Andes*. Philadelphia, PA: University of Pennsylvania Press.

Woites, Ana María. 2020. 'Especialistas en bioética reflexionan sobre los desafíos que se afrontan ante el nuevo coronavirus'. *Télam*, 17 April 2020. Accessed 19 November 2020. https://www.telam.com.ar/notas/202004/453069-bioetica-salud-coronavirus-pandemia.html.

Yates-Doerr, Emily. 2015 *The Weight of Obesity: Hunger and global health in postwar Guatemala*. Berkeley, CA: University of California Press.

Zuñiga, Francisco. 2020. 'Personas con obesidad, niños y adultos mayores no podrán entrar al parque Fundidora'. *Milenio*, 4 July 2020. Accessed 19 November 2020. https://www.milenio.com/ciencia-y-salud/sociedad/coronavirus-personas-obesidad-entrar-parque-fundidora.

15
Scarcity and resilience in the slums of Dhaka city, Bangladesh

Sabina Faiz Rashid, Selima Sara Kabir, Kim Ozano, Sally Theobald, Bachera Aktar and Aisha Siddika

Bangladesh reported its first confirmed case of COVID-19 on 8 March 2020; thereafter infection spread significantly. However, with inadequate testing, the statistics fail to capture the extent of coronavirus infections and deaths. Public health restrictions, such as the national lockdown – loosely referred to as a 'general holiday' deliberately to avoid mentioning coronavirus – meant that many poor people returned to their villages from cities, thus spreading the virus widely. Those who remained in Dhaka and other cities, where the cost of living was already very high, experienced catastrophic economic consequences. Moreover, despite government and private sector responses, the pandemic overburdened the country's fragile and under-resourced health system (Anwar et al. 2020).

Bangladesh, a country of 165.6 million (2.2 per cent of the global population) (BBS 2020), is currently the eighth most populous country in the world; 27 per cent of this population (41 million) lives in cities (BBS 2016). United Nations International Children's Education Fund (UNICEF) Bangladesh estimates that around 3.5 per cent of the population migrates internally every year, mostly to urban areas (UNICEF Bangladesh 2020). Further, between 1996 and 2005, the Centre for Urban Studies estimated that the total population of Dhaka's slums more than doubled, from 1.5 to 3.4 million people (Gruebner et al. 2014), and given the rate of migration into the capital, an estimated 5.3 million now live there (Hossain 2020). Many urban migrants live in slums with heterogenous communities, with varying structures and services. Slums are often squeezed around the periphery of the city or along railway lines, under bridges and elsewhere near factories or near waste dumps, and are characterised by congested living spaces, poorly maintained housing, vulnerability to monsoon rains and floods, and lack access to sufficient water and sanitation facilities, and little rubbish collection, street cleaning or related services (UNICEF Bangladesh 2020). With few rights and agency, and weak informal governance structures, slums tend to be hidden spaces for crime, gang violence and drug trade. Life is precarious, with sudden evictions and thousands of families often displaced overnight (Rashid 2004; Islam et al. 2009). In addition, although Bangladesh has improved the availability of food due to increased production over recent decades, 40 million people – one-quarter of the population – remain food insecure, and 11 million people suffer from acute hunger (WFP Bangladesh 2018). These figures will worsen with the impact of COVID-19 (bdnews24.com 2020).

The closure of businesses between 26 March and 31 May led to huge income losses for the working poor, with hardships continuing even after many businesses re-opened in June (Shawon 2020). Around 86 per cent of the workforce in Bangladesh, the majority women, depends on informal sector activities (ILO 2013). Around 3,596 garment factories actively operate in Bangladesh, employing 3.5 million people (Ovi 2018). Another 3.5 million work as construction workers on sub-contracts, and thousands as domestic workers on monthly or no-contracts (Double Repression 2020). Millions of these informal workers – street peddlers, domestic workers, factory and construction workers, and more, the majority women – lost their jobs during lockdown (Ovi 2018; Double Repression 2020). Most of those who lost employment live in Dhaka's slums.

Adolescents from poor urban slums are vulnerable because of their age, gender, lack of life experiences and other vulnerabilities which result in exploitation and abuse. The proportion of adolescents in secondary schools in Bangladesh is the lowest in South Asia (Haider 2019). Young adult and adolescent boys from very poor households are more likely than girls to start earning to contribute to their families (Ovi 2018). They start working informally, with short-term or no contracts, in order to support their families, rather than going to school or college. They often work in the most hazardous jobs, conditions and circumstances (UNICEF 2020), in work that is mainly unregistered and outside of state regulation and labour laws. Adolescent women also drop out or cannot continue their studies because of the complex interplay of poverty, crime and social pressures to marry early (*The Daily Star* 2014). As we describe, poor adolescents and young adults working in the informal sector have been directly and adversely affected by the pandemic and state policies (Acharya et al. 2020).

Methodology

In this chapter we draw on narrative phone interviews collected from 12 individuals (5 males, 7 females; adolescents and youth) living in urban slums, conducted from late March to the end of June 2020. The first author has long-term and trusting relationships with the respondents through volunteering, support and research interactions since 2006, and has a critical understanding of their contexts and relationships. This addressed any challenges emerging from phone interviews with respect to positionality, building trust and the mediation of power (Au 2019).

Qualitative inductive thematic analysis was conducted drawing on multiple theoretical frameworks based on critical medical anthropology (Singer 2004), structural violence (Farmer 2009) and intersectionality (Tolhurst et al. 2012). We examined affect as the mental and physical response to the emergency, while we considered how resulting emotions are externalised through relational social practices and materiality; we view feelings as a product of the interactions between self and the world. By understanding how emotions or affect can have practical implications for the lives of urban youth, we were able to deeply consider the impact of distress and persistent worry caused by the pandemic. The analytic frameworks on which we drew supported analysis of the interactions of varying forms of violence (physical, economic, political and social), which, as illustrated by intersectionality theory, are often mediated by more 'micro' level characteristics. These are in turn shaped by meso and macro structures of power, making visible the levels of social injustice faced by young people in slums. We discuss how the materiality experienced by poor people is not simply one of a materiality of poverty: adolescents and young people in the slums use material forms to creatively make and remake their social identities and communities, and try to transform their socioeconomic situations and lives. As in many places where poverty is endemic, the situation is complex and nuanced, and young people are not a passive homogenised group; they exert agency despite the structures and constraints of their environments (Bönisch-Brednich and Trundle 2010). We need to see beyond the view of low-income residents as oppressed in power relations, and instead, as Cresswell argues (2004, 27), appreciate the 'entangled processes relating to power' that occur in slums, where people may act in ways to resist, change and challenge existing spaces, in 'subversive ways,' in order to survive.

The sudden loss of income with economic contraction as a consequence of the lockdown brought a sense of desperation and panic about impending hunger, and distress associated with the pressures of providing for one's family and household. The enforcement of lockdown by the police, who are greatly feared, and constant insecurity of the future, resulted in much trauma and anxiety. Unlike in rural areas, where most people own their own homes, renting is common in urban slums. Basic services are erratically available, and utilities are shared among numerous families in different areas of the slums. Below, we illustrate the everyday lived experiences, emotions and feelings of young people, and show how their existing precarity and the struggles that they face were magnified by the lack of state support in response to COVID-19.

Where are the jobs? Desperation sets in

With lockdown, adolescents and youth who sold wares on the street were suddenly left without work, generating emotions of desperation, fear, frustration and powerlessness. Among some of the adolescents interviewed, the uncertainty of the lockdown resulted in sleeplessness, lack of appetite and palpitations, and arguments in the household with family members.

Shiuli's life on the streets, selling small towels, books and paper fans, began nearly 10 years ago. She now has 3 children, after eloping at the age of 14 with her unreliable husband, who is in and out of jail and frequently disappears. While Shiuli (21) has the support of her mother, the pandemic has left her helpless and she was increasingly apprehensive about her children's future. In April and May, despite lockdown, Shiuli and other street peddlers, wearing masks, surrounded the few cars still on the streets, begging. 'I am surviving on what people give when they come outside to buy something; not every day they can give me money or food'. Most passers-by did not hand out any cash for fear of contact and consequent transmission. As lockdown continued, Shiuli increasingly felt hopeless, 'begging on an almost empty road, when everything is closed ... when you have no other source of getting money or food and you have no idea when the situation will improve or become normal like before. I pass every single minute thinking, when will someone come and give me something?'

Similarly, Hanif (17) had previously sold flowers on a busy road in Dhaka city, but overnight, his income disappeared and he had no savings. He lives with his mother, siblings and a cousin in a one-room space in Badda, where most accommodation is less than 45 square feet with occupancy of up to six family members. Many mothers of respondents lost their jobs as housemaids in the homes of middle class and wealthy residents, due to their own fears of transmission and infection. All members of Hanif's household, except for his mother, had work prior to lockdown, earning small amounts of money from informal jobs. When flower selling was no longer possible, Hanif was disheartened, but one day, taking matters into his own hands, he convinced his neighbour to rent him a rickshaw on credit so that he could work as a taxi driver. Within a few days, however, local regulations related to the lockdown were changed to prohibit rickshaws from operating. While adolescents in solvent families adjusted to remote learning and spent the rest of their time with their families, young people like Hanif carried the entire weight of managing households on their shoulders: 'My life is not like others who are staying in their flats and maintaining physical distance. I have to find a means of earning to look after my family'. Paying the rent (approximately US$35 per month) was a constant reminder to Hanif of his responsibility as a son, so out of desperation he borrowed money from the owner of a neighbouring electronics shop, an informal loan provider. He now has the additional stress and ongoing anxiety of repaying this money with interest.

Meena (19), whose husband was ill and unemployed, worked up to 10 hours every day without any weekend breaks, even during the initial stage of the nationwide lockdown, as they relied on her income as a domestic aid to manage the household and meet the needs of her two children. She spoke of constant exhaustion due to her long hours at work, but it was regular income and provided her with a level of security. When she saw the police patrolling the streets, she was frightened and asked for temporary leave, but was only given a few days off. However, as the lockdown continued, her employers fired her, forcing her to manage on loans. She defied the lockdown and walked to nearly 30 houses and flats in affluent residential areas in search of a new job. She explained that the guards would turn her away, because 'no one is employing anyone now because of the pandemic. Everyone is too scared of transmission of the virus (from poor people)'.

Adhering to public health restrictions and the lockdown put adolescents in a precarious economic situation. Faruq (19), who lost his informal job, spent the first week of lockdown sitting inside the room he shared with his mother, attempting to maintain physical distance despite the fact that this was a near impossibility for him and others living in an extremely congested slum. During the second week his mother asked him to get some rice. Faruq, quite despondent, reflected: 'If I stay at home sitting idle, I risk facing starvation, and if I go outside I risk contamination. I finally decided to go outside and pull a rickshaw'. On his first day of pulling Faruq earned BDT 400 (c. US$4.73), but soon after the police confiscated the rickshaw. Faruq regained it a few days later by bribing the police.

Mukta (21) and her work colleagues experienced momentary hope in April when announcements were made that garment factories would re-open in May, but their hopes were dashed when, instead, lockdown was extended until 31 May. The closure of factories also meant that promised unpaid salaries could not be accessed. Like her colleagues, Mukta knew the risks of crowding together to claim her unpaid salary, but she had run out of money and as fears of hunger and panic grew, she had no option: 'If the factory remains closed, how will we manage our rent, buy food for the rest of the days? We now eat twice a day. The rice we have will run out soon'.

Research in Mumbai has revealed how the middle classes depict slums as 'filthy, dirty and noisy' to justify the segregation and exclusion of and discrimination against slum residents (Chandola 2010). As we have already illustrated, Meena was turned away by guards in well-to-do suburbs for fears of spreading the virus, and police confiscated rickshaws and harassed poor people who broke the rules of wearing masks and defied lockdown. These acts of everyday exclusion reveal how young people's lives were constantly under scrutiny and threat. However, they were determined to manage and were entrepreneurial in trying to find alternative sources of income, exhibiting certain levels of agency and resistance to the obstacles and challenges faced.

The Bangladesh government announced a stimulus package of US$8.657 billion in April to compensate people for economic losses caused by COVID-19 (Foyez 2020). This included US$595 million for salaries and allowances for garment workers and employees (Hossain 2020). However, adolescents, young people and adults living on the margins did not get any benefits from this social safety net as the programme targeted elderly populations; widows, destitute and deserted women; and people with disabilities (World Bank 2019). Workers who labour on the streets, in office buildings and factories, in grocery shops and households, rickshaw pullers and daily labourers, were all excluded. Those younger than 18 years old did not have access to a NID (identity card) and so were not entitled to support, and participants older than 18 years with ID cards also often felt betrayed when they did not receive any relief materials, such as rice and other dry foods, if they fell into other categories of exclusion. Young women were especially vulnerable, as most were employed in the informal sector with low pay, and had less security and protection in their jobs than their male counterparts. They were also more likely to live in working poverty before the pandemic (Rashid et al. 2020a).

Informal networks (both reciprocal and supportive, and exploitative) are a key part of settlement life, and it was through these networks that young people from poor households were able to gain access to informal credit in the absence of formal systems of support. Little is known yet about how the pandemic has impacted on money-lending and borrowing behaviour; however, from past crises such as sudden floods, we know that Dhaka slum-dwellers rely on social capital and networks to survive. The congested living conditions in slums create diverse close-knit communities, within which members have strong trusting relationships with each other. This allows members to request financial support from each other, simply and informally, in the form of small credits (Aßheuer et al. 2013). Among the 51 participants reported in our March 2020 study, 'residents mentioned that they had received food from different non-government organizations, local politicians, some well-off families in the locality, and from their employers' (Rashid et al. 2020b). However, 16 of the 51 did not receive food support at all. However, as the pandemic continued and insecurity increased in many households, there was an increasing risk that support would wane, and residents were increasingly worried about how to pay rent, pay back loans, purchase food and feed their families. Uncertainty of how long the situation would last added a new level of powerlessness, frailty and a sense of vulnerability: 'We have lost control of everything. Our lives remain in God's hands now'. Despite these statements of despair, most persisted in exploring options to manage their livelihoods and support their families.

Hunger, insecurity and panic: a bleak future lies ahead

For adolescents and young people, including most of our respondents, the fear of having no money at all, going without food and losing their homes, was very real; hunger, not the pandemic, was the greater concern. This was experienced most harshly in slums where vulnerable and low-income groups like food vendors, the majority women and youth, were disproportionately affected by lockdown with massive job losses and income constraints affecting access to food (Corburn et al. 2020). To add to these worries, they had to manage and placate younger children, including siblings, who were unaware of the full impact of the pandemic. Their anxiety and despair were palpable in interviews.

Rubel (18) lives with his mother, younger brother and several others in a one-room space in one of the largest slums in Bangladesh. He used to work in a plastics factory before lockdown, and, like others, he received no salary following the unexpected shutdown of the business. He does not know when he can return to work, or how he and his family will deal with the economic crisis they are already in. They are on the brink of starvation: 'We have already run out of our supply of rice. I am panicking! I have no idea how we will manage if things go on like this.' Rubel, as a male, with no father in the household, is responsible for providing for his family but feels incapable of doing so.

Poverty also means that many women are taking on these responsibilities in the slums. For example, Meena, with no job, no money and a sick husband, was desperately hungry. She broke lockdown to walk one mile with her baby to receive a relief package from her mother. 'I can't afford a mask, so I used my scarf to cover my mouth and walked with my baby because my mother called me to say she had some rice to share with me.' She was stopped by police, but they felt sorry for her and did not reprimand her as she was female and they realised she was hungry.

Many adolescents and young people interviewed for this research had heard about government relief materials being distributed and were hopeful that this would tide them over until the country opened up. There were reports that government officers had gone around slum areas collecting information about NID (national identification cards), but, as noted above, no respondents received food aid. Although Kabir, Jewel, Meena and Shirin (21, 20, 19 and 20, respectively) placed their names on the official list as entitled to food support, internal bureaucracy and corruption within these local offices prevented them from receiving aid. 'My landlord gets relief for himself and his tenants, but he doesn't distribute anything to us.' Numerous reports have detailed the mismanagement of the distribution of resources, which favoured certain groups, and there is limited coordination between different bodies responsible for distributing state-funded food and/or cash aid programmes (Rashid et al. 2020a).

When Khokon (18) and his colleagues were not paid their wages from various informal jobs, for example in shops and garment factories, they took to the streets to demand food and relief. Law enforcement officers had anticipated such action and were ready to punish protestors, but even so, protests continued in various parts of the city through April (Arab News 2020). Chance (2015) refers to this as a 'public drama', in which poor residents collectively mobilise and identify with each other, creating a form of 'living politics', thereby moving beyond the boundaries between the home and city to make themselves seen and heard, in a place hostile to their needs. Through these demonstrations poor people try to gain rights, resources and recognition of their plight.

When the lockdown ended in May, people rushed back to their jobs, placing themselves at possible risk of infection. For many, the trade-off was either death from the virus or death from starvation. Nearly all respondents made repeated phone calls to people in their social networks, trying everything they could to gain access to cash to buy food. Young people turned to informal social connections to learn of sporadic labour opportunities, and drew on existing relationships to buy food on credit from street vendors, to negotiate with their landlords for waivers, and to sell various goods in the city, despite the lockdown. Kabir and Jewel spoke about selling their wives' and sister's only jewellery (one gold chain and two silver chains). Loans were taken out in the early stages of the pandemic, sometime in May, only two months into lockdown, as people began to exhaust their networks and as their anxiety escalated about being caught in a cycle of debt.

Many of the adolescents, despite their age, continued to experience enormous pressure to provide for their families as heads of households (Figure 15.1). Kabir, for example, had taken on the responsibility of looking after his unmarried younger sister and younger brother after they lost their parents at a young age. His brother recently passed year 10 school, and Kabir reflected: 'Now with this corona, we are in a bad way. No one is happy and I couldn't even feed the neighbourhood sweets to celebrate that my brother did so well in his exams'. For poor people, education is valued greatly and is seen as an eventual path out of poverty, although the reality is quite different. Kabir was unable to continue to support his brother's education, and this 'left him restless and awake most nights'. Shirin (20) recalled how she and her sister had recently relocated from one slum to another with better housing and facilities. Before COVID-19 and lockdown, both young women were working in a garment factory and their mother was a housemaid. However, soon after lockdown, all three became unemployed, forcing them to live on their meagre savings. When their landlord came to demand cash for rent, they used their savings to pay him for the month of April. Shirin worried that she did not have any income to pay him in May. During Eid (religious festival), Shirin bought her younger siblings some clothes as per the customary

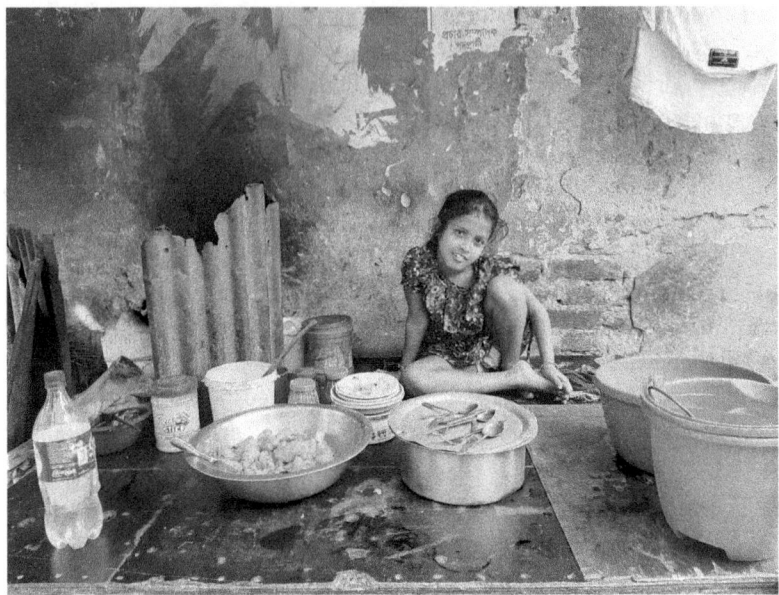

Figure 15.1 An adolescent prepares snacks in a slum in Dhaka city, Bangladesh. Photo: Farzana Manzoor/BRAC JPGSPH

rituals of Eid. She wanted them to have nice things and was distressed to see them unhappy. 'They are young and don't understand … we couldn't deny them, although we didn't buy anything for ourselves'. Kellett (2002, 28) states that those who are poor are conscious of their low social position, and their attempts to aspire for more and to live better suggest that 'their efforts can be interpreted as a "striving for dignity and respect"'. As Perlman argues (1976, 242–3), contrary to the assumptions of the urban poor as 'disorderly' (as is commonly portrayed in Bangladeshi media and narratives), 'most are socially well organised', and aspire to better lives, education, housing and upward mobility in employment. However, they face insurmountable barriers to realise their dreams.

The narratives of young people living in Dhaka indicate the depth of suffering that many urban residents experienced and the adversity they faced, even though they managed to survive. Despite their ingenious ways of trying to manage the world of social, economic and political hierarchies, the situation placed large amounts of stress on adolescents and youth. They have had to shoulder enormous burdens by taking on the responsibilities of adults. Most of those interviewed were already married, had children and were supporting their siblings and other family members financially, despite their youth and that they struggled emotionally, mentally and physically to take on these expectations. The emotional toll and feelings of distress impacted on the young respondents, particularly as their situation became increasingly uncertain.

Gatekeepers and fear

As the above examples indicate, adolescents and young slum residents had to deal with various gatekeepers and powerful individuals, inside and outside the slums, including angry and demanding landlords and aggravated law enforcement officers.

In Meena's case, the tenants in her block of slums decided to confront the landlord with examples of other landlords waiving rent for residents. Yet, when the landlord arrived, most tenants got cold feet and pleaded for more time instead. Kabir and Shiuli were fortunate, as their landlord knew them as long-time tenants and he did not insist on payment. While the situation varied therefore based on people's (pre-pandemic) relationships with their landlords, all of them experienced heightened anxiety and panic, as they worried about convincing their landlord to give them more time for rent payments. At the same time, landlords whose sole income came from rent were also beginning to struggle. With around 50,000 slum-dwellers returning to their villages to avoid paying rent, landlords faced the constraints of demanding rent and risking the tenant leaving, or giving tenants extended time to pay so that they remained (BRAC 2020). At the same time, most adolescents were born in Dhaka or had lived in the city for most of their lives, and did not consider that returning to their natal or parents' village was an option. Further, options to return to a rural village were limited with the introduction and enforcement of a government travel ban on passenger travel via water, rail and on domestic air routes from 24 March, and restrictions on road public transport from 26 March until 31 May (Kamruzzaman and Sakib 2020a; Kamruzzaman and Sakib 2020b).

The police and army patrol officers acted as another set of gatekeepers, causing terror among residents if they left the slums during lockdown. Kabir spoke with us of breaking the lockdown rules and selling mangoes in the streets: 'A crowd was gathering near us ... the police started coming at us with sticks to beat us. I ran and hid in a corner ... We grabbed a few of our mangoes and just ran. Luckily I was not hit by the police.' Likewise, Jewel explained his panic when being confronted by the police: 'I was walking to work (when lockdown restrictions had eased up) and I had my mask with me, but not over my face/mouth. The police started yelling at me, asking why I didn't have my mask on properly. I just put on my mask quietly and didn't say anything.' Shahnaz explained some of the contradictions of interacting with the law:

> Usually the police come to our area and take money from the local shopkeepers and smaller drug stores. Now with the coronavirus they harass us to stay inside, but over the last few months, we see them less and less. In a way it's good because they don't take money from our local people anymore. They are scared of the virus.

Newspapers reported that police threatened low-income people who had to defy lockdown to earn their livelihoods (Sajid 2020), beating them and enforcing humiliating punishment, for instance, forcing men to do sit-ups while holding their ears. Many people view the police as the 'enemy', as holding excessive power, and as corrupt and abusive. Crime and insecurity tend to be rampant in slum settlements, and usually the police are paid off, with little recourse to justice for poor residents. For adolescents, being confronted by a police officer is traumatic and a stark reminder of their lack of power. However, in this chapter, we follow Lombard's (2014) call to focus on 'the everyday' and analyse adolescents and youth as 'more or less autonomous actors who creatively engage with, and shape', and give meaning, to the places and spaces they inhabit. This allows us to see young slum residents not simply as passive subjects with little agency in the face of overwhelming poverty; in both subtle and overt ways many challenged the regulations imposed by the state.

Distrust and fear of the police, and general lack of trust in law enforcement bodies, has been documented in other epidemics, such as Ebola (Van Belle et al. 2020). Effective and transparent urban governance that enables and promotes trust in communities is needed for effective emergency responses. In slums this is absent. Without formal governance, non-state organisations and resident-led informal governance mechanisms stepped in. For example, in Dhaka, the few landlords who owned their own compounds introduced rules to increase physical distancing as much as feasible among the tenants when using shared facilities (Rashid et al. 2020b).

Faith in times of pandemic

For most participants, religion offered some solace. In late March and early April, despite the lockdown, many people were still congregating for prayers. Rubel (18), Hanif (17) and Faruq (19) went to the mosque on a regular basis during the early weeks of lockdown, and explained: 'COVID-19 is a consequence of people's sin and a punishment from Allah, because people no longer pray as much as they should'. The pandemic, they argued, was evidence of wrath from the divine for peoples' perceived lack of morality and sin. Hanif informed us that he had heard that those who perform ablutions five times before prayers were protected from the virus, because it 'keeps them clean'. Meena shared how in her despair, she needed immediate comfort and went to pray in the woman's section of the mosque; when leaving, she placed 10 BDT (UA$0.12), not a small amount for her, into the box for donations. As poor as she was, she felt compelled to donate a small amount, hoping that her prayers for salvation from her current circumstances would be heard.

Where institutions, systems, communities and even families failed to provide the required support, and trust was shaken, many residents were left with only their faith to cope with overwhelming feelings of helplessness. Places of worship also became sites of temporary solidarity and meeting places in the slums, although primarily for men. Local mosques encouraged people to continue to attend Friday prayers until 6 April 2020. Until then, according to those interviewed, soap was available for hand washing and people practised some physical distancing inside the prayer rooms. Moreover, for most people, the mosque was viewed as safer than other sites such as crowded markets, because it was considered a sacred space, leaving some to assume divine protection against transmission of the virus. The comfort and security of meeting others in the mosque also overrode any fears of infection. Religious beliefs and faith in the divine were viewed as a protection against COVID-19, and this theme was repeated by the majority of our respondents (Rabbani 2020).

Conclusion

Deep structures of vulnerability and structural violence shaped the conditions of everyday life during lockdown for young people living in slums, and produced multilevel challenges. As we have illustrated, an intersectional approach highlights how, during the pandemic, different social axes (here, youth, gender, class, poverty, sources of livelihood) intersected with social location (here, Dhaka's slums) through time, and were shaped by interconnected systems, structure and processes of power, oppression and domination to shape all aspects of people's lives. We have also illustrated the importance of affect: that is, people experienced emotional vulnerabilities in response to the economic and social constraints that characterised the COVID-19 pandemic and its unfolding.

We have described the heterogeneity of slum residents and depicted how young people's lives were (and are) enmeshed in struggles with powerful and diverse interest groups, yet their narratives attest to their continued resilience and inventiveness to manage multiple constraints. When officials declared a state of emergency and imposed sudden restrictions, young people, already in a precarious situation, were affected emotionally and materially by the scarcity in their lives. The rules, imposed by the state and the police who were regulating spaces and COVID-19 related behaviours, receive limited attention in public health discourses. The lockdown threatened people with starvation, and addressing this required that they acted in ways that contravened with the precautions to prevent the spread of the pandemic – staying at home and maintaining physical distance. The role of the police force, the extensive curtailing of employment opportunities, restricted movement, and economic and home insecurities, disrupted social relationships and gendered expectations. All presented challenges beyond the control of individuals, and required resources and infrastructure to mitigate them (Coetzee and Kagee 2020).

However, within conditions of deprivation, young people immediately tried to remake their local and social worlds. They made independent decisions in the light of the limited options that were available. They frantically explored all kinds of existing and new networks for support to cope, irrespective of restrictions, looking for alternate income sources, taking loans, exploring social relationships, negotiating and navigating with powerful actors, and turning to faith to manage anxiety and distress. Driven by panic, desperation and the need for quick action for survival, as they grappled with physical hunger and daily mental anxiety, adolescents took risks with the police, landlords and loan agents, when normally they might be fearful or reluctant to engage with them. Their actions showed resilience as they attempted to create a semblance of normalcy in a world turned upside down. We do not wish, here, to romanticise or overstate the agency of adolescents and young people in slums in Dhaka, but most young people tried to transform or navigate, in whatever ways were possible, existing relationships of domination, oppression and exploitation (Cresswell 2004, 29). Sharp and colleagues (2000, 20) argue that power is messy and not simply one of a binary model of domination/resistance. It must be understood as 'an amalgam of forces, processes, practices and relations, all of which spin out along the precarious threads of society and space' (Sharp et al. 2000, 20).

The narratives of adolescents and young people show us how slums are sites of complex social interactions. Cresswell (2004, 11) states that the focus on the everyday, lived experiences of the poor highlights the complicated 'interplay of people and the environment' as it is continually constructed and co-constructed. Simone (2004, 14) argues that by highlighting the struggles and negotiations in which people in poor communities actively engage, these narratives make 'visible urban possibilities that have been crowded out or left diffuse or opaque' in debates that often essentialise the identities of settlement dwellers.

COVID-19 brings new challenges to existing structural violence, deepens this violence, and sharpens the vulnerability of young people and their families. The structural, social, economic and political realities interact to leave young people and their families marginalised and at risk, not only from hunger and malnutrition, but at risk of catastrophic economic losses with long-lasting repercussions. As their lives unfolded during the pandemic, it became clear that the unequal distribution of power and wealth across class, gender, age and location created and perpetuated power inequalities and inequities. Critical medical anthropology combined with intersectionality can help make visible varying forms of structural violence (physical, social, economic, political), and illustrate how these are often mediated by more 'micro' level characteristics and unique circumstances of identity and lack of power and privilege. Poverty and patriarchal gender norms shaping early marriage, norms related to male rice-winners, and lack of voice, for example, interact to shape individual experiences in varying ways.

Definitions of vulnerability tend to exclude young people as they are often viewed as resilient and able to recover, and so they remain among the 'invisible' poor. But in our research, the lives of many young people have been ones of missed dreams and lost opportunities as they transition into social adulthood quickly, taking on roles and responsibilities while still very young. The reality is that they do not lament this loss, for they have no choices or options. Their micro worlds are ones of survival and resilience, and this is the familiar terrain they have navigated since they were very young. They are pragmatic about the circumstances of their lives. Being confronted with illnesses and death is an everyday reality for many poor adolescents living in Dhaka's slums. In this context, COVID-19 was yet another addition to an already long list of health and other challenges that they faced (Rashid et al. 2020a).

There has been limited discussion on the impact of COVID-19 on youth in marginalised contexts, and our research makes visible the experiences of adolescents and young people in urban slums, amplifying the urgency to address the levels of social injustice that exist. Authorities must rethink their engagement with young people living in slums, and respond and recognise the links between governance, health and equity (Arab News 2020). Young people in slums can support mitigation strategies for the short- and long-term impacts of COVID-19, if they are engaged with and participate in shaping responses. The voices and perspectives of adolescents and youth presented here are common among most urban poor populations in the city. Their struggles, however, are largely invisible.

It is not enough to understand why young people live in such deprivation and how they manage and cope. We need to closely examine who is most affected by this pandemic and how to promote justice. The distribution of wealth in the country, and the discrepancies in resources within the population, shape the risk of infection and its outcomes. But it would be myopic to create a national policy to mitigate the impact of COVID-19 without also addressing the unique challenges faced by younger populations. We need to critically reflect not only on the failures of the local state, but also on existing global policies and politics. All combine to impact adversely on the lives of those who are most vulnerable.

Acknowledgements

All research activities were reviewed and approved by the Institutional Review Board (IRB) at BRAC James P. Grant School of Public Health (JPGSPH), BRAC University. Cash incentives of 200 taka were provided at the time of each interview. Data were recorded with consent from the participants, transcribed and translated. Informed consent took place over the phone. All names used are pseudonyms. We thank the participants for so readily sharing their experiences. The research was supported by the core fund of the BRAC JPGSPH, BRAC University; we received no additional external funding for the research, authorship and/or publication of this chapter. Time for some authors to input was supported by the UKRI GCRF Accountability for Informal Urban Equity Hub (also known as ARISE); a UKRI Collective Fund award, RC Grant reference, ES/S00811X/1. ARISE is a research consortium aiming to enhance accountability and improve the health and wellbeing of marginalised populations living in informal urban settlements in Kenya, Sierra Leone, Bangladesh and India. We are grateful to Aisha and Sumona, colleagues at the school, who collected some of the data at different points of the research project, and to the editors of this volume for their positive and constructive comments.

References

Acharya, Rajib, Mukta Gundi, Thaoi Ngo, Neelanjana Pandey, Sangram Kishor Patel, Jessie Pinchoff, et al. 2020. 'COVID-19-related knowledge, attitudes, and practices among adolescents and young people in Bihar and Uttar Pradesh, India: Study description'. April 2020. Accessed 5 July 2020. https://knowledgecommons.popcouncil.org/cgi/viewcontent.cgi?article=2007&context=departments_sbsr-pgy.

Anwar, Saeed, Mohammad Nasrullah and Mohammad Jakir Hosen. 2020. 'COVID-19 and Bangladesh: Challenges and how to address them'. *Front Public Health* [Internet], 30 April 2020, 8:154. Accessed 5 August 2020: https://www.frontiersin.org/article/10.3389/fpubh.2020.00154/full.

Arab News. 2020. '"Starving" Bangladesh garment workers protest for pay during lockdown'. *Yahoo News* [Internet], 13 April 2020, 1–6. Accessed 5 July 2020: https://www.arabnews.com/node/1658186/world.

Aßheuer, Tibor, Insa Thiele-Eich and Boris Braun. 2013. 'Coping with the impacts of severe flood events in Dhaka's slums – The role of social capital'. Erdkunde 67(1): 21–35.

Au, Anson. 2019. 'Thinking about cross-cultural differences in qualitative interviewing: Practices for more responsive and trusting encounters'. *Qualitative Report* 24(1): 58–77. https://www.researchgate.net/publication/330369756.

Bangladesh Bureau of Statistics (BBS). 2016. *Statistical Pocketbook Bangladesh, 2015*. Dhaka, Bangladesh: Statistics & Informatics Division (SID), Ministry of Planning Government of The People's Republic of Bangladesh.

Bangladesh Bureau of Statistics (BBS). 2020. *Statistical Yearbook Bangladesh 2019*. Dhaka, Bangladesh: Statistics & Informatics Division (SID), Ministry of Planning Government of The People's Republic of Bangladesh.

bdnews24.com. 2020. 'BRAC survey finds 14pc of low income people do not have food at home during shutdown'. bdnews24.com, 10 April 2020. Accessed 10 June 2020. https://bdnews24.com/economy/2020/04/10/brac-survey-finds-14pc-of-low-income-people-do-not-have-food-at-home-during-shutdown.

Bönisch-Brednich, Bridgette and Catherine Trundle. 2010. *Local Lives: Migration and the politics of place*. London: Routledge.

BRAC. 2020. '95pc people suffer losses in income'. 10 June 2020. Accessed 10 June 2020. https://www.brac.net/latest-news/item/1284-95pc-people-suffer-losses-in-income.

Chance, Kerry Ryan. 2015. '"Where there is fire, there is politics": Ungovernability and material life in urban South Africa'. *Cultural Anthropology* 30(3): 394–423.

Chandola, Tripta. 2010. Listening in to others: In between noise and silence'. PhD thesis, Queensland University of Technology, Brisbane, Queensland, Australia.

Coetzee, Bronwyné Jo'sean and Ashraf Kagee. 2020. Structural barriers to adhering to health behaviours in the context of the COVID-19 crisis: Considerations for low- and middle-income countries. *Global Public Health* 15(8): 1093–102. https://doi.org/10.1080/17441692.2020.1779331

Corburn, Jason, David Vlahov, Blessing Mberu, Lee Riley, Waleska Teixeira Caiaffe, Sabina Faiz Rashid et al. 2020. 'Slum health: Arresting COVID-19 and improving well-being in urban informal settlements'. *Journal of Urban Health* 97(3): 348–57. https://doi.org/10.1007/s11524-020-00438-6.

Cresswell, Tim. 2004. *Place: A short introduction*. Oxford, UK: Blackwell.

Double Repression. 2020. *Lockdown Measures in Bangladesh and Its Impact on Informal Sector Workers*. Bangkok, Thailand: Heinrich Böll Foundation, Southeast Asia Regional Office. Accessed 5 July 2020. https://th.boell.org/en/2020/05/13/double-repression-lockdown-measures-bangladesh-and-its-impact-informal-sector-workers.

Farmer, Paul. 2009. 'On suffering and structural violence: A view from below'. *Race/Ethnicity: Multidisciplinary Global Contexts* 3(1): 11–28.

Foyez, Ahammad. 2020. 'Bangladesh PM unveils Tk 72,750cr stimulus packages. *New Age Bangladesh*, 5 April 2020. Accessed 5 July 2020. https://www.newagebd.net/article/103845/bangladesh-pm-unveils-tk-72750cr-stimulus-packages.

Gruebner, Oliver, Jonathan Sachs, Anika Nockert, Michael Frings, Md Mobarak Hossain Khan, Tobia Lakes and Patrick Hostert. 2014. 'Mapping the Slums of Dhaka from 2006 to 2010'. Dataset Papers in Science 2014: 172182 | https://doi.org/10.1155/2014/172182.

Haider, Abu Asfarul. 2019. 'Ending child marriage is good economics'. *The Daily Star*, 27 April 2019. Accessed 5 July 2020. https://www.thedailystar.net/opinion/society/news/ending-child-marriage-good-economics-1735297.

Hossain, Md Shahadat. 2020. 'Covid-19 stimulus package – a critique'. *The Financial Express*, 7 April 2020. Accessed 5 July 2020. https://thefinancialexpress.com.bd/views/covid-19-stimulus-package-a-critique-1586274943.

ILO. 2013. *Decent Work Country Profile – Bangladesh*. Available from: https://www.ilo.org/wcmsp5/groups/public/—dgreports/—integration/documents/publication/wcms_216901.pdf.

Islam, Nazmul, A.Q.M. Mahbub and Nurul Islam Nazem. 2009. 'Urban slums of Bangladesh'. *The Daily Star*, 20 June 2020. https://www.thedailystar.net/news-detail-93293.

Kamruzzaman, Md. and Sakib S. Nazmus. 2020a. 'Bangladesh imposes total lockdown over COVID-19'. Accessed 5 July 2020. https://www.aa.com.tr/en/asia-pacific/bangladesh-imposes-total-lockdown-over-covid-19/1778272.

Kamruzzaman, Md. and Sakib S. Nazmus. 2020b. 'Bangladesh reports record deaths as it lifts lockdown'. Accessed 5 July 2020. https://www.aa.com.tr/en/asia-pacific/bangladesh-reports-record-deaths-as-it-lifts-lockdown/1860274.

Kellett, Peter. 2002. 'The construction of home in the informal city'. *Journal of Romance Studies* 2(3): 17–31.

Lombard, Melanie. 2014. 'Constructing ordinary places: Place-making in urban informal settlements in Mexico'. *Progress in Planning* 94: 1–53.

Ovi, Ibrahim Hossain. 2018. 'Women's participation in RMG workforce declines'. *Dhaka Tribune*, 3 March 2018. Accessed 8 October 2020. https://www.dhakatribune.com/business/2018/03/03/womens-participation-rmg-workforce-declines/.

Perlman, Janice. 1976. *The Myth of Marginality: Urban poverty and politics in Rio de Janeiro*. Berkeley, CA: University of California Press.

Rabbani, Atonu. 2020. 'Awareness and knowledge about COVID-19 during the early onslaught of the pandemic'. Accessed 8 October 2020. https://www.sonar-global.eu/covid-19-projects/awareness-and-knowledge-about-covid-19-during-the-early-onslaught-of-the-pandemic/.

Rashid, Sabina Faiz. 2004. 'Worried lives: Poverty, gender and reproductive health of married adolescent women living in an urban slum in Bangladesh', PhD thesis. The Australian National University. Accessed 8 October 2020. https://www.researchgate.net/publication/320923801_Worried_lives_poverty_gender_and_reproductive_health_of_married_adolescent_women_living_in_an_urban_slum_in_Bangladesh.

Rashid, Sabina Faiz, Sally Theobald and Kim Ozano. 2020a. 'Towards a socially just model: Balancing hunger and response to the COVID-19 pandemic in Bangladesh'. *BMJ Global Health* 5(6): e002715.

Rashid, Sabina Faiz, Bachera Aktar, Nadia Farnaz. Wafa Alam, Samiha Ali, Farzana Manzoor, et al. 2020b. 'Impact of COVID-19: Lived experiences of the urban poor in slums during the shutdown'. BRAC JPGSPH Covid-19 Rapid Mini-Research Reports. Accessed 8 October 2020. https://www.ariseconsortium.org/wp-content/uploads/2020/05/Urban-Poor-Lived-Experiences-in-Slums-ARISE_April-19.pdf.

Sajid, Eyamin. 2020. 'Bangladesh coronavirus update: Police enforce social distancing through humiliation, harassment'. *The Business Standard*, 27 March 2020. https://www.tbsnews.net/coronavirus-chronicle/coronavirus-bangladesh/police-enforce-social-distancing-through-humiliation.

Sharp, Joanne P., Paul Routledge, Chris Philo and Ronan Paddison. 2000. *Entanglements of Power: Geographies of domination/resistance*. London: Routledge.

Shawon, Ali Asif. 2020. 'Covid-19: Bangladesh likely to end general holiday on May 31'. *Dhaka Tribune*, 27 May 2020. Accessed 8 October 2020. https://www.dhakatribune.com/bangladesh/2020/05/27/state-minister-update-of-lockdown-coming-soon.

Simone, AbdouMaliq. 2004. *For the City Yet to Come. Changing African life in four cities*. Durham, NC and London: Duke University Press.

Singer, Merrill. 2004. 'Critical medical anthropology'. In *Encyclopedia of Medical Anthropology: Health & illness in the world's cultures*, edited by Carol R. Ember and Melvin Ember, pp. 23–30. New York: Springer-Verlag US.

The Daily Star. 2014. 'Rise of youth'. *The Daily Star*, 19 November 2014. Accessed 8 October 2020. https://www.thedailystar.net/rise-of-youth-51048.

Tolhurst, Rachel, Beryl Leach, Janet Price, Jude Robinson, Elizabeth Ettore, Alex Scott-Samuel, Nduku Kilonzo, et al. 2012. 'Intersectionality and gender mainstreaming in international health: Using a feminist participatory action research process to analyse voices and debates from the global south and north'. *Social Science & Medicine* 74(11): 1825–32.

UNICEF Bangladesh. 2020. *Education for adolescents*. Dhaka: UNICEF Bangladesh. Accessed 8 October 2020. https://www.unicef.org/bangladesh/en/more-opportunities-early-learning/education-adolescents.

Van Belle, S., C. Affun-Adegbulu, W. Soors, Prashanth N. Srinivas, G. Hegel, W. Van Damme, et al. 2020. 'COVID-19 and informal settlements: An urgent call to rethink urban governance'. *International Journal for Equity in Health* 19(1): 81. https://equityhealthj.biomedcentral.com/articles/10.1186/s12939-020-01198-0.

WFP Bangladesh. 2018. 'World Food Programme'. Accessed 8 October 2020. https://www.wfp.org/countries/Bangladesh.

World Bank. 2019. 'Social safety nets in Bangladesh help reduce poverty and improve human capital'. The World Bank. Accessed 8 October 2020. https://www.worldbank.org/en/news/feature/2019/04/29/social-safety-nets-in-bangladesh-help-reduce-poverty-and-improve-human-capital.

Part IV
The reach of care

16
Making do

COVID-19 and the improvisation of care in the UK and US

Ellen Block and Cecilia Vindrola-Padros

COVID-19 has disrupted all aspects of healthcare delivery across the globe. The novel coronavirus has upended both the expectation of relative stability in care and service delivery in the Global North and the assurance that providers and patients will have access to – and knowledge about – the best ways to treat disease. The pandemic has forced healthcare workers (HCWs) to contend with limited knowledge about a disease, uncertainty about the best treatments and practices available and a crisis of faith in the system and in their own ability to provide care. As a result, significant improvisation has occurred at both an institutional level and at a microlevel of everyday practice. Based on data from qualitative interviews with healthcare workers in the United States (US) and United Kingdom (UK), in this chapter we examine the striking similarities in improvisational strategies and techniques that healthcare systems and HCWs have employed during the COVID-19 pandemic. Such improvisation has resulted in structural institutional changes as well as microlevel changes as a response to resource shortages, risk reduction strategies and lifesaving techniques. This improvisation in the UK and the US demonstrates the flexibility of seemingly rigid institutions. At first, the crisis conditions that led to such improvisation appeared to flatten inequalities by mimicking the precarity and uncertainty of practising medicine in resource-poor contexts. Ultimately, however, the COVID-19 pandemic – like all catastrophes – merely serves to reveal the fault lines of inequality and the fractures of healthcare systems.

Context and methods

The COVID-19 pandemic set unprecedented demand on healthcare systems globally. Emerging research from multiple countries has included reports of HCW fatigue, distress and anxiety as well as positive emotional responses (e.g. 'growth under pressure') and helpful coping mechanisms (Liu et al. 2020; Song et al. 2020; Sun et al. 2020). In the US, the largely inadequate response to COVID-19 has been widely publicised, and as of this writing (December 2020), the country continues to lead in both cases and number of deaths globally. Responses to the pandemic, however, vary widely by state, by city and by hospital system, everywhere deeply entrenched in local politics. Because there is no national healthcare system in the US, there is no centralised system of personal protective equipment (PPE) acquisition, no standard way to deal with suspected COVID-19 patients when they show up at the emergency room (ER) and no formal coordination of communication channels to share emerging research and best practices. Instead, each hospital or hospital system, sometimes based on directives from the local and federal government and sometimes based on directives by hospital administrators, has developed its own strategies to manage patient flow and the reorganisation of hospital space, COVID-19 testing, medical student and junior doctor[1] training and PPE acquisition. HCWs have learned from others' experiences through informal channels and grassroots movements.

In the case of the UK, the COVID-19 pandemic impacted a public healthcare system, the National Health Service (NHS), already struggling with workforce issues including high vacancy and low retention rates of staff, limited bed capacity and funding cuts (Dayan et al. 2018). In March 2020, the UK went into lockdown with social distancing policies implemented across the population to reduce the transmission of COVID-19 and the burden on the healthcare system. By April, the NHS had put in place protocols across the system to manage the flow of COVID patients and reduce the volume of non-COVID patients in their hospitals, including suspending a range of services. While there was some variation in how different hospitals responded, national-level recommendations on the expansion of critical care capacity, cancellation of elective care and workforce redesign were made available and followed in most cases (NHS 2020).

Hospitals and HCWs in both countries were unprepared for the needs of patients and staff as a result of the COVID-19 pandemic. Early in the pandemic, it became clear that there would be a need for improvisation both at the institutional level and at the level of everyday practice in order to manage the changed flow of patients and reduce risks to patients, families and frontline workers. Despite vast differences between the US and the UK, the kinds of responses in institutional structures and healthcare practices were strikingly similar in both contexts, indicating a similar sense of uncertainty, global sharing of knowledge and a disease which applies pressure in similar ways, resulting in similar improvisational strategies.

Both studies were designed as rapid appraisals (Vindrola-Padros et al. 2020). The US-based study consisted of 55 hour-long semi-structured interviews conducted between April and September 2020 with healthcare workers from 18 different states, including doctors, nurses and advanced care providers.[2] Findings were analysed using MAXQDA. The UK study combined a review of UK healthcare policies (n=70 policies), mass media and social media analysis of frontline staff experiences and perceptions (n=101 newspaper articles, n=146,000 posts) and in-depth (telephone) interviews with frontline staff (n=123 interviews). The findings from all streams were analysed using framework analysis.

Improvisation and instability

The uncertainty of COVID-19 lies both in its emergence and its complexity. The rapid appearance of COVID-19 created many uncertainties socially, economically and medically. For HCWs treating COVID-19 patients, medical uncertainty centred on the unknowns surrounding infectiousness risk, treatments, symptoms and COVID-19-induced complications. Treatment recommendations for COVID-19 and best practices for supportive care changed rapidly during the first year of the pandemic, especially during the first few months. The widely publicised early hopes for the benefits of drugs such as hydroxychloroquine were quickly dismissed (Self et al. 2020) as clinical trials for more effective drugs such as remdesivir were underway (Beigel et al. 2020). In Wuhan, China, Italy and New York City, three places hit hard by early waves of COVID-19, poor patient outcomes quickly led to changing supportive care practices such as more consistent use of proning (placing the patient on their stomach) and delaying intubation (Coppo et al. 2020; Rola et al. 2020). However, in the early stages of the pandemic, while HCWs gained a better sense of supportive ventilation strategies and gained confidence in the approach to hypoxia in COVID-19 patients, adaptations were largely anecdotal, and did not address uncertainty about long-term outcomes. This led to constantly changing guidelines on the clinical management of patients, the reorganisation of the infrastructure for care delivery (from acute care to rehabilitation) and, considering the use and reuse of PPE in the context of fluctuating equipment stock, the establishment of adequate standards for infection control (Hoernke et al. 2020; Vindrola-Padros et al. 2020).

Additionally, at the beginning of the pandemic very little was known about COVID-19 complications, as countries rapidly battled to save lives as a first priority. Some months into the pandemic, it became clear that COVID-19 is a multisystem disease, affecting the gastrointestinal, nervous, musculoskeletal, endocrine and cardiac systems (Kakodkar et al. 2020; Zhang et al. 2020). However, knowledge about long-term outcomes has been gradual as clinicians and scientists have had to wait for complications to manifest within their patients and for research results to be published. This has caused considerable uncertainty surrounding the delivery of rehabilitation care for the varying and complex needs of patients.

As a result of the rapidly changing information and availability of resources, healthcare workers and hospital administrators have adapted both by changing institutional protocols and structures at the macro level and improvising at the micro level to improve patient outcomes and keep frontline workers safe. For institutions that are typically rigid in both their organisational structure and their daily practices, the level of uncertainty, the rapid pace of change and the need for improvisation was both unprecedented and unsettling. In many ways, the provision of care in the early days of the pandemic mimicked care provision in resource-poor contexts, where healthcare providers have to contend with a lack of evidence-based treatments, limited resources including both drugs and PPE, and the need to shift, tinker and adapt to rapidly changing and unpredictable contexts.

It is not surprising, then, that comparison can be made between the challenges of providing care during the COVID-19 pandemic and ethnographies of medicine stemming from the Global South where resources, space and human capital are habitually limited. Such resource-poor hospitals often show the 'fluid, experimental, and improvised nature of biomedicine' (Street 2014, 16). At first, the COVID-19 pandemic resembled these contexts in how they wrought uncertainty and necessitated improvisation. In writing about improvisation in a public cancer ward in Botswana, Julie Livingston observes the 'daily imperative' to 'improvise new options from the resources available – material and social' (Livingston 2012, 181). The urgency and precarity that requires such improvisation was felt by HCWs in the US and the UK, particularly at the start of COVID-19 before best practices had been established and when it was uncertain how long resources would last. While, as Gawande (2002) points out, doctors have always had to contend with a gap between what they know and what they aim for, HCWs in the US and the UK are unaccustomed to having to improvise at the speed or scale that COVID-19 required.

Many healthcare workers said that meetings and communications noting changes were occurring daily, and they had trouble keeping up. HCWs were patching together information and supplies, from making their own PPE, to joining social media platforms with doctors from all over the world to learn about emerging best practices. For doctors in the Global South, decision making has long been constrained by structural and resource limitations, and such improvisation and flexibility is standard. In Malawi, Wendland shows how doctors cobble together 'social networks, material goods, short-term opportunities and ideas to craft ad hoc solutions to the problems they faced' (2010, 154). In Dewachi's powerful ethnography of post-war Iraq (2017), after years of United Nations sanctions, healthcare infrastructure was crumbling and HCWs could not access the supplies they needed to treat their patients and care for themselves. Doctors reused PPE, improvised by replacing catheters with nasal tubes and sterilised disposable gloves, strategies strikingly similar to those used by our interlocutors. As in the context of COVID-19, while not ideal, these 'improvised practices became essential to saving lives' (Dewachi 2017, xxi). However, unlike those contexts of entrenched poverty, protracted post-war situations and chronic structural vulnerability, the need for improvisation in responding to the uncertainties of COVID-19 in the US and the UK are temporary. And yet, many of the HCWs in this study alluded to the hospitals feeling like a war zone. The difference between the experience of practising medicine – and receiving care – in the US and UK early during the COVID-19 pandemic, and in these other contexts of precarity and war in the Global South, is that the war-like conditions or long-term structural conditions that lead to entrenched precarity do not resolve quickly. Nonetheless, COVID-19 reveals how improvisation can become necessary in a time of crisis, even among wealthier nations and relatively resource-rich healthcare contexts. Given the high likelihood of future pandemics or disasters that require nimble healthcare responses, much can be gained from analysing the efficacy of improvisational strategies employed by HCWs in response to COVID-19.

Improvisation at the institutional level

One of the most surprising areas of improvisation and adaptation during the COVID-19 pandemic has been at the institutional level. Large institutions tend towards both homogeneity and intractability (DiMaggio and Powell 1983). Hospitals and health systems have historically been extremely rigid and slow to change. While HCWs are typically able to nimbly respond to changes in medical practice, such as new treatments, hospital and healthcare reform is notoriously challenging, particularly in public hospital settings (Edwards and Saltman 2017). Yet, as a result of massive global disruption, hospitals and health systems have had to adapt quickly. In both the US and the UK, hospitals and healthcare systems have made massive shifts in organisational structure and protocols, putting into place new systems and changes that might normally take a decade to implement.

As healthcare workers and hospital administrators in the US and the UK watched COVID-19 devastate parts of China and Italy, they began to prepare for the inevitable onslaught on their shores. In both locales, one of the first changes to be implemented was to restructure the physical space of the hospital. Elective surgeries were suspended, emergency departments quickly altered their triage processes to identify those who might have COVID-19, and many hospitals chose to segregate those patients until their infection status was confirmed. In the US, different hospitals had vastly different approaches: some kept patients for longer in the ER until they knew their infection status; some sent any patient suspected of COVID-19 or with respiratory issues to COVID-designated floors until their status was confirmed. In the UK, in order to increase capacity across hospitals, in April 2020, the NHS announced the prioritisation of cancer treatments and suspension of all non-urgent elective surgery for three months. Operating rooms were repurposed and private facilities were commissioned for NHS services (Willan et al. 2020). Strategies to address workforce gaps included: the redeployment of staff; the reintegration of recently retired staff into the active workforce; and early graduation of medical students (Song et al. 2020). In addition, changes were rapidly made to the hospital infrastructure, as critical care units needed to expand to other areas of the hospital and staff improvised space to set up new beds and equipment and the electrical sockets and connections required to power the ventilators.

These changes not only required changing the triaging system, but also required considerable physical changes in the space of the hospital. While some hospitals created zones for COVID and non-COVID patients, converting paediatric intensive care units (ICUs), surgical wards and private facilities into spaces for COVID patients, others tore down walls, erected tents and installed HEPA filters to the windows creating negative pressure rooms. In the UK, the Nightingale Hospitals (referred to by the general public as 'pop-up' hospitals as they were built in a matter of days) were created to help London hospitals deal with the surge in patients requiring hospitalisation. In New York City, one of the hardest hit locales in the US, a Navy ship was parked in New York's harbour to handle patient overflow, the convention centre was converted into a field hospital, and a pop-up tent hospital was erected in Central Park to accommodate coronavirus patients. One hospital system in a midwestern city in the US converted a long-term acute care facility into a COVID hospital in less than a week and began sending COVID patients from all of their partner hospitals to that location. Kieran, a doctor and quality officer for that hospital system, reflected on that time: 'It was very intense. Within, you know, literally a week or two we got that whole thing up and running and that provided a mental model for how we could co-locate all our COVID patients into one location and really begin to standardise our approach to their management'. The completion of the physical rearrangement, which required intensive work by construction workers, engineers, infectious disease experts and environmental service specialists, was necessary before the work of figuring out how to care for patients could really begin.

One of the most frustrating things for healthcare workers was the pace of change. Daily calls, system-wide email directives and meetings after hours informed HCWs of a new approach to patient care or a new way of organising hospital space, only to be changed again a week later. This occurred in relation to testing guidelines in the UK, as Rachel, one of the nurses working in the ICU, indicated, 'at one point we were told we might not get tested even though one person in the team had confirmed COVID-19, which seemed to go against previous suggestions'. Some hospitals tried out a cohort model, segregating COVID-patients to a certain area, but quickly realised there was too much spill over of COVID patients into non-COVID units. Because of the experimental nature of improvisation at a structural level, the guidelines were not always evidence based, and sometimes they simply did not work. Dave, a chief medical officer for a large urban public hospital in the US said, 'Just the tolerance for change, and, you know, basically shutting an entire ambulatory and surgical system down to only essentials and trying to restart it for 7000 employees … it's been challenging. It's been a lot of long hours and I would just say it's been emotionally draining'. Laughing, he added, 'It's like change management on steroids'.

While the pace of change was stressful, it was not impossible, as hospital administrators might have guessed. Some changes were borne out of necessity. For example, in the US and UK, telemedicine implementation and adoption ramped up very quickly (Car et al. 2020; Alexander et al. 2020), and thus avoided some of the bureaucratic slowdowns that would occur under normal circumstances. In the UK, the NHS implemented telemedicine in order to support patients and avoid them visiting their general practitioners or coming into hospital, so reducing the risk of the spread of COVID-19 (Leite et al. 2020). Telemedicine in the UK was also used to monitor patients waiting for surgical procedures and identify any potential cases of deterioration that would need to be escalated to emergency care. John, a cardiothoracic surgeon in the UK who was redeployed to critical care, explained: 'One change we had to make is that every patient who has been deferred an [elective] operation will receive a phone call each week to monitor symptoms and triage patients at home. We can then see who is deteriorating and ask them to come to the emergency department'. William, a nurse practitioner in the US, said: 'The nice thing that COVID did was instead of slowly implementing telehealth and trying to work through all the kinks in it slowly over months at a time, kind of all the resources got put into it'. While these kinds of rapid systemic changes created overwhelming waves of new protocols and procedures for HCWs to learn, they were grateful for the extra communication.

Additionally, several HCWs said the difficulty of the situation brought their colleagues closer together. Dave, a chief medical officer in the US, described in detail some conflict he was having with colleagues over PPE directives. But, he added:

> Despite these interactions, overall, we were much more on the same page. I could have never gotten thirty-five senior leader physicians to get on a call every night. There's no way in hell. I couldn't even get them on a call one night, and now they're calling in every night, faithfully. And everybody's pitching in to try to help each other out. And I'm like, oh, my God, this is great. We can leverage this success onward.

Robert, a chief information officer in the US, was also surprised by the flexibility in implementing massive structural changes at his hospital, and noted: 'So that's good to learn that we can be pretty nimble, we can make adjustments pretty quickly and succeed'. David, a doctor in the UK, associated the speed of changes with the reduction of barriers encountered pre-COVID-19. He said, '[The pandemic] demonstrated that change can be done quickly, what normally takes a year can be done in [a]week, less red tape. We are able to do more in a short time'. Whether these changes are lasting beyond this pandemic is of course unknown.

Improvisation as resource scarcity

Much improvisation also occurred as a result of scarcity or the fear of future scarcity, particularly regarding personal protective equipment. In the UK, HCWs reported several adaptations to delivering care in order to preserve PPE, such as the use of verbal prescriptions, open bays with multiple COVID-19 patients, limiting visitors and fewer HCWs seeing patients on ward rounds. Some HCWs resorted to privately purchasing PPE and some NHS units received donations of PPE, including 3D printed masks and visors. Extreme examples from the media analysis included HCWs improvising PPE out of children's safety goggles, cooking aprons and bin liners.

In the US and the UK, PPE shortages varied from place to place, as did administrators' and HCWs' responses to shortages. In some places, HCWs were directed to use a certain number of masks, gowns and face shields per shift. In others, PPE was used for a certain number of patients or certain types of patients. For example, Julie, a paediatric ICU nurse in Chicago, received one N95 mask per shift but a new surgical mask to put on top of it with each patient. In addition, each room had a designated face shield which nurses shared when they entered the room, which, Julie noted, 'was kind of gross'. Melissa, an ER doctor in the US, explained how she tinkered with the order of patients to preserve PPE:

> We didn't have enough of the outer yellow gowns, so we were trying to use them in a wise way. If I had a COVID rule-out patient, I saw them first. And I could put another gown on for anyone that had COVID plus MRSA or Pseudomonas, one of these other contagious infections. And then I'd get rid of those. And then I would have a new set that I'd wear for COVID only patients but since they already had COVID you could just wear the same gown in each room. In the end it meant that you're wearing this yellow gown for eight patients or ten in a row trying to preserve it because the floor was running out of them, and was trying to keep them for the nurses who had to go in and give medications and bring meals and all these other moments of contact.

Melissa's creative strategy was not implemented as policy, but providers shared such strategies with each other in order to ensure adequate PPE for the whole team. In the UK, there were similar examples of rationing and individual processes of negotiation led by HCWs who believed the measures implemented in their hospital were not safe. Janet, a healthcare assistant, explained:

> They were saying that we were the ones that really should be using [PPE] and anyone who was in the room but is further away doesn't need it, because they're not at the mouth of the patient ... you were begging to have more ... you'd have to really make a stand and say well, 'everybody in my team is wearing it'.

In both countries, several HCWs mentioned that this type of coordination and communication brought their team closer, and in some instances broke down hierarchies between doctors, nurses and other frontline workers.

One of the most frustrating and disconcerting things about PPE shortages were the constantly changing recommendations, which were both hard to keep track of and undermined HCWs' confidence that they were able to protect themselves adequately. At first, some HCWs were told they only needed to use a surgical mask when seeing a COVID-19 patient, unless performing an aerosolising procedure such as an intubation. However, as Quinn, an ER doctor in one of the early US hotspots noted, the HCWs pushed back on this recommendation because it felt unsafe: 'Everyone was like, that's total bullshit and not based on science but just based on the lack of supplies. And that's not appropriate'. After HCWs organised in protest, their hospital changed its recommendation to allow use of N95 masks with all COVID-19 patients. In the UK study, frontline staff found it difficult to follow national-level PPE guidance when there were shortages, leading to re-use and improvisation of personal protective equipment (Hoernke et al. 2020). Linda, a charge nurse, said:

> Some staff felt messages of what PPE is required, in what situations, that there was a little bit of distrust ... If the advice keeps changing, are we getting the right message? And is this message safe? Which caused a bit of worry and anxiety for some of the staff because at the same time they were hearing on the press that colleagues in other hospitals were getting sick.

Josh, a junior doctor in his last year of training in the southern United States, reflected on the fact that he was being told to use PPE in ways contradictory to everything he had learned in medical school:

> I gotta say, it was really funny to have something that the infection prevention people have always trained you so very well on and then all of a sudden we're in this pandemic, and the masks are no longer one time use, right? Because they anticipated that if we did that, we would run out of masks. I think some places around the country did run out of masks. Now, we didn't. But if you consider the fact that we were reusing masks, I kind of consider that as having run out of the masks because they weren't being used the appropriate way they were initially intended.

In other words, the only reason hospitals had not completely run out of PPE is because they were using it inappropriately. While most interviewees in both countries said they had not yet completely run out of PPE, HCWs' experiences with PPE protocols provides a stark reminder that inappropriate PPE usage is a dangerous form of shortage as well, because its effectiveness is unknown.

To preserve PPE, healthcare workers also had to creatively improvise storage, preservation and cleaning techniques. HCWs stored N95 masks in paper bags or rested them on styrofoam cups so they would not touch anything while not in use, while some treated them with UV lights or hydrogen peroxide to try and kill any virus particles on them. In some cases, hospital administrators came up with a system for sending PPE away to be cleaned. But, as Josh noted, clean does not necessarily equate with effective: 'Maybe it comes back clean but there's also a question of does it lose effectiveness? Its filtration, does that lose effectiveness? Because, even if it comes back clean, great it's clean. But after how many uses does the material itself start allowing more stuff through?'. In both countries, HCWs reported foregoing food and water during their shifts in order to preserve PPE and avoid risk of infection. In the UK, there were several cases of dehydration among HCWs who were using full PPE; in many cases, this was because HCWs were not taking the recommended hydration and bathroom breaks because they did not want to 'waste' PPE. Peter, a junior doctor explained: 'So, there were times, for instance, where you needed to go to the loo, but you didn't want to waste PPE'.

While PPE was the primary target of resource scarcity management, HCWs in the UK and the US feared a shortage of ventilators as well, which led to the redistribution and improvisation of machines. In some cases, HCWs used backup ventilators and transport ventilators normally used in ambulances when supplies were low. In most places, hospitals restricted the use of non-invasive ventilation strategies that utilise positive airway pressure such as CPAP and BPAP machines, due to the risk of aerosolising particles (Pirzada et al. 2020; Arulkumaran et al. 2020). However, HCWs made creative adjustments to use these non-invasive strategies in order to make use of them. Leo, a junior doctor in the US, explained how his colleagues adjusted bag valve masks to avoid release of aerosolising particles:

> Technically we're not allowed to use a bag valve mask right now. Some of my colleagues have come up with some clever ways to insert a viral filter into the rest of the system and use these one-way valves and shut off different pieces so you can say, look, you could probably use this as a bag valve mask, and this is probably compliant with the wishes of those above us.

These tactics both avoided intubating patients for whom intermediate positive air support was sufficient and preserved ventilators for patients who needed them. In the UK, HCWs used anaesthetic machines for ventilation because, although these were not fit for the purpose, they felt that they had to 'make do with what they had at the time'. Like many tactics used to address resource shortages, these stopgap measures and improvisations were informal and their effectiveness unexamined.

Improvisation as risk reduction strategy

In addition to PPE, HCWs and hospitals implemented many micro and macro changes to reduce the risk of acquiring and transmitting COVID-19 between patients, themselves and their families. In both the US and the UK, most hospitals administered temperature checks and symptom monitoring for all HCWs arriving at work (although the consistency of these practices varied by hospital). HCWs also reported taking additional precautions upon entering and leaving the hospital to protect their family members at home. Kristen, a nurse working in a COVID unit in the eastern US, was particularly diligent because her husband, who worked from home, was fearful she would contract the virus and bring it home to him and their three young children. She explained:

> On the way to work, I put everything in the canvas washable tote bag. I only bring my wallet in. I leave for work in my scrubs, but when I'm coming home, I take my scrubs off at the hospital, put on pants and a t-shirt. I have a tracker thing where my husband has me share my ETA on my way home. He likes to get the washing machine

going, and the thing is already open and the water and soap already in so I don't touch anything. The basement door is open, everything's ready to go. So I leave my shoes in the car I come inside. I put the t-shirt, the pants, my scrubs and the canvas tote all right in the wash. I have a bleach spray for my phone. And then I have to run upstairs naked, take a shower and then he's fine.

While on the extreme end of cautiousness, most HCWs in both the US and the UK had some kind of rigorous routine, which added a significant amount of time and effort to their already long workday.

One primary strategy that both served to preserve PPE and reduce risk of infection was to limit the number of people and times one entered the room of a COVID-19 patient. In the UK, to reduce the risk of infection and respond to concerns about mask shortages, HCWs were told 'if a member of staff does not need to go into the risk area, they should be kept out'. Leo, a junior doctor in the US, said:

> For a while there we were having some shortages of PPE. So we tried to come up with clever ways of getting around that. Let's count one person and put them in the room and then we're just going to pass you in stuff, you're just going to sit in there for an hour, because we're just going to see if there's anything else we need to do.

Leo also described what he called an intubation box, a plexiglass box some doctors had made, which they would place over the patient's head and reach into to perform intubations. He marvelled, 'The level of ingenuity of emergency room doctors, I think, is very, very high. They're always looking for clever things to do to solve problems that don't have easy solutions and I definitely have seen that kind of stuff'. Jeff, an American ER doctor, and his colleagues developed similarly creative strategies:

> Pretty early on we realised we had to try to minimise the number of times you have to go into a room so we were trying to batch care. So, don't trickle in orders for labs like that so the nurse has to go in once an hour to get new lab draws. We tried do all that at once so they just have to go in one time … I've heard of pretty innovative things in ICUs where instead of putting the IV pumps on the bed right next to the patient, they'll actually run a really long IV line through the door to the nurse's station. So it probably looks crazy, just huge long IV lines running across the floor but it keeps the nurse from having to go in.

The combination of PPE shortages and uncertainties around the transmission of COVID-19 created a scenario ripe for innovation. The constant need for innovation and the uncertainty of these measures created both a sense of solidarity among HCWs and an ever-present reminder that the infection could be anywhere, which was also a source of stress (Block 2020).

Improvisation as a lifesaving technique

At the start of the COVID-19 pandemic, in particular in places hit hard early on, case fatality rates were high and severely ill patients had poor outcomes (Fan et al. 2020; Horby et al. 2020). In the absence of evidence-based approaches, HCWs improvised based on anecdotal experience, communication with personal networks and social media message boards aimed at medical professionals (Chan et al. 2020). While it takes time for randomised controlled studies and clinical trials to go from study design to publication, healthcare providers sought ways to share information, including improvisation strategies. At first, HCWs were troubled by their own lack of knowledge about managing COVID-19. For example, Jonathan, a senior clinical site manager in the UK interviewed early in the pandemic, said:

> The thing with COVID that's, I think, been troubling the most people, and definitely for me, is the lack of knowledge, and so you can read everything and I've been listening to the NHS podcast every week, I've been reading everything that's available online. I've been doing everything I can to keep myself as up to date as possible but there's just not a lot out there. And so that's been quite scary, as a healthcare professional, certainly for me, you arm yourself with as much knowledge and practical application as possible. But when the knowledge is in deficit all you've got is some kinds of application and very little knowledge.

Matt, an ER doctor in the US, expressed similar sentiments in June 2020, just as the first infection peak was subsiding:

> Doctors like to think we're so damn smart, we have all these tricks up our sleeve that we can do to get people better ... And we just do not have that with this virus. It's like, we don't know why some people get so sick and others don't. We don't know if any of the

things we're doing are working or have no impact or are harming people. So I think that's the most infuriating thing about the virus … I just feel totally powerless.

As HCWs gained experience caring for COVID-19 patients, they shared anecdotal information about supportive care practices that seemed to be working to support the patient through the disease (as opposed to treating it). Some key practices, including delaying intubation, which has now been studied (Rola et al. 2020), were first communicated through these informal networks. Jeff, an American ER doctor, described how this information improved his approach to patient care:

It's definitely been a boom of creativity in terms of how we can do this more efficiently and safer, a big sea change, and I think probably it will be seen later in clinical studies that the mortality has gone down. Initially they were saying, you need to put a breathing tube down and intubate the patient once they hit a certain threshold of oxygen, which is pretty standard for most of our patients. But we found, [COVID patients] kind of paradoxically tolerate a lot lower oxygen saturations than most people. So the clinical decision to intubate them was really pushed further down the line over the last couple of months, and those patients have actually done pretty well. So it turned out that, for whatever reason, keeping them off the ventilator as long as we can has really hopefully saved a lot of lives. Initially I'm not sure what was going on in Italy and China, but that wasn't recognised. So that the fact that that could be recognised and changed within about a month was pretty amazing. And that was from a lot of the work in New York. So, just that kind of flexibility to change practice patterns and change what people have been doing for the last 50 years was pretty impressive because medicine can be pretty intransigent in terms of, you know, taking 20 years to change and things have been changing week by week, especially early on.

The medical research on COVID-19 is being published at a feverish pace, and HCWs' experience in caring for and treating COVID-19 patients has also increased. As a result, the need to improvise as a lifesaving technique is becoming less necessary. However, managing long-term complications for COVID-19 patients and the complex needs of patients with particular co-morbidities will require creativity and ingenuity for some time.

Improvisation and inequality

During the early phase of the COVID-19 pandemic in the US and the UK, improvisation – and the conditions that have necessitated it – in many ways flattened inequalities between wealthy and poor communities, nations and healthcare systems. Healthcare workers were overwhelmed with patients, lacked evidence-based treatments and supportive care practices, and experienced acute shortages of PPE and medical devices needed to treat severe respiratory illnesses. COVID-19 patients in wealthy nations, such as Italy and the US, have had astonishingly high mortality rates and deaths (Livingston and Bucher 2020; Johns Hopkins Coronavirus Resource Center 2020). Yet, as the first acute crisis phase of the virus passed, and HCWs learned from each other and from emerging studies, patient outcomes improved (Fan et al. 2020). As the war-like conditions subsided, it became clear that COVID-19 disease and all the reverberating effects, like other major disasters, only served to reveal the fault lines of inequality both for HCWs and for patients. While in theory, anyone is at risk of contracting and dying of COVID-19, in reality race, poverty, occupation and living conditions are risk factors for both infection and death (Patel et al. 2020; Bowleg 2020; El-Khatib et al. 2020; Pan et al. 2020; Abedi et al. 2020).

Josh, an ER junior doctor in the US, explained the living conditions and working conditions that might lead to poor patient outcomes:

> It's a lot easier to social distance when you have a family of four in 4000 square feet in your suburb and have a bunch of yard space between you and your neighbour, than when you are in a row home in an urban area with a multi-generational household. And there's also an economic strain where you might have to go out in the community to do the work you have to do … And you know there's baseline health status even with chronic disease … It's honestly a structure of racism that persists, that is really apparent and really disheartening.

Matt, an ER doctor in the US, described a Latinx woman who was intubated for COVID-19. Upon being extubated, she learned that her husband and son had died of COVID while she was hospitalised. He added, 'We are not seeing that from wealthy white folks in the suburbs going through that problem'.

Inequality also exists for healthcare workers, both in terms of workplace conditions and vulnerability to COVID-19. In the UK study, research participants highlighted that HCWs of lower seniority, females and ethnic minorities faced greater barriers accessing PPE than their colleagues during times of shortages. Female HCWs expressed concerns regarding the lack of small-sized masks and reported having to deliver care despite failed fit-tests for N95 masks. During the 2015 MERS outbreak in Korea, female HCWs experienced similar difficulties, with oversized coveralls impairing clinical skills and large masks not adequately sealing around their faces, raising concerns about both patient and HCW safety (Kang et al. 2018). Despite only making up 21 per cent of the NHS workforce, Black, Asian and Minority Ethnic (BAME) HCWs have been overrepresented in the proportion of HCW deaths from COVID-19 in the UK, accounting for 63 per cent of nurses and 95 per cent of medical staff deaths (Cook et al. 2020). Supporting the concerns raised by our participants, lack of access to PPE was perceived by BAME HCWs as a major contributing factor to the higher death rates (see also Gamlin, Gibbon and Calestani, this volume Chapter 6).

Conclusion

In the US and the UK, the COVID-19 pandemic necessitated improvisation both at the institutional level and at the microlevel of everyday clinical practice. In a matter of days and weeks, hospitals rearranged their physical spaces and drastically changed their flow of patients to deal with the influx of people and the insidious infectiousness of COVID-19. In light of the uncertainty they were facing, healthcare workers tinkered and adapted to improve patient outcomes, protect themselves and their patients, preserve PPE and respond to broader resource shortages in providing supportive care for COVID-19 patients. While in the early stages of the pandemic, as tropes about being 'in it together' and emphasising everyone's susceptibility to COVID-19 abounded, rates of infection and clinical outcomes clearly demonstrated the ways that pre-existing and intersecting structures of inequality play out in this context as well.

Ethnographies of medical improvisation have typically been located in resource-poor contexts where protracted conditions of poverty and conflict necessitate creative tinkering and adjustments (Livingston 2012; Street 2014; Dewachi 2017; Wendland 2010). Yet, the flexibility and adaptability demonstrated here suggests that perhaps improvisation is not merely a reflection of the conditions brought about by war or intractable poverty. The ingenuity and creativity of healthcare workers in both the US and the UK speaks to their ability to adapt to extremely challenging situations and reveals the surprisingly versatile nature of healthcare institutions and healthcare workers to effectively mobilise at both the institutional level and in everyday care in response to a crisis.

Perhaps healthcare as practised always requires improvisation – a constant working around the exigencies and emergencies of the present – from the prioritisation that occurs on the fly during ordinary triaging, to the constant titration and experimentation that occurs with treatments, dosages and prescriptions. As many of our interlocutors noted, particularly those who work in emergency medicine, a high level of uncertainty and the need to respond to people in crisis is precisely the job they signed up for. As Josh, an American ER doctor, explained, '[COVID] probably has just highlighted things that were already there… I think people who are drawn to emergency medicine like the idea that they feel that they're able to help people no matter what their complaint is with limited to no information.' Quinn, another ER doctor in the US, said, 'For me [COVID] just kind of reaffirms my identity of, you know, when there's an emergency, you're there. And you have the skill set to be there and help out.' Healthcare workers always have to think on their feet and to quickly act on their best judgement when faced with a person in crisis. Yet, healthcare systems in the US and the UK typically mask this improvisation through protocols, procedures and evidence-based practices in an attempt to homogenise treatment and minimise risk, adverse events and litigation. Unlike most emergencies, HCWs had not initially internalised the appropriate series of steps they needed to take with this novel coronavirus, so acting on their judgement and expertise felt like a novel form of improvisation. But the fact that such nimble change was possible is noteworthy and undermines the supposed rigidity of such institutions and provides important lessons for future medical crises.

Notes

1   In the UK, a junior doctor is the equivalent to a resident.
2   Advanced care providers include nurse practitioners and physicians' assistants.

References

Abedi, Vida, Oluwaseyi Olulana, Venkatesh Avula, Durgesh Chaudhary, Ayesha Khan, Shima Shahjouei, Jiang Li and Ramin Zand. 2020. 'Racial, economic, and health inequality and COVID-19 infection in the United States'. *Journal of Racial and Ethnic Health Disparities*: 1–11. https://doi.org/10.1007/s40615-020-00833-4.

Alexander, G. Caleb, Matthew Tajanlangit, James Heyward, Omar Mansour, Dima M. Qato and Randall S. Stafford. 2020. 'Use and content of primary care office-based vs telemedicine care visits during the COVID-19 pandemic in the US'. *JAMA Network Open* 3(10): e2021476. https://dx.doi.org/10.1001%2Fjamanetworkopen.2020.21476.

Arulkumaran, Nishkantha, David Brealey, David Howell and Mervyn Singer. 2020. 'Use of non-invasive ventilation for patients with COVID-19: A cause for concern?' *The Lancet. Respiratory Medicine* 8(6): e45. https://dx.doi.org/10.1016%2FS2213-2600(20)30181-8.

Beigel, John H., Kay M. Tomashek, Lori E. Dodd, Aneesh K. Mehta, Barry S. Zingman, Andre C. Kalil, Elizabeth Hohmann et al. 2020. 'Remdesivir for the treatment of Covid-19'. *New England Journal of Medicine* 383(19): 1813–26. https://dx.doi.org/10.1056%2FNEJMoa2007764.

Block, Ellen. 2020. 'Exposed intimacies: Clinicians on the frontlines of the COVID-19 pandemic'. *Anthropology in Action* 27(2): 63–7. https://doi.org/10.3167/aia.2020.270209

Bowleg, Lisa. 2020. 'We're not all in this together: on COVID-19, intersectionality, and structural inequality'. *American Journal of Public Health* 110: 917. https://ajph.aphapublications.org/doi/abs/10.2105/AJPH.2020.305766.

Car, Josip, Gerald Choon-Huat Koh, Pin Sym Foong and C. Jason Wang. 2020. 'Video consultations in primary and specialist care during the Covid-19 pandemic and beyond'. *BMJ* 371: m3845. https://doi.org/10.1136/bmj.m3945.

Chan, Albert K.M, C.P. Nickson, J.W. Rudolph, A. Lee and G.M. Joynt. 2020. 'Social media for rapid knowledge dissemination: early experience from the COVID-19 pandemic'. *Anaesthesia* 75(12): 1579–82. https://doi.org/10.1111/anae.15057.

Cook, Tim, Emira Kursumovic and Simon Lennane. 2020. 'Exclusive: Deaths of NHS staff from Covid-19 analysed'. *Health Services Journal*, 22 April 2020. Accessed 20 July 2020. https://www.hsj.co.uk/exclusive-deaths-of-nhs-staff-from-covid-19-analysed/7027471.article.

Coppo, Anna, Giacomo Bellani, Dario Winterton, Michela Di Pierro, Alessandro Soria, Paola Faverio, Matteo Cairo et al. 2020. 'Feasibility and physiological effects of prone positioning in non-intubated patients with acute respiratory failure due to COVID-19 (PRON-COVID): A prospective cohort study'. *The Lancet Respiratory Medicine* 8(8): 765–74. https://doi.org/10.1016/S2213-2600(20)30268-X.

Dayan, Mark, Deborah Ward, Tim Gardner and Elaine Kelly. 2018. 'The NHS at 70: How good is the NHS?' Accessed 7 December 2020. https://www.health.org.uk/publications/nhs-at-70-how-good-is-the-nhs.

DiMaggio, Paul J. and Walter W. Powell. 1983. 'The iron cage revisited: Institutional isomorphism and collective rationality in organizational fields'. *American Sociological Review* 48(2): 147–60. https://doi.org/10.2307/2095101.

Dewachi, Omar. 2017. *Ungovernable Life: Mandatory medicine and statecraft in Iraq*. Redwood City, CA: Stanford University Press.

Edwards, Nigel and Richard B. Saltman. 2017. 'Re-thinking barriers to organizational change in public hospitals'. *Israel Journal of Health Policy Research* 6(1): 1–11. https://doi.org/10.1186/s13584-017-0133-8.

El-Khatib, Ziad, Graeme Brendon Jacobs, George Mondinde Ikomey and Ujjwal Neogi. 2020. 'The disproportionate effect of COVID-19 mortality on ethnic minorities: Genetics or health inequalities?' *EClinicalMedicine* 23. https://doi.org/10.1016/j.eclinm.2020.100430.

Fan, Guihong, Zhichun Yang, Qianying Lin, Shi Zhao, Lin Yang and Daihai He. 2020. 'Decreased case fatality rate of COVID-19 in the second wave: A study in 53 countries or regions'. *Transboundary and Emerging Diseases*: 1–3. https://doi.org/10.1111/tbed.13819.

Gawande, Atul. 2002. *Complications: A surgeon's notes on an imperfect science*. London: Profile Books.

Hoernke, Katarina, Nehla Djellouli, Lily Jay Andrews, Sasha Lewis-Jackson, Louisa Manby, Sam Martin, Samantha Vanderslott and Cecilia Vindrola-Padros. 2020. 'Frontline healthcare workers' experiences with personal protective equipment during the COVID-19 pandemic in the UK: a rapid qualitative appraisal'. *medRxiv*. https://doi.org/10.1101/2020.10.12.20211482.

Horby, Peter, Wei Shen Lim, Jonathan R. Emberson, Marion Mafham, Jennifer L. Bell, Louise Linsell, Natalie Staplin et al. 2020. 'Dexamethasone in hospitalized patients with Covid-19-preliminary report'. *The New England Journal of Medicine*. https://doi.org/10.1056/NEJMoa2021436.

Johns Hopkins Coronavirus Resource Center. 2020. 'Mortality analysis'. Accessed 1 December 2020. https://coronavirus.jhu.edu/data/mortality.

Kakodkar, Pramath, Nagham Kaka and M.N. Baig. 2020. 'A comprehensive literature review on the clinical presentation, and management of the pandemic coronavirus disease 2019 (COVID-19)'. *Cureus* 12(4): e7560. https://dx.doi.org/10.7759%2Fcureus.7560.

Kang, JaHyun, Eun Jin Kim, Jeong Hwa Choi, Hae Kyung Hong, Si-Hyeon Han, In Soon Choi, Jae Geum Ryu, Jinwha Kim, Jae Yeun Kim and Eun Suk Park. 2018. 'Difficulties in using personal protective equipment: Training experiences with the 2015 outbreak of Middle East respiratory syndrome in Korea'. *American Journal of Infection Control* 46(2): 235–7. https://doi.org/10.1016/j.ajic.2017.08.041.

Leite, Higor, Ian R. Hodgkinson and Thorsten Gruber. 2020. 'New development: "Healing at a distance" – telemedicine and COVID-19'. *Public Money & Management* 40(6): 483–5. https://doi.org/10.1080/09540962.2020.1748855.

Livingston, Julie. 2012. *Improvising Medicine: An African oncology ward in an emerging cancer epidemic*. Durham, NC: Duke University Press.

Livingston, Edward and Karen Bucher. 2020. 'Coronavirus disease 2019 (COVID-19) in Italy'. *JAMA* 323(14): 1335. https://doi.org/10.1001/jama.2020.4344.

Liu, Qian, Dan Luo, Joan E. Haase, Qiaohong Guo, Xiao Qin Wang, Shuo Liu, Lin Xia, Zhongchun Liu, Jiong Yang and Bing Xiang Yang. 2020. 'The experiences of health-care providers during the COVID-19 crisis in China: A qualitative study'. *The Lancet Global Health* 8: e790–98. https://doi.org/10.1016/S2214-109X(20)30204-7.

NHS. 2020. 'Clinical guide for the management of surge during the coronavirus pandemic: Rapid learning'. Accessed 7 December 2020. https://www.england.nhs.uk/coronavirus/wp-content/uploads/sites/52/2020/03/C0167-specialty-guide-surge-based-on-current-hospital-experience-v2.pdf.

Pan, Daniel, Shirley Sze, Jatinder S. Minhas, Mansoor N. Bangash, Nilesh Pareek, Pip Divall, Caroline ML Williams, Marco R. Oggioni, Iain B. Squire, Laura B. Nellums, Wasim Hanif, Kamlesh Khunti and Manish Pareek. 2020. 'The impact of ethnicity on clinical outcomes in COVID-19: A systematic review'. *EClinicalMedicine* 23: 100404. https://doi.org/10.1016/j.eclinm.2020.100404.

Patel, J.A., F.B.H. Nielsen, A.A. Badiani, S. Assi, V.A. Unadkat, B. Patel, R. Ravindrane and H. Wardle. 2020. 'Poverty, inequality and COVID-19: The forgotten vulnerable'. *Public Health* 183: 110–111. https://dx.doi.org/10.1016%2Fj.puhe.2020.05.006.

Pirzada, Abdul Rouf, Salih A. Aleissi, Aljohara S. Almeneessier and Ahmed Salem BaHammam. 2020. 'Management of aerosol during noninvasive ventilation for patients with sleep-disordered breathing: Important messages during the COVID-19 pandemic'. *Sleep and Vigilance*: 1–6. https://doi.org/10.1007/s41782-020-00092-7.

Rola, Philippe, Joshua Farkas, Rory Spiegel, Cameron Kyle-Sidell, Scott Weingart, Laura Duggan, Marco Garrone and Adam Thomas. 2020 'Rethinking the early intubation paradigm of COVID-19: Time to change gears?' *Clinical and Experimental Emergency Medicine* 7(2): 78–80. https://doi.org/10.15441/ceem.20.043.

Self, Wesley H., Matthew W. Semler, Lindsay M. Leither, Jonathan D. Casey, Derek C. Angus, Roy G. Brower, Steven Y. Chang et al. 2020. 'Effect of hydroxychloroquine on clinical status at 14 days in hospitalized patients with COVID-19: A randomized clinical trial'. *JAMA* 324(21): 2165–76. https://doi.org/10.1001/jama.2020.22240.

Song, Xingyue, Wenning Fu, Xiaoran Liu, Zhiqian Luo, Rixing Wang, Ning Zhou, Shijiao Yan and Chuanzhu Lv. 2020. 'Mental health status of medical staff in emergency departments during the Coronavirus disease 2019 epidemic in China'. *Brain, Behavior, and Immunity* 88: 60–65. https://doi.org/10.1016/j.bbi.2020.06.002.

Street, Alice. 2014. *Biomedicine in an Unstable Place: Infrastructure and personhood in a Papua New Guinean hospital*. Durham, NC: Duke University Press.

Sun, Niuniu, Luoqun Wei, Suling Shi, Dandan Jiao, Runluo Song, Lili Ma, Hongwei Wang et al. 2020. 'A qualitative study on the psychological experience of caregivers of COVID-19 patients'. *American Journal of Infection Control* 48(6): 592–8. https://doi.org/10.1016/j.ajic.2020.03.018.

Vindrola-Padros, Cecilia, Georgia Chisnall, Silvie Cooper, Anna Dowrick, Nehla Djellouli, Sophie Mulcahy Symmons, Sam Martin et al. 2020. 'Carrying out rapid qualitative research during a pandemic: Emerging lessons from COVID-19'. *Qualitative Health Research* 30(14): 2192–2204. https://doi.org/10.1177%2F1049732320951526.

Wendland, Claire L. 2010. *A Heart for the Work: Journeys through an African medical school*. Chicago, IL: University of Chicago Press.

Willan, John, Andrew John King, Katie Jeffery and Nicola Bienz. 2020. 'Challenges for NHS hospitals during covid-19 epidemic'. *BMJ* 368: m1117. https://doi.org/10.1136/bmj.m1117

Zhang, G., C. Hu, L. Luo, F. Fang, Y. Chen, J. Li, Z. Peng and H. Pan. 2020. 'Clinical features and short-term outcomes of 221 patients with COVID-19 in Wuhan, China'. *Journal of Clinical Virology* 127: 104364. https://doi.org/10.1016/j.jcv.2020.104364.

17
Carescapes unsettled

COVID-19 and the reworking of 'stable illnesses' in welfare state Denmark

Sofie Rosenlund Lau, Marie Kofod Svensson, Natasja Kingod and Ayo Wahlberg

On 11 March 2020, Denmark's Prime Minister Mette Frederiksen addressed the nation through a televised press conference. Flanked by Health Minister Magnus Heunicke and infectious disease experts, she announced that Denmark would be going into lockdown. Images of overflowing hospital wards and overworked healthcare workers in Italy, and an expected spike in COVID-19 cases as people returned from skiing holidays in the Alps, prompted Frederiksen to be one of the first heads of state in Europe to send everyone home from work and school and to close national borders. Armed with a cardboard prop, Heunicke animated why 'flattening the curve' was necessary by contrasting the (by now) internationally recognisable red peak that inevitably bursts through a black dotted line representing national hospital capacity with the smoother green hill that remained within capacity (see Figure 17.1). For Denmark to remain green, strict stay-at-home measures, physical distancing, sneezing and coughing into elbows, and scrupulous hand hygiene were essential. Drawing on what was becoming clear from outbreaks in China, Italy and Spain, the prime minister emphasised that people living with a range of chronic conditions and older people were especially 'at risk' of hospitalisation and death from COVID-19. These groups were advised to self-isolate, while others would be allowed to leave their homes for shopping, pharmacy visits and outdoor leisure, albeit while adhering to strict physical distancing and hygiene requirements.

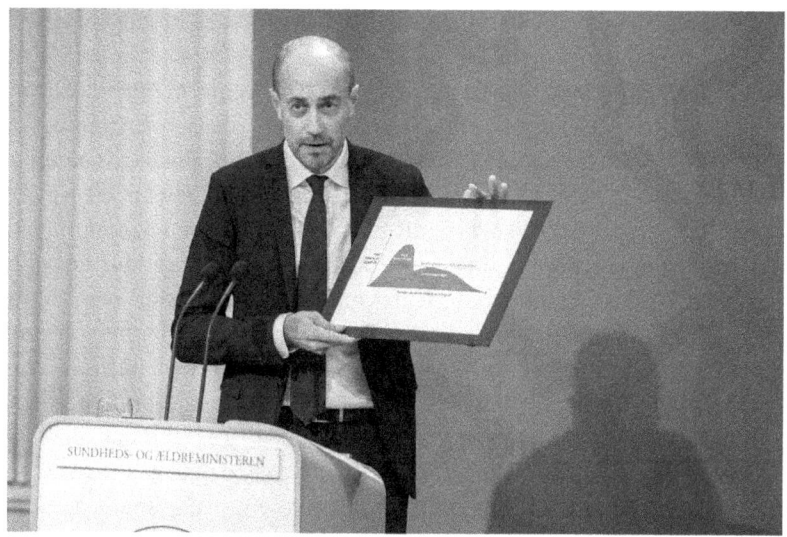

Figure 17.1 Health Minister Magnus Heunicke urging Danes to 'flatten the curve'. Photo: Martin Sylvest/Ritzau Scanpix

In the meantime, behind the scenes, the National Health Board was instructed to urgently devise a plan to ensure that Danish hospitals were ready for an influx of COVID-19 patients who might require intensive oxygen therapy and in some cases respiratory care. While time was of the essence, it was imperative to raise the dotted black line on the Health Minister's 'flatten the curve' chart as high as possible in order to avoid overwhelming the healthcare system. The Prime Minister insisted that this was one of the most important objectives of Denmark's national lockdown:

> We need to prevent the collapse of our healthcare system. Should that happen, it would have consequences for everyone's lives. ... We are demonstrating our *samfundssind* [Danish; 'social solidarity mentality']. And we stand together in looking after those who are most vulnerable. Yes, in fact, we are standing together in caring for our society. ... Right now we are seeing the value of the strong social contract that we Danes have with each other (Statsministeriet 2020a).[1]

Two days later, on 13 March 2020, the National Board of Health drew up a 'Memo on reduction of hospital activity in connection with COVID-19' (Board of Health 2020), and sent it to all hospitals in the country.

Alongside plans for how to increase numbers of beds in intensive care units, hospitals were instructed to free up staff to look after an expected influx of hospitalised COVID-19 patients: 'The Board of Health deems that this can be achieved by reducing outpatient activities in a number of clinical specialities [since] all forms of outpatient check-ups for patients with *a stable illness* can be postponed or redirected' (Board of Health 2020, our emphasis). Likewise, diagnostic and treatment 'guarantees', which had been enshrined in law in 2002 to ensure that serious diseases were detected earlier and treatments commenced as quickly as possible, were suspended in order to reroute resources (see Manderson and Wahlberg 2020). In these ways, Denmark's healthcare agenda was transformed overnight from a decades-long focus on chronic conditions to a focus on a singular infectious disease. While this exceptional focus on COVID-19 subsided during the summer with fewer confirmed cases, with winter approaching, by late 2020, doctors were warning that a 'second wave' influx of patients was leading to cancelled elective operations and fewer outpatient visits (Møller and Goos 2020).

In this chapter, we explore the ways in which COVID-19 unsettled not only Denmark's universal, tax-funded healthcare system, but also the lives of those living with chronic medical conditions. Although fears of an overwhelmed hospital system never came close to materialising in spring 2020, and we have yet to see the full effects of Denmark's 'second wave', the knock-on consequences of shifting resources and political attention to a single infectious disease has already and will continue to impact on the lives of those with chronic conditions, not least since, as the prime minister commented, Danes will have to 'learn to live with the virus' (Frederiksen 2020).

Chronic conditions emerged as the premiere focus of Danish healthcare policy from the early 2000s. We describe how a series of 'carescapes' (policies, services and programmes determined by nation-state, local government and employers, aimed at providing care for 'deserving citizens') coalesced and stabilised around some of the most prevalent chronic conditions within Denmark's welfare state, in conjunction and at times in tension with various 'caringscapes' (forms of informal care carried out by family members and loved ones) (Bowlby and McKie 2019). Henriette Langstrup (2013, 1010) has argued that it is exactly through and around both formalised and informal forms of care that 'chronic care infrastructures' arise, encompassing the medications, knowledge and equipment that allow for the work required to manage disease over time and distribute it between various actors and locations. Within such infrastructures of chronic care, the emphasis has been on encouraging and teaching patients to 'live with' their (multiple) medical condition(s) in order to ensure that they remain as independent as possible and able to lead 'normal' lives. Danish healthcare and interrelated eldercare has come to promote self-care and rehabilitation together with enabling treatment and support interventions under slogans like 'help for self-help' and 'as long as possible in one's own home' (Kjellberg et al. 2011; Christensen 2020). At the same time, however, a string of reports from healthcare authorities in the past decade (most recently in September 2020) have drawn attention to glaring health inequalities in a welfare state that claims to provide universal healthcare for all: People with limited education experience more illness, suffer greater consequences from their illnesses, and die earlier than people with a higher education (Board of Health 2020). Reflecting this, in Denmark's fourth largest city, Aalborg, people living in well-off neighbourhoods in the western part of the city live a staggering 13 years longer on average than those living just a few kilometres to the east (Board of Health 2020). Despite declared goals of universal access to and equal provision of high quality care to all citizens, socioeconomic inequalities continue to shape both 'carescapes' and 'caringscapes' in Denmark in ways that render chronic care infrastructures more or less accessible and relevant for those living with long-term conditions.

Only a few weeks into the national lockdown, general practitioners, cardiologists and oncologists began warning that the 'massive corona-focus can cost lives' (Nielsen 2020), as clinicians experienced a worrying fall in numbers of appointments and referrals.[2] These numbers might well reflect the result of government officials' appeal to Danes' *samfundssind*, which for some meant 'holding off' on using the healthcare system for routine purposes (GP visits, dental care and outpatient check-ups), albeit others were wary of infection risks in hospital and clinic settings. Whatever the cause, healthcare providers felt a need to use national media outlets to appeal to the general public to not refrain from seeing a doctor if experiencing symptoms that could indicate any serious condition, not least since early detection was essential for the best possible outcomes.

But what of those already living with and managing a known chronic condition? In this chapter, we build on our long-term fieldwork engagements in Denmark, well before the COVID-19 pandemic, with families living with congenital heart defects, persons living with type 1 diabetes and 'frail' seniors. We explore the kinds of disruptions and concerns experienced by people living with medical conditions other than COVID-19 during Denmark's national lockdown, calls to self-isolate and shifts of healthcare resources away from 'stable illnesses'. In addition, we explore how these families experienced receiving information and advice on being particularly 'at risk'.

Over the past six years, though engaged in individual ethnographic projects, we have collectively explored how novel forms of chronic living have been taking shape in welfare state Denmark. Working together with the Danish Heart Foundation, Marie Svensson has carried out fieldwork among families living with congenital heart defects to gain insights into the everyday challenges they face in the years following the birth of a *hjertebarn* (heart-child) (Svensson et al. 2020). Based at the Steno Diabetes Center Copenhagen, Natasja Kingod has developed new forms of online–offline ethnography to explore how people living with type 1 diabetes use peer-to-peer online platforms – especially the Facebook groups function – to exchange experiences and tips with people who share the same diagnosis (Kingod 2018; Kingod and Cleal 2019; Kingod and Grabowski 2020). Sofie Rosenlund Lau has worked with home carers to examine how multimorbidity and resultant polypharmacy are managed in home settings through regular visits by healthcare professionals (Lau 2020). In addition, Ayo Wahlberg has been leading a five-year collaborative ethnographic study of chronic conditions, designed to characterise chronic living in the twenty-first century (Wahlberg 2018).[3] While the pandemic continues to progress at time of writing (December 2020) with hospitals experiencing a second influx of COVID-19 patients and numerous restrictions currently being reimplemented in Denmark, our empirical insights were gathered in spring 2020 as COVID-19 disrupted the everyday lives of Danes for the first time.

The birth of 'kronikere' in Danish healthcare

In the 1980s and 1990s, Danish healthcare authorities were preoccupied with what was considered a somewhat embarrassing vital statistic: on average, Danes were living significantly shorter lives than citizens in neighbouring countries like Sweden or Norway (Juel and Kamper-Jørgensen 1989). In response to this anomaly, in 1992 then Health Minister Ester Larsen established a Life Expectancy Commission to investigate why 'Danish life expectancy is not advancing as gainfully as in other countries' (Ministry of Health 1994, 1). Two years later, their conclusion was clear: lifestyle – especially smoking – was to blame. Consequently, a series of public health initiatives were developed under a collective banner of KRAM (an acronym for the Danish words for diet, smoking, alcohol and exercise, which also means 'hug', an important part of pre-COVID-19 Danish sociality when meeting friends and family). Sine Knudsen and Peter Triantafillou have argued that these developments amounted to a 'lifestylisation of the social' in Denmark, leading to the consolidation of an extensive 'lifestyle dispositive' (2020, 3). Within such a dispositive, 'although health and illness are the products of the sum of social and environmental influences, it is our lifestyle – made up by our consumption of tobacco, alcohol, accidents, physical exercise and diet – that constitutes the primary cause of … disease' (Frandsen and Triantafillou 2011, 212). To address this, a series of initiatives targeting individual health behaviours (KRAM campaigns) were launched (Vallgårda 2011). By the turn of the millennium, healthcare officials had proclaimed success as life expectancy was again catching up with neighbouring countries, albeit unequally so, not least because Denmark's record in diagnosing and effectively treating cancers continued to lag behind neighbouring welfare states (see Bergeron-Boucher et al. 2019). At the same time, as elsewhere in the world, increasing life expectancy had ushered in a new challenge – how to improve the lives of those who were now *living with* lifelong chronic conditions:

> In recent years, average life expectancy has increased significantly more in Denmark than in those countries we normally compare ourselves to. … But health is not only about length of life. At least as important is quality of life. … We [must] focus much more than hitherto on *both* length and quality of life, not least quality of life in the years after working life when major diseases are more prevalent (Government of Denmark 2002, 6).

And so, alongside the 'lifestylisation of the social' in Denmark, we have over the past two decades witnessed what Ayo Wahlberg and Nikolas Rose have described as a *governmentalisation of living* 'in the course of which the social and personal consequences of living with disease come to be an object of political concern, and made knowable, calculable and thereby amenable to various strategies of intervention' (2015, 60). As a direct consequence of these more recent developments in Denmark's universal, tax-financed healthcare system, the figure of the 'kronikere' (a Danish neologism used to designate those living with a chronic condition) has emerged as an object of concern (Wind and Vedsted 2008, 7–8) around whom chronic care infrastructures have coalesced. In Henriette Langstrup's work on chronic care, such infrastructures are defined as 'made up of various inconspicuous elements (medication, standards, control visits, doses, daily routines, sheets of article for registration and more) that tend to sink into the daily practices of patients and professionals' (2013, 1010).

These chronic care infrastructures allow for what the Board of Health, in its COVID-19 instructions to hospitals, described as 'patients with a stable illness'. Yet, as we consider below, describing people in this way unwarrantably overlooks the many forms of 'illness work' (Corbin and Strauss 1985, 1988) or 'chronic homework' (Mattingly et al. 2011) involved in keeping an illness stable, the costly resources that make chronic care infrastructures possible (not to mention extending these to people across the community), and the grave inequalities that can render such illness work more or less impossible 'independently'. In what follows, we show how, by identifying those living with chronic medical conditions as particularly at risk and by asking them to self-isolate, Denmark's efforts to control the COVID-19 pandemic amplified and highlighted the often laborious work involved in keeping illnesses 'stable', the challenging ways risk is negotiated by those already ill, and the often unrecognised efforts of individuals, families and 'auxiliary' care workers to (self-)manage chronic conditions. We now turn to three ethnographic descriptions of how families experienced their new-found and unsolicited status as 'particularly at risk' of COVID-19 and its complications.

In and out of risk – living with a complex congenital heart defect in a pandemic

'I think the guidelines on what *hjertebørn* [heart-children] should do have been confusing and conflicting ... one day almost isolate and the next day not at all', Anita wrote in an email at the beginning of May 2020, when asked how her heart-child, 10-year-old Mikael, and the rest of the family, were coping during the COVID-19 pandemic. In Denmark, around 16,000 children and youth under 18 years live with a congenital heart defect (CHD) (Hjerteforeningen n.d.); worldwide, this is the most common major birth defect (Linde et al. 2011, 2241). CHDs encompass a broad spectrum of defects from 'simple' (without symptoms or need for treatment) to 'complex' and life-threatening (requiring surgery soon after birth coupled with lifelong follow up) (National Heart, Lung, and Blood Institute 2017). In Denmark today, as in other countries with well-resourced healthcare systems, even some of the most complex CHDs have been transformed into chronic conditions (Jacobsen et al. 2010, 40; Lüscher 2017, 2021).

However, as children with CHDs live longer, it is becoming increasingly clear that many live with risks of complications, deteriorations, further surgical interventions and reduced long-term survival compared to the background population (Larsen et al. 2017; Lüscher 2017, 2021).

For Anita and Mikael's father, Ole, risks related to Mikael's CHDs have been all too clear since his birth. Anita and Ole thought they had welcomed a healthy baby boy to the world, only to learn that Mikael had a complex CHD, needed surgery urgently and might not survive. Mikael has so far undergone three heart surgeries that have completely rebuilt his heart, but this is a temporary solution, and he may require a heart transplant in the future. The risks and high stakes of Mikael's CHD have taken a detrimental toll on Ole, who has struggled with his mental health since the diagnosis, leaving it very much up to Anita to care for Mikael and his younger sister, Maja, as well as provide an income for the family.

Like most families living with CHDs in Denmark, Mikael's family try to de-emphasise the risks of CHDs in their everyday lives. This is encouraged by healthcare providers who urge families to focus on the positives of the present rather than on their children as sick, limited and with a future full of risks. For Mikael's family, living with his health risks is a routine aspect of everyday life. He is vaccinated against influenza and pneumonia and is kept at home if there is much illness in his school, and Mikael, according to his mother, pointed out to a classmate visiting for a playdate, 'in this house, we sanitise our hands!' The outbreak of COVID-19 accentuated such risks and moved them to the forefront of everyday life. It was, in fact, the hand sanitiser that made Anita aware that 'there are actually people who are starting to panic', as the pharmacy was unable to fulfil her routine order of hand sanitiser at the end of February. Fourteen days later, the Danish government announced a national lockdown, which was, as we noted above, to a large extent directed at so-called 'vulnerable groups' such as people with chronic conditions and the elderly.

In the following weeks, it became apparent to Anita that she needed to find out whether Mikael was 'particularly vulnerable', and especially whether he could return to school once the lockdown ended. This proved difficult, as it was for many parents. Calls to The Danish Heart Foundation's 'heart-line' doubled during March–May 2020, and many sought peer advice on the Facebook page of the Foundation's children's club in the same period (around 50 posts with over 1,200 comments). In these early weeks of the pandemic, families came to rely on and expand their caringscapes, as priorities within the national healthcare system shifted towards COVID-19. At first, Mikael's GP deemed him 'at particular risk', much like Anita had interpreted the general guidelines. However, things changed rapidly, and Anita 'panicked when one day it was said [in the guidelines] by both the pediatric cardiologists and the Board of Health that he was at 'particular risk', and then the next day he wasn't!' More phone calls ensued, first unsuccessfully to Mikael's current cardiologist, and then to his former cardiologist, who agreed with the GP. However, Mikael's social worker decided that the decision on whether Anita would be granted compensation for lost earnings, so that she could home-school Mikael, had to be made by a medical consultant who did not know Mikael. As the family had previously experienced collaboration with municipal social workers as rather cumbersome, like many other Danish parents to disabled or chronically ill children (For Lige Vilkår 2019, 2), Anita was quite surprised when she was granted financial compensation.

Each month a new assessment arrives, and Mikael could suddenly fall out of risk in the eyes of the Danish welfare system. As sole provider, this would force Anita to assess whether Mikael's risk of infection from COVID-19 would outweigh the financial risks were she to take unpaid leave from her job as a nursery teacher, which Anita felt made her 'particularly exposed' to infection. Coupled with stories of doctors' experiences of complications from COVID-19 flooding the media, such as blood clots, she and Ole were left extremely confused and worried.

Yet, keeping Mikael at home was not without risks either. Anita had already been forced to defend to colleagues why Ole's mental health problems meant that he could not home-school Mikael. Anita and Ole also had to leave conversations about the pandemic until moments where 'small ears are not listening', as Anita phrased it, because 'it is just difficult for him, when it is something that makes him feel sick'. Mikael's checkups, for example, would cause such unwanted attention to his heart defect every six months. Now, the reminders were daily. One and a half weeks into isolation, Mikael got sick – out of fear Anita thinks. While he vomited, he told her that he was scared. Unfortunately, Mikael's therapy sessions, originally initiated to help him deal with psychological and social problems at school, were also paused. Furthermore, the risks he had so far evaded concerning his 'underlying' CHD now surfaced. When he started therapy again after the lockdown, he told his mother bluntly on the way home that 'you are super lucky that I have survived all of this [e.g. three heart surgeries], because there are not many who do!' Home-schooling, however, relieved Mikael of long school days that often left him physically exhausted. He was also comfortable with less socialising, as his social interactions with peers after school were already limited due to exhaustion but also because he struggled with forging friendships. Yet, Anita realised while home-schooling Mikael, 'he is fine with just sitting on his own. It's not because there is anything wrong with that, but you can get a little weird by just being on your own'. So, although she feared the consequences were he to contract COVID-19, Anita realised that keeping Mikael at home was a 'balancing act'. It involved '[keeping] several balls in the air in terms of when you are doing the wrong or the right thing, and it is the kind of thing you can only know in the future'.

For Mikael's family, this balancing act had to be done in the midst of a dramatic shaking up of the carescapes and chronic care infrastructures on which they normally leaned. Mikael's current cardiologist was impossible to reach; previously routine precautions to avoid infections now caused panic (hand sanitiser) or proved impossible (staying home from school sporadically when there were bouts of influenza); the struggle for compensation for lost earnings was an everyday (uncertain) reality rather than a short-term solution during hospitalisations for surgery; therapy was paused when Mikael perhaps needed it more than ever; and guidelines on CHDs were constantly changing. Their situation exemplifies how depending on what struggles already surround the chronic condition, COVID-19 affects families differently. For this family, exacerbated social isolation, financial problems and mental health issues posed a particular risk that added to those related to Mikael's physical health.

Many children with CHDs were, unlike Mikael, placed outside of risk groups, or were categorised as 'at risk' but still advised to attend kindergarten and school. However, for those 'at risk' isolated at home, the Danish government's attempts to shield people with chronic conditions created a heavy extra burden of risk. Ina, mother of Julie, aged 15 and with a moderate CHD, reflected on the consequences of the COVID-19 pandemic, writing:

> I don't think that the fear will ever recede. ... Now it is not just the congenital condition that is a risk, now there are also external risks that I cannot regulate or control. No matter how much I look after my child and keep distance, it can come to us and ruin an entire family. We cannot shut ourselves in for the rest of our lives, but how do we move on?

Navigating noise in online type 1 diabetes communities during COVID-19

As with congenital heart defects, uncertainty surrounding COVID-19 has been evident within several Danish Facebook communities for people living with type 1 diabetes. News about the unfolding pandemic made it to Danish television in early 2020 and gave rise to new communities on Facebook, where people shared their fears and concerns in the wake of the global lockdown. To meet rising demand for information from the public, doctors created their own Facebook community to take the pressure off clinics and to provide reliable and evidence-based answers to the many questions on COVID-19 from the public. Offshoots within the larger patient-driven Danish online diabetes communities emerged around COVID-19 where interpretations of the government's guidelines were shared and debated: are we at higher risk of contracting COVID-19? Do we experience more severe complications if infected by COVID-19? The flood of information from both news media and from peers within Facebook communities made it difficult for lay people to distinguish between health misunderstandings and facts.

With the rise of social media in the 2000s, and the opportunity to create interest groups on Facebook in 2010, the classical 'field site' has become ever more fragmented and its boundaries fluid (Hine 2015). At the same time, although they are a convenient 24/7 space to share important information, tips and knowledge on how to live with a chronic condition, online peer-to-peer communities have not replaced traditional 'in real life' conversations (Kingod et al. 2017; Borkman 1976). In times of uncertainty and despair when living with a chronic condition that involves complex self-care management regimes, mobile technologies are a valuable part of everyday chronic care infrastructures that enable patients to seek out peer knowledge through a single tap on their smartphone. Hence online caringscapes have come to supplement the support of loved ones through their offers of reciprocal informal care (Kingod 2020).

In Denmark, people living with diabetes co-create and tinker with different types of knowledge both from peers within communities on social media channels and from more conventional authoritative guidelines (Kingod 2018). Tinkering occurs to fit self-care technologies to bodies and medical guidelines to daily living with type 1 diabetes. With the complex chronic homework that goes into keeping type 1 diabetes 'stable', patients seek inspiration from peers online on how to interpret and adjust medical guidelines with the purpose of living a better life with the disease (see also Mattingly et al. 2011). This type of patient-to-patient knowledge is based on everyday embodied experiences that reach into all corners of daily life.

Lisa, mother to an 8-year-old daughter with type 1 diabetes, was confused by the initial authoritative statements in relation to COVID-19 risk for those living with type 1 diabetes. As she explained in a text-based conversation in a restricted Facebook community for mothers of children with type 1 diabetes:

> I don't know if I should let her [daughter] go out at all. I talked to the Danish Diabetes Association and they told me that I should keep her at home and not send her to school. They even wrote that as a relative to a person with diabetes you can work from home to reduce the risk of catching the virus. But then I can see within other Facebook communities that there are great misunderstandings and differing understandings about these guidelines. First, the Ministry of Health said that people with diabetes were at high risk, then they changed it to people with poorly regulated blood sugar and then they were suddenly not at risk at all. Now the Diabetes Association has suggested my girl is at risk again. What should I believe in and do?!

Lisa is referring to contradictory information from Danish health authorities and other government spokespeople that flooded news channels and were recirculated on Facebook in the early weeks and months of the pandemic. Initial information placed people with diabetes in a category of 'high risk' in relation to catching COVID-19. While all citizens are at risk of contracting COVID-19, people with diabetes were given a double 'at risk' status, not only in relation to catching the virus but also to developing severe complications. For many people self-managing type 1 diabetes, being at health risk while immunologically and clinically vulnerable does not necessarily create feelings of being sick (see also Jauho 2019). Still, although the risks were unclear, many people with diabetes self-isolated at home during the first months as the pandemic spread. Lisa's daughter has lived with type 1 diabetes for several years, and Lisa sees her as perfectly normal and capable of doing the same everyday life things as her friends. This is confirmed at quarterly check-ups at the clinic where her daughter receives her long-term blood sugar measurement, a haemoglobin A1c test that indicates her average blood sugar level over the past two to three months. Lisa uses this number as an indication of how well her daughter is managing her type 1 diabetes; for several years, this number has been within the 'normal' range.

Lisa is an active member of several Facebook communities. These have become an important part of her family's caringscapes and have enabled her to emotionally cope with the heavy burden of receiving her daughter's diagnosis years ago. She remembers that she was terrified and devastated, harbouring 'forbidden feelings' about her daughter as 'broken and fragile'. By lurking in a larger community on Facebook and belonging to a smaller private group, she experienced support from like-minded mothers with children at the same age. For years, Lisa was a member of a closed community targeting the specific insulin pump brand her daughter uses. She is also a member of a community that encourages and advises people on how to 'hack' their insulin pumps with complicated algorithms in order to fit the technologies to bodies and daily lives (Gavrila et al. 2019).

With the first cases of coronavirus, the government quickly closed institutions and schools; only grocery stores and pharmacies remained open. Lisa found a good rhythm in home-schooling her daughter, and she felt safe with the recommendation to distance her family from other people. When the government announced that primary schools would be the first institutions to re-open, Lisa felt unsure what to do. Confused about the different categories of risk in relation to diabetes, she joined a newly established Facebook community, 'My child should not be a guinea pig for COVID-19',[4] which quickly gained more than 38,000 members. She checked the online activities of this community several times a day to receive support and guidance in her own decision-making processes about whether or not to send her child to school. Navigating an online sea of information was not easy, as posts turned into long threads with contradictory answers on governmental restrictions and guidelines. Online noise is a side effect of the bombardment of information on news and social media channels (whether contradictory or not) that people living with type 1 diabetes in Denmark must process, interpret and attune their lives to (Kingod and Cleal 2019). With the strength of aligned voices of parental fear, Lisa concluded that her daughter should stay home for another 14 days, so she could see whether the situation in Denmark had stabilised, with infections and hospitalisation rates declining. Lisa would lurk within the large community, and then discuss answers from this community with members in the closed group. Members of this smaller group have known each other for several years and they meet offline, and Lisa feels safest in expressing her concerns among peers that she knows and trusts. Lisa and peer mothers remain unconvinced about the safety of the situation. They keep themselves and each other updated online, share news feeds within the group, and discuss school and governmental guidelines. The category and presence of double risk will stay with them for a long time. Further, they have become increasingly exposed to the noise of massive amounts of health information. With changes in caringscapes and carescapes, in terms of the growing availability of peer-to-peer exchanges on social media between quarterly check-ups at the clinic and the shifting of resources towards COVID-19, many forms of type 1 diabetes care, formal and informal, moved online. Lisa and her peers were placed in yet another 'at risk' category – the uncertainty of how to evaluate health information they found online – and so she devised a strategy of discussing it with other mothers in a smaller Facebook group.

Cancelled appointments – disrupted social care among 'frail' seniors

'Up we go', announced Wicky, the home care worker, as she raised Viggo's elevation bed to her hip level. It was 8:15 a.m. on a cold Monday morning in February 2020 as news of a 'mystery virus' that had devastated Wuhan and since spread to Italy and Spain was making headlines in Denmark. Wicky was there to wake Viggo and help him get washed and dressed. Viggo contributed as best he could by taking off his shirt and following Wicky's guidance. They chatted a bit during the work. 'So, did your family visit this Friday?' Wicky asked. 'Yeah, my son was here. He brought *fastelavnsboller* [cream buns]', Viggo recalled with a wide smile. 'Haha, you should have seen the blood sugar', he continued. Wicky laughed. She helped him get dressed and moved his 100 kg body to the wheelchair.[5] Viggo was diagnosed with diabetes in 1991. Years of uncontrolled blood sugar had damaged the nerves in his feet, and eventually a wound on his heel resulted in untreatable gangrene. Four years ago, he lost the leg. He stayed for a short time at a rehabilitation centre, and had difficulty adapting after he returned home. His house was not fit for a wheelchair, and, despite daily home care visits, he was alone and had no one to help him on a regular basis. One morning, struggling to reach something on a shelf, he fell and broke his remaining leg. Afterwards, he was granted the penthouse senior apartment in a new multi-storey building and received more intensive home care.

Viggo had grown up, with four siblings, in a small apartment in a rough neighbourhood of southern Copenhagen. After primary school, he joined the Danish Railway Network and worked for 40 years as a train conductor. When he was diagnosed with diabetes, he was, in train terminology, 'dropped off', and took early retirement. Besides the diabetes, Viggo suffered from chronic pain and depression, and took medicines for raised blood pressure, raised cholesterol, oedema and vitamin deficiency. In total, to manage his various conditions, he took 17 pills per day.

During the last two decades, therefore, as with nine other interlucotors in a project on 'frail' elderly and medicines, Viggo intimately experienced health inequalities as someone from a particular socio-economic background living with a multitude of illnesses (Lau 2020). As a result of their 'lifestyles' through many decades, these elderly are aging 'unhealthily'; when the COVID-19 pandemic struck, they were already at risk of functional decline and early death. These seniors are all dependent on help from a variety of social and healthcare institutions, including home care – a comprehensive, yet strictly standardised, carescape made possible by the Danish welfare state (Tufte and Dahl 2016) – and, due to high levels of multimorbidity, their daily living is primarily centred around and shaped by chronic homework (Mattingly et al. 2011). For Viggo, as for most seniors receiving daily home care services, every day looked more or less the same. A helper from the home care team woke him up in the morning. Twice a week, Monday and Thursday, he was provided an assisted shower. Afterwards, he ate his breakfast and drank his coffee while listening to the radio. At 10:00 a.m., the nurse called him, or dropped by to monitor his blood sugar and give him insulin injections. Afterwards, Viggo went on an outdoor trip; most days this included some kind of visit to a health clinic. Twice a week, he rolled himself down to the nursing clinic, where the pressure bandages on his leg were replaced. He went for regular checks at a diabetes clinic, an eye clinic and a foot therapist. Some trips included assisted transport, which required a lot of waiting time and often took the entire day. On other days, he brought himself across the parking lot to visit his general practitioner, the physiotherapy clinic or the pharmacy. In the afternoon, he often stopped at the grocery store at the ground level of his apartment building to buy bread, cold cuts and condiments for his breakfast and lunch. Dinner was provided by a private distributor commissioned by the welfare state, responsible for delivering microwaveable meals twice weekly. He ate most meals alone at home, but occasionally his daughter and her partner would drop in and prepare dinner, or his sister would take him out to eat at a local cafe. In the evening, Viggo called his children or sister and watched a movie while waiting, first for the nurse and his nightly insulin shot, then for the home care worker to help him back to bed.

In summing up these daily routines of chronic living that shaped his everyday life, Viggo's caringscape seemed mainly connected to the chronic care infrastructures related to addressing his medical conditions and preventing decline. But it would be a great mistake not to include the social interactions embedded in these infrastructures: it was exactly these interactions which constituted enough *enacted togetherness* (Nyman et al. 2012) to create meaning in Viggo's daily life, hence to keep a lurking social death at bay. Viggo thrived in the company of others and suffered in his homely solitude. To counteract feelings of loneliness, the radio or the TV was constantly turned on. Viggo used his phone frequently and, despite deteriorating sight and fine motor skills, used Facebook and other social media. However, what counted most in 'keeping up spirits', as he framed it, were the daily trips out of the apartment. He always dressed up, even for the short strolls down to the nursing clinic. His hair was combed and he wore a fancy flat cap, giving him a slightly modern look. Viggo cared about his appearance. For some time, it had bothered him that he wore a slipper on his remaining foot, as it was almost impossible to find a nice and tidy shoe that would fit his oedematous ankle. He was full of joy the day the local shoe store finally brought him a tailored shoe. Appearance was important because Viggo used his outdoor trips to get in contact with other people. These trips meant so much to him, because, as he said, he needed the conversations with others to 'feel alive'. The trips were pivotal to Viggo's everyday life; they allowed social interactions and provided meaningfulness; when returning home in the afternoon, he felt he had accomplished something that day; he had seen and talked to other people.

For Viggo, the lockdown and self-isolation that came into force on 11 March 2020 dramatically altered these daily routines and disrupted his already confined social life. Viggo was, like other so-called vulnerable persons, told to stay at home as much as possible. Previously daily trips out of the apartment were reduced to a minimum, and instead substituted with more movies and, for Viggo, unhealthy solitude. Visits from family and friends were restricted. No more coffee chats or cream buns. His family kept away to minimise the risk of bringing the virus into his home, as an act of caring. Yet, for Viggo, the cancelled appointments changed the foundation not only of his chronic care work but, more essentially, of *social care*. As COVID-19 changed Viggo's carescape in terms of the availability of clinical and social resources in his daily life, it automatically altered his caringscape and subsequently Viggo's ability to care for himself.

Despite these efforts to keep Viggo out of harm's way, on 23 March 2020 Viggo died from coronavirus infection and its complications.

Care interrupted

Three weeks into Denmark's lockdown in late March, just as Viggo's passing had added yet another COVID-19 casualty to the climbing daily mortality numbers published in newspapers and online media, Prime Minister Frederiksen held another of her regular press briefings, this time with a special message for those 'vulnerable groups' who had been advised to self-isolate: 'It pains me to say this to our elderly and most vulnerable: you will need to adjust your lives against your risk of contracting COVID-19. We are asking the weakest to be the strongest. This is a harsh message' (Statsministeriet 2020b). While Denmark emerged out of its 'first wave' relatively unscathed when compared to Italy, Brazil and the United States, we have seen here through the experiences of Mikael, Lisa and Viggo, their families and the healthcare professionals on whom they rely, how COVID-19 has generated new forms of chronic homework, concern, worries and in Viggo's case, his death. As we have shown, in the past two decades, Denmark's healthcare system has come to be reconfigured around *kronikere* who lead lives with what the National Health Board calls 'stable illnesses'. Yet, as the disruptions brought on by COVID-19 have shown, speaking of 'stable illnesses' belies the complex efforts that go into maintaining stability, and masks the genuine concerns that the pandemic brought as families struggled to come to grips with what it meant to be 'particularly at risk'.

The navigation and interpretation of risk in relation to COVID-19 has become an extra burden for people with chronic conditions and their families. These families were already leading lives with many forms of risk related to their medical conditions and their socio-economic conditions, and COVID-19 added to already existing anxieties and difficulties. While the National Board of Health retracted its call for a massive rerouting of resources to address the pandemic, and COVID-19 units were closed down in a number of hospitals due to a lack of patients during the summer months, Denmark's 'second wave' took hold towards the end of 2020, again leading doctors and nurses to warn of the knock-on consequences and necessary reprioritisations that rising hospitalisation rates entail. Likewise, the worries that a circulating novel coronavirus have generated for people living with (multiple) chronic conditions have not dissipated and will not do so any time soon.

Chronic conditions do not disappear because a pandemic arrives. While these 'other' conditions are (however provisionally) moved to the bottom of the healthcare agenda and prioritisation lists within healthcare systems, disrupted treatment and monitoring, calls for self-isolation and designating the chronically ill as 'vulnerable groups' who are 'particularly at risk', all serve to move 'stable' chronic conditions to the forefront of everyday life for patients and their families, much more so than in 'non-pandemic' times. The chronic care infrastructures, carescapes and caringscapes that had coalesced around people living with conditions like congenital heart defects, type 1 diabetes and multiple chronic conditions have been unsettled by a pandemic that has raised questions about how healthcare systems should be financed and organised in the coming years and decades, not least in the face of looming austerity. In the months and years to come, we will learn how a communicable condition like COVID-19 has reshaped care- and caringscapes, hence complicated and unsettled the chronic care infrastructures and chronic homework routines aimed at keeping chronic conditions 'stable'.

Acknowledgements

Sofie Rosenlund Lau would like to acknowledge Velux Fonden for supporting her research. Marie Kofod Svensson would like to acknowledge the Danish Heart Foundation and Natasja Kingod Steno Diabetes Centre for their continued funding. Ayo Wahlberg acknowledges the European Research Council (grant no. ERC-2014-STG-639275). All authors would like to thank the families who shared their experiences during the first months of the COVID-19 pandemic in Denmark.

Notes

1. Throughout this chapter, we have translated quotes from Danish politicians, policy papers and interlocutors, which originally appeared or were in Danish.
2. A December 2020 study from the Danish Cancer Association confirmed these fears, showing that there were 2,800 fewer cancer diagnoses from March to May 2020; an early indication of knock-on consequences when resources are shifted in such a massive way (Munch 2020).
3. Each project was ethically approved by relevant authorities nationally and at the University of Copenhagen.
4. Original in Danish: *Mit barn skal ikke være forsøgskanin for covid-19*.
5. For empirical insights from Viggo's daily life and passing, see also Lau, Kristensen and Oxlund (2020).

References

Bergeron-Boucher, Marie-Pier, Jim Oeppen, Niels Vilstrup Holm, Hanne Melgaard Nielsen, Rune Lindahl-Jacobsen and Maarten Jan Wensink. 2019. 'Understanding differences in cancer survival between populations: A new approach and application to breast cancer survival differentials between Danish regions'. *International Journal of Environmental Research and Public Health* 16(17): 3093. https://doi.org/10.3390/ijerph16173093.
Board of Health. 2020. Sundhedsstyrelsen Sagsnr. 04-0101-35. Directive no. 04-0101-35. Copenhagen, Denmark.
Borkman, Thomasina. 1976. 'Experiential knowledge: A new concept for the analysis of self-help groups'. *Social Service Review* 50(3): 445–56.
Bowlby, Sophie and Linda McKie. 2019. 'Care and caring: An ecological framework'. *Area* 51 (3): 532–39. https://doi.org/10.1111/area.12511.
Christensen, Loa Teglgaard. 2020. *Crafting Valued Old Lives: Quandaries in Danish home care*, PhD dissertation, Department of Anthropology, University of Copenhagen.
Corbin, Juliet and Anselm Strauss. 1985. 'Managing chronic illness at home: Three lines of work'. *Qualitative Sociology* 8(3): 224–47. https://doi.org/10.1007/BF00989485.
Corbin, Juliet and Anselm Strauss. 1988. *Unending Care and Work: Managing chronic illness at home*. San Francisco, CA: Jossey-Bass Inc. Publishers.

For Lige Vilkår. 2019. 'Undersøgelse blandt forældre til børn med handicap eller kronisk sygdom: Deres samarbejde med kommunen og tilknytning til arbejdsmarkedet'. Copenhagen, Denmark: For Lige Vilkår. Accessed 20 November 2020. https://forlige.dk/images/For_Lige_Vilkaar_survey.pdf.

Frandsen, Martin S. and Peter Triantafillou. 2011. 'Biopower at the molar level: Liberal government and the invigoration of Danish society'. *Social Theory & Health* 9(3): 203–23. https://doi.org/10.1057/sth.2011.2.

Frederiksen, Mette. 2020. 'Skal lære at leve med virus'. Accessed 20 November 2020. https://sport.tv2.dk/video/RjUxSEgybXlQN1R5QVZRVkFLTktXOUNzajF0SFY3T1M.

Gavrila, Valerie, Ashley Garrity, Emily Hirschfeld, Breann Edwards and M. Joyce Lee. 2019. Peer support through a diabetes social media community. *Journal of Diabetes Science and Technology* 13(3): 493–7. https://doi.org/10.1177/1932296818818828.

Government of Denmark. 2002. *Sund hele livet*. Copenhagen, Denmark: Ministry of Health.

Hjerteforeningen. n.d. 'Medfødt hjertefejl'. Hjertetal. Accessed 22 June 2020. https://hjerteforeningen.shinyapps.io/HjerteTal/?_inputs_&outcome_chd=%22Enhver%20medf%C3%B8dt%20hjertefejl%22&navbar=%22chd%22&outcome=%22Alle%20hjerte-kar-sygdomme%22.

Hine, C. (2015). *Ethnography for the Internet: Embedded, embodied and everyday*. London: Taylor & Francis.

Jacobsen, Joes Ramsøe, Keld Sørensen, Jørgen Videbæk and Lars Søndergaard. 2010. 'Arbejdsgruppen for medfødte hjertesygdomme'. Dansk Cardiologisk Selskab. Accessed 17 September 2018. https://www.cardio.dk/dcs-50-ars-jubilaeumsberetning-2014.

Jauho, Mikko. 2019. 'Patients-in-waiting or chronically healthy individuals? People with elevated cholesterol talk about risk'. *Sociology of Health & Illness*. https://doi.org/10.1111/1467-9566.12866.

Juel, Knud and Kamper-Jørgensen, Finn. 1989. *Udviklingen i sundhedstilstanden i 80'erne. Nogle sundhedsmæssige udfordringer for 90'erne*, Copenhagen, Denmark: Dansk Institut for Klinisk Epidemiologi.

Kingod, N. 2018. 'The tinkering m-patient: Co-constructing knowledge on how to live with type 1 diabetes through Facebook searching and sharing and offline tinkering with self-care'. *Health* 24(2): 152–68. https://doi.org/10.1177/1363459318800140.

Kingod, N. 2020. The tinkering m-patient: Co-constructing knowledge on how to live with type 1 diabetes through Facebook searching and sharing and offline tinkering with self-care. Health (London). 24(2): 152–68.

Kingod, N. and B. Cleal. 2019. 'Noise as dysappearance: Attuning to a life with type 1 diabetes'. *Body & Society* 25(4): 55–75. https://doi.org/10.1177/1357034X19861671.

Kingod, N., B. Cleal, A. Wahlberg and G. Husted. 2017. 'Online peer-to-peer communities in the daily lives of people with chronic illness: A qualitative systematic review'. *Qualitative Health Research* 27(1): 89–99.

Kingod, N. and D. Grabowski. 2020. 'In a vigilant state of chronic disruption: How parents with a young child with type 1 diabetes negotiate events and moments of uncertainty'. *Sociology of Health & Illness* 42(6): 1473–87. https://doi.org/10.1111/1467-9566.13123.

Kjellberg, P.K., R. Ibsen and J. Kjellberg. 2011. 'From health care to rehabilitation. Knowledge and recommendations.' (In Danish). Copenhagen, Denmark: The Danish Committee for Health Education.

Knudsen, Sine G. and Peter Triantafillou. 2020. 'Lifestylisation of the social: The government of diabetes care in Denmark'. *Health*. January 2020. https://doi.org/10.1177/1363459319899454.

Langstrup, Henriette. 2013. 'Chronic care infrastructures and the home: Chronic care infrastructures and the home'. *Sociology of Health and Illness* 35(7): 1008–22. https://doi.org/10.1111/1467-9566.12013.

Larsen, Signe H., Morten Olsen, Kristian Emmertsen and Vibeke E. Hjortdal. 2017. 'Interventional treatment of patients with congenital heart disease'. *Journal of the American College of Cardiology* 69(22): 2725–32. https://doi.org/10.1016/j.jacc.2017.03.587.

Lau, Sofie Rosenlund. 2020. 'Like playing Kalaha: Polypharmacy in public home care'. *Tidsskriftet Gerontologi* 36(1): 8–13.

Lau, Sofie Rosenlund, Nanna Hauge Kristensen and Bjarke Oxlund. 2020. 'Taming and timing death during COVID-19: The ordinary passing of an old man in an extraordinary time'. *Anthropology and Aging* 40(2): 207–20. http://dx.doi.org/10.5195/aa.2020.319.

Linde, Denise van der, Elisabeth E.M. Konings, Maarten A. Slager, Maarten Witsenburg, Willem A. Helbing, Johanna J.M. Takkenberg and Jolien W. Roos-Hesselink. 2011. 'Birth prevalence of congenital heart disease worldwide'. *Journal of the American College of Cardiology* 58(21): 2241–47. https://doi.org/10.1016/j.jacc.2011.08.025.

Lüscher, Thomas F. 2017. 'Congenital heart disease: Some progress, but still the challenge of a lifetime!' *European Heart Journal* 38(26): 2021–23. https://doi.org/10.1093/eurheartj/ehx372.

Manderson, Lenore and Ayo Wahlberg. 2020. 'Chronic living in a communicable world'. *Medical Anthropology* 39(5): 428–39. https://doi.org/10.1080/01459740.2020.1761352.

Mattingly, Cheryl, Lone Grøn and Lotte Meinert. 2011. 'Chronic homework in emerging borderlands of healthcare'. *Culture, Medicine, and Psychiatry* 35(3): 347–75. https://doi.org/10.1007/s11013-011-9225-z.

Ministry of Health (1994). Levetiden i Danmark. Middellevetidsudvalget (Publikation 2). Copenhagen, Denmark: Sundhedsministeriet.

Munch, Per. 2020. 'Formand for lægerne: "Folk bruger deres liv på at frygte corona, mens de får kræft"'. *Politiken*, 9 December 2020. https://politiken.dk/forbrugogliv/sundhedogmotion/art8027647/Formand-for-l%C3%A6gerne-%C2%BBFolk-bruger-deres-liv-p%C3%A5-at-frygte-corona-mens-de-f%C3%A5r-kr%C3%A6ft%C2%AB.

Møller, Albert S. and Sebastian Goos. 2020. 'Stigende smitte fører til aflyste operationer på stribe – nu sender læger og sygeplejersker bøn til regeringen'. *TV2 Nyheder*. 11 December 2020. Accessed 20 December 2020. https://nyheder.tv2.dk/2020-12-11-stigende-smitte-foerer-til-aflyste-operationer-paa-stribe-nu-sender-laeger-og.

National Heart, Lung, and Blood Institute. 2017. 'What are congenital heart defects?' Accessed 24 October 2017. https://www.nhlbi.nih.gov/health/health-topics/topics/chd#.

Nielsen, Kasper Buur. 2020. 'Hjerte-og kræftoverlæger i opråb: Massivt corona-fokus kan koste liv'. Accessed 24 September 2020. https://www.tv2fyn.dk/fyn/hjerte-og-kraeftoverlaeger-i-opraab-massivt-corona-fokus-kan-koste-liv.

Nyman, Anneli, Staffan Josephsson and Gunilla Isaksson. 2012. 'Being part of an enacted togetherness: Narratives of elderly people with depression'. *Journal of Aging Studies* 26 (4): 410–18. https://doi.org/10.1016/j.jaging.2012.05.003.

Statsministeriet. 2020a. 'Statsminister Mette Frederiksens indledning på pressemøde i Statsministeriet om corona-virus den 11. marts 2020'. Accessed 24 September 2020. https://www.stm.dk/statsministeren/taler/statsminister-mette-frederiksens-indledning-paa-pressemoede-i-statsministeriet-om-corona-virus-den-11-marts-2020/.

Statsministeriet. 2020b. 'Statsminister Mette Frederiksens indledning på pressemøde i Statsministeriet om corona-virus mandag den 30. Marts 2020'. Accessed 24 September 2020. https://www.stm.dk/statsministeren/taler/statsminister-mette-frederiksens-indledning-paa-pressemoede-i-statsministeriet-om-corona-virus-mandag-den-30-marts-2020/.

Svensson, Marie Kofod, Ayo Wahlberg and Gunnar H Gislason. 2020. 'Chronic paradoxes: A systematic review of qualitative family perspectives on living with congenital heart defects'. *Qualitative Health Research* 30(1): 119–32. https://doi.org/10.1177/1049732319869909.

Tufte, Pernille and Hanne Marlene Dahl. 2016. 'Navigating the field of temporally framed care in the Danish home care sector'. *Sociology of Health & Illness* 38(1): 109–122. https://doi.org/10.1111/1467-9566.12343.

Vallgårda, Signild. 2011. 'Addressing individual behaviours and living conditions: Four Nordic public health policies'. *Scandinavian Journal of Public Health* 39(6): 6–10. https://doi.org/10.1177/1403494810378922.

Wahlberg, Ayo and Nikolas Rose. 2015. 'The governmentalization of living: Calculating global health'. *Economy and Society* 44(1): 60–90. https://doi.org/10.1080/03085147.2014.983830.

Wahlberg, Ayo. 2018. 'The vitality of disease'. In *The Palgrave Handbook of Biology and Society*, edited by M. Meloni, J. Cromby, D. Fitzgerald and S. Lloyd, pp. 727–48. London: Palgrave Macmillan.

Wind, Gitte and Peter Vedsted. 2008. 'Om kronisk sygdom'. *Tidsskrift for Forskning i Sygdom og Samfund* 5(9): 5–16. https://doi.org/10.7146/tfss.v5i9.1324.

18
Care within or out of reach

Fantasies of care and connectivity in the time of the COVID-19 pandemic

Earvin Charles Cabalquinto and Tanja Ahlin

Information and Communication Technologies (ICTs) have become an integral part of contemporary society. They are fundamental in forging and sustaining everyday interactions, as mobile phones and online channels enable a sense of co-presence (Licoppe 2004; Baldassar et al. 2016), intimacy (Vincent and Fortunati 2009) and care practices (Ahlin 2018) across geographic distances. Individuals can choose from a range of mobile devices, online channels and mobile applications, which give shape to different polymedia environments (Madianou and Miller 2012). With the COVID-19 pandemic, smartphones, social media channels and a wide range of mobile applications have served as lifelines. As the ongoing health crisis constrains people's movements and social interactions because of distancing requirements, travel bans and lockdowns, ICTs have been key to sustaining relationships in already networked societies.

During the COVID-19 pandemic, global technology corporations have adopted the language of care to promote digital connectivity. For instance, Facebook launched its spectrum of care-themed reactions, and thematic 'we are all in this together' stickers have been embedded in Facebook Messenger. Instagram, also run by Facebook, introduced a sticker signalling the call to 'stay at home' to encourage people to self-isolate and practise social distancing. The impulse and imperative to care crystallised in the form of a 'care emoji', a smiley face hugging a heart, launched by Facebook in April 2020. Such digital objects reflect one of the many ways through which online platforms highlight virtual connection as a form of self and social care.

In this chapter, we critically examine how selected online platforms appropriate the notion of care and its provision as key in promoting digital communication during a pandemic. We focus on how Facebook, Google, YouTube and Instagram deploy discursive strategies to reiterate the importance of digital practices in the delivery and access of care – individual, social and corporatised. We chose these platforms, which are global, although most popular in Anglo-American and European parts of the world, to provide a snapshot of how commonly used online channels reconfigure and position their services during a crisis.

Our inquiry is guided by three steps. We first consider how online platforms have adopted and framed the rhetoric of care thus far during the pandemic. Second, we describe various digitally mediated activities that online platforms promote and mobilise as a form of care. Lastly, we interrogate how the articulation of 'staying connected and informed' in a health crisis context facilitates digital surveillance, profit accumulation and digital exclusion in a networked society. In the study that informs this chapter, we conducted a textual analysis (Flick 2011) of the community guidelines of online platforms from April to May 2020 by paying attention to how the vocabulary of care was used in online texts and narratives. Scholars have previously used this method efficiently to analyse the deployment of discursive and emotionally charged contents to promote online platform use among dispersed individuals (Peile 2014; Cabalquinto and Wood-Bradley 2020). We then contrasted care-related themes that arise from our textual analysis of the online platforms' community guidelines to several studies on the benefits and limits of digital connectivity as expressions of care.

Social media channels are not only created to facilitate sociality and connectivity. Rather, business protocols and a system of governance established by technology companies shape the operation of online platforms. An individual's online interactions and activities are recorded, segregated, stored and even sold to third parties (Helmond 2015; van Dijck 2012, 2013). Online platforms use convenience and connectivity to conceal the lack of transparency in collecting and manipulating data to amplify profit and individual control (van Dijck 2013). Additionally, through targeted and effective advertising, online platforms become essential tools for profit accumulation and mobility control (Andrejevic 2003). In this chapter, we engage with these key issues on the operations of online platforms, particularly pinpointing how technology companies frame and legitimise digital connectivity during the pandemic.

Overall, our focus is on how social media platforms exploit care to achieve their business goals. We examine how technology companies utilise various mechanisms to promote digital connectivity as a 'lifeline' in enabling a secure and safe way of managing one's wellbeing, and sustaining intimate relationships during the COVID-19 pandemic. We argue that the strategies of the four examined online platforms, in positioning social media use as 'essential' in dealing with the pandemic, necessitates a critical investigation. Such an inquiry is crucial because the practices of technology companies are often embedded in the realms of entrepreneurship, data governance and digital inequalities. In the following sections, we highlight how Facebook, Google, YouTube and Instagram promote a digitally connected, equitable and safe environment – accessible to some but a fantasy to others.

Digital care in pandemic times

ICTs have played an important part in supporting care well before the onset of the pandemic. This includes the role of ICTs in care in studies of transnational families. Baldassar and colleagues (2007, 2014, 2016), for example, have shown how the use of mobile phones and online channels in caregiving at a distance is informed by family obligations, individual (financial, practical and other) capacities and the negotiation of commitments. To explicitly emphasise how technologies influence care at a distance, ICTs in transnational family care have been further analysed through a theoretical approach grounded in science and technology studies. Within this approach, care is described as something that is enacted through practices in which people, social systems and technologies are involved (Mol et al. 2010). Thus, care is enacted within 'transnational care collectives', which include people and non-human actors: mobile phones, webcams and online platforms (Ahlin 2018). The impact of ICTs on family care practices has been described as detrimental in some cases (Turkle 2012; Wajcman 2015) and positive in others, particularly at times of crisis (Horst and Miller 2006; Brown 2016). In the context of crisis, dispersed individuals enact 'crisis caregiving' (Baldassar 2014) by increasing both cross-border mobility and digital communication. Such studies have shown that digital technologies play an essential part in shaping what care comes to mean and how it is practiced when physical distance is introduced among people.

In our analysis here, we add a third party to the mix of people and ICTs in care, namely the technological companies that provide the infrastructure for ICTs to function. We critically interrogate the nuances of mediated care by focusing on how technology companies deploy various strategies in promoting their online services as key in the transfer of care during a crisis. In the context of a global pandemic, how are care practices articulated, represented and deployed by online platforms?

We approach the discursive articulation of mediated care as a by-product of the socio-cultural, economic and political structures of online social platforms (Light et al. 2016). These platforms operate through business protocols and systems of governance that capture, analyse and commodify the personal data of individual users (van Dijck 2013). To ensure the continued use of online platforms by individuals and corporations, companies frame connectedness through digital media as inevitable in maintaining personal relationships (Helmond 2015) and highlight how sharing one's personal experiences on social media is a form of caring for valued individuals (John 2013). At the same time, the architecture of online platforms (which includes easy-to-code likes, shares and emoticons), facilitates the processes of collection, value making and commodification of personal data (Wahl-Jorgensen 2018). Technological companies that own online platforms rationalise their collecting, storing and processing of personal data through the rhetoric of convenience (van Dijck 2013). Yet scholars such as Andrejevic (2003) have critiqued such use of the notions of comfort and connectedness, arguing that enterprises deploy such rhetorical mechanisms to subject individual social media users to commodification and control.

In reflecting on the politics of care rhetoric appropriated by technology companies in their operations during the COVID-19 pandemic, we draw on the conceptual frame of 'fantasy production' (Tadiar 2004). Tadiar (2004) proposes this concept as a fruitful notion for her analysis of various texts, discourses and strategies of the Philippine government in sustaining and advancing its economy through privatisation, international partnerships and global connections. For Tadiar, fantasy production denotes the imaginaries of those in power to reinforce the regime of profit accumulation, domination and marginalisation. For instance, the ideals of modernisation or security are often articulated through the mutual partnerships of an elite and oligarchic government and multinational corporations and international companies. In this arrangement, individuals in privileged positions implement various mechanisms to realise visions of advancement, including the privatisation and deregulation of social welfare services. As a result, these individuals and their institutions accumulate profit while those with limited or no resources struggle to achieve a good life (Tadiar 2004). In the Philippines, people from lower socioeconomic classes often have no access to a stable income due to the privatisation of public services and social welfare systems; consequently, this leads them to migrate abroad in search of work opportunities.

Ultimately, the fantasy of production reveals that the imagination of conditions or outcomes of those in a privileged position remain an aspiration for those with limited resources, living in poor conditions. This proposition, we argue, echoes the contemporary visions, operations and strategies of business-oriented technology companies in promoting digital connectivity as a powerful means for survival and safety, and for sustaining a business-as-usual modality.

The economies of a digital lifeline

The data from the four online platforms that we examined show that technology companies have been consistent in communicating values of connectivity, convenience and support during the COVID-19 pandemic. The language of 'being there' for the consumers serves as a strategy for technology companies to position themselves as supportive and 'caring'. By communicating the relevance of services during challenging times, corporations develop and even improve their ability to sustain the relationship between their services and the target market, leading to the accumulation of profit (Hyken 2017). In our close and critical reading of the community guidelines of Facebook, Google, YouTube and Instagram, we uncovered three key categories through which online platforms communicate care: (1) a space for enacting digital wellness, (2) connected communities and (3) a credible digital resource hub in a pandemic. We found that through the rhetoric of care, the prescribed activities in online spaces link to surveillance, profit accumulation and digital inequalities. Through these findings we flesh out the fantasy of care in the digital realm.

Prescribing digital wellness

The online platforms that we examined each highlighted the importance of staying connected to family members and friends while being at home during the pandemic, framing care in ways that showed how digital corporations articulate 'caring about' their users in turbulent times. To start with, online platforms developed phrases such as 'stay close' (Facebook Messenger), 'keep people safe and informed' (Facebook), 'stay connected and informed' (Google), 'stay home with me' (YouTube) and 'Keeping people informed, safe and supported' (Instagram). Such phrases highlight the vital role that online platforms are seen to play in supporting people to cope, while simultaneously promoting physical distance, safety and knowledge. Further, effective taglines often involved prescribing digital activities for care. For instance, Facebook promoted the importance of chat, voice and videocalls to generate a sense of closeness while practising physical distancing: 'Call friends and family to hear a familiar voice. Make a video call to feel close when you're not together' (Facebook 2020a). YouTube (2020) emphasised physical distancing through a wide range of 'timely tips' in the form of playlists to highlight for various indoor activities, such as working out, cooking, crafting and so on. Here are some examples (YouTube 2020):

Workout with me – At Home #WithMe: Turn your home into your personal gym with these exercises that require just a pair of dumbbells or no equipment at all.
Cook with me – At Home #WithMe: Join creators in their kitchens to chop, sauté and cook up a feast with these videos made to accompany you during your own meal prep.
Plant with me – At Home #WithMe: Exercise your green thumb by repotting, watering, and online shopping for new plants.

With such campaigns, the online platforms illuminate a broad range of digital activities in which their users could engage from the safety of their homes while physically distanced from others.

Further, online platforms incorporated emotionally laden features (Wahl-Jorgensen 2018) such as care-themed digital artefacts. For instance, Facebook Messenger introduced an augment reality filter, GIFs, stickers, emojis and other features (Facebook Messenger 2020). Facebook (2020b) also allowed individual users to use the #SafeHands profile sticker. Instagram (2020) promoted the stay home sticker for stories and YouTube (2020) introduced the hashtag #WithMe, which content producers could use to categorise recorded videos. Google urged people to 'stay home and save lives' through an especially designed Doodle (Google 2020a). These digital designs primarily promoted ways of managing one's wellbeing and showing care for others by staying at home. Such practices are grounded in the idea of networked connectivity, a notion which suggests that individuals enact an imagined and ambient co-presence with distant others (Madianou 2016). Ultimately, the creative features of Facebook, Google, YouTube and Instagram promoted intimate, personalised and ambient connectivity during the pandemic, in the context of prescribed physical distancing associated with lockdowns and travel bans.

Connected communities

Online platforms commonly employed the word 'community' in promoting digital connectedness, and they specifically referred to education-based communities, business communities and local communities. For instance, Facebook Messenger (2020) promoted the use of group voice and video calls for educators, free messaging tools for business customers, and messenger for communities of faith, civic organisations or activity groups. The following examples are from the Facebook Messenger (2020) website entitled 'Here are some ways that Messenger can help you stay together during the pandemic':

> Educators: Messenger can help you stay connected with your community even when you can't be together in person. Communicate updates or check in on each other with group voice and video calls.
>
> Local community: Whether it's a community of faith, civic organisation or activity group, this climate of uncertainty has made maintaining personal connections with those in our community more important than ever.

Facebook (2020b) also encouraged users to use the hashtag #Healthy AtHome and #SafeHands. For the former, individuals were encouraged to record and upload a video of their healthy household activities to the World Health Organization's social media channels using the hashtag #HealthyAtHome. For the latter, individuals were invited to record themselves while washing their hands and to share their video to social media channels using the hashtag #SafeHands. YouTube (2020) encouraged individual users to engage with a community of 'creators' who presented different skills, activities and performances, and, if they wanted to create a video, to use the hashtag #WithMe (YouTube 2020). Google highlighted the 'Stay Home. Save Lives' campaign, mapping out the five ways to 'help stop coronavirus': (1) Stay home as much as you can, (2) Keep a safe distance, (3) Wash hands often, (4) Cover your cough and (5) Sick? Call ahead (Google 2020b). Google also highlighted the use of training resources and Google Hangout to enable remote working, learning and the development of skills, career or business (Google 2020b). Lastly, Instagram showcased the video chat feature, allowing connectivity among different individuals online (Instagram 2020). Further, the 'Stay Home' sticker was added and users could opt to include this sticker in their Instagram story. The sticker promotes the act of staying at home and performing social distancing (Instagram 2020).

Credible digital resource hub

Digital corporations marketed their online tools and services as credible sources to deal with and combat the effects of the pandemic. Technology companies forged partnerships with health organisations to promote and legitimise social media use. Both Facebook and Google, for example, established partnerships with the World Health Organization (WHO) and national ministries of health across various countries (Facebook 2020a; Google 2020b). Thus, these two companies served as launch pads for the production and circulation of relevant and verified health information. By controlling what kind of information is shared through their platforms, technology companies countered the spread of misinformation and disinformation in an effort to combat a 'coronavirus infodemic' (Ali and Kurasawa 2020; Skopeliti and John 2020). For example, both Facebook (2020a) and Google (2020b) promoted handwashing tips or observing proper hygiene, as evident on Facebook Messenger (2020), Instagram (2020) and YouTube (YouTube Help 2020). Through partnerships with the WHO, United Nations Children's Fund (UNICEF), and national ministries of health, Facebook launched the Coronavirus (COVID-19) Information Centre (Facebook 2020b). Health experts utilised videos to present accurate information produced by the WHO. Further, the Centre alerted people to stay safe and avoid scams online, such as unapproved medical treatments or false fundraisers (Facebook 2020a, Facebook Messenger 2020). Instagram emphasised the 'educational resources' in Instagram search, connecting individuals to resources from the WHO and local health ministries (Instagram 2020):

> People who search for information related to the coronavirus or COVID-19 on Instagram will start to see an educational message connecting them to resources from the World Health Organization and local health ministries. We are working quickly to make this available globally over the coming weeks. … Over the past few weeks we've added a notice at the top of feed for countries affected by COVID-19. The notice includes reliable resources from expert health organisations. In addition, we've been highlighting resources from these organisations when people view related hashtags.

In some cases, online platforms employ strategies to also manage the spread of health misinformation. For instance, Instagram (2020) added special stickers to promote 'accurate information' posted by 'credible' health organisations. Similarly, Facebook Messenger (2020) highlighted 'verified accounts' – particularly WHO as the only credible source of information on COVID-19 – and issued the following instructions on how to recognise misinformation and refrain from spreading it:

> Verify facts with trusted official sources, and watch out for people running scams such as unapproved medical treatments or false fundraisers. If you aren't sure that something's true, don't share it. …
>
> Prevent the spread of misinformation. Verify the facts with other trusted sources such as the World Health Organization or your ministry of health. Look for forward indicators that alert you when you are receiving a forwarded message, which helps you know when a message that you received was not created by the person who sent it. If you're not sure if something is accurate, please don't forward it.

By assuming the role of gatekeeping, online platforms significantly shaped the public discourse on COVID-19. Yet, as the pandemic continues, it remains unclear which sources are more accurate than others and who should make a final decision on this issue. Experts are in continuous open disagreement about measurements such as compulsory face masks, limitations of personal contact and restrictions on various types of events (Nicholds 2020). In imposing measurements, different national ministries draw on different analyses. By contrast, online platforms are transnational, which makes the prescription of one single guideline challenging if not impossible. Organisations such as WHO may base their recommendations on scientific research, but in the past several months, scientific research on COVID-19 has been published faster than usual to solve the many puzzles of the virus. Some of these studies, published in prestigious academic journals, have already been retracted (Boseley and Davey 2020). Moreover, the very notion of an infodemic, which refers to an overabundance of (mis)information, is predicated on social media platforms that are difficult to tame, as they remain a source of all sorts of contradictory information. The effort to provide accurate information on online platforms may thus be little more than lip-service, while technological companies behind them profit from their users engaging in debates that arise from contradictions and controversies.

Framing online platforms as credible sources of information was paired with philanthropic endeavours. Facebook started the COVID-19 Solidarity Response Fund to support the WHO's global efforts to combat the pandemic, support frontline workers, assist patients, and support the fast development of the vaccine and treatment by matching the first

US$10 million donated (Facebook 2020c). Google.org will match up to $10.5 million to benefit the COVID-19 Solidarity Response Fund of WHO (Google 2020c). These practices demonstrate how progress and security are envisioned to be achieved through partnerships on a global scale. The strategies are operationalised by providing medical protective equipment to medical workers and donations to those hit by COVID-19 (Jin 2020). Through such actions, technology companies position themselves as socially responsible and caring. Yet, building on their increasing userbase, these companies simultaneously also reinstate their dominant position in a global and digital market. In the context of fantasy production (Tadiar 2004), positive images of partnerships are highlighted, which may then conceal and reinforce existing hierarchies and divides within and between societies.

Care and surveillance

In the discursive practices of care on social media, technology corporations aim to create an over-arching impression of care. Through the use of stickers related to the prevention of COVID-19, and by sharing health resources deemed credible by online platforms, users are enacted as caring for each other, their families, friends and the wider community. At the same time, through providing healthcare advice, regularly updated information on government regulations and tips on how to survive and thrive during the quarantine, for example through YouTube's (2020) 'At Home #WithMe' campaign, the online platforms appear as caring towards their users.

However, on the online platforms the boundaries between 'we care for you' and 'we are tracking you' are blurred; the practices of care and exploitation are interrelated. Online platforms are operated through business protocols that collect users' data, which may then be sold for various purposes, including data mining for research and targeted marketing based on personal information and captured mediated interactions, and targeted promotion to businesses (Kennedy 2016). For example, Facebook Messenger (2020) issued the following message targeting business owners:

> Messaging helps businesses stay connected to customers when they can't be there in person. Leverage free messaging tools to provide customers with important information and consider setting up automated responses to frequently asked questions such as shop closures, opening hours and more.

Since Facebook receives nearly all its revenue through advertising, such strategies have undoubtedly contributed to increases in profits (Swartz 2020). Through such 'care for business', the users of online platforms are simultaneously enacted as consumers and providers of data that translate into corporation profits. Thus, while encouraging their users in various care activities both online and offline, technology companies generate profit by attracting advertisers and investors. Facebook, for instance, had a daily average of 1.73 billion users for March 2020, which translated into an increase of 11 per cent profit (Facebook 2020d). In the first quarter of 2020, Facebook (2020d) earned more than US$17 billion based on advertising and other sources.

Moreover, the data that users share on online platforms are surveyed with the aim of tracking the spread of COVID-19. The platforms share such data with governments and researchers. Google and Facebook are among the companies with the largest amount of non-public data that can be tapped for disease tracking (DeChiaro 2020). During the COVID-19 pandemic in China, 'sick posts' that users published on Weibo, a popular local social media platform, were used to identify outbreaks (Holder 2020), and content that users post on online platforms can be used for broader law enforcement and control. In Europe, the data shared by users on such platforms has been used to assess whether or not people are abiding the quarantine rules. In Italy, more than 500,000 profiles on Instagram were scraped to identify people violating quarantine (Ng 2020a). This raises privacy concerns, but around the world, privacy commissioners have encouraged such practices, lifting data restrictions to enable more efficient tracking of people (Ng 2020b). Under pressure to reach the end of the pandemic, and despite intense ethical debates of digital tracking (Klar and Lanzerath 2020), government agencies are increasingly allowing technology and private companies to legitimise the harvesting and monetisation of people's data (Manokha 2020).

Exclusive care

The four online platforms that we examined target a particular audience of digitally literate and networked individuals. Who, then, is excluded from the use of online platforms during a pandemic? The most obvious excluded group are those who lack the finances to access a digital technology and a stable internet connection. According to the International Telecommunication Union (2019a), 3.6 billion people in the world are offline, mostly in low income countries. This digital divide results from the inaccessibility of digital devices and services, poor telecommunication infrastructures or nationally regulated access to social media, and limited access to data (Hargittai 2002; Brandhorst 2020; Cabalquinto 2018a, 2020; Ahlin and Li 2019). The divide may also be a result of people's limited technological literacy, including older people and others who have only recently accessed digital technology (Cabalquinto 2018b; Wilding 2006; Ahlin 2018; Baldassar et al. 2007).

In the platforms that we examined, the omission of elderly people was especially obvious in terms of who was addressed through the content promoted on the platforms. The audiences were commonly young adults and families with school-aged children. For example, in its campaign 'Get Digital', Facebook (2020e) provided a range of resources specifically targeting (1) youth, (2) parents and caregivers, and (3) educators:

> Get Digital in your online communities! Bring digital citizenship and wellbeing into your online world. Our engaging activities are expert informed and reinforce and expand on the digital skills you are learning at school and at home.
>
> Get Digital at home! You and your child can improve your digital citizenship with resources created in conjunction with online safety experts. The easy-to-use tips and tools are designed to help you start a conversation with your child to build and reinforce their digital skills.
>
> Get Digital in the classroom! Bring digital citizenship into your classroom with the Get Digital programme. These ready-to-use lessons provide educators with tools and resources to help young people learn digital citizenship and wellbeing skills.

From such content, Facebook emerges as a platform oriented towards young people, especially children and their parents, and those who work with children professionally. By contrast, none of the content we analysed on Facebook and the other three platforms under study addressed digital citizenship and wellbeing for people who do not belong to any of these categories. Older people remain invisible users of online platforms, despite their increased use of digital technologies worldwide (Todd 2018).

Further, in our analysis the users that the online platforms address were presumed to have a home, which indicates specific socioeconomic status. The calls for donations and fundraisers promoted, for example through Facebook Messenger in the form of 'Donation stickers', imagine a user who is able to give away money to others. Yet, around the world, homelessness is a widespread phenomenon and homeless people have been identified as among the most vulnerable populations for COVID-19 (Tsai and Wilson 2020). Even for those with homes, the conditions to safely remain in shelter are shaped by their access to a range of resources. For instance, in the European Union in 2017, more than 20 million workers lived in households at risk of poverty (Eurofound 2017). People from such households may continue living at or fall below the poverty threshold, and such low-waged, often contract workers have been among many 'essential workers' during the COVID-19 pandemic (O'Connor 2020). The structural forces, such as living in inadequate and temporary housing, also contribute to an individual's risk (Team and Manderson 2020).

In many countries across the globe, economic inequalities are strongly shaped by race and ethnicity, which is further reflected in health disparities (van Dorn et al. 2020; Manderson and Levine 2020). This has led to critical anthropological discussions of the 'Stay Home' message (Yates-Doerr 2020). Besides the issue of socioeconomic class, the assumption behind this message is the fantasy of familial and other social relations as essentially 'good' and unproblematic. Through maintaining the particular fantasy of home and family as a safe haven, the online platforms in our study gloss over the dramatic increase of domestic violence and (sexual) abuse across various types of relationships, especially against women and children, during the COVID-19 pandemic internationally (Usher et al. 2020; Khaddari 2020). Yet, the online platforms we examined offer few campaigns to support those who are suffering at home from isolation and violence.

Finally, beyond stickers, the texts published on online websites we examined, dedicated especially to the COVID-19 pandemic, promote a sense of 'digital wellness', particularly through video calling. Facebook (2020a), for example, has published suggestions such as 'Call friends and family to hear a familiar voice. Make a video call to feel close when you're not together'. Calling through digital technologies has been described as a form of care practice available to people who are physically separated from each other (Ahlin 2020; Arnold 2020). However, calls can also create tensions among family members and may be emotionally disturbing. Here, digital media use becomes both a burden and blessing (Horst 2006) in enacting mediated caregiving. For example, Facebook use may help to enact co-presence at a distance, but it also makes people acutely aware of the physical distance between them. This contradiction becomes palpable when physical contact is impossible online or when internet connection is interrupted (Cabalquinto 2018a). Nonetheless, promoting digital connectivity, exclusively in positive terms, is thus another layer that adds to the fantasy of care through digital media.

Conclusion

Social media platforms have appropriated discourses on safety, connectivity, care and social relations during the COVID-19 pandemic. Our examination of four selected online platforms illustrates how care is articulated through digital technologies. First, to enact and experience digital wellness, one must access a wide range of online and credible resources, which relate to personal activities and lifestyle. Second, the notion of care is framed through connectedness in a community, encompassing an education, business or locale setting. Lastly, the online platforms we examined showcase connectivity as crucial for coping with the pandemic. They position themselves as caring for a digitally connected society through their partnership with WHO and national health institutions and through philanthropic projects. This approach contributes to gaining trust among individual users. In a sense, digital corporations embed online platforms as a way to express 'caring about' by prescribing certain practices, such as labelling and posting 'accurate' information, and providing digital tools and resources that enable those practices. Further, the partnership between online platforms and health institutions creates an accessible space for educational or business purposes or managing one's wellbeing.

We have in this chapter presented a snapshot of how selected social media channels frame their services during the pandemic. Future research should also examine how other online platforms promote digital connectivity during and after the pandemic, including perhaps how digital platforms contribute to questions of vaccination. Such an approach would provide a point of comparison on the diverse strategies of social media channels as shaped by economic and political agendas. Further, future studies can explore the implications of the partnership between government agencies and tech companies on data privacy, capitalism and democratic processes in post-pandemic futures.

Online platforms produce and maintain a particular fantasy of care, family and social relations. As we have critically reflected, care is complex and heterogenous, often differentially performed and experienced depending on people, technologies and social structures. As Tadiar (2004) notes, fantasies also create opportunities for profit making, domination and marginalisation along various lines. As the possibility to care is shaped by finances, time, social capital and health, the ideals of safety, security, care and connectedness tend to remain in the imaginaries of those who are in power and/or privileged (Tadiar 2004). The textual and visual deployment of these ideals on online platforms may deepen the gap between people of different socioeconomic status. Those who are relatively privileged remain in the safety of their homes and post 'Stay home' stickers on each other's virtual walls, and they are able to engage with the benefits of connectivity, yet what such practices seem to contribute to is increased disconnection from the realities of many people around the world. By appealing to emotions – as fear and uncertainty become glossed over with fantasies of care – the corporations that own online platforms tap into shared data as a way to enhance their profits and increase surveillance. The crisis of COVID-19 offers an opportunity to reflect on the politics of care embedded in the consumption of online platforms and the consequences that are triggered by their use.

References

Ahlin, Tanja. 2018. 'Only near is dear? Doing elderly care with everyday ICTs in Indian transnational families'. *Medical Anthropology Quarterly* 32(1): 85–102.

Ahlin, Tanja. 2020. 'Frequent callers: "Good care" with ICTs in Indian transnational families'. *Medical Anthropology* 39 (1): 69–82. https://doi.org/10.1080/01459740.2018.1532424.

Ahlin, Tanja and Fangfang Li. 2019. 'From field sites to field events: Creating the field with information and communication technologies (ICTs)'. *Medicine, Anthropology, Theory* 6: 1–24. https://doi.org/10.17157/mat.6.2.655.

Ali, S. Harris and Kurasawa, Fuyuki. 2020. '#COVID19: Social media both a blessing and a curse during coronavirus pandemic'. Accessed 22 March 2020. https://theconversation.com/covid19-social-media-both-a-blessing-and-a-curse-during-coronavirus-pandemic-133596.

Andrejevic, Mark. 2003. 'Monitored mobility in the era of mass customization'. *Space and Culture* 6: 132–50.

Arnold, Lynnette. 2020. 'Cross-border communication and the enregisterment of collective frameworks for care'. *Medical Anthropology* 39(7): 624–37. https://doi.org/10.1080/01459740.2020.1717490.

Baldassar, Loretta. 2014. 'Too sick to move: Distant "crisis" care in transnational families'. *Revue Internationale de Sociologie* 24: 391–405. https://doi.org/10.1080/03906701.2014.954328.

Baldassar, Loretta, Cora Baldock and Raelene Wilding. 2007. *Families Caring Across Borders: Migration, ageing and transnational caregiving*. Basingstoke, UK: Palgrave Macmillan.

Baldassar, Loretta and Laura Merla. 2014. 'Introduction: Transnational family caregiving through the lens of circulation'. In *Transnational Families, Migration and the Circulation of Care: Understanding mobility and absence in family life*, edited by Loretta Baldassar and Laura Merla, pp. 3–24. New York: Routledge.

Baldassar, Loretta, Mihaela Nedelcu, Laura Merla and Raelene Wilding. 2016. 'ICT-based co-presence in transnational families and communities: Challenging the premise of face-to-face proximity in sustaining relationships'. *Global Networks* 16: 133–44. https://doi.org/10.1111/glob.12108.

Boseley, Sarah and Melissa Davey. 2020. 'Covid-19: Lancet retracts paper that halted hydroxychloroquine trials'. *The Guardian*. Accessed 4 June 2020. https://www.theguardian.com/world/2020/jun/04/covid-19-lancet-retracts-paper-that-halted-hydroxychloroquine-trials.

Brandhorst, Rosa M. 2020. 'A regimes-of-mobility-and-welfare approach: The impact of migration and welfare policies on transnational social support networks of older migrants in Australia'. *Journal of Family Research* 3: 1–19. https://doi.org/10.20377/jfr-374.

Brown, Rachel H. 2016. 'Multiple modes of care: Internet and migrant caregiver networks in Israel'. *Global Networks* 16(2): 237–56. https://doi.org/10.1111/glob.12112.
Cabalquinto, Earvin Charles. 2018a. '"We're not only here but we're there in spirit": Asymmetrical mobile intimacy and the transnational Filipino family'. *Mobile Media and Communication* 6: 1–16.
Cabalquinto, Earvin Charles. 2018b. '"I have always thought of my family first": An analysis of transnational caregiving among Filipino migrant adult children in Melbourne, Australia'. *International Journal of Communication* 12: 4011–29.
Cabalquinto, Earvin Charles. 2020. 'Standby mothering: Temporalities, affects, and the politics of mobile intergenerational care'. *Journal of Intergenerational Relationships* 18(3): 358–76. https://doi.org/10.1080/15350770.2020.1787049.
Cabalquinto, Earvin Charles and Guy Wood-Bradley. 2020. 'Migrant platformed subjectivity: Rethinking the mediation of transnational affective economies via digital connectivity services'. *International Journal of Cultural Studies* 23(5): 787–802. https://doi.org/10.1177%2F1367877920918597.
DeChiaro, Dean. 2020. 'Social media data could greatly aid in tracking COVID-19 worldwide'. Accessed 24 March 2020. https://www.rollcall.com/2020/03/24/social-media-data-could-greatly-aid-in-tracking-covid-19-worldwide/.
Eurofound. 2017. *In-work Poverty in the EU*. Luxembourg: Publications Office of the European Union.
Facebook. 2020a. 'Coronavirus (COVID-19) information centre'. Accessed 9 June 2020. https://www.facebook.com/coronavirus_info/.
Facebook. 2020b. 'Coronavirus (COVID-19) information hub for media'. Accessed 9 June 2020. https://www.facebook.com/facebookmedia/solutions/coronavirus-resources.
Facebook. 2020c. 'Global coronavirus resource: Connecting people during the COVID-19 pandemic, a guide for media partners'. Accessed 9 June 2020. https://scontent.fman2-2.fna.fbcdn.net/v/t39.8562-6/10000000_626188491284662_323098655211896881_n.pdf?_nc_cat=106&ccb=1-3&_nc_sid=ae5e01&_nc_eui2=AeHYSaYsKTZemwCpOpTU-jqmvpRASHRHnBO-lEBIdEecE0i-Dd3MmkpgFJgljtS6qoM8vdsjJ3DF3mn943qkknhC&_nc_ohc=vUKqNHzCVdQAX9pfkld&_nc_oc=AQkNA0oMdpYrU-jeZPPaFwZeyfVNsbTJK7ubF-TDajwM3YMHKsIJLpk1hAej0rPJFpE&_nc_ht=scontent.fman2-2.fna&oh=fa9c8133f758dd1fba2d3d021c20c43f&oe=60F9A9EC.
Facebook. 2020d. 'Facebook reports first quarter 2020 results'. Accessed 1 August 2020. https://investor.fb.com/investor-news/press-release-details/2020/Facebook-Reports-First-Quarter-2020-Results/default.aspx.
Facebook. 2020e. Facebook Get Digital. Last modified 1 April 2020. https://www.facebook.com/fbgetdigital.
Facebook Messenger. 2020. 'Here are some ways that messenger can help you stay together during the pandemic'. Accessed 1 August 2020. https://www.messenger.com/coronavirus.
Flick, Uwe. 2011. *Introducing Research Methodology*. London: SAGE Publications Ltd.
Google. 2020a. Doodle archive, Google. Accessed 1 April 2020. https://www.google.com/doodles/stay-home-save-lives.
Google. 2020b. 'Covid-19 information and resources'. Accessed 1 April 2020. https://www.google.com/covid19/.
Google. 2020c. 'COVID-19 solidarity response fund for the World Health Organization'. Accessed 1 April 2020. https://www.google.org/intl/en_us/covid-19/.
Hargittai, Eszter. 2002. 'Second-level digital divide: Differences in people's online skills'. *First Monday* 7(4). https://firstmonday.org/article/view/942/864.
Helmond, Anne. 2015. 'The platformization of the web: Making web data platform ready'. *Social Media + Society* 1: 1–11. https://doi.org/10.1177%2F2056305115603080.
Holder, Kathleen. 2020. '"Sick posts" on social media help early tracking of COVID-19'. Accessed 16 April 2020. https://www.ucdavis.edu/coronavirus/news/sick-posts-social-media-help-early-tracking-covid-19/.
Horst, Heather. 2006. 'The blessings and burdens of communication: Cell phones in Jamaican transnational social fields'. *Global Networks* 6(2): 143–59.
Horst, Heather and Daniel Miller. 2006. *The Cell Phone: An anthropology of communication*. Oxford: Berg.
Hyken, Shep. 2017. 'Social customer care is the new marketing'. Accessed 22 April 2020. https://www.forbes.com/sites/shephyken/2017/04/22/social-customer-care-is-the-new-marketing/#4dfe98b8196c.

Instagram. 2020. 'Keeping people informed, safe, and supported on Instagram'. Accessed 24 March 2020. https://about.instagram.com/blog/announcements/coronavirus-keeping-people-safe-informed-and-supported-on-instagram.

International Telecommunication Union. 2019. 'Measuring digital development: Facts and figures 2019'. Accessed 21 October 2020. https://www.itu.int/en/ITU-D/Statistics/Documents/facts/FactsFigures2019.pdf.

Jin, Kang-Xing. 2020. 'Keeping people safe and informed about the Coronavirus'. Accessed 21 June 2020. https://about.fb.com/news/2020/08/coronavirus/#ad-and-commerce-update.

Khaddari, Raounak. 2020. 'Hulpvraag bij seksueel misbruik onder jongeren steeg explosief tijdens lockdown'. Accessed 10 June 2020. https://www.parool.nl/nederland/hulpvraag-bij-seksueel-misbruik-onder-jongeren-steeg-explosief-tijdens-lockdown~b2003d8e/.

John, Nicholas. 2013. Sharing and Web 2.0: The emergence of a keyword. *New Media & Society* 15(2): 167–82. https://doi.org/10.1177%2F1461444812450684.

Kennedy, Helen. 2016. *Post, Mine, Repeat: Social media data mining becomes ordinary*. London: Palgrave Macmillan.

Klar, Renate and Dirk Lanzerath. 2020. 'The ethics of COVID-19 tracking apps – challenges and voluntariness'. *Research Ethics* 16(3–4): 1–9. https://doi.org/10.1177%2F1747016120943622.

Licoppe, Christian. 2004. '"Connected" presence: The emergence of a new repertoire for managing social relationships in a changing communication technoscape'. *Environment and Planning D: Society and Space* 22(1): 135–56. https://doi.org/10.1068%2Fd323t.

Light, Ben, Jean Burgess and Stephanie Duguay. 2016. 'The walkthrough method: An approach to the study of apps'. *New Media and Society*, 881–900. https://doi.org/10.1177%2F1461444816675438.

Manderson, Lenore and Susan Levine. 2020. 'COVID-19, risk, fear, and fall-out'. *Medical Anthropology: Cross-Cultural Studies of Health and Illness* 39(5): 367–370. https://doi.org/10.1080/01459740.2020.1746301.

Madianou, Mirca. 2016. 'Ambient co-presence: Transnational family practices in polymedia environments'. *Global Networks* 16(2): 183–201. https://doi.org/10.1111/glob.12105.

Madianou, Mirca and Daniel Miller. 2012. *Migration and New Media: Transnational families and polymedia*. Abingdon, UK: Routledge.

Manokha, Ivan. 2020. 'How data-mining companies are set to gain from the COVID-19 pandemic'. Accessed 21 September 2020. https://www.opendemocracy.net/en/can-europe-make-it/how-data-mining-companies-are-set-gain-covid-19-pandemic/.

Mol, Annemarie, Ingunn Moser and Jeannette Pols, eds. 2015. *Care in Practice: On tinkering in clinics, homes and farms*. Bielefeld, Germany: Transcript Verlag.

Ng, Alfred. 2020a. 'Governments could track COVID-19 lockdowns through social media posts'. Accessed 25 March 2020. https://www.cnet.com/health/governments-could-track-covid-19-lockdowns-through-social-media-posts/.

Ng, Alfred. 2020b. 'Coronavirus pandemic changes how your privacy is protected'. Accessed 21 March 2020. https://www.cnet.com/health/coronavirus-pandemic-changes-how-your-privacy-is-protected/.

Nicholds, Alyson, 2020. 'Coronavirus: Why experts disagree so strongly over how to tackle the disease. *The Conversation*, 8 April 2020. Accessed 14 April 2021. https://theconversation.com/coronavirus-why-experts-disagree-so-strongly-over-how-to-tackle-the-disease-135825.

O'Connor, Sarah. 2020. 'It is time to make amends to the low-paid essential worker'. Accessed 1 April 2020. https://www.ft.com/content/2b34269a-73f8-11ea-95fe-fcd274e920ca.

Peile, Cecilia. 2014. 'The migration industry of connectivity services: A critical discourse approach to the Spanish case in a European perspective'. *Crossings: Journal of Migration and Culture* 5: 57–71. https://doi.org/10.1386/cjmc.5.1.57_1.

Skopeliti, Clea and Bethan John. 2020. 'Coronavirus: How are the social media platforms responding to the 'infodemic'?' Accessed 19 March 2020. https://firstdraftnews.org/latest/how-social-media-platforms-are-responding-to-the-coronavirus-infodemic/.

Swartz, Jon. 2020. 'Facebook earnings and user growth miss expectations, but stock still spikes'. Accessed 29 April 2020. https://www.marketwatch.com/story/facebook-earnings-and-user-growth-miss-expectations-but-stock-still-spikes-2020-04-29.

Tadiar, Neferti Xina M. 2004. *Fantasy Production: Sexual economies and other Philippine consequences for the new world order*. Hong Kong: Hong Kong University Press.

Team, Victoria and Lenore Manderson. 2020. 'How COVID-19 reveals structures of vulnerability'. *Medical Anthropology* 39(8): 671–74. https://doi.org/10.1080/01459740.2020.1830281.

Todd, Laura-Jane. 2018. 'The technological skills of the global elderly population'. Accessed 12 September 2020. https://www.openaccessgovernment.org/technological-skils-elderly-population/53518/.
Tsai, Jack and Michal Wilson. 2020. 'COVID-19: A potential public health problem for homeless populations'. *The Lancet Public Health* 5(4): e186–7.
Turkle, Sherry. 2012. *Alone Together: Why we expect more from technology and less from each other*. New York: Basic Books.
Usher, Kim, Navjot Bhullar, Joanne Durkin, Naomi Gyamfi and Debra Jackson. 2020. 'Family violence and COVID-19: Increased vulnerability and reduced options for support'. *International Journal of Mental Health Nursing* 29(4): 549–52. https://doi.org/10.1111/inm.12735.
van Dijck, Jose. 2012. 'Facebook as a tool for producing sociality and connectivity'. *Television and New Media* 13: 160–76. https://doi.org/10.1177%2F1527476411415291.
van Dijck, Jose. 2013. *The Culture of Connectivity: A critical history of social media*. New York: Oxford University Press.
van Dorn, Aaron, Rebecca E. Cooney and Miriam L. Sabin. 2020. 'COVID-19 exacerbating inequalities in the US'. *The Lancet* 395: 1243–4. https://doi.org/10.1016/S0140-6736(20)30893-X.
Vincent, Jane and Leopoldina Fortunati, eds. 2009. *Electronic Emotion: The mediation of emotion via information and communication technologies*. New York: Peter Lang.
Wahl-Jorgensen, Karin. 2018. 'The emotional architecture of social media'. In *A Networked Self and Platforms, Stories, Connections*, edited by Zizi Papacharissi, pp. 77–93. New York, NY: Routledge.
Wajcman, Judy. 2015. *Pressed for Time: The acceleration of life in digital capitalism*. Chicago IL and London: The University of Chicago Press.
Wilding, Raelene. 2006. '"Virtual" intimacies? Families communicating across transnational contexts'. *Global Networks* 6: 125–42. https://doi.org/10.1111/j.1471-0374.2006.00137.x.
Yates-Doerr, Emily. 2020. '"Stay home, stay healthy" is dangerous language'. Accessed March 4. https://msmagazine.com/2020/04/03/stay-home-stay-healthy-is-dangerous-language/.
YouTube. 2020. At Home #WithMe. Accessed 1 April 2020. https://www.youtube.com/c/youtubeANZ/search?query=At%20Home%20%23WithMe.
YouTube Help. 2020. 'Help centre: Coronavirus disease 2019 (COVID-19) updates'. Accessed 20 May 20220. https://support.google.com/youtube/answer/9777243?hl=en.

19
Pandemic times in a WhatsApp-ed nation

Gender ideologies in India during COVID-19

Haripriya Narasimhan, Mahati Chittem and Pooja Purang

In India, going 'viral' is a matter of prestige, attention and popularity. Lots of things go viral, not just COVID-19. YouTube videos, TikTok shots and WhatsApp memes all circulate in the public sphere, virus-like, on and on, with no end in sight. As the nation struggles to deal with the coronavirus pandemic, a look at other 'viral' circulations yields interesting and (sometimes worrying) concerns. In this chapter, we focus on one such phenomenon very specific to COVID-19 experience in India.

A simple search on Google about mobile phone distribution in India illustrates the enormous growth of information technology and internet and cell phone communication in the last two decades. In a country in which less than 1 per cent of the population was covered by landline phones in the late 1980s, the population latched on to cell phones (mobile phones) as soon as they reached India's shores. India today is one of those countries that is perpetually on the phone. Some 15 GB (gigabytes) are consumed per person every month in the country, with some 26 per cent of the population said to own smart phones (Ericsson Corporation 2020, 13). This is a country with a population of 1.2 billion. Working from home during COVID-19 lockdown has only increased this consumption.

The increase in mobile phone usage in India was well documented by Roger Jeffrey and Assa Doron (2013). They had seen the futility of making and receiving phone calls in India through landlines from the

1960s to the 1990s, and keenly recognised the first decade of the new millennium as a revolution in communication. Now one could call another person on a phone and not worry about either the cost of the call or getting cut off. As they discuss in another piece (Jeffrey and Doron 2011), a lot of effort from the state and the corporate world went into making India a cell phone nation. In 1987, only 0.3 per cent of the population had access to phones. By 2010, this increased to an incredible 60 per cent, mostly through cell phones.

In 1991, the Indian government introduced an economic policy to open up the economy; the economic growth stimulated by this has been well documented (Fernandes 2000). So has the emergence of what came to be known as the 'new middle class' in India (see Fuller and Narasimhan 2014). Some of the features that distinguish this middle class from the older 'Nehruvian socialist' middle class include a desire for the consumption of goods and technologies, if not necessarily ideas that challenge inequality and hierarchy, a significant feature of Indian society, as Aditya Bharadwaj illustrates in Chapter 7. Mobile phones were a commodity that captured the attention not only of the upwardly mobile middle classes, but also of a much wider cross section of society.

Projections abound about how smartphone and mobile phone subscriptions will grow exponentially in India. One claim is that by 2026, this will reach 1.2 billion phones (Ericsson Corporation 2020, 13). With a population of over 1.35 billion people at time of writing (December 2020), this is almost one phone per person. Such calculations can be dismissed as the fanciful or ambitious claims of large corporations. Nonetheless, the significance of access to mobile phone technology, particularly in India, cannot be dismissed. We argue that it is essential to understand people's access to and interactions with digital technologies to get a sense of what is happening in contemporary India.

The mobile phone is of course not just a technology. It is an enabler and disruptor of socialities (Nakassis 2014; Venkatraman 2017). As recent anthropological studies illustrate (Jeffrey and Doron 2011, 2013; Venkatraman 2017; Tenhunen 2018; Rangaswamy and Cuttrell 2012), mobile phones take on various meanings beyond their materiality. Tenhunen (2018) showed how women in rural Bengal used the newly arrived mobile phones in the first decade of the millennium to seek support from natal families against violence and other forms of inequality in their affinal residences. The power that mobile phones afforded to women became a point of contention in rural Tamilnadu, where boys and young men had far more access to mobile phones than did their sisters (Venkatraman 2017), and only marriage and the desire to keep a check on their daughters' welfare led parents to buy mobile phones for their married daughters.

Mobile phones became increasingly common not only in rural areas, but also among working class people of urban areas, who used the phones to compete successfully in the highly competitive business environment. Young men used Facebook as a medium to engage in romantic relationships, albeit brief and often unsatisfactory (Rangaswamy and Arora 2016); mobile phones provided access to Facebook for people who still had little access to laptops and personal computers. This contrasts with the US, where young college students have been frustrated with Facebook for leading them to constantly monitor their own and others' lives (and selfhood) online (Gershon 2011). Daniel Miller (2012) some years ago alerted us to the importance of looking at digital technologies as cultural sites. The newly emerged subdiscipline of digital anthropology has until now confined its focus mostly to social network sites, as evident in the vast multi-site project undertaken by Miller and others, 'Why we post'.

WhatsApp is a major form of communication in India, and this motivated us to examine the circulations on that medium more closely. The extended lockdown that India experienced resulted in an already active public sphere going wild with images, videos and texts, including information (often wrong or alarming) about COVID-19, and about its impact on our everyday lives. It is here that we intervene to argue for a closer look at forms of viral circulations, and to pause and engage with cultural notions that emerge anew or are refreshed via mobile phones in a country that is constantly online. The ubiquity of mobile phones in India means that memes circulate in various languages across vast distances, and are talked about in the mainstream press and in people's homes. WhatsApp has come to take such an important place in Indian public discourse that the derisive term 'WhatsApp University' has emerged to discredit spurious and sometimes dangerous information circulating on the medium.

Studying memes in anthropology

In order to understand memes from an anthropological perspective, we have to look to scholarship from the fields of media, communications and journalism (Denisova 2019). Pointing out the inadequacy in Richard Dawkins' 1976 definition of memes, emerging from biological sciences and genetics, Denisova (2019) cites more useful interpretations such as those by scholars Esteves and Miekle (2015), who see memes as a form of story-telling. Denisova herself defines memes as 'context-bound viral texts that proliferate on mutation and replication' (2019, 10). As she elaborates, memes gather meaning only with 'audience' participation. As texts or images, the meaning is only half-done. Those who read, 'forward' and comment when receiving a 'WhatsApp' bestow meaning to the meme. This is related to the context in which the memes are born and sent forward.

Memes related to COVID-19 can be seen as 'biosocial experience of an infectious disease pandemic in the age of internet' (Marcus and Singer 2017, 342). They symbolise the churn happening inside the homes of the middle class in India pertaining to expected gendered behaviours and their (imagined) upending due to the pandemic. In that sense, they are 'cultural artifacts' (2017, 342). To borrow again from Marcus and Singer, memes circulating during the pandemic are a 'noteworthy social response to a lethal epidemic in the digital age' (2017, 342).

In this chapter, we examine memes that emerged in the context of the national lockdown announced by the central government of India, which lasted from 24 March to 31 May 2020. These memes were circulated on WhatsApp and appeared in newspaper articles and online in social media. We juxtapose these with first-hand narratives in two different timelines during the lockdown. The experiences of women with children, both with paid employment and without, against the backdrop of the lockdown, provides an opportunity to separate the 'imagined' realities of lockdown life for men, and the actual ways in which it played out for women.

Our methods were as follows. HN observed memes circulating on WhatsApp from April 2020 onwards. These memes were shared in groups to which she belonged, both of friends and family, and co-residents in the gated community in which she lives. HN also looked at some memes in online newspaper articles. These data were analysed in juxtaposition with interview data, generated by MC as part of a study on mothers' lives during lockdown. We used a longitudinal design with qualitative interviews at three time points: at the start, during and after the lockdown. Interview questions asked at the first time point focused on (i) women's thoughts and views on COVID-19 and the lockdown, (ii) their relationships with household members (e.g., husband, children and elderly relatives), (iii) self-care behaviours, including diet, exercise and sleep), (iv) experiences and challenges of working from home, and (v) their aspirations and concerns for themselves and their families during and after the lockdown. Data from the first time point T1 (i.e.

second week of lockdown) were analysed by all of us and helped frame a semi-structured interview schedule for the second time point during the lockdown (T2 – weeks seven and eight of lockdown). These in turn informed the interviews which were conducted at the third point (T3 – early 2021). Informed consent was collected from every participant for each interview. Demographic data (e.g. age, type of marriage [arranged or love marriage], occupation of mother and father, number of children) were collected during the interviews. Transcribed interviews were analysed using thematic analyses.

Lockdown in India: a brief history

Little was known in India of the SARS-CoV-2 virus – the novel coronavirus – at the beginning of 2020. Through January and February, news about a virus causing numbers of deaths in China appeared here and there, but at least to the larger public, the first indication that something might be seriously wrong came only in March. Holi, the spring festival which occurred in the first week of March, was relatively subdued. On 19 March, the prime minister Narendra Modi addressed the nation, informing people of the dangers of the virus and asking for co-operation for a whole day curfew – a 'Janata curfew' (people's curfew) – on 22 March. On 25 March, an extended lockdown was announced, to take effect four hours later. This lasted through various phases until 31 May. From June onwards, the country was expected to 'unlock' in stages; regulations that guided this were released by the central government and, to an extent, state governments.

The short duration between the announcement of the lockdown and its implementation meant that many people were caught unawares and could not move out of their homes. Many were stranded in places they were visiting. Flights, trains and all forms of intra- and interstate transport were cancelled, as were private cab and bus services. Offices, schools, colleges, restaurants, malls and entertainment centres closed. Economic and social activity came to a complete halt, except for essential services. This was reflected in photographs of millions of labourers, migrants to industrial hubs in western India such as Mumbai and Surat, making their way back to their homes, mostly by foot, in the east and the north, in states like Bihar and Uttar Pradesh. Heartrending scenes of small children walking barefoot with their parents, with little to eat except for biscuits and water, since roadside eateries called *dhabas* were closed, were given front page coverage on newspapers and were broadcast widely on television. This huge wave of internal migration, an unexpected effect of the lockdown, was documented by photographs, videos, cartoons and memes. In this chapter, we do not include memes on migration, but it is impossible to discuss the lockdown related to COVID-19 without referring to this migrant labour crisis.

Among those who could not go to work because of the lockdown were domestic helpers, called 'maids' in middle class India. The majority of these helpers are women, although it is not unusual to find male helpers in some parts of the country. The number of women employed in this sector is hard to estimate. The National Sample Survey Organisation (NSSO) suggest that four million women work as 'domestic workers' (Press Information Bureau 2019); unofficial estimates suggest that the number is closer to 50 million (Viswanath 2020). Many lost their jobs during lockdown because their employers did not feel it necessary to pay them. How these women from very poor households survived through those nine weeks has yet to be described.

Ray and Qayum's seminal study on domestic help in the eastern Indian city of Kolkata (2009)[1] traces the origins of present-day domestic labour in the colonial period. The authors refer to this phenomenon as a 'culture of servitude', to denote the institutionalised and normalised form it takes in the Indian context. It is assumed to be usual for middle class as well as rich households to have 'servants' in India; it is also expected that domestic work is undertaken by others, with the distribution of tasks predicated on inequality and subservience.

Sara Dickey (2013, 2016), in her recent work on domestic workers in south India, points to the heavy dependence of middle class women on their domestic helpers. Helpers who have worked in households for many years are treated at times as part of the family, although at other times they are expected to 'know their place' and observe distance. In either case, both domestic helpers and their employers are acutely aware that the former are indispensable for the functioning of the household. This is particularly so when women work outside of the home, usually in jobs that do not involve manual labour; such women have domestic helpers who come to their houses every day, to sweep and mop floors, wash dishes, and wash and sometimes hang clothes to dry.

Domestic helpers are different from a 'cook', whose job is confined only to the kitchen and to cutting vegetables and meat. Some domestic helpers stay permanently with a family and are referred to as 'live-in maids'. Most women in our respective cities, in Mumbai and Hyderabad, worked in several households in one neighbourhood, where the quantum of work might differ from one household to another. At time of writing

(December 2020), these 'essential workers' still faced problems in returning to pre-COVID levels of employment. In the gated community where HN lives, many domestic workers had been replaced by electric dishwashers, with one dishwasher maker reporting a 400–500 per cent increase in sales (Koshi 2020). Until then seen as a luxury good owned and used only by the rich, COVID-induced lockdown prompted middle class women to turn to electrical appliances for household chores. There was also continuing concern about disease spread by domestic workers, consistent with the concept of lower class and lower caste bodies as polluting (Dickey 2000; Bharadwaj, Chapter 7, this volume; Garimella, Murthy, Whittaker and Tolhurst, Chapter 11, this volume).

Lockdown in meme

Although men and women were both at home during the lockdown, men were not expected to do household chores. In many parts of India, there is a strong taboo against men touching a broom or a mop. However, popular memes circulated during this time showed a parallel universe where men were engaged in backbreaking household work while women were relaxing. The video we discuss below (see Figure 19.1), circulated on WhatsApp, is a perfect example.

A man is seen lying in bed and reading a magazine. Suddenly his hair flays, as happens in movies and TV serials, indicating the appearance

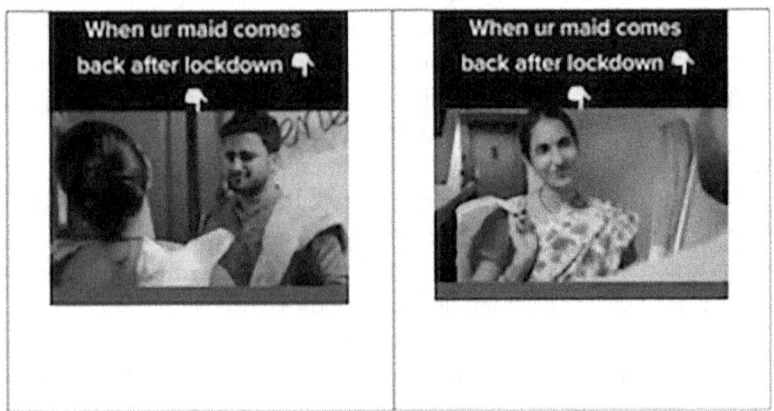

Figure 19.1 When ur maid comes back after lockdown. Facebook, https://www.facebook.com/officialspwrites/videos/2068890199923609/

of a romantic interest nearby. The 'maid' comes running through the streets, with her anklet-adorned feet and slippers, her right hand holding a bag drawn over her right shoulder. The man tosses a towel, in cotton, the kind of usually seen on characters who play 'servants' in movies and comes running towards the front door. In his hand, he holds a bucket of water, a mop stick and a broom. He looks eagerly at the landing and turns away disappointed. Suddenly he stops and turns to see the woman stopping to catch her breath at the landing. She points her fingers at him teasingly. She then asks him … He does an *aarti* (brief welcome ritual) with the bucket, welcoming her home, as one would do to a new bride entering her in-laws' house (*sasuraal*). He gives her the bucket of water and the mop (*jaadu-pocha*), gestures as if to touch her cheeks, and then makes another affectionately dismissive gesture. He has tears of joy in his eyes as he watches the woman go inside.

This video suggests a sexual tension inherent between a male employer and a female worker. It also sexualises and objectifies the woman worker, negating the labour of her work and identity. The same

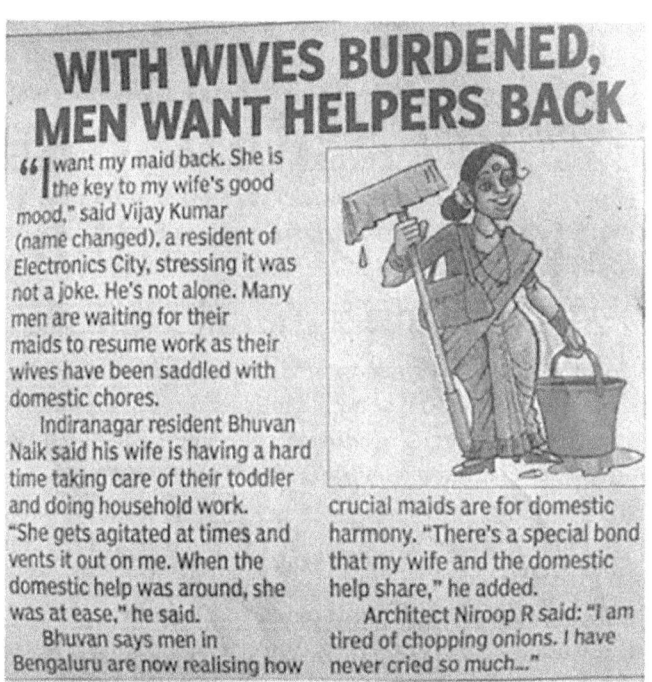

Figure 19.2 With wives burdened, men want helpers back. Twitter feed, Samar Halankar. Accessed 3 May 2020

apparent anxiety with which men wanted domestic workers back in their homes is captured in the newspaper article in Figure 19.2.

In this article, men point to their wives' good mood being dependent on the availability of a domestic help. Without her, the wife is cranky, and she takes it out on her husband. One man complained about having to take on specific household chores, such as cutting onions, which most men did not do, pre-COVID. The comments from men stem not from their realisation of the drudgery, boredom and backbreaking nature of household work, which in India involves considerable manual work. Their woes have more to do with the fact that with a helper around, their wives complain less and allegedly prepare more (and better) food for them. Moreover, when a paid helper – a 'maid' – is available, men are not asked to undertake household chores.

Another characteristic of lockdown was an explosion of images of people cooking, trying out new recipes and resurrecting old ones.[1] This has been remarked upon by many commentators around the world; it is not unique to India. The WhatsApp memes targeted women specifically, however, either as those who should be cooking enormous amounts of food, or as those who have not done so and have therefore abandoned their dutiful wifely behaviour. The meme in Figure 19.3 follows this trajectory of provoking a woman who is clearly not interested in cooking.

The meme in Figure 19.3, using a popular line – *kab khoon khaulega re tera* – from the cult film *Gangs of Wasseypur* (2012), shows the character played by actor Richa Chadha, the wife of gangster Sardar. Her son Faisal (played by actor Nawazzudin Siddiqui) asks her when her blood will boil, that is, when will she get angry and jealous enough to copy other women and cook delicious dishes for her family. During lockdown, without maids and cooks, middle class women took to cooking enthusiastically. While many women (including HN) admitted to searching online and trying out new recipes, these memes articulate something else – an arena of competition among women to outdo each other at a task routinely tied to gendered roles.

In a lengthy article in *The Telegraph*, published in Kolkata, the gendered implications of lockdown were discussed (Sarkar 2020). In households where both men and women had paid jobs, the stress was depicted in a number of cartoons in the piece. A more relaxed atmosphere was said to prevail in those homes where the woman did not have paid employment, and therefore had no meetings to attend on Zoom or phone calls from work to answer. One meme shows a woman informing the prime minister Mr Narendra Modi (referred to using the respectful

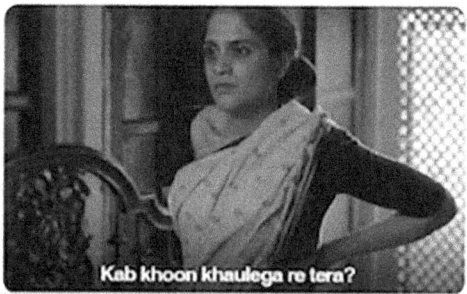

Figure 19.3 When your mother is not cooking various dishes during lockdown. https://humornama.com/memes/when-your-mother-is-not-cooking-various-dishes-during-lockdown/. Meme artwork: Rishav Sen Choudhury

address of 'ji') not to lift lockdown, since she has domestic help from her husband and is under no major inconvenience.

Subarna Ghosh, mentioned in another article, was left angry during the lockdown, when she found herself working a lot more than usual while her husband and children went on with their lives nonchalantly (Pandey 2020). She started a petition on change.org, calling on the prime minister to speak to men about undertaking household chores in his monthly radio address, *Mann ki Baat* (the voice of the heart), which he made to the citizens of India. Pertinent to our discussion here, apart from Ms Ghosh's unhappiness, is the 'maid' whose absence increased her workload and made her realise how little housework was undertaken by others in her home. In her words, 'domestic help also helps maintain peace in our homes'. She is upset with her husband for not sharing in household chores, not only because she believes he should do so, but also because, prior to lockdown, the maid fulfilled a crucial role in keeping the household running. If the lockdown had not prevented people's mobility, especially of maids, then chances are that Mrs Ghosh would not have started the petition. The article refers to a set of memes in Bengali which satirised what lockdown had come to mean.[2] One is as follows:

Lockdown uthe geley, karo jodi kajer meso dorkar hoy amake bolben

Let me know if anyone needs a maid uncle once lockdown is over.

In Bengali, a maid is referred to as *kajer masi*, i.e. working aunt or maid aunt. A man who does household chores now calls himself *kajer meso*, i.e. household help uncle or maid uncle. Biplab Basu of Greenwood Park, New Town, lists his daily chores:

> *Bason maja, ghor jhar dewa, ghor mochha,* washing machine *theke kapor mela.*
>
> Wash dishes, sweep the floor, wipe it dry, take the washed clothes out of the washing machine to dry.

These men present lockdown as a capacity-building exercise in honing specific skills, which has come to define who they are – domestic helpers-in-the-making.

Another popular meme widely circulated on WhatsApp was shared by the noted industrialist Anand Mahindra in April (Jagran Trending Desk 2020). It shows, Vijaykanth, a Tamil actor, popular in the 1980s and 1990s. He is dressed in formal clothing, with a black shirt and trousers and a jacket, a laptop on his lap. He is seated in a chair and speaking (Figure 19.4). The meme is entitled 'expectations', as opposed to the 'reality' of a man cooking. Mahindra, who has millions of 'followers' on social media, and whose words media keenly watch, deftly remarks that he too dressed informally at home during meetings, wearing a formal piece of clothing on top and informal *lungi* not visible in camera. He avoids commenting on the subtext, that of men multi-tasking at home, cooking and attending office work. It is not just the sartorial difference of the two men that informs this meme. The man in lungi is not only pretending to be attending a meeting while dressed informally. He's actually cooking. He's present in the meeting only aurally, with the video clearly switched off.

What's the reality here, and what's the expectation? When a major influencer like Mahindra shares such a meme for laughs, it brings home the fact that lockdown is widely understood as a space for a 'role-reversal' and a shift in gender dynamics in India. One of the comments to Mahindra's 'share' is a simple text: 'Some couples are now MAID for each other'. In cooking for her family, a woman is assumed to be the maid; now the man has become a maid as well. The meme is a pun on the well-known phrase 'made for each other'. It is also a telling commentary on the absence of the usual 'maid' as a result of lockdown.

Another issue often commented on in memes was about weight gain during lockdown, resulting from excessive cooking and eating, with very

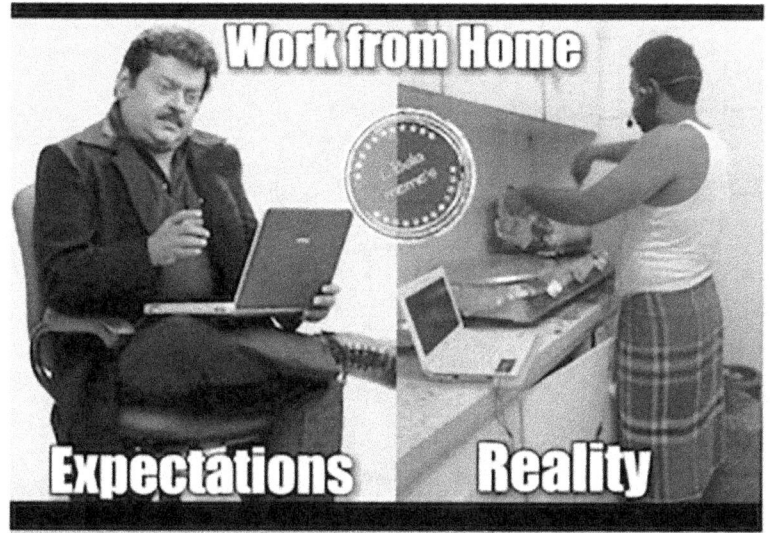

Figure 19.4 Work from home. Shared on Twitter by Anand Mahindra, @anandmahindra, 5 April 2020. Accessed 20 December 2020

little physical exercise. In this context, a number of memes also talked about the danger of obesity (see also Saldaña-Tejeda, Chapter 14). While some target men, a number focused on women's weight gain. The implication is that women put on weight by not doing enough household chores. In the absence of a maid or cook, the conjecture is that the husband had done all the work. The meme in Figure 19.5 features a gender-neutral character talking to its tummy, saying 'should I tell you separately (meaning, once again) that there is a lockdown, and you should not come out?' And in Figure 19.6, a woman goes for a medical consultation thinking she is pregnant; it turns out she's just obese. 'The lockdown is to keep everyone safe and healthy, not to become sweetmakers', says another text meme.

The comments on obesity are ironic given the huge labour crisis that occurred post lockdown. Data continues to emerge of jobs lost and livelihoods severely affected by the pandemic and the resulting economic situation, as many memes reflected (Figure 19.7). Another meme captured the spectre of hundreds and thousands of migrant workers leaving urban areas on foot, back to their villages. Entitled 'The Social Distance', it pictorially renders the wide gap in the lives of middle class and poor people. While the middle classes, who have come to be called

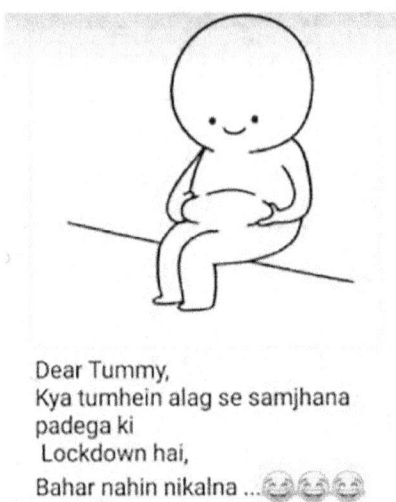

Dear Tummy,
Kya tumhein alag se samjhana padega ki
Lockdown hai,
Bahar nahin nikalna ...😂😂😂

Figure 19.5   Dear Tummy. WhatsApp. Accessed 19 April 2020

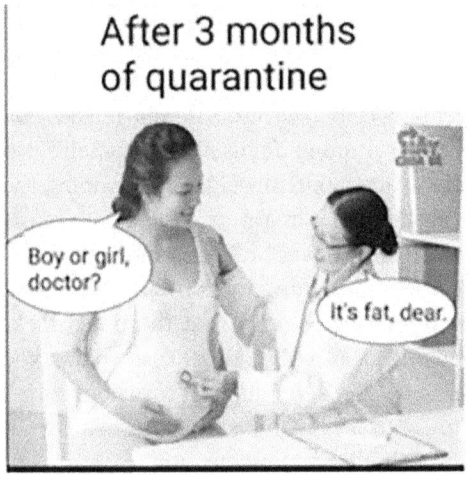

Figure 19.6   After three months of quarantine. WhatsApp. Accessed 19 April 2020

the 'balcony class', gathered on their balconies to show their appreciation for frontline workers on 22 March 2020 (the day of Janata curfew) in a manner reminiscent of Italy and the UK, poor migrants gathered their belongings and started the long walk home (Figure 19.8).

Nonetheless, memes were laughs that were 'forwarded' and 'shared'. These often caricatured women as shrill and shrewish, relishing the

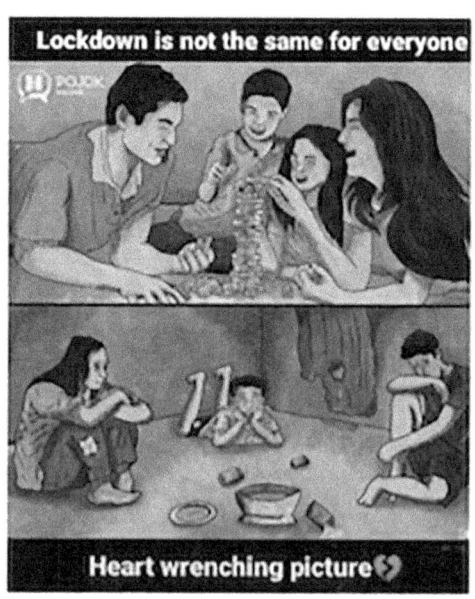

Figure 19.7 The lockdown is to keep everyone safe and healthy. WhatsApp. Accessed 27 April 2020

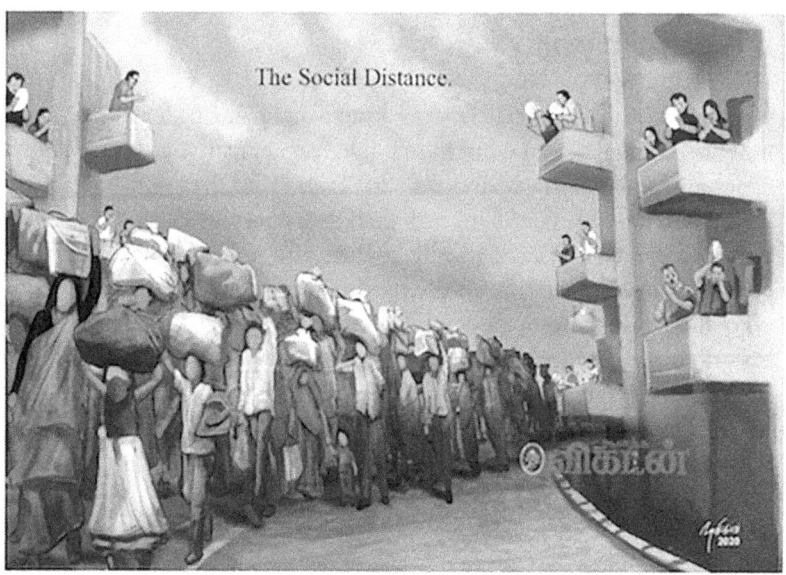

Figure 19.8 The social distance. Artwork: Ananda Vikatan

opportunity provided by the lockdown to lord over their husbands. This 'joke' in Hindi, circulated on WhatsApp, is one example:

पेट पर से बार नीचे सरकते बरमूड़ा को ऊपर चढ़ाते संता ने ख़ुशी ज़ाहिर की !
मुझे लगता है मैं दुबला हो गया हूँ ... देखो ये बरमूड़ा कितना लूज होने लगा है !
किचन से हाथ में बेलन पकड़े उसकी बीबी प्रीतो बाहर आई और बोली !
आइने में अपनी शक्ल देखो ध्यान से ... ! महीने भर से दारू नहीं मिली तुम्हे तो तुम्हारे दिमाग ने भी काम करना बंद कर दिया है ! सुबह से मेरा पेटीकोट पहने घूम रहे हो ! फौरन उतारो उसे !

Santa the husband says he must have lost weight since his 'bermuda' [as shorts are called in India] are very loose. His wife, Preeto, coming with a belan [stick used to make roti], says to him furiously, 'your brain has stopped working because of non-availability of alcohol. Since morning you have been wearing my petticoat and walking around. Remove it immediately'.

Alcohol shops were shut during the lockdown. The meme here stereotypes the man as excessively fond of drinking, without which he cannot think. The woman is portrayed as dominating, the man as an idiot who has lost his thinking capacity. Santa is a popular Sikh character, usually portrayed as a dimwit in jokes.

Lockdown in reality

We now move to empirical vignettes from women during lockdown, to see how these images played out in real life. A recent survey by well-known economist Ashwini Deshpande (2020) found that there was a marginal increase in the time that men spent on domestic work. The memes shared through WhatsApp seem to reflect this, either with mild or extreme exaggeration. But we turn to the narratives of women, especially those who had paid employment and were mothers, and examine their experiences of the lockdown. As mentioned above, this study had three stages, of which two are completed. The third stage will look at the same women in January 2021. We provide some excerpts from interviews, before moving to the analysis.

> I don't enjoy doing all this domestic stuff. So, I have been feeling so lucky and so grateful that I have somebody helping me out with all this. Because trust me, if I had to do the household work, I would be in a very shitty mood. Like snapping at everybody, because oh my

god! You know. The kind of a mess these kids make, the mess I make um ... there is really no way I would be so (laughing) happy. So, I am very, very grateful and so lucky that I am in this situation. And from the beginning of the lockdown, I have been thinking, oh my god! I am so lucky that I have got this girl along with me. You know, because I was coming here only for four days, and I am like what is the point of spending all this money on a flight ticket, why should I bring her? Then I thought let me see you know, she will get out of the house, what is the big deal? So, I am so grateful to her, that she is here, baba.

Malati is a 38-year-old upper caste, stay-at-home mother of two young children (9 and 4 years old). She had a love marriage with a man from another caste. A resident of Hyderabad, she had recently moved to Mumbai, and had come on a visit to Hyderabad when the lockdown happened. She found herself 'stuck' in the city. She had brought with her a 'live-in maid' whose presence she deeply appreciated. About her husband, Malati had this to say:

So I do the cooking, and you know Kishore [husband] can't cook to save his life. So, he goes out and buys whatever groceries I need. He has actually begun to learn the name of vegetables, and learn the name of you know, *dals*. He had no idea about these things, absolutely no idea. So, he has totally impressed me with the knowledge of how to pick the right vegetables, how to get stuff and all these things ... he has become more domesticated ... after he is done with his meal, he takes up the plate and takes it to the kitchen which he would normally not do. He ... after his shower he picks up his clothes and puts them in tub to be washed and all that. You know, it sounds really spoiled, but um ... (laughing)

For Malati, with two small children and a full-time paid helper, it still mattered a lot that her husband was doing some tasks at home, even if some of them were his own, and she appreciated the learning curve he had negotiated.

Both working women and those who were at home full time commented at length in interviews on the loss of maids and cooks due to lockdown. One of their 'lockdown memories', as was the case for middle class women across India, was the sudden non-availability of maids. The revelation that from now on for the foreseeable future, at least before constraints due to COVID-19 were lifted, women were expected to sweep, mop floors and wash dishes, came to many as a rude jolt. This was particularly so for working women, who simultaneously had to manage housework, answer calls and be available to their superiors at work. One of the 'positives' women took from this was not waiting for the maid to turn up. The maids do not have fixed hours of work, although a maid and her employer might agree on an approximate time. Being able to work at home at one's own pace without depending on another person was also liberating for some women. But some of them also mentioned that maids helped them to achieve 'peace' in a personal sense, by taking away stress, as well as to ensure the smooth running of the household.

Shailaja, one of the respondents, commented that the lockdown did not initially have particular impact on her, because she expected it would last only for a few weeks, from late March to April, although it was then extended until May and then June. Like many others, Shailaja assumed that sooner or later, her life, and that of her family, would return to normal. But the lockdown was extended again and again, and life seemed to be in limbo, with husband and children at home, and this hit women hard. Some women working as maids returned to their native villages, fearing infection were they to remain in the city. For women like Shailaja, it became essential that she find household help. She had two children aged 10 and 5. As a stay-at-home mother, she managed to enlist her husband and older daughter in household work.

> I do the cooking and cleaning, Karthik [husband] does the dishes. I think yeah, Karthik does the dishes. Ribhav [son], shower, and whatever ... he takes care of it. Nandini [daughter] helps me with the laundry. Ah ... Ribhav I think is too small so I won't count him. But yeah, Karthik and Nandini yeah. So, dishes part and all Karthik is taking care of, cooking and cleaning I am doing, laundry me and Nandini together we do it. Again Nandini's room and all is up to her. She has to clean it and dust it off.

Working mothers emphasised the importance of 'structure' in their lives. This was a struggle to locate and put in place, at least in the initial days of the lockdown. Malini, aged 36 with two children, found it extremely difficult to run a school virtually. As she explained, the first week of the lockdown was especially hard:

> That week was difficult because, everything, my home has changed. My husband is working all the time, even on Sundays many times. I suddenly have him all the time in home. So, that was a big, big shift in our entire family structure. So, you know, plus with my children

being home all the time. And they are not used to – they have like physical activities in the evening. So, I think, for me, the difficult part was to manage my work. And yet make sure, that ah … my presence is equally felt at home. That was one, one challenge that I had to overcome. The other challenge was that to help everybody at home, realised that while I am at home, I am still doing my work. So to respect that time and space, that okay I am on a call or when I am working, I am working. I can't be available to you.

Far from feeling in charge, women mentioned the struggle to find 'balance' between being at home and engaged for their family, and attending to all the household requirements, while also, as in this case, continuing their paid work. After a few weeks, Malini managed to establish some structure to the way her household functioned. But her husband was always at work, and her mother-in-law was staying with them, and Malini felt the pressure to ensure that the household did not collapse. She explained that she took the lead to organise tasks and delegate duties, lest, in her words, 'if I don't do it, or if I didn't do it, we would be living on Maggi [instant noodles] or something, yaar. We would not have food on the table [laughing]. Our clothes won't be [washed] big time I guess'. In addition to her established career in the field of education, which kept her very busy, during the lockdown Malini also tried many dishes and felt extremely happy with her family's response to her cooking.

Shabari, in her mid-thirties and a manager in an IT firm, had calls to take from 9 p.m. since her clients are based in the US. She has an inter-caste marriage – what is termed a love marriage in India – which means that she and her husband knew each other much better before marriage than do couples whose marriages are arranged. She often mentioned her husband's cooperation with her in managing the home. A self-confessed 'control freak', Shabari said the lockdown taught her not to bother if her garden wasn't tidied up for several days. As a secretary in charge of the housing society which administered the complex where she lived, she was involved in the decision to stop maids and cooks from entering the building, and in keeping lockdown protocol, facing wrath from fellow residents. Without help, she found it very difficult to keep her huge bungalow (a 'villa' in Indian real estate terminology) tidy all the time. She spent nearly five hours on weekends just cleaning the house. It was therefore essential for her to have a 'cooperative' husband prepared to vacuum and help in other ways.

Cooking took a toll on her even though she insisted she enjoyed it and her husband, Madan, also helped in the kitchen. Perhaps the 'love marriage' gave her a little more leeway than women in arranged marriages had. However, as a working woman, it was difficult to manage both the household and the people in it, and demands from work:

> I think home, as I said ... because there is no house help ... and we ... we have ... like a considerable-sized place ... and this just means that you need to be aware ... If you have to plan for lunch, then you have to cook in the morning, which also means that you know, plan ahead. Like usually what happens is when I cook the lunch itself I think ... what should I cook for dinner. *Toh* my plan is ready at that point in time. And when I cook the dinner, I know that okay what I am gonna do tomorrow. Which is, you see, in the mind is stressful right? Because you are always constantly thinking.

Conclusion

The four women whose narratives we summarised above were very clear about who was responsible for the running of the household – they were. They sought help from spouses in the absence of maids, in one case, even with a domestic helper also present. In our sample of 14 women, 6 of them also had elderly parents or parents-in-law staying with them. They felt a strong sense of duty in ensuring that they were taken care of. In the extended interviews, women voiced their worries about their own physical and mental health, not having time for themselves, lack of exercise for their children, and their children's school work. Those with paid work felt under even more pressure.

The interviews were conducted only with women, but questions were asked about their spouses and their participation in household activities. Interviews with men might have offered different perspectives on lockdown and its impact on households. Almost all women observed that their husbands did share in some tasks, whether it had to do with children or doing minor chores in the kitchen. Women did not complain much, unlike Mrs Ghosh who started a petition demanding the intervention of the prime minister. However, they did not acquiesce quietly, batting for the home and the kitchen as their exclusive domain. Contrary to popular assumptions that women who stayed at home would have an easier transition to life in lockdown, they were emphatic that they made sure that their husbands and young children stepped up to the situation and did their bit.

However, the man with the broomstick and a mop, a towel on his shoulder wiping his forehead of sweat, as seen in the video that went viral, did not manifest. Women admitted to 'training' their husbands to undertake various tasks at home. Men featured in memes and newspaper articles, attending meetings in informal clothing while cooking, squatting on the floor and washing dishes while their wives chatted away on the phone (including with the PM), and being woolly headed enough to not realise what they were wearing. These images did not emerge in women's narratives. A time-use survey conducted in 2019 across India (for the first time) showed that urban men spend 94 minutes per day on 'unpaid domestic service for household members', while urban women spend 293 minutes doing the same 'service' (Time Use Survey 2019). The question then arises as to why the memes showed women lazing around and men hard at work in the kitchen. Was this wishful thinking, a 'could have been this' scenario? If so, whose wishful thinking was it? Does the sheer presence of such memes reflect a 'nightmare' scenario dreamed up largely by men?

Where the identity of the creators of such memes is unknown, given the fact that more men than women own mobile phones in India, it is possible that these memes were a doomsday version playing out. Nevertheless, mere speculation does not help situate where contemporary India stands in its approach to the home, and to changing gender dynamics as increasing numbers work from home. Articles touting the benefits of working from home appear with increasing frequency online. The Indian IT industry is a flagship project for the urban middle class. News of more and more IT companies, looking at working from home as a serious option, not only for health and safety reasons but also to save costs on renting huge office space, percolates the public space (TNM 2020). Washing dishes or cutting vegetables may not remain a dream (or nightmare) for men for long.

For an anthropological take on various dimensions to COVID-19 and its impact on our lives, memes such as the ones described in this chapter call for more serious attention. Blevins (2020) argues that memes are to be seen from three angles – as revelation, critique and ideation. As Marshall McLuhan (1964) pointed out long ago, we have to ask what this medium does, and how crucial a given medium is in transmitting a message. What does it reveal and what does it hide? Who does it exclude and who does it suddenly allow to emerge? In line with Blevins' (2020) argument, we propose that these memes appeared to 'imagine new futures'. Daniel Miller (2020) suggests that memes can be serious or humorous depending on the situation. In Irish memes, he detected a moral undertone about the right behaviour to observe during the pandemic.

In this line, what might we say about the memes shared in India through WhatsApp? Devoid of (female) domestic helpers, women attempted to involve men in household work, with varying degrees of success. The memes reflect the animated discussion of this shift in domestic relations and labour. But if our empirical data are any indication, the man who had supposedly completely transformed into a 'maid uncle' by the end of the lockdown has not yet made his appearance. With one more cycle of interviews to do, we could say 'watch this space!'. What is certain at this stage is that the pandemic-induced lockdown has inaugurated a vibrant debate on men's participation in household tasks, at least among urban, middle class, Indians.

Acknowledgements

The authors wish to acknowledge the support of Indian Council of Social Science Research (ICSSR), Government of India, for its support to this research. Our thanks also to Akash Rajoria, Sravya Vallala and Shoban Babu Dharavath for transcribing the interviews.

Notes

1 This Facebook group called 'Quarantine Cooking' also calls itself a mental health support group. Most members appear to be Bengali-speaking. https://www.facebook.com/groups/560796447893450.
2 We thank Saloka Sengupta for this translation.

References

Blevins, Kai. 2020. 'The poetics of internet memes'. Accessed 18 December 2020. https://thegeekanthropologist.com/2020/08/03/the-poetics-of-internet-memes/.
Dawkins, Richard. 1976. *The Selfish Gene*. Oxford, UK: Oxford University Press.
Denisova, Anastasia. 2019. *Internet Memes and Society: Social, cultural and political contexts*. New York: Routledge.
Deshpande, Ashwini. 2020. 'The COVID-19 pandemic and gendered division of paid and unpaid work: Evidence from India'. IZA Institute of Labour Economics Discussion Paper Series, October. Accessed 28 December 2020. http://ftp.iza.org/dp13815.pdf.
Dickey, Sara. 2000. 'Permeable homes: Domestic service, household space, and the vulnerability of class boundaries in urban India'. *American Ethnologist* 27(2): 462–9.
Dickey, Sara. 2013. 'Apprehensions: On gaining recognition as middle-class in Madurai'. *Contributions to Indian Sociology* 47(2): 217–43.
Dickey, Sara. 2016. *Living Class in Urban India*. New Delhi: Permanent Black.
Ericsson Corporation. 2020. *Ericsson Mobility Report*. Stockholm, Sweden: Ericsson Corporation. Accessed 2 January 2021. https://www.ericsson.com/4adc87/assets/local/mobility-report/documents/2020/november-2020-ericsson-mobility-report.pdf.
Esteves, Victoria and Graham Meikle. 2015. '"Look @ this fukken doge": Internet memes and remix cultures'. In *The Routledge Companion to Alternative and Community Media*, edited by Chris Atton, pp. 561–70. New York: Routledge.

Fernandes, Leela. 2000. 'Structuring the new middle class in liberalizing India. *Comparative Studies of South Asia Africa and the Middle East* 20(1&2): 88–104.

Fuller, C.J. and Haripriya Narasimhan. 2014. *Tamil Brahmans: The making of a middle class caste*. Chicago, IL: University of Chicago Press.

Gershon, Ilana. 2011. 'Un-friend my heart: Facebook, promiscuity, and heartbreak in a neoliberal age'. *Anthropological Quarterly* 84(4): 865–94.

Jagran Trending Desk. 2020. 'WFH "Reality vs Expectation": Anand Mahindra shares hilarious meme, confesses he wore "lungi" during video calls'. 6 April 2020. Accessed 20 December 2020. https://english.jagran.com/trending/work-from-home-reality-vs-expectation-anand-mahindra-shares-hilarious-meme-confesses-he-wore-lungi-during-video-calls-see-pic-10010410.

Jeffrey, Robin and Doron, Assa. 2011. 'Celling India: Exploring a society's embrace of the mobile phone'. *South Asian History and Culture* 2(3): 397–416.

Jeffrey, Roger and Assa Doron. 2013. *The Great Indian Phone Book: How the cell phone changes business, politics and daily life*. Cambridge, MA: Harvard University Press.

Koshi, Luke. 2020. 'Dishwasher sales suddenly shoot up in India'. thenewsminute.com, 29 May 2020. Accessed 31 May 2020. https://www.thenewsminute.com/article/dishwasher-sales-suddenly-shoot-india-125497.

Marcus, Olivia R. and Merrill Singer. 2017. 'Loving Ebola-chan: Internet memes in an epidemic'. *Media, Culture & Society* 39(3): 341–56.

McLuhan, Marshall. 1964. *Understanding Media*. New York: McGraw-Hill.

Miller, Daniel. 2012. 'Social networking sites'. In *Digital Anthropology*, edited by Heather A. Horst and Daniel Miller, pp. 146–62. London: Berg.

Miller, Daniel. 2020. 'Memes – the moral police of the internet in the time of Covid-19'. 24 April 2020. Accessed 18 December 2020. https://anthrocovid.com/2020/04/24/memes-the-moral-police-of-the-internet-in-the-time-of-covid-19/.

Nakassis, Constantine. 2014. 'Suspended kinship and youth sociality in Tamil Nadu, India'. *Current Anthropology* 55(2): 175–99.

Pandey, Geeta. 2020. 'Coronavirus in India: "PM Modi, please make men share housework!"' BBC News online. Accessed 17 December 2020. https://www.bbc.com/news/world-asia-india-53469696.

Press Information Bureau, Government of India, Ministry of Labour. 2019. National Policy on Domestic Workers. 7 January 2020. Accessed 13 December 2020. https://pib.gov.in/Pressreleaseshare.aspx?PRID=1558848.

Rangaswamy, Nimmi and Edward Cuttrell. 2012. 'Anthropology, development and ICTs: Slums, youth and the mobile internet in urban India'. Proceedings of the Fifth International Conference on Information and Communication Technologies and Development, Atlanta, GA, 85–93.

Rangaswamy, Nimmi and Payal Arora. 2016. 'The mobile internet in the wild and every day: Digital leisure in the slums of urban India'. *International Journal of Cultural Studies* 19(6): 611–26.

Ray, Raka and Seemin Qayyum. 2009. *Cultures of Servitude: Modernity, domesticity and class in India*. Redwood City, CA: Stanford University Press.

Sarkar, Brinda. 2020. 'Two states of being'. *The Telegraph Online*, 23 April 2020. Accessed 18 December 2020. https://www.telegraphindia.com/west-bengal/calcutta/coronavirus-lockdown-in-west-bengal-two-states-of-being/cid/1767426.

Tenhunen, Sirpa. 2018. *A Village Goes Mobile: Telephony, mediation, and social change in rural India*. New Delhi: Oxford University Press.

TNM staff. 2020. 'Infosys to allow employees to work from home or office from 2021'. Thenewsminute, 16 December 2020. https://www.thenewsminute.com/article/infosys-allow-employees-work-home-or-office-2021-139717.

Time Use Survey. 2019. 'Time use in India'. Government of India, Ministry of Statistics and Programme Implementation, 2019. http://mospi.nic.in/sites/default/files/publication_reports/Report_TUS_2019_0.pdf.

Venkatraman, Shriram. 2017. *Social Media in South India*. London: University College London Press.

Viswanath, Kalpana. 2020. 'It is time to stop seeing domestic workers as COVID-19 "carriers"'. Thewire.in, 27 May 2020. Accessed December 2020. https://thewire.in/labour/covid-19-lockdown-domestic-workers.

Writes, Sp. 2020. 'When your maid comes back after lockdown'. Facebook, 8 April 2020. Accessed 18 December 2020. https://www.facebook.com/officialspwrites/videos/2068890199923609/.

20
Purity's dangers
At the interstices of religion and public health in Israel
Tsipy Ivry and Sarah Segal-Katz

In *Purity and Danger,* Mary Douglas (1966, 30) argued that materialist explanations of biblical rules concerning the body, such as in relation to diet and sex, as beneficial to health, are insufficient. By pointing out the semiotic rationale of these rules within a sorting system that classifies conditions of pollution and purity, she insisted that even if some of Moses' rules were 'hygienically beneficial it is a pity to treat him as an enlightened public health administrator, rather than as a spiritual leader' (1966, 30). Douglas never conceived of hygiene/contamination versus purity/defilement classification systems as mutually exclusive, but the COVID-19 pandemic provides a sharp perspective on their interplay and on the institutional division of labour between religious and public health experts. In this chapter, we look at how a purification ritual risks becoming a site of infection and how spiritual leaders take on public health responsibilities.

Toward the end of March, the Israeli media reported that religious centres in Israel, particularly those with ultra-orthodox populations, were registering high coronavirus infection rates. Community members were accused of transgressing governmental lockdown restrictions and endangering public health, thus reigniting stereotypes of faith-based communities as resistant to state and public health rationales. By mid-March, however, rabbinic authorities affiliated to the full range of Jewish religious observance – ranging from ultra-orthodox to modern orthodox – had already invested in restructuring communal and family life in order to facilitate adherence to public health measures.

This entailed a deep transformation, particularly given the intensive sociality of Jewish faith-based communities, including large families which, in densely populated urban settings, means overcrowded housing. The restructuring of long-standing religious styles of worship and sociality – the social configuration of praying, religious learning and the scale of Passovers meals – involved innovative negotiations of rabbinic laws. Marital sexuality became a locus of particular tension, as the halachic (rabbinic legal) requirement that women immerse in a *mikveh* (ritual bath) before resuming sexual relations after menstruation was seen to place women, and their families and communities, at risk of infection. For observant couples comprising women of fertility age who are not pregnant, this meant the imminent disruption of the rhythm of marital intimacy, namely, the recurrent cycle of sexual abstinence and complete 11–14 day physical distance upon the onset of menstrual bleeding followed by reunion after the woman's immersion in the mikveh.

In mid-March, swimming pools and men's *mikvehs* were closed, along with gyms, shopping malls, restaurants and more.[1] However, women's mikvehs remained open. The state-authorised chief rabbinate assured the public that women's mikvehs were safe and under state supervision and encouraged women to continue their immersion practice. Yet, at the same time, the public was informed of cases of women who tested positive soon after visiting the mikveh, although in no cases was the mikveh identified as the source of infection. In response to ensuing public anxiety, halachic opinions suggesting alternatives to immersion in a public mikveh were published in social and public media by rabbis who were not part of the state-authorised religious establishment. These alternatives were condemned by various rabbinic figures. The debate intensified when two women rabbinic scholars, Sarah Segal-Katz and Dr Chanah Adler-Lazarowitz, a gynaecologist by profession, published a public statement on the lack of institutional supervision and general uncertainty about the sanitary condition of mikvehs. Their statement encouraged women to consider not immersing if they were unsure about hygienic standards and claimed that there were halachically appropriate ways to uphold abstinence if the risk of infection was to linger. The statement led to a heated public debate on the safety of mikvehs, the observance of family purity laws (FPL) and kosher ways to negotiate their observance.

On 1 April, a few days before the Passover holiday and in the midst of an almost complete lockdown in Israel, Rabbanit[2] Malka Piotrokowski, a prominent modern-orthodox scholar of rabbinic law, participated with three other women rabbinic scholars in a public Zoom panel discussion on the mikveh (Karish-Hazony 2020). The panel, organised by *Makor Rishon*, a newspaper with a wide readership among various orthodox and traditional Jewish communities, received 13,000 views as of 30 September 2020. Piotrokowski opened with a direct attack on the established rabbinic authorities:

> I have been waiting to hear, for once, in an unusual reality, that a cohort of rabbis have gathered and strained their brains [to find a halachic solution] … because until Sarah [Segal-Katz] and Chanah [Adler-Lazarowitz] came out bravely, and it was clear they are going to pay for it personally, there was no clear guidance. Much worse, I know that an unequivocal demand by the Ministry of Health to close the mikvehs was silenced; no one considered it (Karish-Hazony, 2020, Hebrew, translated by Ivry).

Piotrokowski thus condemned the macro politics of religion and health, according to which health concerns are overridden by religious considerations (see Ivry 2013). Yet, drawing on her own experience as a halachic instructor, Piotrokowski admitted that, 'Personally, when women consulted me … about whether to go to the mikveh, I couldn't bring myself to say "don't go", because I am acutely and painfully aware of the implications of not going to the mikveh' (Karish-Hazony 2020). Thus, prioritising religious obligations over public health concerns can be traced to the micro politics of intimacy.

COVID-19 offered an opportunity to challenge this order of priorities by asking how the pandemic entered the macro and micro politics of religion, health and marital intimacy. We examine the suggestions emerging from public debates on women's mikvehs among religious scholars and lay people, paying particular attention to the interaction between two bodies of authoritative knowledge, rabbinic law and biomedicine and public health, in challenging the structure of rabbinic authority and illuminating relations between state and religion. We consider two specific kinds of threats: the risk of infection by COVID-19 and other pathogens – as negotiated by references to biomedical and public health discourses – and, in line with Mary Douglas (1966), the danger associated with pollution, with references to rabbinic discourse about the spiritual consequences of violating FPL. We heed the political interplay between these risks and dangers while exploring the tensions between public health initiatives and communities of faith.

Religion, state and public health

Religious belief systems and social structures emerge in the public health literature as being potentially either impediments or incentives to health promotion (Chatters 2000; Idler 2014; Van Ness 1999). Affiliation to a faith community has been identified as influencing a range of health outcomes throughout the life cycle including longevity, depression, cancer survival, suicide (Li et al. 2016), reproduction (Gaydos et al. 2010) and child health (Bramadat et al. 2017). The involvement of religious leaders and organisations in public health initiatives, and their accompanying tensions, has also been noted (e.g. Murray et al. 2011).

In Israel, representatives of orthodox Jewish communities are involved in shaping health policies as part of their general political participation. At the level of legislation, tensions gather around issues at both the beginning of life (e.g. abortion (Ivry 2015)) and the end of life (e.g. the legal definition of brain death (Gabbay and Fins 2019)). Ultra-orthodox Jewish communities are often perceived as presenting challenges to maternal and child health. For example, there is higher vaccine hesitancy among ultra-orthodox (16 per cent) and orthodox (9.5 per cent) Jews than among secular Jews and Arabs (Velan 2016), and ultra-orthodox women use state-funded prenatal care services selectively (Sher et al. 2003). Yet, ethnographic work has complicated notions of 'compliance' (Ivry 2015; Ivry et al. 2011), and orthodox Jewish communities tend to be eager consumers of healthcare and medical services, particularly community tailored programmes (Ivry 2010; Ivry and Teman 2019).

Such public health programmes echo an institutional imperative, authorised as Ministry of Health (MH) formal guidance since February 2011, to make public health services culturally and linguistically accessible to all ethnic and cultural minorities in Israel. Nonetheless, the expectation that medical care providers cultivate sensitivity to religious commitments may have questionable consequences. In one specific rabbinic organisation, FLOH (a pseudonym of Fertility in Light of Halacha), in which rabbis negotiate halachically appropriate routes to reproductive medicine with doctors on behalf of religious patients, they may also use their authority to pressure medical experts into compromising safety standards (Ivry 2013). A similar prioritisation of religious concerns emerged from the debates over women's mikvehs, albeit on a larger scale at the level of government ministries. Unlike the rabbis documented by Ivry (2013), the women rabbinic scholars whose public statement ignited the current debate advocated against the exemption of religious medical services from full adherence to state safety standards. We now explore the debates as a collaboration between Tsipy Ivry, a medical anthropologist, and one of the leading figures in the public debates, Sarah Segal-Katz, a rabbinical scholar and long-term mikveh attendant volunteer.

Methodology

Ivry had studied the intersection between medicine, rabbinic Judaism and women's reproductive health (Ivry 2010, 2015; Ivry et al. 2011; Ivry and Teman 2019), and was drawn to the debates over women's mikvehs. After conducting a few short, informal telephone conversations with former informants, she collected over 100 texts including articles published in the public and religious media on the subject from mid-March to mid-April 2020, statement papers and formal instructions issued by the MH and the Ministry of Religious Services (MRS) and watched Zoom panel discussions. Ivry then embarked in a dialogical collaboration with Sarah Segal Katz, bringing together the medical anthropological perspective of a non-participant online observer (Ivry) and the rabbinical scholar/activist perspective of a deeply involved participant observer (Segal-Katz). This was an opportunity, for Ivry, to rethink a decade-long exploration of the politics of medicine and religion from the vantage point of a pandemic; for Segal-Katz, it was an opportunity to reflect on the consequences of a debate in which she is deeply involved.

We discussed how best to bring the responses of observant women and men into our analysis and decided, due to ethical considerations, not to opt for seeking permission to quote (anonymously) from conversations in the exclusive social networks in which Segal-Katz participates as a leader, respondent and observer. Rather, Segal-Katz retrieved a range of responses from the open public Facebook network, that, she believes, allows for a preliminary mapping of responses. Our combined collection of data thus includes a wide variety of responses from women and men, religious and non-religious people, healthcare providers and mikveh attendants who participated in the debates between mid-March and mid-April. Excerpts from four Zoom panel discussions were transcribed verbatim in Hebrew and selected quotations, along with posts from the public Facebook discussions, were translated into English by Ivry. Both authors analysed the materials in light of four orienting questions: which discourses – religious and/or public health – are used, by whom, on what scale and to what effect? We applied these questions to the dataset described above, noticing how different contestants negotiated their religious and/or public health rationales, and the political consequences of this.

A short history is now required of transformations in FPL over the last two millennia – laws that have often served as the battleground for struggles over rabbinic authority, thus echoing Foucault's (1990) notion of sexuality as a dense transfer point of power relations.

Family purity laws

According to Leviticus 15, the onset of menstrual bleeding places a woman in a state of ritual impurity which renders her a *niddah* (separated, removed from the community of the pure) for seven days. Leviticus 17–26 warns twice that sexual relations and other forms of physical closeness with a niddah are strictly forbidden and violators are punished by being cut off from the people of Israel (*karet*). Menstrual impurity lapses on the eighth day. Bleeding beyond the seven days or a resumption of spotting is deemed an abnormal impurity (*zavah*) and requires women to count seven more days before they may perform purification rituals.

The collapse of Jewish national sovereignty, the destruction of the Second Temple in 70 CE, and the subsequent development of rabbinic Judaism wrought a change in the niddah laws. The period of sexual abstinence was extended, arguably for fear of confusing irregular bleeding (*zavah*) with normal menstrual blood (Rosenak 2011; Wasserfall 1999). The extension received the status of a full-fledged rabbinic law in the second century CE and has since retained its authority in orthodox and ultra-orthodox communities around the world. Whereas biblical law assumed a simple timeline to ritual purity, from the second century women were instructed to systematically inspect their menstrual flow and all genital discharges. Only after ascertaining seven 'clean' days via pieces of cloth and daily check-ups, may a woman immerse in a mikveh. While biblical law had held women accountable for self-diagnosing, the Mishnah allocated this authority to rabbis, and women were expected to bring samples of their vaginal discharges to rabbis for their ruling (Fonrobert 1999). This still occurs in many ultra-orthodox communities. There is extensive discussion in contemporary rabbinic literature about the correct observance of FPL, including the appropriate length of sexual abstinence and how to count it (Ivry 2013). There are both historical (Cohen 1999; Wasserfall 1999) and contemporary accounts (Avishai 2008) of women choosing to lengthen the period of abstinence for contraceptive purposes or as a means of empowerment (Wasserfall 1999). In addition, the

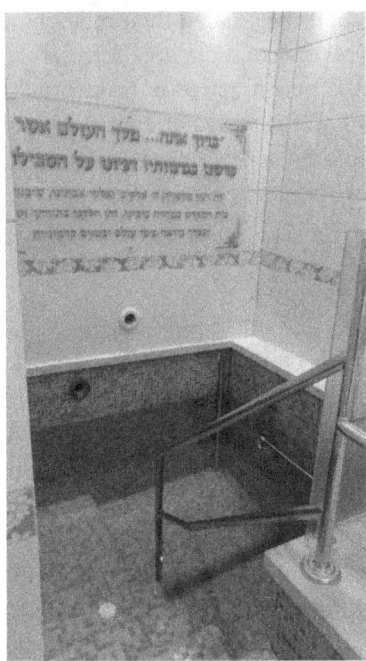

Figure 20.1 Immersion pool in a mikveh in Haifa. During outbreaks mikveh attendants are expected to sterilise the railings and tiles leading to the pool after each immersion. A blessing is recited by women before immersion: 'Blessed are You, our G-d, Who has sanctified us with His commandments, and commanded us concerning the immersion'. This is written in Hebrew on the sign over the pool. Photo: Merav Fenigstein Gizbar

architectural structure and dimensions of a mikveh were specified to ensure that a person of average size is completely covered by the water; only rain water collected without direct human intervention can purify menstrual impurity and a woman's body must be fully immersed in the water. This led to the requirement that the immersion be witnessed by another woman.

Contemporary mikvehs in Israel are designed to meet orthodox rabbinic requirements, as represented by MRS, and sanitation standards set by MH. They are, accordingly, built as a complex of private preparation rooms, each equipped with a bathtub, cleansing paraphernalia, a mirror to confirm that no object remains that might separate the woman's body from the water (a single hair is considered a separation), and a door leading to a common immersion pool (Figure 20.1). Until the outbreak of Covid-19, a woman was expected to conduct lengthy preparations inside one of these private rooms according to detailed rabbinic instructions, which include soaking for 30 minutes in a hot bath, washing her entire body with soap, shampooing her hair, cutting her nails and more. She then calls the woman mikveh attendant, who confirms that she has done all the necessary preparations, leads her to the immersion pool and supervises her immersion. 'Secular' cleanliness (to use Douglas' [1966] idiom) is only a prerequisite to the purification ritual, and it was precisely the fear that 'secular' public health standards of hygiene were compromised that ignited the women's mikveh crisis.

The mikveh as a state service

In contemporary Israel – a state constituted to be both democratic and Jewish – mikveh immersion is a personal choice as part of the freedom to practise religion granted by the state. Mikvehs are a state-funded religious service that operate under the mandate of MRS and according to MH regulations. These regulations, issued in 1999, require that to operate legally, mikvehs must hold a business licence, which is conditional on fulfilling MH health and safety standards. According to an MRS report from 22 April 2020, over 700 mikvehs operate throughout Israel and around 130,000 women immerse in them each month (Ministry of Religious Services, 2020).

The use of mikvehs extends beyond self-defined religiously observant Jewish women (Cicurel 2000). Of Israel's six million Jewish citizens, 30 per cent identify themselves as religiously observant and 25 per cent as traditional (Central Bureau of Statistics 2018). The observant communities are divided into various categories according to theological orientation, attitudes and commitment to Halacha, styles of observance, ethnic origin and political inclination (Ivry and Teman 2019). Orthodox Judaism maintains a powerful and controversial legal standing within the apparatus of state governance with state-sanctioned religious courts ruling on matters of personal status and family laws and the orthodox rabbinate having full authority over citizens registered as Jewish. Jewish Israelis can only marry under the authority of the chief rabbinate; one prerequisite for marriage is that the woman, regardless of her self-definition, brings a certificate testifying that she has immersed in a mikveh. Israel endorses freedom of religion, but freedom from religion is a contested issue (Ferziger 2008; Neuberger 1999).

Orthodox Jewish representatives also play an important role in policy making. For example, Ya'akov Litzman, the minister of health who handled the Covid-19 outbreak until his resignation on 25 April, is an ultra-orthodox Jew. Despite popularity associated with the implementation of several health reforms, Litzman was criticised for his handling of the pandemic and accused of using his position to prevent senior MH executives from closing women's mikvehs. Decades earlier, senior MH executives had also refrained from closing mikvehs that failed to meet MH standards of safety, arguing that 'closing the mikvaot without providing an alternative solution would cause the religious public, for whom this service is vital, great distress' (Adler-Lazarowitz and Segal-Katz 2020).[3]

Underlying this is the notion that religious obligations are non-negotiable and the rules unchanging. This does not conform with either the history of contestation over FPL or recent gendered challenges to rabbinic authority. While FPL were deemed throughout history the epitome of a woman's Jewish identity and a source of pleasure and empowerment (e.g. Cicurel 2000; Waserfall 1999), women continued to negotiate and resist the rabbinic laws of niddah and to foster their own private versions of observance, sometimes despite explicit protests (Cohen 1999). However, for the past four decades, women's initiatives to reclaim authority over the observance of FPL have increasingly been made public.

The rise of women's rabbinic authority

Orthodox commentators and scholars of Jewish orthodoxy have claimed that observant Judaism is undergoing a 'women's literacy revolution' (El-Or 2002; Ross 2004). Orthodox women can now become halachically proficient through a variety of institutional routes, and women rabbinic scholars, such as Piotrokowski, are becoming more prominent. The majority of institutional opportunities for women to qualify and become certified as halachic experts lie in the realm of FPL. Avishai (2008, 209) pointed out a 'cultural industry surrounding niddah' that began in the 1980s, and the list of formally certified women professionals now includes premarital educators who teach FPL to brides and niddah consultants who are trained to answer women's questions on the observance of the niddah laws and to serve 'as quasi marriage counsellors, medical professionals and sex educators' (Avishai 2008, 210; see also Zimmerman 2001). Women halachic experts are advancing new kinds of knowledge that is simultaneously traditional and modern, religiously committed and emancipatory (Avishai 2008).

These experts also offer new venues of consultation that almost bypass direct engagement with male rabbis, thus steadily transforming the structure of authority while emphasising their full commitment to traditional structures. Feminist religious women's movements with their commitment to both Halacha and feminist ideals exerted important influence over these developments (Irshai 2014; Irshai and Zion-Waldoks 2013). Observant women's advocacy groups have struggled with gender inequality in religious marriage and divorce and with sexual harassment and abuse perpetrated by rabbinic figures. Social networks have given these struggles considerable momentum. Segal-Katz and Adler-Lazarowitz are both rabbinic scholars and instructors, co-leaders and participants in large closed Facebook groups dedicated to discussions on the halachic lives of women.[4] Segal-Katz, an orthodox feminist activist on issues of religion and state, has been active in Advot, a group that was involved in a successful petition to the high court submitted by ITIM,[5] granting women the right to immerse in the mikveh without supervision. COVID-19 rode on the wave of women's efforts to reclaim authority over FPL and, with health at stake, pushed them forward.

Sanctified state regulations and halachic alternatives in 'times of distress'

From mid-March 2020, the numbers of confirmed infection cases were rising and lockdown restrictions were tightening. Businesses were closed by state order and citizens were warned to wear masks, to refrain from gathering, to keep a minimum of two metres from other people, and not to go more than 100 metres from their homes. On 12 March, Ashkenazi Chief Rabbi Lau issued guidance that sanctified state regulations, emphasising that 'these restrictions are halachically binding' (Berger 2020). The guidance included detailed instructions limiting various gatherings in synagogues including learning, prayer quorums, weddings, funerals and other religious celebrations. The instructions concerning women's ritual immersion were comparatively brief and vague, stating that 'the routine of "home purity" should be continued and there is no place for apprehension. A woman who, according to MH instructions, must self-quarantine, should act as her situation necessitates'. What her situation necessitated remained unclear.

In the ensuing days, 15 women who had immersed in various mikvehs around the country and two mikveh attendants tested positive, two mikvehs were closed and women who had visited the mikveh on the same day as those infected went into self-quarantine. The MRS issued instructions for the operation and use of mikvehs, including that women wash and prepare in their homes to shorten their visit and that mikveh attendants monitor the chlorination of the water in the immersion pool more often and change the water once a day. Tiles, railings and all surfaces were to be sterilised after each immersion, and women's visits to the mikveh were to be scheduled in advance to ensure 15-minute intervals between each immersion. The media reported that rabbis abroad had issued instructions to close women's mikvehs for fear of infection. By 16 March, the MH had negotiated plans to issue a full lockdown during and possibly beyond the week of the Passover holiday, leading to the closing of all public institutions excluding mikvehs.

On 17 March, Rabbi Haim Amsalem, a rabbinic scholar, former member of parliament, and Mizrahi social activist, uploaded a post on Facebook suggesting that in 'times of great distress' (*she'at dechak*) women be permitted to immerse in their own bathtubs on condition that this fulfils rabbinic requirements concerning the structure, dimensions, and volume and quality of water. His post, quoting the halachic literature, addressed men – the traditional audience of halachic texts – occasionally insinuating the difficulty of sexual abstinence. Immediate responses on Facebook ranged from women's assertions that the mikveh is 'the practice that has protected us [spiritually and physically] for generations', doubts by both women and men about Amsalem's qualifications as a rabbi, and, more specifically, requests for a simpler clarification of the dimensions of an appropriate bathtub.[6] The chief rabbinate published unequivocal condemnation of Amsalem's solution, explicitly addressing women and praising their devoutness to FPL. Women were encouraged to proceed with the practice and not 'lend their ears to lies, because [proper observance of the FPL] is crucial to the well-being of our souls'.

On 18 March, 100 new COVID-19 cases were reported. The following day, after more women tested positive after immersing in the mikveh, Kolech, the leading orthodox feminist movement, published a handwritten halachic opinion (not a ruling) by Rabbi Dr Daniel Sperber, an authority in Israeli modern-orthodox circles and a supporter of orthodox feminism. Sperber cited the Mishna to argue for 'leniency on the prohibition against physical closeness for women who choose not to immerse'. Soon after, the Sephardi Chief Rabbi Eliyahu Bakshi-Doron published his opposition, reinforcing the danger of breaking FPL and invoking the traditional notion of death as a consequence of breaking a taboo (Douglas 1992, 16). Both rabbis avoided any detailed discussion of the sanitary condition of the mikvehs.

Evidence-based halachic statement

On 20 March, as new lockdown restrictions were implemented, Segal-Katz and Adler-Lazarowitz published a public statement addressed to women entitled, 'Women, be very careful for your souls/lives (*venishmarten lenaphshoteichen*)'.[7] The two women authors identified themselves as halachic instructors who had received 'a flood of questions' about the safety of immersion and were striving to provide responsible answers:

> We felt that it was preferable to obtain a clear picture of the actual reality before issuing a halachic response. We therefore wish here to inform the public of what we have learned regarding the mikveh system over the years. In so doing, we hope to allow the public to make an informed decision about observing the mitzvah of immersion as long as the MH refrains from ensuring proper standards in every mikveh (Adler-Lazarowitz and Segal-Katz 2020).

Unlike the previous rabbinic statements, this one recognised the difficulty of giving halachic instructions, highlighted the contingency of halachic decisions on empirical realities and, importantly, called for personal 'evidence-based halachic decision-making'. Segal-Katz and Adler-Lazarowitz (2020) informed the public of repeated institutional warnings about the non-implementation of MH standards in the mikvehs long before the outbreak of COVID-19. For example, the state comptroller in 2004 had criticised the 'unsatisfactory and undersupervised' conditions of mikvehs, but recommendations for increased sanitary supervision and increased training of mikveh attendants had been ignored. A report from 2015 (Achrak-Wein et al. 2015) stated that only 75 per cent of mikvehs actually held a valid business licence. In a parliamentary discussion in 2017, the director-general of MRS admitted that 'they simply lack the means or ability to enforce the business licenses of mikvehs'. Segal-Katz and Adler-Lazarowitz reported that MH supervision was infrequent and mikveh attendants monitored sanitation alone. Public swimming pools, by comparison, are monitored by MH on a fortnightly basis for chlorine and bacteria levels, and pools that deviate from standards are closed. Following the outbreak of COVID-19, MRS updated mikveh instructions; however, according to Segal-Katz and Adler-Lazarowitz, 'not all mikvehs have been supplied with all the means for disinfecting the mikveh and protecting mikveh attendants, some of whom are in a high risk group because of their age'.

Segal-Katz and Adler-Lazarowitz wrote as citizen scientists (Conrad and Hilchey 2011), quoting institutional reports, their own research and their own experiences. But they also drew on rabbinic scholarship, claiming that 'it is forbidden by Halacha to put oneself in potential danger if there is no safe immersion option'. They encouraged women observing FPL and their spouses to be 'stringent in matters of life and death', reminded readers that many couples contend with long periods of abstinence after birth, miscarriage and irregular bleeding, and stressed the importance of couples cultivating 'emotional and spiritual affinity'. In their evidence-based attitude, neither health risks nor halachic obligations are taken for granted. Their statement provoked an immediate response signed by 46 community rabbis, reasserting that physical touch between spouses was forbidden according to Halacha, that mikvehs under MRS responsibility were safe and that the virus cannot survive in water chlorinated according to MH instructions. However, MRS data indicated a 16.8 per cent decrease in the number of women using mikvehs since the outbreak of COVID-19.

On 1 April, the head rabbi of FLOH addressed observant women in a special broadcast on Arutz 7, a popular religious news channel (Arutz 7 2020). He suggested that women take contraceptive pills continuously to prevent menstruation and so delay the need to visit the mikveh as long as possible. Reassuring them of the safety of long-term contraception, he asked women who resisted this for ideological reasons 'to make as much effort' to prevent menstruation for the sake of *shalom bayit* (marital harmony) and to ask their gynaecologists to prescribe them several packages of contraceptives. Consistent with its strategic approach to technology to advance the observance of religious duties (Ivry 2010, 2013, 2015), FLOH thus advocated a hormonal solution to a halachically aggravated problem, dismissing considerations of safety (Bartz et al. 2020; Huber et al. 2020). While there were intense discussions in 2006 about FLOH's hormonal solution to delay ovulation for women with 'halachic infertility' due to the length of observance required by FPL (Ivry 2013), this 2020 solution raised few responses. Instead, women complained about the shortage of contraceptive pills in pharmacies, implying the wide use of contraceptives by women in religious communities to work around mikveh requirements both with and without rabbinic permission.

Negotiating uncertainties

Segal-Katz and Adler-Lazarowitz's statement prompted a heated debate, not only because of their explicit call for couples to take halachic decisions into their own hands. Their description of the infrastructure of mikvehs attempted to achieve a somewhat paradoxical feat: to clarify the uncertainty about the sanitary conditions while appealing to MH for supervision and transparency. This attempt to demystify various interrelated uncertainties seems to have challenged the public.

Most participants in the open Facebook discussions on the topic were women, including medical doctors, an epidemiologist, the head of a local religious committee, mikveh attendants, niddah consultants and pre-marital instructors. Initially, participants tended to reduce the message, in particular questions of uncertainty, potentiality, and contingency of the halachic and medical systems. Many interpreted the statement as either an (unsolicited) rabbinic ruling – rather than a confession about the inability to give halachic answers – or as an unequivocal proclamation of all mikvehs as dangerous places – rather than an attempt to alert the public to potential health risks and to advocate for systematic state supervision, clarity and transparency. Participants' acknowledgement of uncertainty in one arena, Halacha or public health, often led to statements of certainty in the other. See, for example, an exchange on Facebook between Segal-Katz and RT:

RT: [The solution is] simply not to immerse. That's what I've written as a medical doctor in two other discussion groups. The discussion should proceed to consider the halachic question of where the limit of distancing between spouses should be.
Segal-Katz: I hinted at such space of halachic discussion. If this is indeed all that is left to us, these will be the questions. The question is though: is this indeed all that is left?
RT: Unfortunately, that is what's left.

RT interpreted the statement as an unequivocally negative assessment and concluded that immersion was unsafe by default. Segal-Katz attempted to emphasise uncertainty, but this did not change RT's conviction that the public health aspect was non-negotiable. Other participants conveyed the opposite, namely, that halachic obligation was non-negotiable even if there was uncertainty about safety:

> I am so ambivalent ... I immersed in the mikveh a short while ago, I was trembling from fear, and then I heard that a mikveh attendant in Maale Adumim tested positive ... This can happen in other mikvehs as well, clearly there is no way not to immerse, especially

since [the pandemic] is here for a long time ... It was the first time I really wanted to cry my heart out after immersion, only from the stress that my body accumulated during the long days before immersion.

Anxiety notwithstanding, many participants insisted that even doubts about their hygiene would not open the mikveh to negotiation. N stated: 'This is all very important but we must immerse, we shall not remain without [the option] to immerse'. Segal-Katz then reminded participants of the contingency of halachic considerations on public health assessments and of the negotiability of Halacha on even the most binding obligations: 'If there is a danger to life here, if not for an individual woman but for the general public, then the halachic consideration will not necessarily reach the same conclusion'. Faced with the negotiability of Halacha, N returned to the public health arena to doubt the severity of the sanitary condition of mikvaot and the potential health risk; 'some (public health) professors' she wrote, 'claim that there is needless public panic and that statistically more people die of influenza'.

Several trajectories thus emerged. The first echoed the criticisms of several Israeli health professionals: 'There are professors who claim that much of the current crisis is due to anxiety ... statistically more die of flu, so I am not sure I understand'. The second draws on participants' own experiences of the cleanliness and aesthetics of mikvehs. Y wrote: 'I have never seen a dirty mikveh. The most I have seen is a mikveh operating in an old building but always clean and sterile'. S, on the other hand, described how filthy her local mikveh was, reminding the participants that 'not all the mikvehs are clean'. The participants used cleanliness and sterility as interchangeable terms, while Segal-Katz repeatedly pointed out that cleanliness was not the same thing as sterility. A third trajectory of scepticism related to MRS instructions.

L: I know that they doubled the quantity of chlorine stated in the instructions ... I spoke yesterday to the mikveh attendant who told me they sterilize the rooms between women.

Segal-Katz: Implementation and strict adherence to the instructions are wonderful, but are you sure this is really happening? According to Halacha, can a woman who works in the mikveh and receives her salary from the religious local authority, testify to the condition of the water and the sanitation as a whole? She has not taken an MH course that qualifies her to supervise and assess the level of sanitation, and if she says there's a problem, isn't she endangering her employment? Can she really testify to everything being excellent, or is it, halachically, a conflict of interest? Everybody's intentions are good, but it is necessary to establish order and professional supervision in the mikvehs.

Women responded with testimonies about having their temperature taken before entering the mikveh and the diligence with which mikveh attendants cleaned between immersions: 'I doubt whether the virus can survive more than three minutes'. Others noted, however, that even people with no temperature can later test positive and that little is known about the virus.

Mikveh attendants themselves depicted their meticulousness in following MRS instructions. One even scolded Segal-Katz: 'What do you think? That there is lawlessness here? There are water checks, there is chlorine in the water automatically and tablets are added, we change the water frequently, I have to report the number of towels used ... this is sacred work (*avodat kodesh*)'. While Segal-Katz attempted to transfer responsibility for safety standards to MH, the attendants sanctified their work and MRS instructions and saw themselves as responsible for ensuring safety. Segal-Katz responded:

> I am familiar with the instructions and the heavy load that mikveh attendants carry ... what you witness around you cannot be a reflection of everything that happens in all mikvehs. There are mikveh attendants who are willing to follow the instructions but lack the necessary equipment or there is a problem with the frequency of changing the water. So please enjoy the good that you witness, but understand that I am raising awareness about the sanitary conditions in places where the instructions are not applied fully because more test tubes are needed now than usual and ... there are even sometimes problems ... ensuring a 15-minute gap between immersions.

Both mikveh attendants and women who defended the safety of mikvehs attempted to establish certainty. However, depictions of mikvehs that 'smell of bleach' also raised ironic responses such as: 'There is chlorine in the water, it is changed twice a week, it's really revolting but sacred' and 'the mikveh is so sterilized that you can get bleach poisoning from corona'.

Women thus expressed the paradox of a purification ritual that had become potentially infectious.

Facing uncertainty about the sanitary conditions of mikvehs

When uncertainty about the state of sanitation was acknowledged, some participants tried to measure the risk against similar risks in other public arenas – 'People can sneeze on you in the supermarket too' – leading some to compare general health risks with the dangers of non-compliance with religious obligations: 'The mikveh is within the category of *pikuach nefesh* [meaning it endangers one's life not to immerse in a mikveh]; it is as necessary to religious people as food'. The participant thus reversed the meaning of the halachic idiom of *pikuah nefesh*, which allows for temporary violations of Halacha when a life is endangered, echoing MH avoidance of closing mikvehs that do not meet safety standards and rabbis' difficulties telling women not to immerse due to health risks (Piotrokowski cited in Karish-Hazony, 2020, Hebrew, translated by Ivry).

Segal-Katz was accused of 'a cold halachic discourse', of misunderstanding the 'sacred value of the spousal union', and of overlooking the stressful real-life struggles of couples during the pandemic. One head of a local religious authority accused her of causing needless anxiety and reassured women of the safety of the mikvehs under his jurisdiction. Other participants protested MRS strategies. They reported feeling 'offended as a woman and a person' or 'cheated – they endanger my life for immersion' and asked how 'the health of religious women is being discarded?' After discussing and rejecting alternatives to mikveh (bathtubs, natural springs, the sea), some participants declared immersion during a pandemic as irresponsible.

Some women demanded clarification of the uncertainty. S asked Segal-Katz directly: 'I would be grateful for a focused and clear answer. Your writing takes many directions. For those who are halachically committed, please write an answer to the point ... to immerse or not to immerse?' Segal-Katz answered: 'I am trying to say that I cannot give halachic answers in a situation where it is unclear whether the necessary conditions in the mikveh are fulfilled'. Participants continued pleading for an unequivocal (male) rabbinic ruling in the face of the uncertainty. The rabbinic authorities answered this plea to an extent when, on 6 April, FLOH and the Association of Community Rabbis in Israel published a list of mikvehs that adhered to MH standards and the names of the responsible rabbis. However, the supervision procedures remained unclear. Segal-Katz continued to update the public on her personal website about women who had tested positive, sharing women's reports on safety standards in mikvehs.

By 11 May, after the first wave of COVID-19 was deemed contained, the MRS cancelled the requirement for a 15-minute interval between immersions. Following the outbreak of the second wave, with thousands of new cases each day and new lockdown instructions, including strict limits on mobility, for at least three weeks starting from 18 September, MRS published a statement allowing women to walk further than the permitted one kilometre to visit a mikveh. MH was silent.

Segal-Katz's preliminary mapping of observant women's choices during the second wave suggests great diversity. Some women continue to immerse in public mikvehs (where health and safety is now being monitored more strictly by MRS) and they see attempts to question the sanitation of the mikveh as heresy. Others are foregoing immersion and reducing their commitment to FPL. Between these poles, women continue to immerse after checking the state of sanitation and sharing their findings, travelling, when possible, to well-maintained and less crowded mikvehs in remote areas, or immersing in natural springs or the sea. Finally, some women have deferred immersion and remain fully committed to the halachic rules of physical separation and some take long-term contraception.

Purity's dangers and risks

What, then, can controversies over the potential infectiousness of a purification ritual during a pandemic teach us about the intersection between religion and public health? What can religious scholars' negotiations over public health responsibilities show about the role of a pandemic in challenging state and religious structures of authority?

The women's mikveh crisis demonstrates that an event such as a pandemic can illuminate long-standing institutional dysfunctions and intensify ongoing inter-communal and inter-institutional strife. The outbreak of COVID-19 loaded onto the macro and micro politics of religion, health and gender, particularly women's ongoing efforts to reclaim authority over rabbinic laws organising sexuality and question rabbinic authority. The statement that ignited the debates entangled public health discourse with rabbinic scholarship, calling for MH intervention to ensure the safety of a religious ritual and drawing public attention to the issue at hand. This call for both public and institutional attention was made in the name of women's health, the health of their communities and the entire public.

Significantly, rabbis incorporated biomedical knowledge into rabbinic considerations. Yet, as work on FLOH illustrates, biomedical knowledge and technologies are often presented as progressive ways of assisting religious commitments while downplaying risks (Ivry 2010, 2013). In contrast, Segal-Katz and Adler-Lazarowitz pursued a powerful public health risk discourse in the context of rising morbidity and mortality rates.

In 1966, Douglas pointed out the role of danger in guarding 'the ideal order of society' (1966, 3), noting that 'pollution beliefs can be used in a dialogue of claims and counter-claims to status' (1966, 3). If dangers are to risks as pre-modern is to modern, then negotiating a matrix of contingencies around dangers, risks, pollution and viral contagion at the interstices of two authority systems – a state public health governance of risk and a religious system of authority – seem to have the dramatic potential to reorganise the social order.

However, in addressing the moral implications of risk discourse, Douglas argued that being '"at risk" is not an equivalent but the reciprocal of being "in sin". To be "at risk" is equivalent to being sinned against, being vulnerable to the events caused by others, whereas being "in sin" means being the cause of harm' (1992, 28). By pointing out both purity's risks and dangers, Segal-Katz and Adler-Lazarowitz tried to remind observant women, their spouses and mikveh attendants of their matrix of religious and citizenship rights and obligations while advocating against religious exceptionalism. Yet, the introduction of a matrix of contingencies and contradictions stimulated attempts to separate the systems and declare one of them non-negotiable.

Such separations are 'useful' for policymakers to draw on when prioritising religious obligations over health concerns. Underlying the prioritisation of religion in the name of cultural sensitivity or commitment to Halacha, religious obligations are presented as a non-negotiable set of rules. However, the debates over women's mikvehs illustrate what medical anthropologists have argued for decades, namely, that any consideration of health policy should take into account the open-ended, power-ridden, and multivocal diversity of cultures and religious communities. Specifically, intercommunal structures of meaning and governance and gendered challenges carry simultaneously conservative and transformative powers, thus opening up many spaces for negotiation.

Acknowledgements

Tsipy Ivry is grateful to Aviya Lensky for her dedicated assistance with the collection and organisation of the database on which this article is grounded.

Notes

1. Men also immerse in the mikveh, but this is rendered a custom and not a commandment.
2. 'Rabbanit' designates a woman rabbinic scholar (not the wife of a rabbi). An appeal to the high court to make women elegible to attend state exams is pending.
3. Names by alphabetical order.
4. Segal-Katz is co-leader of 'Tranquil Immersion' (Tovlot benachat) with 1,400 participants, and Adler-Lazarowitz is co-leader of 'Halachic Feminists' with 11,000 participants.
5. ITIM is an 'advocacy organization working to build a Jewish and democratic Israel' https://www.itim.org.il/en/
6. Segal-Katz published on her internet site the halachic opposition of Rabbanit Tikochinski (2020).
7. The title converts the famous verse from Deuteronomy quoted previously, which is originally phrased in the second person male plural, into the second person female plural.

References

Achrak-Wein Michal, Ariel Finkelstein and Dvir Schwartz. 2015. *The Mikveh System in Israel*. Jerusalem, Israel: The Institute for Zionist Strategies. [Hebrew]

Adler-Lazarowitz, Chanah and Sarah Segal-Katz. 2020. *Public Statement on Tevila in Mikvaot – 'Take good heed of yourselves'*. March 2020. Accessed 18 April 2021. https://gluya.org/wp-content/uploads/2020/03/coronavirusmikvaot.pdf?fbclid=IwAR0-Vrh0gnO153kv3Gq_sYok7r3eTMRydgFA4mr7o_XH9S8tGjMBIe1JRa8.

Arutz 7. 2020. 'Special broadcast: Passover and purity during COVID-19 outbreak'. 1 April 2020. Accessed 18 April 2021. https://www.inn.co.il/news/432589. [Hebrew]

Avishai, Orit. 2008. 'Halakhic niddah consultants and the orthodox women's movement in Israel: Evaluating the story of enlightened progress'. *Journal of Modern Jewish Studies* 7(2): 195–216.

Berger, Mandy. 2020. 'Protection from the corona virus: The chief rabbi's halachic instructions'. *COL*, 12 March 2020. Accessed 18 April 2021. https://col.org.il/news/123594. [Hebrew]

Bramadat, Paul, Maryse Guay, Julie A. Bettinger and Réal Roy, eds. 2017. *Public Health in the Age of Anxiety: Religious and cultural roots of vaccine hesitancy in Canada*. Toronto, Canada: University of Toronto Press.

Central Bureau of Statistics. 2018. *Religion and Self-Definition of Extent of Religiosity. Selected data from the Society in Israel Report No. 10*. Jerusalem, Israel: Central Bureau of Statistics. https://www.cbs.gov.il/he/mediarelease/DocLib/2018/195/32_18_195b.pdf. [Hebrew]

Chatters, Linda M. 2000. 'Religion and health: Public health research and practice' *Annual Review of Public Health* 21(1): 335–67.

Cicurel, Inbal E. 2000. 'The rabbinate versus Israeli (Jewish) women: The mikvah as a contested domain'. *Nashim: A Journal of Jewish Women's Studies & Gender Issues* 3: 164–90.

Cohen, Shaye J.D. 1999. 'Purity, piety, and polemic: Medieval rabbinic denunciations of "incorrect" purification practices'. In *Women and Water: Menstruation in Jewish life and law*, edited by Rahel Wasserfall, pp. 87–100. Hanover and London: Brandeis University Press.

Conrad, Cathy C. and Krista G. Hilchey. 2011. 'A review of citizen science and community-based environmental monitoring: Issues and opportunities'. *Environmental Monitoring and Assessment* 176 (1–4): 273–91.

Douglas, Mary. 1966. *Purity and Danger: An analysis of concepts of pollution and taboo*. London: Routledge.
Douglas, Mary. 1992. *Risk and Blame*. London: Routledge.
El-Or, Tamar. 2002. *Next Year I Will Know More: Literacy and identity among young orthodox women in Israel*. Detroit, MI: Wayne State University Press.
Ferziger, Adam S. 2008. 'Religion for the secular: The new Israeli rabbinate'. *Journal of Modern Jewish Studies* 7(1): 67–90.
Fonrobert, Charlotte Elisheva. 1999. 'Yalta's ruse: Resistance against rabbinic menstrual authority in talmudic literature'. *Women and Water: Menstruation in Jewish life and law*, edited by Rahel Wasserfall, pp. 60–81. Hanover and London: Brandeis University Press.
Foucault, Michel. 1990. *The History of Sexuality: An introduction, Vol. 1*. Translated by Robert Hurley. New York: Vintage.
Gabbay, Ezra and Joseph J. Fins. 2019. 'Go in peace: Brain death, reasonable accommodation and Jewish mourning rituals'. *Journal of Religion and Health* 58(5): 1672–86.
Gaydos, Laura M., Alexandria Smith, Carol J.R. Hogue and John Blevins. 2010. 'An emerging field in religion and reproductive health'. *Journal of Religion and Health* 49(4): 473–84.
Huber, D., S. Seitz, K. Kast, G. Emons and O. Ortman. 2020. 'Use of oral contraceptives in BRCA mutation carriers and risk for ovarian and breast cancer: A systematic review'. *Archives of Gynecology and Obstetrics* 4: 1–10.
Idler, Ellen L., ed. 2014. *Religion as a Social Determinant of Public Health*. New York: Oxford University Press.
Irshai, Ronit. 2014. 'Judaism, gender, and human rights: The case of orthodox feminism'. *Religion and the Discourse of Human Rights*, pp. 412–38. Jerusalem, Israel: Israel Democracy Institute.
Irshai, Ronit and Tanya Zion-Waldoks. 2013. 'Modern-orthodox feminism in Israel: Between nomos and narrative'. *Mishpat Umimshal* 15(1–2): 1–94. [Hebrew]
Ivry, Tsipy. 2010. 'Kosher medicine and medicalized Halacha: An exploration of triadic relations among Israeli rabbis, doctors, and infertility patients'. *American Ethnologist* 37(4): 662–80.
Ivry, Tsipy. 2013. 'Halachic infertility: Rabbis, doctors, and the struggle over professional boundaries'. *Medical Anthropology* 32 (3): 208–26. https://doi.org/10.1080/01459740.2012.674992.
Ivry, Tsipy. 2015. 'The predicaments of koshering prenatal diagnosis and the rise of a new rabbinic leadership'. *Ethnologie Française* 45(2): 281–92.
Ivry, Tsipy, Elly Teman and Ayala Frumkin. 2011. 'God-sent ordeals and their discontents: Ultra-orthodox Jewish women negotiate prenatal testing'. *Social Science & Medicine* 72(9): 1527–33.
Ivry, Tsipy and Elly Teman. 2019. 'Shouldering moral responsibility: The division of moral labor among pregnant women, rabbis, and doctors'. *American Anthropologist* 121(4): 857–69.
Karish-Hazony, Hodaya. 2020. 'Watch: Family purity in the shadow of corona: A special panel'. *Makor Rishon*, 1 April 2020. Accessed 18 April 2021. https://www.makorrishon.co.il/judaism/217539/. [Hebrew]
Li, Shanshan, Olivia I Okereke, Shun-Chiao Chang, Ichiro Kawachi and Tyler J. VanderWeele. 2016. 'Religious service attendance and lower depression among women: A prospective cohort study'. *Annals of Behavioral Medicine* 50 (6): 876–84.
Mavhunga, Clapperton Chakanetsa. 2011. 'Vermin beings: On pestiferous animals and human game.' *Social Text* 29 (1): 151–76. https://doi.org/10.1215/01642472-1210302.
Ministry of Religious Services. 2020. *The Spread of COVID-19 – An interim update about the state of operation of women's mikvehs*, 22 April 2020. Accessed 18 April 2021. https://www.gov.il/BlobFolder/generalpage/the_mikvah_service_during_the_corona_period/he/%D7%A2%D7%93%D7%9B%D7%95%D7%9F%20%D7%A1%D7%98%D7%90%D7%98%D7%95%D7%A1%20-%20%D7%AA%D7%A4%D7%A2%D7%95%D7%9C%20%D7%9E%D7%A7%D7%95%D7%95%D7%90%D7%95%D7%AA%20%D7%91%D7%97%D7%A8%D7%95%D7%9D%20%D7%A7%D7%95%D7%A8%D7%95%D7%A0%D7%94%2004.20.pdf. [Hebrew]
Murray, Laura R., Jonathan Garcia, Miguel Muñoz-Laboy and Richard G. Parker. 2011. 'Strange bedfellows: The Catholic church and Brazilian national AIDS program in the response to HIV/AIDS in Brazil'. *Social Science & Medicine* 72(6): 945–52.
Neuberger, Benyamin. 1999. 'Religion and state in Europe and Israel'. *Israel Affairs* 6(2): 65–84.

Roe, Andrea, Deborah A. Bartz and Pamela S. Douglas. 2020. 'Combined estrogen-progestin contraception: Side effects and health concerns'. *UpToDate*. Accessed 12 October 2021. https://www.uptodate.com/contents/combined-estrogen-progestin-contraception-side-effects-and-health-concerns?search=Combined%20estrogen-progestin%20contraception:%20side%20effects%20and%20health%20concerns&source=search_result&selectedTitle=1~150&usage_type=default&display_rank=1 (Sist oppdatert 26).

Rosenak, Daniel. 2011. *To Restore the Splendor: The real meaning of severity in applying Jewish marital traditions*. [In Hebrew.] Miskal: Tel Aviv.

Ross, Tamar. 2004. *Expanding the Palace of Torah: Orthodoxy and feminism*. Waltham. MA: Brandeis University Press.

Segal-Katz, Sarah. 2000. March 18 Facebook. Accessed 18 April 2021. https://www.facebook.com/photo.php?fbid=10157424354044926&set=a.10150923566434926&type=3&theatre. [Hebrew]

Segal-Katz, Sarah. 2000. 'The fight against corona: Do the mikvehs endanger life?' *Yisrael Hayom*, 19 March 2000. https://www.israelhayom.co.il/article/743415. [Hebrew]

Sher, Carron, Orly Romano-Zelekha, Manfred S. Green and Tamy Shohat. 2003. 'Factors affecting performance of prenatal genetic testing by Israeli Jewish women'. *American Journal of Medical Genetics* Part A 120(3): 418–22. https://doi.org/10.1002/ajmg.a.20047.

Tikochinski, Michal. 2020. 'Is immersion in a home-bath halachically kosher?' 30 April 2020. Accessed 18 April 2021. https://gluya.org/detailed-answer-is-immersion-in-bath-home-is-halachic/. [Hebrew]

Van Ness, Peter H. 1999. 'Religion and public health'. *Journal of Religion and Health* 3(1): 15–26.

Velan, Baruch. 2016. 'Vaccine hesitancy as self-determination: An Israeli perspective'. *Israel Journal of Health Policy Research* 5(1): 1–6.

Wasserfall, Rahel. 1999. 'Introduction: Menstrual blood into Jewish blood'. In *Women and Water: Menstruation in Jewish life and law*, edited by Rahel Wasserfall, pp. 1–18. Hanover, MA and London: Brandeis University Press.

Zimmerman, Deena R. 2001. 'The Nishmat taharat hamishpacha hotline: Women helping women'. *Le'ela: A Journal of Judaism Today* 5: 17–20.

Part V
Lessons for a future

21
Fracturing the pandemic
The logic of separation and infectious disease in Tanzania
Rebecca Marsland

As COVID-19 unfolded, a stark picture of global health inequalities emerged. This invites reflection on the 'pan' in pandemic, for as anthropologists know all too well, when it comes to infectious disease, we are certainly not 'all in it together'. Instead, public health measures require us to isolate ourselves from other human beings, and other forms of life – viruses, bacteria, and insect and animal vectors. Pandemics fragment; they do not create unity.

In this chapter, I reflect on the pandemic via another globalised infectious disease – malaria – which, in contrast with COVID-19, is experienced as part of ordinary life. I consider how public health measures used to interrupt the transmission of malaria, COVID-19 and many other infectious diseases frequently depend on what I call a 'logic of separation'. This logic, in which it is assumed that humans can be separated from each other and from other forms of life, informs the protective barriers that we try to put in place between humans and pathogenic microbes. Interrogating this logic may help us understand responses to COVID-19 – not just in relation to the lockdowns that have taken place across the world, but because this new virus is considered to have crossed the 'species barrier'. It is likely that future disease prevention efforts will focus with renewed intensity on relations between humans and nonhuman species, through the One Health approach to control and surveillance.

In African countries, COVID-19 has not been so severe as in the Americas, Europe and South-East Asia (WHO n.d.). This has been attributed to a swift response by African health ministries, the greater experience of individuals and public health systems with infectious disease in contrast to the Global North, and the younger population. African countries have had to weigh up the economic costs of lockdown, and so in general have imposed fewer restrictions. The situation in Tanzania is less clear. The late Tanzanian president, John Magufuli, closed schools and universities, but did not enforce a lockdown or social distancing, citing economic danger to life. Controversially, he instead encouraged Tanzanians to attend church to pray. No data have been published since 29 April 2020, when the number of confirmed cases had reached 509 (BBC News 2020a).[1] In May, Tanzanians crossing the borders into Zambia and Kenya were tested, found positive and turned back. In June, President Magufuli announced that the virus had been defeated. President Magufuli died on 17 March 2021, and a month later his successor, President Samia Suluhu, announced that an expert committee would advise her on COVID-19.[2] Given reports of the detention of journalists who have criticised Magufuli (BBC News 2020b), I have assumed that Tanzanian friends and colleagues cannot speak freely about COVID-19. Instead, the research on which I draw in this chapter comes from fieldwork in Kyela District, in the southwest of Tanzania, originally conducted from 2000 to 2002, and since then, through multiple return visits. I understand that there was no upsurge in funerals in Kyela in 2020, as there was during the peak of the HIV pandemic, but this is not evidence of the absence of infections or deaths from coronavirus.

My long engagement with people who live in Kyela allows me to reflect on some of the limits to interventions that depend on the logic of separation. Kyela, located on the north shore of Lake Nyasa, is low-lying and malaria is holoendemic. In the early 2000s, people trod an uneasy line in their efforts to separate themselves from the causes of malaria in order to avoid risk of infection. Their use of and sometimes reluctance to use insecticide-treated mosquito nets (ITNs) in order to inhabit separate spaces to mosquitoes to protect themselves from malaria were tied up with moral concerns about sociality at funerals and overlapping ontological worlds. I draw on this experience to illustrate how the logic of separation can puncture multispecies and social worlds, and requires people to produce pluriversal solutions, if they are to hold these worlds together. I relate this to the indifference, as manifested in their resistance to ITNs, of mosquitoes to this logic and the reluctance of global health science to debate the associated risk of the loss of a partial immunity to malaria that could, in theory, result when transmission is temporarily interrupted. To conclude, I argue that it is important to acknowledge the complex relations between humans, nonhumans, social structures, biology and political agendas that the logic of separation ignores, and consider lessons for responses to COVID-19, in particular One Health.

Pandemic/polydemic?

What is a pandemic? Does this word adequately reflect the ways that people everywhere experience a pathogen with global reach? A pandemic is defined loosely as a disease that spreads over two (or more) continents and is destructive of human life. Its etymology (pan – all, demos – a population of people in a democracy) reveals a once deprecatory term that in the seventeenth century referred disapprovingly to a 'political system in which all the people govern equally' (Oxford English Dictionary, n.d.) and to 'vulgar forms of love' (Harrison 2016, 130). As European imperialism intensified and hastened the spread of pathogens through the forced movement of people through slavery, colonial rule and impoverishment, the word's negative connotations were linked to disease.

Despite the imperial and post-imperial role of Europe and North America in spreading disease to the global south, an 'outbreak narrative' (Wald 2008) has formed in which it is imagined that new diseases emerge in the 'global south' and travel to the economic centres of the 'global north'. In this narrative, the African continent is prominent. Viruses, themselves seen as ancient life forms (Wald 2008, 33), emerge out of a place which in the western imagination is also positioned back in time (Fabian 1983). The colonial 'heart of darkness' image of Africa still conjures up an antediluvian zone where humans are part of a fecund 'nature' that brings forth disease. China, despite its technological sophistication and superpower status, occupies a similar place in the western imagination; it, too, is thought to be a place located in primordial time, where 'spillover' across the species barrier is likely to occur (Lynteris 2020a; Zhan 2005). The US and Europe do not feature in this imagined geography of disease emergence (Wald 2008, 44), even though swine flu originated in the US and BSE ('mad cow disease') in the UK. The fact that in Africa COVID-19 has not caused the devastation that was predicted further indicates the blind spots that the outbreak narrative produces (Chigudu 2020).

Malaria shares with pandemic disease its prevalence and high mortality rates across more than two continents. However, it is understood to be endemic rather than pandemic. This endemicity is linked to the distribution of the *Anopheles* mosquitoes which spread malaria. *Anopheles* once transmitted malaria in England, Italy, North America and Siberia, and its present-day prevalence in the tropics is an outcome of the history of human ecology, rather than a straightforward relationship with geographical place (Packard 2007). In 2018, malaria caused 405,000 deaths in the Americas, sub-Saharan Africa, South and East Asia (Medicines for Malaria Venture n.d.).

The meanings of pandemic, epidemic and endemic are, as historian Mark Harrison notes, highly 'elastic' (2016, 139), with distinctions in meaning mirroring their social and emotional significance. Plague is still framed as a pandemic, even if its prevalence is insignificant (Lynteris 2020b). The historian Charles Rosenberg points out that in the nineteenth century tuberculosis 'did not elicit the sense of crisis that accompanied epidemics of yellow fever and cholera' (1992, 285). The everyday quality of an old disease like malaria contrasts with the fear and urgency generated by the new disease COVID-19, and the global social, economic and political upheaval associated with what is unknown about the virus SARS-CoV-2. The distinction between crisis and the everyday is a political matter, raising questions about how different human lives are valued (Marsland and Prince 2012).

Pandemics are not equal in their effects. The risks of infection, serious disease and fatality are higher in some socio-economic groups than others. Social divisions are firmed up as the borders around nation-states are policed and quarantines put into place, and while pathogens hold the same biological forms (give or take mutations) wherever they go, they are not, to use Nading's (2013) phrase, 'entangled with' the same socio-economic groups, political systems, economies, social structures or geographical locations. A disease can manifest differently in different bodies or as time passes, and there can be a range of ways of interpreting the symptoms. Within biomedicine, different specialisms produce alternative understandings of a disease, and create new kinds of social relationships (Berg and Mol 1998). We can extend these ideas about multiplicity to pandemics: Mignolo (2018), challenging the western concept of the universal as assumed to be a universal, encourages us to think in terms of a pluriverse. In acknowledging the pluriversal nature of pandemics, I propose here the idea of polydemics and highlight the 'interconnected diversity' (Mignolo 2018, x) of the effects of, and responses to, the same pathogen. Thinking about polydemics acknowledges that disease outbreaks are filtered through 'many cosmologies, [and there is] no longer one that subsumes and regulates all the others' (Mignolo 2018, x) and so allows us to see that different versions of a pandemic can coexist.

The logic of separation

We can examine the 'interconnected diversity' of a global outbreak by considering a key component of infectious disease control, elimination and eradication: that is, in the absence of a vaccine, the cycle of transmission is broken by separating humans from each other or from nonhumans. This is a 'contagionist' view of infectious disease (Rosenberg 1992), within which 'barriers to transmission and contamination become the main technology through which health is delivered' (Hinchliffe 2015, 30). With this logic of separation, single disease interventions from control measures to eradication campaigns are orchestrated from the top. The emphasis is on technological innovation, at the expense of primary healthcare and improvements to standards of living. In this way, social inequality is allowed to continue – life is promoted under conditions that might otherwise cause death. The approach medicalises politics because it sidesteps questions about the distribution of wealth and discrimination based on 'race' and gender.

Techniques of separation such as quarantine, social distancing and cordons sanitaires focus on humans, their susceptibility to pathogens and their role in facilitating the movement of microorganisms. But vectors and microbes do not recognise human social borders, and the public health response to this is to understand and implement borders that take nonhumans into account. And so other forms of life, often not considered as part of our society (Latour 2004), are also singled out for separation.

Anxieties about the hazards of nonhuman life crossing over into human spaces are central to outbreak narratives. New pathogens are considered to 'spillover' when the pristine zone of nature is entered by humans, or creatures from it encroach on human 'territory' (Quammen 2013; Wald 2008). 'Spillback', the transmission of disease from humans to other species, rarely features in outbreak narratives even though it can establish new reservoirs of disease and zoonotic cycles (Guth et al. 2020, 3). That spillback is marginal to this narrative reveals the anthropocentricity of the logic of separation. The wild places where spillover is predominantly thought to take place are cast in the media as dangerous, exotic and uncivilised. Humans local to them are often racialised as animal-like, with discriminatory discourses of race projected onto hierarchies that distinguish between human and nonhuman (Haraway 1989; Mavhunga 2011). These pejorative racial hierarchies combine with fears about boundary-crossing pollution (Douglas 1966), as evident in the association of outbreaks with the consumption of wild animals. The hunting of bats and bushmeat

(Ebola), and sale of civet cats as food in China (SARS) confound the western category of 'food'; pangolins (COVID-19) used in Chinese Traditional Medicine likewise fall outside of the western category of 'medicine' (Lynteris 2020a; Zhan 2005). Thus, nonhuman forms of life are incorporated into biomedical understandings of hygiene, and the management of 'inappropriate' human contact with animals becomes a matter of medical concern (Keck and Lynteris 2018, 9).

The separation of humans and nonhumans in biomedical thinking about outbreaks has been incorporated into pandemic preparedness; with COVID-19 this is likely to intensify. The One Health idea has been taken up by the WHO, the World Organization for Animal Health and the Food and Agriculture Organization to address the threat of emerging zoonotic diseases. The western division between the human and nonhuman world is fundamental to One Health projects, which understand interactions between human, animal and environmental health in terms of the historical distinctions between these categories (MacGregor and Waldman 2017; Wolf 2015). The geographer Steve Hinchliffe argues that One Health is 'one world-ist' because it aims to generate a 'single biosecure planet' where 'good' and 'bad' forms of life are separated out. In practice, biosecurity predominantly exists in the Global North, whereas the Global South is potentially dangerous because of 'interspecies intimacy' (2015, 30). This logic of separation of humans and nonhumans is also at the centre of malaria control. Attending to this may offer clues to thinking about the response to COVID-19.

The emphasis in malaria control has been on separating humans from nonhumans (mosquitoes and the parasitic *Plasmodia* that cause malaria) rather than separating humans from humans. Still, in colonial settings, 'native' humans were seen as a reservoir of infection and a danger to colonising humans (Litsios 1996; Manderson 1996; Packard 2016; Packard and Brown 1997). Public health measures were intended to protect colonial settlers from local populations, and towns were segregated accordingly. Homes for Europeans were often located in elevated land (where there were fewer mosquitoes), at a distance from areas designated for the residence of local populations and immigrant labourers (Curtin 1992; Goerg 1998; Harrison 2016, 137). In 1930s South Africa, assumptions about 'malaria tolerant Africans' justified segregation, and health officials claimed that Africans did not need to live in areas provided with malaria control services (Packard 2016). The segregation of colonised humans reflects the fact that they were not considered to be fully human; they were rarely distinguished from an environment that harboured diseases harmful to Europeans (Vaughan 1992, 42).

The logic of separation depends on a western cosmology in which humans occupy a separate space to nonhumans. In this world, humans, and some domesticated nonhumans, are assigned places marked out by culture; other forms of life are designated to places of nature (Descola 2013). In this understanding of the world, foundational to western thinking although not universal, nature is seen to be subdued and exploited by humans (DeMello 2012, 36–40). As this logic of separation travels and interacts with different cosmologies, it becomes pluriversal. This is how polydemics proliferate. The ethnography that follows illustrates how efforts to separate humans from mosquitoes can generate a pluriverse.

A world without mosquitoes?

The *Plasmodia* parasites that cause malaria are transmitted by *Anopheles* mosquitoes – the vectors of malaria. Since this link between mosquitoes and malaria was discovered by Ronald Ross in 1897, the separation of humans from mosquitoes has been a major component of malaria control: killing adult mosquitoes using insecticide, killing mosquito larva with larvicide, using repellents and sleeping under bed nets. In the 1990s, ITNs were found to be effective at reducing transmission, and have been promoted since then. The *Plasmodia* can also be targeted with antimalaria drugs either as treatment or prophylaxis. Malaria has been eliminated from some parts of the world with improved socioeconomic conditions, referred to by Packard as 'growing out of malaria' (2007, 65).[3]

Mosquito control is part of the logic of separation in global health (Beisel 2015). It originated with the goal of eradication, a possibility that has fallen in and out of sight. In the 1950s, the Global Malaria Eradication Programme (GMEP) used the insecticide dichlorodiphenyltrichloroethane (DDT) to kill mosquitoes and interrupt the transmission cycle (Stepan 2011). DDT had been developed during the Second World War, and was used primarily in parts of Asia to protect troops from mosquitoes. This led to a new era of confidence in the use of a single technology to control malaria (Packard 2007, 143). In the context of the Cold War, the GMEP fell into the US strategy to demonstrate its superiority to socialist regimes. It was known that mosquitoes would develop resistance to DDT, but eradication work went ahead (Packard 1997; 1998). The consequences were disastrous: DDT lost its efficacy, and there were large epidemics of malaria in the 1960s and 1970s (Litsios 1996, 83).

These epidemics were a result of the 'rebound effect'. Those who survive childhood without dying of malaria develop partial immunity.

They may still experience mild symptoms if infected, but they are unlikely to develop severe or fatal malaria. Partial immunity relies on 'endemic stability' in which there are high levels of infection but little disease (Coleman et al. 2001). Immunity is also lost during pregnancy, and is not acquired at all when malaria transmission is unstable. The risk of death is higher for nonimmune adults than it is for infants.

After the failure of the GMEP, malaria control was neglected. Eradication had never been seriously attempted in Africa because there was insufficient infrastructure and resources to support it; hence here there was no rebound effect. However, the burden of malaria continued to grow with reduced spending on malaria control, increased poverty and parasite resistance to chloroquine – the most affordable antimalarial treatment. This resurgence led to the launch of Rollback Malaria (RBM) in 1998; a partnership between the WHO, malaria-affected countries, development agencies, donors, researchers, non-governmental organisations and the private sector. RBM's target was to halve the burden of malaria by 2010 with the use of ITNs, effective treatment and early warning systems to control epidemics.

In 2000, I watched a health education film with about two hundred other people in a bus station in Kyela. I'd travelled there with a team of Tanzanians who worked for the social marketing NGO, Population Services International (PSI), and were promoting ITNs as part of the RBM campaign. They were touring the country and teaching people how to use *ngao* (shield), a tablet of insecticide that could be dissolved in water, in which a mosquito net could be soaked, then hung up in the shade to dry. Afterwards, the ITN would kill any mosquito that landed on it for a period of about three months; it would then have to be treated again. The film, which I described in my fieldnotes from February 2000, was part of their road show:

> A young woman is sleeping fitfully, raising her hand to swat away the mosquitoes which are filling the air with their remorseless high-pitched hum. When she wakes, she has a high fever and is very ill indeed. When her parents discover her, they have a heated argument about where to take her for treatment. Her mother wants to take her to see the medical officer at the nearest health facility. Her father argues that she should go to see a *mganga* (a traditional healer) to get some herbs and to divine in order to find out which spirit has made her sick. Her mother gives in reluctantly and they go to see the *mganga*. However, after the *mganga*'s administrations, the girl is still ill, and her father then angrily accuses an elderly neighbour of

bewitching her. In the midst of all this, the young woman starts convulsing, and her father leaves his quarrel to help his wife give their daughter more of the herbs from the *mganga*. It is at this point that his wife's brother appears on the scene and he insists that the sick woman is taken to hospital. At first her father is angry, and complains that he is head of the household, and cannot listen to decisions made by the brother of his wife. But, in the end they all go to hospital.

A few days later, the woman is much better, and not only that, her father has learnt at the hospital that her illness was malaria. There he was advised that to prevent malaria, his family should sleep under a mosquito net, and he also learnt to treat the net with insecticide so that it can kill and repel mosquitoes. The father left his superstitious ways and made up the quarrel with his family. Peace and happiness reigned in the household.

The film was faithful to a genre of colonial health education films which commonly depicted two opposing characters. One would demonstrate moral failings by seeking help from a traditional healer, believing in witchcraft and exhibiting personality flaws such as argumentativeness. The other would follow the directions of biomedicine, and would be rewarded with 'health, fertility and prosperity' (Vaughan 1992, 183). In the PSI film a message intended to reshape people's relationship to mosquitoes was tied into this moral lesson. The film aimed to teach people to use bednets and to treat them with insecticide. The message, consistent with the logic of separation, was that a division must be created between the spaces of human and insect life.

ITNs are more effective than untreated nets. Their repellent effect reduces the number of mosquitoes in the environment and discourages them from biting. ITNs also kill other insects that disturb sleep or spread disease, such as bed lice, fleas and other species of mosquito. In the early days of RBM, *Anopheles* mosquitoes tended to bite at night when people were sleeping, and so ITNs afforded protection at a time when malaria transmission is highest. Trials in Tanzania demonstrated that their use led to a clear reduction in mortality from malaria (Lengeler 2001).

The challenge was to persuade people to use them. Research was carried out to identify beliefs about malaria – it could be caught by sitting in the hot sun, getting caught in the rain, working too hard or drinking dirty water – that might be corrected through education, and replaced with knowledge of the role of mosquitoes and parasites (Winch et al. 1996). Between 1997 and 1999, the Ifakara Health Research and Development Centre trialled social marketing to provide ITNs at near cost price with relative success. ITNs were popular when people could afford them: according to Renggli and colleagues (2013), 72.7 per cent of Tanzanian households were using ITNs by 2012. However, people were not always able to pay for ITNs, and often the sole ITN was used by the head of household – the man, not women and children who are more vulnerable to severe malaria. Local health officials had underestimated the market for the largest nets, because they thought that people in villages did not sleep in large beds (Marsland 2006). The large nets are used by women and children who share sleeping mats. People were less likely to buy insecticide to re-treat nets (Armstrong Schellenberg et al. 2001), and so long-lasting insecticidal nets were introduced.

Another 'barrier' (to use the public health jargon) in Kyela was widespread acceptance that humans and non-domestic creatures inhabit the same spaces. Mosquitoes can be avoided in great density if one sits in the smoke of a fire, but this is uncomfortable and inconvenient. Mosquitoes fly in and out of houses and latrines, and bite people when they are resting in the shade under cocoa bushes and mango trees. They are part of a way of living that includes other wild creatures: termites must be dug out of kitchens, and bat manure scraped from roofs. Long-legged spiders span the surfaces of walls, scorpions hide in beds and clothing, rats and mice run across the rafters and chew their way into stored sacks of grain, monkeys steal the cocoa crop, and at night pods of hippopotamus trespass and feast on the rice paddy and green mamba snakes suddenly drop out of trees. People, domestic animals and wild creatures muddled along together. The notion that somehow people might erect a permanent barrier between themselves and these various insects and animals seemed unthinkable and unrealistic.

The everyday presence of wild creatures in human spaces challenged the notion that pests are unwanted forms of life that enter human spaces (Knight 2000). Nobody particularly liked mosquitoes, but their presence was rarely questioned. And so, an important part of RBM's work was to instil the idea that mosquitoes should not be tolerated: they are enemies because they spread malaria. ITNs divided space up into zones where mosquitoes could circulate freely with people, and human sleeping places that they could not enter. This was quickly accepted, and applied to ordinary, night-time, indoor sleeping arrangements.

In conversations with people in Kyela, it became clear to me that because mosquitoes were ubiquitous, part of the everyday mundane world, and despite the suffering and nuisance they caused, it had not occurred to people to regard their presence as a problem that could be acted upon.[4] Unlike entomologists (Kelly 2012) and public health workers, they did not know the mosquito in microscopic detail. Instead, the female mosquito, which feeds on blood to provide nutrition for her eggs, made herself known through her irritating whine, the itchy lumps that she left on ankles, and the satisfying smear of blood left on the wall if someone successfully swatted her. Most people knew that mosquitoes caused malaria in some way, but they were not that interested in knowing any more. They would say things like 'they say malaria is caused by mosquitoes, but I don't know if it is', or 'the scientists say it is caused by mosquitoes, but I can't comment on that'. This 'not knowing' reflected a 'combination of secrecy, uncertainty, and skepticism' (Last 2007, 9) in relation to medical knowledge.

Those willing to expand commented on mosquitoes as a reflection of the poor state of the environment in which they lived (see also Kelly and Lezaun 2014; Nading 2014, 17). They told me that mosquitoes were a product of rain, living in a valley or close to standing water, leading to complaints about the conditions in which people live. Many people lived in homes constructed from mud bricks and bamboo with thatched roofs. Even those who could afford burnt bricks and corrugated iron roofs usually had open eaves, and screens on windows or doors were rare. Homes were not mosquito proof, hence the advantage of the ITN, as it formed a mosquito-free zone where people slept. For the poorest people in Kyela, mosquitoes were emblematic of their poverty: they had no choice but to live in mosquito-ridden environments.

Despite 'not knowing' about mosquitoes, ITNs featured in some local bylaws that had been passed against 'misleading traditions of the Nyakyusa'. One of the clauses in the bylaws pertained to malaria, and stipulated that during funerals and the subsequent mourning period, 'the relatives of the deceased (women folk) with small children are forbidden to be at a funeral without a mosquito net'. This acknowledged a problem that RBM had not adequately taken into account – that people do not always sleep inside, and when they sleep outside they rarely use an ITN (see also Moshi et al. 2017; 2018). Unofficially, by making it compulsory to sleep under nets at funerals, the bylaw undermined the moral authority of the community to complain about women who slept under nets and so, in a roundabout way, protected people from the murmurs of dissatisfaction that led to a form of witchcraft called *imbepo sya bandu* (the breath of the people). This operates as a form of indigenous law, whereby members of the community mutter about a person who has committed an offence against them. These words manifest a collective breath with the power to cause magical harm (Marsland 2015; Wilson 1951).

At funerals, female relatives and neighbours of the bereaved sleep at her home in order to take part in the mourning songs, to help with cooking and to collect firewood and water. Houses are not big enough to accommodate all these women overnight, and so they sleep outside. The mosquitoes would bite them so much that they could not sleep, and afterwards my exhausted neighbours came to show me their arms, covered in mosquito bites as evidence of their suffering. It was unthinkable to sleep under a mosquito net on these occasions, because suffering was an important element of the work of mourning (see also Moshi et al. 2018). Women were both literally and symbolically close to mosquitoes at funerals, because they left a mark which could be shown to others as a sign of wretchedness in their grief. Building on Monica Wilson's ethnographies, mosquitoes act as a 'prophylactic against the effects of death' (1957, 89), that is, the madness that is part of grief. Wilson described how mourners would associate themselves with dirt as would a mad person. Mosquitoes are not dirt, but only a mad person would sleep outside and proudly show others their mosquito bites. To sleep under a mosquito net would invite the disapproval of others, and therefore *imbepo sya bandu*. It would be seen as 'showing off', an act of individual self-preservation at a time when group solidarity was required.

In 2000–02, it was possible to imagine a world in which separating humans and mosquitoes from each other made sense and seemed achievable, despite people's apparent resignation to the presence of mosquitoes and local notions of the immorality of protecting oneself against mosquitoes at funerals. But women in Kyela were anxious that they would be seen to be guilty of failing to protect human relations, which were essential to protect against witchcraft. 'Knowing or not knowing the mosquito', I wrote in my fieldnotes, 'was a moral matter'. For scientists working in the field of global health, knowing the mosquito meant that it was essential to live apart from it and save millions of lives. For women in Kyela, not knowing and tolerating the mosquito was essential to live healthy social lives. One mosquito could be eradicated or separated out from human worlds; the other mosquito was entangled in human social lives.

Over time, however, women in Kyela supported each other to make use of ITNs at funerals. They clubbed together to buy enough mosquito nets to take with them and hang up under trees. By making sure that everyone had access to ITNs, it was possible to maintain healthy social connections while separating themselves from mosquitoes at night. By 2008, ITNs were a normal feature of funeral arrangements. For them, malaria control required they prevent witchcraft and mosquito bites at the same time. This takes us back to the idea of the pluriversal polydemic. In Kyela, people were able to hold together these contradictory understandings of being in the world and to resolve them.

A decade later, *Anopheles* mosquitoes were developing resistance to the pyrethroid insecticide used to treat bed nets, and changing their behaviour to feed during the day and evening (Finda et al. 2019; Moshi et al. 2017). Mosquitoes have not signed up to the logic of separation, which is based on a cosmology that sees nonhumans as inert or at best tractable. They are not biddable to human agendas, and through their resistance to our chemical challenges and nets, they bind us closer to them. Malaria is shaped by multispecies co-existences (Kelly and Beisel 2011).

This resistance of mosquitoes means that malaria could be transmitted even when ITNs were used. This raises the question of the rebound effect. If ITNs successfully interrupted the transmission of malaria, people might lose or never acquire immunity to malaria. With mosquito resistance, malaria could resurge. Studies conducted in the 1990s to examine the relationship between ITNs and immunity (Guyatt et al. 1999) concluded that it was too difficult to make any predictions. ITN programmes should continue 'in the absence of other tools to control malaria adequately', but they should be carefully monitored (Mathanga and Molyneux 2001, 1220). One team of researchers recommended that improvements in health services, and better use of antimalarials, would be preferable to the risks of the rebound effect (Trape and Rogier 1996).

Between 2000 and 2002, I asked health workers in Tanzania about this, and they were clear that 'bed nets should not be withheld when so many children are dying from malaria'. Prior to this, questions about the link between acquired immunity and the use of ITNs had been dismissed by prominent scientists as 'irresponsible'; one commented that any intervention in the host-parasite life cycle was bound to lead to 'surprises', but that 'this is not a reason to deny anyone the protective measures that are available' (Brown 1997).[5] Randall Packard (2007, 242) describes a similar conversation with the Director of the Malaria Control and Evaluation Partnership in Africa. These responses are reminiscent of the tendency of those advocating vertical, technical, public health interventions to dismiss critique (Parker and Allen 2014, 227). The mainstream view was that the combination of available technology, cautiously optimistic scientific evidence and moral urgency were sufficient to dispel any lingering doubts about acquired immunity and to press on. Debate was suppressed with the claim that critique could endanger the good that ITNs promised.

The current response to the resistance of mosquitoes to insecticide is to invest in the development of new insecticides along with integrated vector management led by the Innovative Vector Control Consortium.[6] If vector control were to fail, the remaining technologies would be diagnostics, antimalarial treatment and the distant prospect of a vaccine. Beyond one paper (Griffin et al. 2015), it is hard to find published evidence that the rebound effect is taken seriously. There is, however, still a debate to be had. Vaccines are generally accepted as a means to confer immunity to disease, but acquired immunity is not. This is for good reason; it would require that a number of deaths should be tolerated – in effect a sacrifice.

Immunity is solely conceived of in biological terms, but it operates in a social context. Could we extend it to 'biosocial immunity'? This might allow us to move beyond the logic of separation and open up the debate. We could consider anthropologist Uli Beisel's (2015, 153) recommendation to take seriously the possibility that people may have to coexist with mosquitoes and 'slowly rework the complex knots of mosquito-human-parasite entanglements'. Currently, social immunity is used to describe the efforts of social insects – honeybees, ants, termites – to collectively cooperate to reduce the risk of disease (Cremer et al. 2007, 693). Could local, collective collaborations take this up by finding ways to make the acquisition of immunity to malaria safer through better healthcare, or by working to understand how social inequalities, poor standards of living and multispecies communities are tied up with the bodily immune response to malaria parasites?

Conclusions: lessons for COVID-19

These reflections on malaria – a global disease with high mortality, but one which is experienced as ordinary – invite us to consider how the logic of separation is shaping responses to the globalised spread of COVID-19. This logic has fractured our everyday worlds into unfamiliar pieces, and finds danger in nonhuman life 'spilling over' into what we perceive to be our separate human world. The outbreak narrative imagines this is more likely in African countries, and COVID-19 is likely to increase One Health efforts on the continent. The pandemic so far has turned out to be not so devastating in most countries in Africa as it has in the Global North, but they are likely to be required to prioritise the prevention of emerging zoonotic diseases. There are multispecies and pluriversal lessons here for One Health, which, despite its holistic aspirations, is based on the logic of separation – of humans, animals and the environment. Resistant mosquitoes have exposed the categories of nature and culture on which this logic is based for the 'fictive, man-made arbitrary creations that they are' (Douglas 1966, 200). If this logic is not questioned, we risk ignoring the tightening human–nonhuman entanglements that currently threaten the viability of ITNs and other vector control measures.

This takes us to the suppressed debates about acquired immunity to malaria, which provide a clue to the public disgust at proposals to mitigate COVID-19 by permitting herd immunity to develop without a vaccine. Herd immunity is a multispecies concept originating in veterinary science (Jones and Helmreich 2020), and it assumes that sacrificing human lives is acceptable to control the disease and to protect others. But as with malaria, there has been no discussion about a biosocial approach to immunity, that is, how collective care and social forms of protection might promote an immune response.

The term pandemic suggests that the events that follow in the wake of a pathogen are the same across the world, and it has generated an outbreak narrative that is based on a particular, western medical, cosmology. Unpacking the logic of separation through the example of malaria control in Tanzania highlights how a pluriversal response was required to accommodate this cosmology, enforced through the biomedical measure of the ITN and based on non-universal, historically shaped categories of nature–culture, human–nonhuman, and biological–social. People in Kyela at once acknowledged the logic of separation, but also worked out how to maintain multispecies and social relationships that would ordinarily be incompatible with this logic. To be successful, One Health responses to COVID-19 will also need to work their way through a multispecies pluriverse, and pay attention to the interconnected diversity of this, in anticipating and responding to future polydemics.

Acknowledgements

Many thanks to James Staples, Lenore Manderson, Ayo Wahlberg and Nancy Burke for feedback on this chapter.

Notes

1   In 2019 Tanzanian authorities were criticised for not providing sufficient information to the World Health Organization (WHO) about a suspected Ebola case (WHO 2019).
2   https://www.theeastafrican.co.ke/tea/news/east-africa/tanzania-covid-19-expert-committee-formed-3368024, accessed on 19 April 2021.
3   'Horizontal' interventions, such as those carried out in the 1930s by the Tennessee River Valley Authority (Carter 2014) and in colonial Malaya (Manderson 1996, 154–57, 164–65) deliberately attempted to bring this about, but during and after the Cold War, this was associated with socialism, and thus became politically unacceptable in northern capitalist countries, most notably the US (Packard 2007, 149).

4   In contrast, Nading (2014) describes how women carrying out dengue control work in Nicaragua take great pleasure in getting to know mosquitoes.
5   After the Brown article, a small controversy played out on the pages of *New Scientist*. Lengeler and Tanner (1997) claimed that Snow and Marsh's findings would dissuade donors from funding nets. Snow and Marsh's response (1997) was that they had never suggested that nets should not be used; they simply wanted to examine the long-term effects of using ITNs.
6   https://www.ivcc.com/, accessed 29 October 2020.

References

Armstrong Schellenberg, Joanna R.M., Salim Abdulla, Rose Nathan, Oscar Mukasa, Tanya J. Marchant, Nassor Kikumbih, Adiel K. Mushi, et al. 2001. 'Effect of large-scale social marketing of insecticide-treated nets on child survival in rural Tanzania'. *Lancet* 357: 1241–47.

BBC News. 2020a. 'Coronavirus in Tanzania: What do we know?' 19 June 2020. Accessed 4 December 2020. https://www.bbc.com/news/world-africa-52723594.

BBC News. 2020b. 'Tanzania journalist Erick Kabendera freed after seven months'. 24 February 2020. Accessed 6 December 2020. https://www.bbc.com/news/world-africa-51619618.

Beisel, Uli. 2015. 'Markets and mutations: Mosquito nets and the politics of disentanglement in global health'. *Geoforum* 66: 146–55.

Berg, Marc and Annemarie Mol. 1998. *Differences in Medicine: Unravelling practices, techniques and bodies*. Durham, NC and London: Duke University Press.

Brown, Phyllida. 1997. 'Picking holes in the net'. *New Scientist* 16 Aug: 16–17.

Carter, Eric D. 2014. 'Malaria control in the Tennessee Valley Authority: Health, ecology and metanarratives of development'. *Journal of Historical Geography* 43: 111–27.

Chigudu, Simukai. 2020. 'The politics of pandemics in Africa'. Presented at the Oxford Development Talks, 25 June 2020. Accessed 3 December 2020. https://www.youtube.com/watch?v=IlbUEe-YK8s.

Coleman, P.G., B.D. Perry and M.E.J. Woolhouse. 2001. 'Endemic stability – a veterinary idea applied to public health'. *The Lancet* 357 (21 April): 1284–86.

Cremer, Sylvia, Sophie A.O. Armitage and Paul Schmid-Hempel. 2007. 'Social immunity'. *Current Biology* 17(16): R693–702.

Curtin, Philip D. 1992. 'Medical knowledge and urban planning in colonial tropical Africa'. In *The Social Basis of Health and Healing in Africa*, edited by Steven Feierman and John M. Janzen, pp. 235–55. Berkeley, CA: University of California Press.

DeMello, Margo. 2012. *Animals and Society: An introduction to human-animal studies*. New York: Columbia University Press.

Descola, Philippe. 2013. *Beyond Nature and Culture*. Chicago, IL: Chicago University Press.

Douglas, Mary. 1966. *Purity and Danger: An analysis of the concepts of pollution and taboo*. London and New York: Routledge.

Fabian, Johannes. 1983. *Time and the Other: How anthropology makes its object*. New York: Colombia University Press.

Finda, Marceline F., Irene R. Moshi, April Monroe, Alex J. Limwagu, Anna P. Nyoni, Johnson K. Swai, Halfan S. Ngowo, et al. 2019. 'Linking human behaviours and malaria vector biting risk in South-Eastern Tanzania'. *PLOS ONE* 14(6). https://doi.org/10.1371/journal.pone.0217414.

Goerg, Odile. 1998. 'From hill station (Freetown) to downtown Conakry (First Ward): Comparing French and British approaches to segregation in colonial cities at the beginning of the twentieth century'. *Canadian Journal of African Studies* 32(1): 1–21.

Griffin, Jamie T., T. Déirdre Hollingsworth, Hugh Reyburn, Chris J. Drakeley, Eleanor M. Riley and Azra C. Ghani. 2015. 'Gradual acquisition of immunity to severe malaria with increasing exposure'. *Proceedings of the Royal Society B: Biological Sciences* 282 (1801): 20142657.

Guth, Sarah, Kathryn A. Hanley, Benjamin M. Althouse and Mike Boots. 2020. 'Ecological processes underlying the emergence of novel enzootic cycles: Arboviruses in the neotropics as a case study'. *PLOS Neglected Tropical Diseases* 14(8). https://doi.org/10.1371/journal.pntd.0008338.

Guyatt, H.L., R.W. Snow and D.B. Evans. 1999. 'Malaria epidemiology and economics: The effect of delayed immune acquisition on the cost-effectiveness of insecticide treated bednets'. *Philosophical Transactions: Biological Sciences* 354(1384): 827–35.
Haraway, Donna J. 1989. *Primate Visions: Gender, race, and nature in the world of modern science*. New York: Routledge.
Harrison, Mark. 2016. 'Pandemics'. In *The Routledge History of Disease*, edited by Mark Jackson, pp. 129–46. London: Routledge.
Hinchliffe, Steve. 2015. 'More than One World, more than One Health: Re-configuring interspecies health'. *Social Science & Medicine* 129 (March): 28–35.
Jones, David and Stefan Helmreich. 2020. 'A history of herd immunity'. *The Lancet* 396(10254): 810–11.
Keck, Frédéric and Christos Lynteris. 2018. 'Zoonosis: Prospects and challenges for medical anthropology'. *Medicine Anthropology Theory* 5(3): 1–14.
Kelly, Ann H. 2012. 'The experimental hut: Hosting vectors'. *Journal of the Royal Anthropological Institute*, s145–s160.
Kelly, Ann H. and Javier Lezaun. 2014. 'Urban mosquitoes, situational publics and the pursuit of interspecies separation'. *American Ethnologist* 41(2): 368–83.
Kelly, Ann H. and Uli Beisel. 2011. 'Neglected malarias: The frontlines and back alleys of global health'. *Biosocieties* 6(1): 71–87.
Knight, J. 2000. *Natural Enemies: People-wildlife conflicts in anthropological perspective*. London: Routledge.
Last, Murray. 2007. 'The importance of knowing about not knowing'. In *On Knowing and Not Knowing in the Anthropology of Medicine*, edited by Roland Littlewood, pp. 1–17. Walnut Creek, CA: Left Coast Press.
Latour, Bruno. 2004. *Politics of Nature: How to bring science into democracy*. Cambridge, MA and London: Harvard University Press.
Lengeler, Christian. 2001. 'Insecticide-treated bednets and curtains for preventing malaria'. *Cochrane Database of Systematic Reviews* 2. https://pubmed.ncbi.nlm.nih.gov/10796535/.
Lengeler, Christian and Marcel Tanner. 1997. 'Nets work'. *New Scientist* 155(2100, 20 Sept): 61.
Litsios, Socrates. 1996. *The Tomorrow of Malaria*. Kaori, NZ: Pacific Press.
Lynteris, Christos. 2020a. 'Sinophobia, epidemics, and interspecies catastrophe'. *Hot Spots, Fieldsights*, 23 June 2020. Accessed 29 June 2020. https://culanth.org/fieldsights/sinophobia-epidemics-and-interspecies-catastrophe.
Lynteris, Christos. 2020b. 'Covid-19 as pandemic mystery'. Accessed 25 October 2020. https://www.theasa.org/conferences/asa2020/panels#9479.
MacGregor, Hayley and Linda Waldman. 2017. 'Views from many worlds: Unsettling categories in interdisciplinary research on endemic zoonotic diseases'. *Philosophical Transactions: Biological Sciences* 372: 1–9.
Manderson, Lenore. 1996. *Sickness and the State: Health and illness in colonial Malaya. 1870–1940*. Cambridge, UK: Cambridge University Press.
Marsland, Rebecca. 2006. 'Community participation the Tanzanian way: Conceptual contiguity or power struggle?' *Oxford Development Studies* 34(1): 65–79.
Marsland, Rebecca. 2015. 'Keeping magical harm invisible: Public health, witchcraft and the law in Kyela, Tanzania'. In *The Clinic and the Court: Law, medicine and anthropology*, edited by Ian Harper, Tobias Kelly and Akshay Khanna, pp. 27–48. Cambridge, UK: Cambridge University Press.
Marsland, Rebecca and Ruth Prince. 2012. 'What is life worth? Exploring biomedical interventions, survival, and the politics of life'. *Medical Anthropology Quarterly* 26(4): 453–69.
Mathanga, Don and Malcolm E. Molyneux. 2001. 'Bednets and malaria in Africa'. *The Lancet* 357 (April 21): 1219–20.
Medicines for Malaria Venture. n.d. 'Malaria facts & figures | Medicines for malaria venture'. Accessed 7 December 2020. https://www.mmv.org/malaria-medicines/malaria-facts-figures.
Mignolo, Walter D. 2018. 'Foreword. On pluriversality and multipolarity'. In *Constructing the Pluriverse: The geopolitics of knowledge*, edited by Bernd Retier, pp. ix–xvi. Durham NC: Duke University Press.
Moshi, Irene R., Halfan Ngowo, Angel Dillip, Daniel Msellemu, Edith P. Madumla, Fredros O. Okumu, Maureen Coetzee, Ladslaus L. Mnyone and Lenore Manderson. 2017. 'Community perceptions on outdoor malaria transmission in Kilombero Valley, Southern Tanzania'. *Malaria Journal* 16(1): 274.

Moshi, Irene R., Lenore Manderson, Halfan S. Ngowo, Yeromin P. Mlacha, Fredros O. Okumu and Ladislaus L. Mnyone. 2018. 'Outdoor malaria transmission risks and social life: A qualitative study in South-Eastern Tanzania'. *Malaria Journal* 17(1): 397.

Nading, Alex M. 2013. 'Humans, animals and health: From ecology to entanglement'. *Environment and Society: Advances in Research* 4: 60–78.

Nading, Alex M. 2014. *Mosquito Trails: Ecology, health, and the politics of entanglement*. Berkeley, CA: University of California Press.

Oxford English Dictionary Online. 2020 'Pandemic, Adj. and n'. Oxford University Press. Accessed 9 December 2020. https://www.oed.com/view/Entry/136746?redirectedFrom=pandemic.

Packard, Randall M. 1997. 'Malaria dreams: Postwar visions of health and development in the Third World'. *Medical Anthropology* 17(3): 279–96. https://doi.org/10.1080/01459740.1997.9966141.

Packard, Randall M. 1998. '"No other logical choice": Global malaria eradication and the politics of international health in the post-war era'. *Parassitologia* 40(1–2): 217–29.

Packard, Randall M. 2007. *The Making of a Tropical Disease: A short history of malaria*. Baltimore, MA: The Johns Hopkins University Press.

Packard, Randall M. 2016. 'Indexing immunity to malaria in South Africa in the 1920s and 1930s'. *Anthropology Southern Africa* 39(2): 116–30.

Packard, Randall M. and Peter J. Brown. 1997. 'Rethinking health, development, and malaria: Historicizing a cultural model in international health'. *Medical Anthropology* 17(3): 181–94. https://doi.org/10.1080/01459740.1997.9966136.

Parker, Melissa and Tim Allen. 2014. 'De-politicizing parasites: Reflections on attempts to control the control of neglected tropical diseases'. *Medical Anthropology* 33(3): 223–39. https://doi.org/10.1080/01459740.2013.831414.

Quammen, David. 2013. *Spillover: Animal infections and the next human pandemic*. London: Vintage Books.

Renggli, Sabine, Renata Mandike, Karen Kramer, Faith Patrick, Nick J. Brown, Peter D. McElroy, Wilhelmina Rimisho, et al. 2013. 'Design, implementation and evaluation of a national campaign to deliver 18 million free long-lasting insecticidal nets to uncovered sleeping spaces in Tanzania'. *Malaria Journal* 12(1): 85.

Rosenberg, Charles E. 1992. *Explaining Epidemics and Other Studies in the History of Medicine*. Cambridge, UK: Cambridge University Press.

Snow, Robert W. and Kevin Marsh. 1997. 'Yes, use the nets'. *New Scientist* 156(2105, 25 Oct): 57.

Stepan, Nancy L. 2011. *Eradication: Ridding the world of diseases forever?* London: Reaktion Books.

Trape, Jean-François and Christophe Rogier. 1996. 'Combating malaria morbidity and mortality by reducing transmission'. *Parasitology Today* 12(6): 236–40.

Vaughan, Megan. 1992. *Curing Their Ills: Colonial power and African illness*. Cambridge, UK: Polity Press.

Wald, Patricia. 2008. *Contagious: Cultures, carriers, and the outbreak narrative*. Durham, NC: Duke University Press.

WHO. 2019. 'Cases of undiagnosed febrile illness – United Republic of Tanzania'. World Health Organization. 21 September 2019. Accessed September 2020. http://www.who.int/csr/don/21-september-2019-undiag-febrile-illness-tanzania/en/.

WHO. n.d. 'WHO coronavirus disease (COVID-19) dashboard'. Accessed 6 December 2020. https://covid19.who.int.

Wilson, Monica. 1951. *Good Company: A study of Nyakyusa age villages*. London, New York, Toronto: Oxford University Press for the International African Institute.

Wilson, Monica. 1957. *Rituals of Kinship among the Nyakyusa*. Oxford, UK: Oxford University Press.

Winch, P, A.M. Makemba, S.R. Kamazima, M. Lurie, G.K Lwihula, Z. Premji, J.N. Minjas and C.J. Shiff. 1996. 'Local terminology for febrile illness in Bagamoyo District, Tanzania and its impact on the design of a community-based malaria control programme'. *Social Science & Medicine* 42 (7): 1057–67.

Wolf, Meike. 2015. 'Is there really such a thing as "One Health"? Thinking about a more than human world from the perspective of cultural anthropology'. *Social Science & Medicine*, 129 (March): 5–11.

Zhan, Mei. 2005. 'Civet cats, fried grasshoppers, and David Beckham's pajamas: Unruly bodies after SARS'. *American Anthropologist* 107(1): 31–42.

22
Living together in precarious times
COVID-19 in the Philippines
Gideon Lasco

Ostrich

On 4 August 2020, just as Metro Manila, Philippines, was living through a newly reimposed lockdown, two ostriches escaped from a gated upper middle-class village, running through streets made deserted by the restrictions on public transportation and stay-at-home mandates. Within hours, the footage of the ostriches had gone viral on social media, giving rise to numerous memes, celebrity reactions and even political commentary. 'The absurdity of the runaway ostriches – which are not native to the Philippines – made them an Internet sensation and a welcome distraction during one of the world's longest and most stringent lockdowns', a report from *The Washington Post* observed (Cabato 2020).

Just like the other animals – fake and real – that went viral throughout the world at the height of the pandemic (see, for example, Daly 2020), the ostriches were a reminder, foremost, that this is a more-than-human world. In my own house in Los Baños – some 50 kilometres away from Manila – olive-backed sunbirds have taken up residence in the small garden. Like dogs, sunbirds can live up to 12, even 15 years. Without the pandemic and the quarantine, I surely would not have had the opportunity – and the perspective – to notice my nonhuman *companions*.

Of course, the ostrich is something else: not only is it relatively rare, it is also relatively big for a bird. In the viral videos, one notable aspect was how people actually talked to the ostriches. In their *macro*-ness, they seemed amenable to conversation. 'You need a quarantine pass!', a village guard jokingly shouted after them, referring to the slip of paper issued to one member of each household that served as a requirement for going out of one's house. Adding to the birds' appeal was the fact that their mad dash through the streets of Quezon City was a transgression of the world as we knew it: roads are for people; ostriches belong to the zoo, or in the wild. Seeing these birds on the streets had some subversive quality, especially at a time when humans themselves were confined to their houses.

In the end, one of the ostriches died and was cooked into a local dish called *adobo*, eliciting some outrage because such a 'cute' animal – an animal that belongs to a 'more charismatic species who are "big like us"' (Greenhough 2012, 291) – should not have been eaten. Anthropologists, of course, would have immediately bracketed such responses in terms of cultural norms of what is good to eat. Elsewhere, there were questions about the legalities of keeping an ostrich in a subdivision.

Framework

This is all in keeping with the turn towards multispecies anthropology and the conceptualisation of the Anthropocene (for example, Chakrabarty 2009; D'Souza 2015), falling under the rubrics of science, technology and society studies that see humans as enmeshed, entangled and imbricated in networks with nonhuman actors (Latour 1993). I will not rehearse the literature, for as the cultural geographer Hayden Lorimer (2005, 84) puts it, 'To do so would very likely bore the most devoted and risk baffling the uninitiated'. However, it is important to stress that today, as we live through a pandemic – or more aptly, a syndemic (Singer et al. 2017) – a multispecies perspective is not just a fancy theory but an ecological and even existential necessity.

Indeed, a multispecies perspective is upon us whether we like it or not. Ten years ago, 'living with a virus' may have been a title of a conference, a panel or an academic paper, but today it is a catchphrase used by politicians and physicians alike. We are learning, via the hard and painful way, what Donna Haraway calls the 'foolishness of human exceptionalism' (2008, 244), for, as Jane Goodall averred back in April, 'it is our disregard for nature and our disrespect for animals that has caused this pandemic' (Burton 2020).

Moreover, and relevant to COVID-19, a 'public health optimism' that imagined a world free from disease – borne of the Pasteurian belief in antibiotics and vaccines – has not aged well. Not only are humans becoming increasingly affected by non-communicable diseases like hypertension and diabetes; microbes have adapted to antibiotics, and today antimicrobial resistance is a growing threat (Chandler et al. 2016). Viruses have proven particularly difficult to diagnose and treat, as they, too, can mutate, especially when they cross species. Consequently, the pandemic has forced humans to grapple with a world where we are vulnerable, even through the air we breathe, a world where microbes pose an existential threat.

How, then, can anthropology account for the interspecies encounters in the time of COVID-19? One approach – one that I follow in this chapter – entails following species as they travel amid the milieu of the pandemic and expanding conceptions of their trajectories beyond the individual level (e.g. 'How did the ostrich *qua* species reach the Philippines in the first place?'). Analytically, it also involves moving nonhumans from the level of *zoe* or 'bare life' to that of *bios* – 'with legibly biographical and political lives' (Agamben 1998, in Kirksey and Helmreich 2010, 545), and foregrounding them in our ethnographies. In the oft-cited language of Eduardo Kohn (2013, 4), we must move towards 'an anthropology that is not just confined to the human but is concerned with the effects of our entanglements with other kinds of living selves' – and just as importantly, recognise that such a perspective is as valid and vital in highly urbanised cities like Manila as it is in the Amazonian rainforest – or the Philippines' own lush tropical jungles. If not more so: after all, the world has never been more urbanised and has brought species together in unprecedented proximity and intimacy, and this is why pandemics are closely linked with urbanisation (Santiago-Alarcon and MacGregor-Fors 2020).

For the purpose of this chapter, what is more useful is to highlight that this perspective, or set of perspectives, has long animated the 'national anthropology' in the Philippines, albeit often implicitly. For instance, at the 2018 conference of Ugnayang Pang-Agham Tao (UGAT), the country's association of anthropologists, the theme was 'Our Interconnectedness: Doing Anthropology in Times of Environmental Crisis'. The conference featured presentations that ranged from human–seaweed relations in the Tawi-Tawi Islands and human–elephant communications in a zoo, to living with crocodiles in Palawan Island and with cats in urban settings. Taken together, these papers underscored that far from linear, let alone vertical, our encounters with nonhumans are best characterised as 'rhizomatic' (Deleuze and Guattari 1988) – that is, non-hierarchical and relational (see also Ogden et al. 2013).

This ecological consciousness comes to us not just as part and periphery of global anthropological currents, but also from our interlocutors who have always thought along these lines, not as a way of thinking, but as a way of living. As our wealth of ethnography, folklore and cultural history shows, local notions of ecology have always seen the world as animated by more-than-human actors. When the Mindanao indigenous leader Bae Inatlawan performed a ceremony in April to pray amid the pandemic, she mentioned the trees, the birds and the eagle in the same breath as humans and the virus, unknowingly, as she spoke of humans belonging to the forest as much as the forest belonging to humans, endorsing the tenets of 'biophilia' (Kellert and Wilson 1993).

Such knowledge is vital not just in asserting the local character of our anthropology but also in tempering our own aspirations as to what this way of thinking might mean for the world. Writing on human–pig relations among the Pala'wan, Will Smith (2020) rightfully warns against a 'post-environmentalism' that assumes 'affective relationships' will always be based on loving and caring. His warning echoes the insight of Padmapani Perez (2018) in her work on conservation in Benguet and Borneo – we cannot idealise indigenous peoples as 'noble green savages'.

As for microbes, while little – if any – local research has been in terms of characterising human relations with them, the above warning is likewise useful, for, while we can either view them as noxious germs that must be killed with antibiotics – or as 'good bacteria' to be cultivated and consumed, it is more insightful to view them in terms of what Paxson (2008, 18) calls 'microbiopolitics', or the 'recognition and management, governmental and grassroots, of human encounters with the vital organismic agencies of bacteria, viruses, and fungi'.

My own thinking in this direction was inspired by my fieldwork with forest guards in Mindanao, but also by my childhood experiences of growing up near Mt Makiling in the university town of Los Baños, southeast of Manila, and by my travels to ecotourism destinations of the world. Before the pandemic, I had the opportunity to visit the Amazon rainforest and the Galápagos Islands. In the former I saw the intimacy with which people lived with wildlife. In the Galápagos I glimpsed the world without humans, although within a few centuries of human settlement on Isabela Island, guava trees had invaded hectares upon hectares of land, while Darwin's finches approached humans with evolutionary innocence, unaware of the havoc we have wrought throughout much of the planet.

My visit to the Galápagos – weeks before the first cases of COVID-19 were reported in the Philippines – reminded me of environmental writer Robert Macfarlane's (2016) call to imagine ourselves as 'inhabitants not just of a human lifetime or generation, but also of deep time'. Can we approach the pandemic in those same terms – not as a singular moment in human history, but as event in longer processes? And, following Anna Tsing (2013), can we analyse how nature comes into being rather than seeing it as a backdrop for this account?

Coronavirus

First, of course, we need to attend to the encounter between humans and microbes, including bacteria and the coronavirus itself. Technically, viruses are not a 'species' because they don't fulfil the criteria of 'organism'. Anthropologists, however, have labelled them as quasi-species, and, in any case, part of a multispecies perspective is to question the ontology and validity of our biological categories.

Microbes have been around for billions of years. Scientists tell us that they're the earliest organisms, hardy enough to survive in the depths of the earth, the deepest parts of the oceans, perhaps even in space, as the recent brouhaha over possible life on Venus showed (see Lasco 2020a). But as far as humans are concerned, viruses are a recent phenomenon. People never viewed illness as caused by microbes prior to their discovery. For example, the Filipino national hero and polymath Jose Rizal, whose medical practice came at the twilight of humoral theory, opined that *El aire, el calor, el frio, el vapor de tierra y la indigestion, son las unicas causas patogenas que se admiten en el pais* ('Winds, heat, cold, vapors of the earth, and indigestion are the main causes of illness in the country') (Bantug 1953, 12).

The Pasteurian worldview – which today remains the dominant mode of thinking on illness – sees the world as made up of noxious microbes against which humans must battle through antibiotics or vaccines. According to anthropologist Heather Paxson (2008, 15), this view explains why people 'blame colds on germs, demand antibiotics from doctors, and drink ultra-pasteurized milk and juice, while politicians on the campaign trail slather on hand sanitizer'. Likely, it explains the appeal of Filipino soap commercials from the 1970s onwards that depict germs on the body as being eliminated '99 per cent of the time'. Although, as mentioned above, this view has been shattered by the failure of medicine to eradicate pathogens, it remains at the fore of people's consciousness.

In some ways, however, the pre-Pasteurian worldview is still upon us, with microbes and wind melding in people's conceptions, as when President Rodrigo Duterte interpreted airborne transmission to mean that COVID-19 is *nasa hangin*, even as the outdoor *hangin* does not correspond with biomedical understandings of airborne transmission (for instance, as occurring in poorly ventilated, indoor spaces) (see Tan and Lasco forthcoming). Similarly, people's 'germ consciousness' may not correspond with Pasteurian notions of virus. As Michael Tan (2008, 91) noted:

> Concepts about microorganisms vary, sometimes with amusing variations. The idea that food dropped on the floor isn't necessarily dirty if it hasn't been on the floor for a certain time (varying between 30 seconds and 5 minutes) is tied to childhood concepts that the dropped food 'scares' off germs ... Germs are often given qualities of humans, if not the supernatural. Women fear toilet seats, believing that the germs lie waiting, ready to pounce on the vulnerable. Terms such as *kumakapit* (sticking on) show that the germs' mode of infection [is] not often understood. I have found villagers speaking of intestinal parasites (*bulate*) as 'adult germs' (*mikrobyong naging laki*).

These insights resonate today when people talk about '*madapuan*' *ng virus* and '*matamaan*' *ng* COVID. When Duterte joked, back in February, just as the threat of a pandemic was emerging, that he wanted to slap the virus, he was reaching for an object. The microscopic, transcending our sensory faculties in terms of scale, is semantically transposed to language that facilitates our ability to visualise and conceptualise the virus, on top of technologies that render the virus visible. Unlike colonial plagues that did not localise onto a tangible object, COVID-19 has acquired an *objecthood*. Thanks to our technologies of imagination, we visualise the virus as this red pathogen with spikes, even though viruses actually do not have colour and the red is merely the human attempt at visualisation. But such is the certitude of the virus' existence as this red, spiked object that food writers have even compared it to the rambutan, much to the outcry of many Southeast Asians (Estrada 2020).

Beyond the processes of visualisation, there are also the politics of association, as when certain groups of people and places get lumped together with the virus – from Chinese tourists, returning overseas Filipino workers (and returning Senegalese workers, see Onoma, Chapter 10), to Donald Trump referring to the coronavirus the 'China virus' or the 'Wuhan virus'.

Yet already before the pandemic, anthropologists had documented a shift to a post-Pasteurian view that considers microbes not as harmful but in some ways potentially useful (Paxson 2008). From the Yakult and yoghurt to keffir and kombucha, we have become patrons of microbial *goodness*. Now more than ever, we recognise microbes and macrobes alike as what Donna Haraway (2006) terms 'companion species'.

The microbial presence in the human body is actually even more profound. Year after year, scientists continue to chart the full extent of so-called 'normal flora'. As the Human Microbiome Project of the National Institutes of Health (2012, n.p.) revealed:

> The human body contains trillions of microorganisms – outnumbering human cells by 10 to 1. Because of their small size, however, microorganisms make up only about 1 to 3 percent of the body's mass (in a 200-pound adult, that's 2 to 6 pounds of bacteria), but play a vital role in human health.

Additionally, and contrary to popular imagination, 50 per cent of the oxygen we utilise comes from microbes. At one point, this recognition led to questions over the necessity of handwashing, while Japanese doctors voiced concerns that 'hygiene addiction' might actually remove good microbes (Uranaka 2001).

The pandemic has at least temporarily suspended – or superseded – this paradigm, renewing our suspicion of microbes, helping make sense of the 'rituals of disinfection' of our time (Lasco 2020b) regardless of their biomedical efficacy. Suddenly, people are potential vectors of a virus, despite the fact that we have long been exchanging all kinds of microbes not just among ourselves but also our nonhuman companions (Rillig et al. 2015). And while this exchange with every handshake, hug or huddle has largely been unwitting, it is worth mentioning that once upon a time, human vectors of a virus arrived in the Philippines not as a threat, but as salvation, as when orphan boys from Mexico came to the country, their blood containing the weakened viral strains of smallpox as part of the Balmis expedition (Mark and Rigau-Perez 2009).

The divergence between local and biomedical knowledge of microbes can have public consequences, and when this tension is adjudicated by the powers that be – as when Duterte decided that one metre physical distancing was good enough (Reuters Staff 2020) – we see, often painfully, what is truly at stake with the 'microbiopolitics' of COVID-19. Indeed, the contested knowledge claims about the virus – whether it is airborne, whether masks are enough, whether face shields are needed – all rest on our understandings of the virus and how it is mediated. But, ultimately, it is political actors who make the decision with life-and-death consequences for their constituents.

Of course, it's not like other microbes have disappeared. Floodwaters still pose the risk of leptospirosis infection, and tuberculosis has not left us. Neither have HIV and other venereal diseases, or the myriad other viruses in and around us that are harmless and perhaps even beneficial – to say nothing about the viruses and bacteria that afflict nonhumans and can potentially cause zoonoses and human pandemics (Levitt 2020). We have always been exchanging microbes, from one community to another, but microbiopolitics foregrounds the ways in which some viruses are visible and others, invisible.

Finally, we see this microbiopolitics in the conceptualisation of vulnerability and resistance, as when people say, *Ang tibay ng mga mahirap* ('The poor are strong'). In my ongoing ethnographic research on local health knowledge and how it has affected how people make sense of the pandemic (see Tan and Lasco 2021), I have encountered people saying that the poor – particularly those in urban areas – cannot be infected by the coronavirus because they are exposed to a lot of bacteria and, therefore, have higher *resistensya* to viruses. *Resistensya* is to the physical as resilience is to the social, and both have been used to justify health and social disparities in the time of COVID-19. To borrow from Stawkowski's (2016, 155) account of marginalised communities living in the aftermath of radioactive pollution in Kazakhstan, it seems that for the urban poor in Manila and elsewhere, 'their only option is to become (or believe themselves to be) enhanced human beings who can survive in toxic environments'.

Nonhuman animals

Beyond and alongside the virus, other animals have been involved in the pandemic in various ways. As Deleuze and Guattari (1988, 11) write: 'We form a rhizome with our viruses, or rather our viruses cause us to form a rhizome with other animals'. Animals figure in the purported genesis of the virus' jump to humans; they figure in the way humans cope with the virus, in entanglements that range from abuse to affection. And I refer not just to the ability of dogs to detect the presence of a virus, even though this is an amazing reminder that our sensory universes hardly overlap.

At the start of the pandemic, animals figured in two major ways. First, there was the question of which animals served as vectors or hosts, that is, which animals were to *blame* for the pandemic. Pangolins were proposed as intermediate hosts, which struck a chord among Filipino environmentalists, given that the pangolin is poached heavily in Palawan.

Eventually, suspicion fell on bats; this remains the current view. But bats have always had coronaviruses. In the Philippines, a study found that among bats from two campuses of the University of the Philippines, 55 per cent had coronaviruses of some sort (Watanabe et al. 2010). The question is how the virus jumped from bats to humans, why and how bats have come to be in such close proximity to humans, and why this particular strain of coronavirus is so virulent and effective.

The indictment of certain species as disease carriers – potential or real – is a matter of life and death for them. When millions of chickens were culled in Indonesia as a result of avian flu, Celia Lowe (2010) described those chickens as part of a 'viral cloud' of H5N1 in the country. Similarly, in November 2020, millions of minks were killed in Denmark over fears of spread and potential mutation of the coronavirus through them. To quote one report: 'Mass graves have appeared in the Danish countryside filled with the slaughtered animals' (Murray 2020). Farmers were in tears, although their concern was more over their lost livelihoods than the lost lives of the animals whose fur is used to make luxury garments and fake eyelashes. Evidently, unlike the ostrich, which, when turned into adobo, sparked outcry in the Philippines, certain species do not attract as much human sympathy: a further reminder of our local moral taxonomies.

Another major way in which animals have figured in the pandemic is via the narrative of 'nature's revenge' – or of a healing planet. In the early months of the pandemic, the news media repeatedly circulated images of animals roaming and 'reclaiming' the streets: from deer in Japan and monkeys in Thailand to wild goats in Wales and wild boar in Spain (Kretchmer 2020). But as environmental scientists have pointed out, COVID-19 is actually not 'good' for the environment. Discarded personal protective equipment is contributing to plastic waste, while economic deprivation has led people to hunt down and poach endangered species. Zoos and wildlife parks are losing revenue and funding, leaving their animals vulnerable both to hunger and the virus itself (Wang et al. 2020). Two months into the lockdown, Filipinos were greeted by the pitiable sight of an emaciated lion in the privately owned Malabon Zoo, its owner appealing for cash donations (for which he felt embarrassed because 'the focus should be on humans'):

> [Some were] apologizing that during this time, the focus has been on human beings and somehow the animals seem to have been forgotten. And I had to assure them that [they were right; the focus should be on] people, especially the poor and the hungry people.

So I myself am ashamed to be asking for help for the animals during these trying times (Valenzuela 2020).

Beyond the material consequences of the pandemic to animals, social scientists have warned that such narratives simplify the discourse and reinforce the 'apart-ness' of humans from so-called 'nature' (Searle and Turnbull 2020). Of course, animals do not just figure as part of the etymology of the virus and its ecological impacts, but also in the phenomenological experience of the pandemic. Dogs and cats have served as quarantine companions, immune to the rules of physical distancing. Already, there is emerging literature from various countries on how human–dog relations were also disrupted during lockdowns (Morgan et al. 2020; Tomé 2020); how the presence of pets became more important than ever; and how the constant presence of humans in their houses has endangered intimacy between households of humans and nonhumans.

Plants

All of the above point to the pandemic as a more-than-human event. But it is also more-than-animal. One fascinating development during the pandemic is the ersatz 'botanic boom'. Biking in my hometown in Laguna, I would see tricycles packed with potted plants, plants being sold on the highways, people traveling all the way from Manila just to buy plants. Social media, too, has become overgrown with monsteras and carnivorous plants. And not just for the upper and middle classes. I see people in low-income neighbourhoods walking with plants they just purchased, tending to their recently refurbished gardens.

Filipinos have long cared for and nurtured plants; the Spanish priest and chronicler Antonio Morga described the first bonsai seen by westerners on his visit to Manila in 1603. These seemingly mundane houseplants actually come from different places, finding their way from colony to metropole and back to colony – a reminder that just like the pandemic, colonialism, too, was a multispecies process that involved uprooting and transplanting different species. The irony now is how 'plants are able to travel much more freely than humans in the time of the pandemic', as a friend pointed out.

Another notable observation is the growing trend of naming houseplants. To name is to confer importance, and humans only give names to people and things that matter to them. While mostly said in jest, being 'plant parents' – *plantito, plantita* – establishes a form of kinship that is arguably new, at least among the many who have recently discovered the joys of nurturing houseplants. And with this, there is growing concern about the commodification of plants. What happens when something taken for granted suddenly has value, and when that value can be quantified in monetary terms? Plants hold immense value, but they have to be literally uprooted for such value to be realised, like trees in a forest that are more valuable dead than alive. Given that ferns can now sell for far more than rice, how will this phenomenon shape our mountains, and transform our ways of living?

At the personal level, of course, plants matter differently to different people. Some may see them as a project to be shared with others. Others may see nature in them, even as they are far from 'natural' given all the artificial interventions from breeding and transportation to potting and cultivation. And then there are those who perceive the health benefits of plants, an inkling increasingly supported by the notion of 'biophilia' (Ulrich 1993).

But the plants thriving in our homes cannot be dissociated from their ecological entanglements. For instance, their popularity has prompted cries of alarm from environmentalists who fear its impacts on biodiversity (Lim and Lasco 2020):

> Some of the plants on sale are sourced from our mountains and other unique ecosystems, disrupting habitats and potentially further endangering plant species and the wild fauna that depend on them for food and shelter. With rarity and 'exotic-ness' being valued characteristics in plant collecting, this craze might drive unscrupulous entrepreneurs deeper into our forests in search of plants that will command high prices in both local and international markets. Already, Department of Environment and Natural Resources offices in many parts of the country are reporting encroachments driven by the demand for these plants.

They also warn that 'plants can also bring along with them pests and diseases that can infest, infect, and kill other plants in one's collection' (Lim and Lasco 2020), further underscoring the limits of thinking in terms of individual species. Although plants are thought to be immune to coronaviruses, it is also worth adding that they are not without their own viral nemeses, not to mention all kinds of pests – as consequence of their participation in our lifeworld – even as they can also forge alliances with microbes (Wilkinson et al. 2019).

My own thinking about plants (Lasco 2020c) is that they link us to the past by serving as enduring lifelong companions. My mother has held on to her bonsai since she was in her early twenties, taking the plants with her from apartment to apartment until, when my parents had the money to buy their own land, the bonsai, too, were allowed take root in the ground. 'They've been around for much longer than you, and unlike *human* children, they never leave', she told me, showing that trees are 'portable companions' that can follow humans – not just in the sense of Lucia Monge's *planton movil* (Vich 2016; see also www.luciamonge.com). Perhaps beyond the COVID-19 pandemic, the plants we have today will hold a special place as companions through a difficult moment. Moreover, at a time when life itself seems most precarious, perhaps plants offer an alternative vision of life, one of growth and regeneration, with each new leaf signifying hope and positive change.

But regardless of the entanglement of motivations that have allowed plants to take root in our households, and mindful of the threats to plant life that the pandemic has exacerbated, the question remains: Can our newfound affection for plants translate to heightened concern for the planet?

Living together

In light of the necessity of multispecies ways of thinking about the world, our mandate is clear: we must act on the implications, from the personal to the political, of our more-than-human togetherness amid the precarities of our time. At a personal level, this can simply mean a greater appreciation for the world-at-large, perhaps making us less lonely, wherever we are. Here in Los Baños, I have not welcomed a single guest since March, but the sunbirds, our two dogs, the narra trees and even the *Stephanie erecta* that I have been nurturing, all keep me company. They also raise the stakes of whom – and what – we are responsible for.

At a professional level, thinking of and about interspecies connections should enrich our praxis and broaden our conceptions of the 'field' to include what these connections actually do, and what they mean, for the people with whom we engage. At the outset, I already argued for the methodological necessity of following species as they travel, and foregrounding them in our ethnographies. But in light of COVID-19 and its aftermath, we need to go back to our interlocutors, human and nonhuman, and see how they are living, and living together, in a pandemic. Given our current constraints, we need methodological innovations and research ethics adaptations that facilitate and support these changes. Surely, many anthropologists are already working on this, and we will hopefully see the fruits of their labours in the coming years.

Logistically, this can also lead to engagements with people from other disciplines –microbiologists, horticulturists, zoologists, farmers, physicians – and a host of other fields, advocacies and activisms. If the task at hand is 'thick description', and if it entails long-term observation, then we have a lot to offer in helping people understand their own work, especially among those dealing with other species. While resisting the urge to view terms of *engagement* solely as terms of *endearment*, we need to trace the connections – from affectionate to antagonistic – that make up the 'convivium' of organisms to which we belong.

Finally, at a political level, it entails recognising the power relations that underwrite, disrupt, destroy and render antagonistic our relations with nonhumans – the structural violence that not only exposes humans to harmful species, but exposes other species to human harm. Although those at the forefront of thinking about post-human politics are suggesting an attention to land and indigenous peoples as priorities (see Panelli 2010), this is something we in the Philippines have always known.

It also entails challenging the neoliberal order that renders vulnerable not just humans, but the whole planet, from the rising incidence of diabetes among our pets, global warming that threatens animal habitats and, of course, the pathogenic viruses that result from habitat destruction, illegal wildlife trade and industrial farming. On the local scale, we see this unfold in what Wolfram Dressler (2011) calls 'nature as capital', as when national parks protecting immense biodiversity are viewed in terms of their 'market value'. Surely, anthropologists can speak to debates on valuing and expanding our time-honoured notions of reciprocity and kinship to 'natureculture' (Fuentes 2010) around us. It may even lead us to interrogate our symbolic taxonomies – how some species are seen as more worthy of compassion than others – as well as rethinking our unsustainable ways of life. After all, do we really need millions of rodents in farms just so humans can have fur coats and fake eyelashes?

I conclude with three questions. The first one, raised in the 2018 UGAT conference, remains salient as ever. In light of our interconnectedness, how do we live together in precarious times, in times of environmental, medical and political crises? Mindful that structural violence and state violence (see Tandog 2020) necessarily extend to nonhumans, we should also ask: How can we bear witness to forms of more-than-human togetherness, from abuse to affection, in ways that lead to action, in ways that do justice to both humans and other species? Finally, returning to anthropology's core mission: How do we do all this in ways that allow us to deepen our understanding of what it means to be human in a more-than-human world?

References

Bantug, José Policarpio. 1953. *A Short History of Medicine in the Philippines during the Spanish Regime, 1565–1898*. Manila: Colegio Médico-Farmacéutico de Filipinas.

Burton, Bonnie. 2020. 'Jane Goodall: "Without hope, there's no point in continuing on"'. *CNET*, 23 April 2020. Accessed 1 November 2020. https://www.cnet.com/news/jane-goodall-without-hope-theres-no-point-in-continuing-on/.

Cabato, Regine. 2020. 'Forget bird flu – ostrich fever is gripping the Philippines'. *The Washington Post*, 11 August 2020. Accessed 2 November 2020. https://www.washingtonpost.com/world/asia_pacific/ostrich-escape-manila-coronavirus-lockdown/2020/08/11/e10f4d64-db90-11ea-b4f1-25b762cdbbf4_story.html.

Chakrabarty, Dipesh. 2009. 'The climate of history: Four theses'. *Critical Inquiry* 35(2): 197–222.

Chandler, Clare, Eleanor Hutchinson and Coll Hutchison. 2016. *Addressing Antimicrobial Resistance Through Social Theory: An anthropologically oriented report*. London: London School of Hygiene and Tropical Medicine.

D'Souza, Rohan. 2015. 'Nations without borders: Climate security and the South in the epoch of the Anthropocene'. *Strategic Analysis* 39(6): 720–28.

Daly, Nastasha. 2020. 'Fake animal news abounds on social media as coronavirus upends life'. *National Geographic*, 4 March 2020. Accessed 22 December 2020. https://www.nationalgeographic.com/animals/2020/03/coronavirus-pandemic-fake-animal-viral-social-media-posts/.

Deleuze, Gilles and Félix Guattari. 1988. *A Thousand Plateaus: Capitalism and schizophrenia*. London: Bloomsbury Publishing.

Dressler, Wolfram H. 2011. 'First to third nature: The rise of capitalist conservation on Palawan Island, the Philippines'. *The Journal of Peasant Studies* 38(3): 533–57.

Estrada, Olivia. 2020. 'FYI: We could have done without comparing rambutan to a virus'. *Philippine Daily Inquirer*, 25 June 2020. Accessed 2 November 2020. https://lifestyle.inquirer.net/365024/fyi-we-could-have-done-without-comparing-rambutan-to-a-virus/.

Fuentes, Agustín. 2010. 'Naturalcultural encounters in Bali: Monkeys, temples, tourists, and ethnoprimatology'. *Cultural Anthropology* 25(4): 600–24.

Greenhough, Beth. 2012. 'Where species meet and mingle: Endemic human-virus relations, embodied communication and more-than-human agency at the Common Cold Unit 1946–90'. *Cultural Geographies* 19(3): 281–301.

Haraway, Donna. 2006. 'Encounters with companion species: Entangling dogs, baboons, philosophers, and biologists'. *Configurations* 14(1–2): 97–114.

Haraway, Donna J. 2008. *When Species Meet*. Minneapolis and London: University of Minnesota Press.

Kellert, Stephen R. and Edward O. Wilson, eds. 1993. *The Biophilia Hypothesis*. Washington, DC: Island Press.

Kirksey, S. Eben and Stefan Helmreich. 2010. 'The emergence of multispecies ethnography'. *Cultural Anthropology* 25(4): 545–76.

Kohn, Eduardo. 2013. *How Forests Think: Toward an anthropology beyond the human*. Berkeley, CA: University of California Press.

Kretchmer, Harry. 2020. 'These locked-down cities are being reclaimed by animals'. *World Economic Forum*, 17 April 2020. Accessed 23 December 2020. https://www.weforum.org/agenda/2020/04/covid-19-cities-lockdown-animals-goats-boar-monkeys-zoo/.

Lasco, Gideon. 2020a. 'What if there *is* life on Venus?' *Sapiens*, 22 October 2020. Accessed 5 November 2020. https://www.sapiens.org/column/entanglements/anthropology-extraterrestrial-life/.

Lasco, Gideon. 2020b. 'The Severe Acute Respiratory Syndrome (SARS) outbreak in the Philippines in 2003'. *Philippine Studies: Historical and Ethnographic Viewpoints* 68(3/4): 337–69.

Lasco, Gideon. 2020c. 'How COVID-19 is changing people's relationships with houseplants'. *Sapiens*, 17 September 2020. Accessed 5 November 2020. https://www.sapiens.org/column/entanglements/covid-19-houseplants/.

Latour, Bruno. 1993. *We Have Never Been Modern*. Cambridge, MA: Harvard University Press.
Levitt, Tom. 2020. Covid and farm animals: Nine pandemics that changed the world. *The Guardian*, 15 September 200. Accessed 23 December 2020. https://www.theguardian.com/environment/ng-interactive/2020/sep/15/covid-farm-animals-and-pandemics-diseases-that-changed-the-world.
Lim, Theresa Mundita and Gideon Lasco. 2020. 'Plantitos, plantitas, and the environment'. *Philippine Daily Inquirer*, 6 October 2020. Accessed 23 December 2020. https://opinion.inquirer.net/134199/plantitos-plantitas-and-the-environment.
Lorimer, Hayden. 2005. 'Cultural geography: The busyness of being "more-than-representational"'. *Progress in Human Geography* 29(1): 83–94.
Lowe, Celia. 2010. 'Viral clouds: Becoming H5N1 in Indonesia,' *Cultural Anthropology* 25(4): 625–49.
Macfarlane, Robert. 2016. 'Generation Anthropocene: How humans have altered the planet for ever'. *The Guardian*, 1 April 2016. Accessed 3 November 2020. https://www.theguardian.com/books/2016/apr/01/generation-anthropocene-altered-planet-for-ever.
Mark, Catherine and José G. Rigau-Pérez. 2009. 'The world's first immunization campaign: The Spanish Smallpox Vaccine Expedition, 1803–1813'. *Bulletin of the History of Medicine* 83(1): 63–94.
Morgan, Liat, Alexandra Protopopova, Rune Isak Dupont Birkler, Beata Itin-Shwartz, Gila Abells Sutton, Alexandra Gamliel, Boris Yakobson and Tal Raz. 2020. 'Human-dog relationships during the COVID-19 pandemic: Booming dog adoption during social isolation'. *Humanities and Social Sciences Communications* 7: 155.
Murray, Adrienne. 2020. 'Coronavirus: Denmark shaken by cull of millions of mink'. BBC, 11 November 2020. Accessed 20 December 2020. https://www.bbc.com/news/world-europe-54890229.
National Institutes of Health. 2012. 'NIH Human Microbiome Project defines normal bacterial makeup of the body'. Accessed 6 November 2020. https://www.nih.gov/news-events/news-releases/nih-human-microbiome-project-defines-normal-bacterial-makeup-body.
Ogden, Laura A., Billy Hall and Kimiko Tanita. 2013. 'Animals, plants, people, and things: A review of multispecies ethnography'. *Environment and Society* 4(1): 5–24.
Panelli, Ruth. 2010. 'More-than-human social geographies: Posthuman and other possibilities'. *Progress in Human Geography* 34(1): 79–87.
Paxson, Heather. 2008. 'Post-Pasteurian cultures: The microbiopolitics of raw-milk cheese in the United States'. *Cultural Anthropology* 23(1): 15–47.
Perez, Padmapani L. 2018. *Green Entanglements: Nature conservation and indigenous peoples' rights in Indonesia and the Philippines*. Quezon City: University of the Philippines Press.
Reuters Staff. 2020. 'Philippines' Duterte keeps one meter social distancing rule'. *Reuters*, 19 September 2020. Accessed November 3, 2020. https://www.reuters.com/article/us-health-coronavirus-philippines/philippines-duterte-keeps-one-meter-social-distancing-rule-idINKBN26A07N.
Rillig, Matthias C., Janis Antonovics, Tancredi Caruso, Anika Lehmann, Jeff R. Powell, Stavros D. Veresoglou and Erik Verbruggen. 2015. 'Interchange of entire communities: Microbial community coalescence'. *Trends in Ecology & Evolution* 30(8): 470–76.
Santiago-Alarcon, Diego and Ian MacGregor-Fors. 2020. 'Cities and pandemics: Urban areas are ground zero for the transmission of emerging human infectious diseases'. *Journal of Urban Ecology* 6(1): juaa012.
Searle, Adam and Jonathon Turnbull. 2020. 'Resurgent natures? More-than-human perspectives on COVID-19'. *Dialogues in Human Geography* 10(2): 291–5.
Singer, Merrill Charles, Nicola Bulled, Bayla Ostrach and Emily Mendenhall. 2017. 'Syndemics and the biosocial conception of health'. *The Lancet* 389(10072): 941–50.
Smith, Will. 2020. 'Beyond loving nature: Affective conservation and human-pig violence in the Philippines'. *Ethnos*: 1–19.
Stawkowski, Magdalena E. 2016. '"I am a radioactive mutant": Emergent biological subjectivities at Kazakhstan's Semipalatinsk Nuclear Test Site'. *American Ethnologist* 43(1): 144–57.
Tan, Michael L. 2008. *Revisiting usog, pasma, kulam*. Quezon City: University of the Philippines Press.
Tan, Michael L. and Gideon Lasco. Forthcoming. '"Hawa" and "resistensya": Local health knowledge and the COVID-19 pandemic in the Philippines'. *Anthropology and Medicine*. https://doi:10.1080/13648470.2021.1893980.

Tandog, Thea Kersti Condes. 2020. '"Bigas hindi dahas": COVID-19 and state violence'. *Fieldsights*, 30 April 2020. Accessed 5 November 2020. https://culanth.org/fieldsights/bigas-hindi-dahas-covid-19-and-state-violence.

Tomé, Pedro. 2020. 'Walking the dog in Madrid during the pandemic'. *Anthropology Today* 36(5): 24–25.

Tsing, Anna L. 2013. 'More-than-human sociality: A call for critical description'. In *Anthropology and Nature*, edited by Kirsten Hastrup, pp. 27–42. New York: Routledge.

Ulrich, Roger S. 1993. 'Biophilia, biophobia, and natural landscapes'. In *The Biophilia Hypothesis*, edited by Stephen R. Kellert and Edward O. Wilson, pp. 73–137. Washington DC: Island Press.

Uranaka, Taiga. 2001. 'Parasitologist says excess hygiene threatens Japan'. *The Japan Times*, 4 February 2001. Accessed 3 November 2020. https://www.japantimes.co.jp/news/2001/02/04/national/parasitologist-says-excess-hygiene-threatens-japan/.

Valenzuela, Nikka G. 2020. 'Malabon Zoo owner seeks donations for 'No. 1 love". *Philippine Daily Inquirer*, 20 May 2020. Accessed 4 November 2020. https://newsinfo.inquirer.net/1277768/malabon-zoo-owner-seeks-donations-for-no-1-love#ixzz6g6wYMxLu.

Vich, V. (2016). '¿ Qué es el pueblo?¿ Qué son las plantas? El "plantón móvil" de Lucía Monge'. *Las humanidades por venir: políticas y debates en el siglo XXI*: 289-382. Accessed 22 December 2020. http://209.177.156.169/libreria_cm/archivos/pdf_2297.pdf#page=289.

Wang, Leyi, Patrick K. Mitchell, Paul P. Calle, Susan L. Bartlett, Denise McAloose, Mary Lea Killian, Fangfeng Yuan et al. 2020. 'Complete genome sequence of SARS-CoV-2 in a tiger from a US zoological collection'. *Microbiology Resource Announcements* 9(22). https://doi.org/10.1128/mra.00468-20.

Watanabe, Shumpei, Joseph S. Masangkay, Noriyo Nagata, Shigeru Morikawa, Tetsuya Mizutani, Shuetsu Fukushi, Phillip Alviola, Tsutomu Omatsu, Naoya Ueda, Koichiro Iha, Satoshi Taniguchi, Kiharu Fujii, Shumpei Tsuda, Maiko Endoh, Kentaro Kato, Yukinobu Tohya, Shigeru Kyuwa, Yasuhiro Yoshikawa and Hiroomi Akashi. 2010. 'Bat coronaviruses and experimental infection of bats, the Philippines'. *Emerging Infectious Diseases* 16(8): 1217–23.

Wilkinson, Samuel W., Melissa H. Magerøy, Ana López Sánchez, Lisa M. Smith, Leonardo Furci, T.E. Anne Cotton, Paal Krokene and Jurriaan Ton. 2019. 'Surviving in a hostile world: Plant strategies to resist pests and diseases'. *Annual Review of Phytopathology* 57: 505–29.

23
COVID-19 in Italy

A new culture of healthcare for future preparedness

Chiara Bodini and Ivo Quaranta

When the first autochthonous cases of COVID-19 were diagnosed in Lombardy in late February 2020, the whole country went into a shock (Raffaetà 2020). Both the virus and the effect it elicited quickly spread to the rest of Europe. Suddenly, what had been described as a 'Chinese virus', a threat confined to far away countries perceived as 'less developed', was inside our borders, in the very heart of a rich and productive region in Northern Italy. The severe underestimation of the pandemic in Italy, that was already rapidly spreading worldwide, resulted in the slow and chaotic reaction of Italian authorities facing the diffusion of the virus. The lack of preparedness, and fragmentations in governance between central government and the regions, led to contradictory messages being communicated to the public and incoherent and inconsistent measures being adopted. This led to the exposure of large numbers of people, including many 'essential services' workers. Huge numbers of critically ill patients required hospital care in a healthcare system that had suffered from budget cuts and privatisation over the past decades, particularly in its primary care and public health components. It was a very long time since hospitals in Europe had been overwhelmed in the way that they were in Lombardy, and this was seen as a wake-up call for other European countries and a portent of how COVID-19 might impact other settings. Measures to contain the epidemic, including a two-month national lockdown, were introduced.

However – as we argue in this chapter – the response to COVID-19, consistent with the culture and the organisation of health and medicine in Italy, was largely biomedical, and so failed to incorporate the social dimensions of the disease. This response was inadequate to build future preparedness.

COVID-19 in Italy

In late January 2020, two Chinese tourists visiting Rome were diagnosed with COVID-19. The news was alarming as it showed that the virus had entered the country, but not too disturbing as it fitted the stereotype of a foreign-borne virus that could be controlled by closing the borders. In what appeared to be strategic timing, the day before these cases were diagnosed, the government had blocked all flights to and from China; this measure was later labelled as detrimental as it made it impossible to test and trace people coming from China who chose other indirect routes to reach Italy. For two more weeks, no other measures were taken, until – on 21 February – the first Italian case of COVID-19 was diagnosed in Lombardy. To the shock of many, the 38-year-old man, labelled as 'patient 1', had not travelled to China, and all efforts to find 'patient 0' and trace the origin of the virus failed. From then on, the situation rapidly escalated, with new diagnoses concentrated in the same geographical area. Lombardy became the first 'red zone' under lockdown. Still, the belief was that the virus came from abroad and, if contained where it had first been found, the rest of the country would be spared (Horton 2020a). Unfortunately, the data later showed that the virus had been circulating in Lombardy since at least a month before, with hundreds of cases of infection – including severe ones – that had not been tested and therefore not diagnosed.

The period that followed was intense and confusing. The central government and regional authorities took decisions in an uncoordinated way, and messages to the population were openly contradictory. While the people in Codogno were locked in their homes, neighbouring cities such as Milan and Bergamo launched a media campaign to emphasise that life there was going on as usual – 'Milan does not stop' (#milanononsiferma) – and that there was no reason to panic. Similar messages appeared on social media, posted by key political figures from different parties.

Less than a week later, on 4 March, schools and universities were closed across the country and, on 8 March, a national lockdown was imposed. It was an unprecedented measure for Italy and for the world. People could not go out of their homes unless they carried a self-declaration that stated the reason to do so – for health, work or to assist relatives in need – and few were so permitted. The (rather arbitrary) application of this norm resulted in thousands of fines ranging from 400 to 3,000 euros, many of which have been contested.

Many praised the Italian government for acting decisively. However, the delay in implementing lockdown measures are, at time of writing, under investigation: this applies especially in the province of Bergamo, the hardest hit by the epidemic. Government documents, made public over the northern summer 2020, showed that on 3 March the National Scientific Committee had called for a 'red zone' in the area, and an investigation is ongoing to find out why this had not been applied, although allegedly motivated by the desire to avoid the economic consequences of a lockdown. At the same time, for several weeks, even under the lockdown, so-called 'essential services' continued to function, exposing health providers, transport workers and cleaners, among others, to a higher risk of infection.

The daily report issued by the Civil Protection from early March was dominated by the escalating number of new cases, hospital admissions, patients in intensive care units (ICU) and deaths. The National Health System (NHS), although still considered as one of the best in Europe, soon became insufficient to admit and adequately treat all patients, especially in Lombardy. Despite a referral system which included all public and some private facilities throughout the country, there were increasing reports by physicians in Lombardy that patients were being told to stay at home because hospital facilities were overloaded, and that patients could not be ventilated – despite meeting the clinical criteria for such action – because there were not enough ventilators available. These reports were so shocking that they were silenced or openly contested by public authorities, but they circulated widely, particularly among health professionals. A few weeks later, the army trucks moving coffins of coronavirus victims from Bergamo because there were no spaces available in local cemeteries could not so easily be concealed.

The lack of preparedness and insufficient human and material resources, combined with an elderly population and a high level of air pollution in the areas most affected, likely contributed to a particularly high mortality rate in the first wave of the pandemic. Delays in admitting patients to the hospitals and inappropriate approaches to both antimicrobial and intensive care treatment were particularly called into question by public health officials and health activist networks; so too was the approach to test and trace in Italy in ways that did not follow the recommendations of the World Health Organization (WHO).

As of 22 December 2020, Italy had recorded 1,977,370 cases and 69,842 COVID-19 deaths. One quarter of the cases and almost one third of the deaths were recorded in Lombardy (Ministry of Health 2020).

A healthcare response to a public health emergency

Interviewed in early April, the president of the Medical Board of Bergamo, the city in Lombardy that became the symbol of the COVID-19 crisis in the country, declared:

> The National Healthcare Service (NHS) has been dramatically dismantled, hospitals and community services ... A public health emergency has been mistakenly considered as an emergency of intensive care units. At the beginning, COVID cases were not isolated, epidemiological investigations were not done, patients were not tested, doctors did not have personal protective equipment (Marinoni 2020).

In a few words, Dr Marinoni summarised the failure of the initial response to the crisis and identified its root causes.

It is now clear that Italy was not prepared for the epidemic, and its preparedness plan, drawn up in 2006 and unknown to most health professionals, has been judged 'old and inadequate' (Giuffrida and Boseley 2020). In addition to this, since the early 1990s the NHS has been subject to reforms and budget cuts that severely altered its capacity to react to a sudden increase in health needs (Geddes da Filicaia 2020). As in many countries across the globe, privatisation affects the capacity of public state-funded and government-run health systems to coordinate large-scale preventive campaigns, and limits their capacity to expand curative services in crisis situations, while eroding the broad public's confidence in the health system as a whole (De Ceukelaire and Bodini 2020). Moreover, the regionalisation of healthcare – very much part of a broader design to progressively dismantle and privatise the NHS – significantly delayed the adoption of coherent measures to contain the disease and strengthen the health system. While the Italian public health authorities at regional and national levels tried to cope with the growing epidemic, the highly fragmented health system resulted in a complex situation that became difficult to manage (Villa et al. 2020).

The area that suffered the most from these processes, now considered the weakest link of the NHS, is primary healthcare (PHC), particularly at the intersection of public health, primary care departments and family doctors. Structural weaknesses date back to the healthcare reform of 1978, when, under pressure from the physicians themselves, legislators decided that family doctors would not be employed by the NHS, but would be contracted as private professionals under a national agreement. A decade after, what were initially called 'local social and healthcare units' (Unità Sanitarie Locali, USL) became 'local healthcare enterprises' (Aziende Sanitarie Locali, ASL), with a double shift: the removal of the word 'social' and the shift from 'unit' to 'enterprise'. This change marked the inauguration of the managerialisation of the NHS, which coincided with the progressive reduction of the national public healthcare budget. The participation of citizens at different levels of the system's governance, included in the original reform, was never developed.

The region that most aggressively pursued privatisation, and that developed secondary and tertiary-level hospitals to the detriment of primary care, is Lombardy. This has been repeatedly used as (part of) the explanation of why the region was hit harder by coronavirus and why the region failed to implement a coherent and effective strategy in an effort to contain it. To date, the problems of primary care and public health organisation have not been addressed, and professionals in the field are still left alone to face a new wave of infections.

As a critical situation, the pandemic revealed the impact of austerity and market-oriented reforms in undermining the capacity of the NHS to perform its biopolitical duties of health promotion, prevention and care (Basu et al. 2017). It also made explicit the cultural values informing national health policy: the pandemic was mainly dealt with at the hospital level, with a reactive approach that focused on acute care, infection control and virology, rather than a proactive public health approach grounded on epidemiological surveillance and health promotion. Moreover, although the spread of the virus began to be contained mainly through lockdown and people's willingness to modify their social behaviour, the NHS did not act through its community-based local articulations such as primary care health facilities and professionals. These were, in fact, rather inaccessible to the public, as either closed down (as in the case of many primary care facilities) or overwhelmed (as in the case of GPs). It was not until late April that special 'home care units' were established, in order to assist and monitor patients who did not meet the criteria for hospitalisation. However, their implementation has been uneven across the country in terms of both capacity and timeliness.

The inadequate management of the COVID-19 epidemic, particularly evident in the region that invested the most in a privatised, market-oriented and hospital-centric healthcare system, draws attention to the failures of such an approach in dealing with a complex public health emergency. More intensive care beds and ventilators, although necessary at the beginning of the crisis, soon became a technical fix that was ineffective at the source of the problem. In the community, the virus was circulating, undetected by an inadequate public health effort.

Cultural values informing national health policy

These preliminary considerations help us understand how human agency contributes to shaping the local configuration of COVID-19 in a specific context. In order to further develop the analysis, we now examine the implicit cultural assumptions that guided the Italian response to the pandemic.

The initial underestimation of the pandemic was clearly rooted in the fallacious idea that highly contagious infectious diseases are a medical reality confined to low-income countries in the Global South (Kleinman and Watson 2006). Consistent with this, the initial tracing operations focused on 'Chinese contacts' of the first cases. Rather than engaging in collaborative and cooperative actions with Chinese (and other national) authorities, the government decided to stop flights arriving in Italy from the risk regions, ignoring the most basic global health assumptions on the collective nature of any local phenomenon (Biehl and Petryna 2013; Farmer et al. 2013). Looking at the patterns of its distribution and at the different national responses to it, we can certainly consider COVID-19 as an indicator of our *glocal* (Kearney 1995) (dis-)order: an assemblage by which the viral pathogen mingles with specific social configurations within which people's actions unfold at the local and global level. Infectious viruses are about social networks and cultural norms, as much as about microbes. As virological research makes clear, viruses are inert, sometimes for thousands of years, unable to attack us. We transmit viral data though our social networks and cultural pathways. We give viral information to each other by how we live and what we do. Understanding cultural contexts is therefore just as important as sequencing genomes in tackling viral outbreaks (Napier and Fischer 2020).

The very absence of an adequate pandemic plan testifies the lack of a global health perspective in the Italian institutional response, that might have been able to explicitly address the social nature of the virus agency. The Italian response reduced COVID-19 to its aetiology: SARS-CoV-2. Even the National Scientific Committee, appointed on 5 February

2020 by the government to manage the emergency, has been mainly informed by a reductionist medical perspective with little acknowledgement of socially-oriented approaches including public health, epidemiology and the social sciences. In so doing, the complex reality of COVID-19 was stripped of its social dimensions, limiting the possibility for action (Rajan et al. 2020).

A behavioural approach to prevention

Such reductionism was also present in the preventive strategy adopted by the state, rooted in a well-known behavioural approach geared around the spread of information for the adoption of individual practices such as avoiding contact, frequently washing hands, wearing masks and gloves and so on. Such campaigns, as they unfolded in Italy, have a number of limitations and side effects which were not adequately considered.

In the first place, in general behavioural campaigns fail to address possible structural constraints impacting on individual behaviour. This was particularly evident when trying to halt the transmission of coronavirus in the cases of homeless people, asylum seekers and refugees living in overcrowded centres, seasonal migrant workers living in informal settlements, Roma people living in camps (see also Pop, Chapter 8) and detainees in prisons. Despite vibrant protests by people who were imprisoned, and different advocacy actions by groups, associations and networks working with vulnerable populations, very little was done to improve the structural conditions contributing to their risks for contagion. On the contrary, rather than highlighting such constraints, people's culture and values tended to be presented as obstacles in health promotion, leading to forms of blaming of different groups of people. Depending on the phase of the emergency and the lockdown, these included migrants who were alleged to bring the virus from abroad (as Onoma, Chapter 10, also describes), even if at the time – given the situation in Italy – the risk was rather that they would become infected upon arrival. Blame was also directed at people walking or jogging in parks, who were accused of placing individual interest above everything else; and youth, who were charged with returning too quickly to socialising after the lockdown was eased. Both public authorities and the social media accused these groups of people of deliberately ignoring public health norms and so of being responsible for the spread of infection.

Framing the issue of responsibility in individual terms undermined the very possibility for a representation of the crisis as a collective condition to be dealt with in cooperative terms. Even now, rather than imagining new forms of sociality as a collective response to the perduring emergency, we are facing increasing sanitisation of sociality, with the risk of its very criminalisation. To strip COVID-19 of its social dimensions inevitably precludes the possibility of acknowledging the importance of looking at people's perspectives, and of considering how to promote their wellbeing. Paraphrasing Napier and colleagues (2014, 1611), if we ignore what brings value and meaning to another's life, it becomes difficult to make it better when it is necessary to do so.

Yet little room was left for an approach capable of taking into consideration people's understandings of their needs and how to meet them. Unless we look at health as a cultural construct and equip our healthcare services with the proper competence to foster the participation of people in the very definition of their best interests, we are always at risk of producing ineffective interventions. Again, we have a cultural issue here, related to the biomedical devaluation of the cultural dimensions of health and wellbeing.

People as a resource

If there is one lesson from social science analysis of past epidemics, it is that people's behaviours make a difference and, therefore, the ability to actively involve them in the processes that concern them can be decisive (Packard 2016; Richards 2016). Yet, to address people's behaviours implies the need to consider their capabilities, for example, to negotiate the terms of their social engagement and circumstances in a given local reality. Despite the fact that it was only through a lockdown that the emergency was kept under control, people's behaviours were never assumed as a possible resource in managing the crisis. Yet these behaviours made a difference also by attending to the needs of those who were most affected by the economic and relational consequences of lockdown.

At the grassroots level, many initiatives took shape. In the Municipality of Bologna, for example, formal and informal civil society groups organised themselves to support those in need, delivering to them food supplies, medical equipment and pharmaceuticals. This effort largely came from below, as in many other places throughout the country, while public services were shut down and public officials were discussing what should be done in endless online meetings. Well-established charity organisations linked to churches, political parties, trade unions and private foundations were joined (or, at times, were preceded) by many new and often informal networks, largely composed of students and people who, due to the lockdown, suddenly had a lot of spare time and felt the urge to help others. New needs also appeared and were rapidly addressed by grassroots solidarity networks, such as the need for laptops and tablets for families with children who – with all schools closed – had to follow distance learning programmes.

Even in the City of Bologna, with a centuries-old tradition of good governance and progressive welfare policies, it took several weeks, even months, for the public system to acknowledge, support and finally regulate such efforts. Meanwhile, this activity remained fully voluntary and largely autonomous of public institutions, and was hyperlocal in nature, involving people at the level of buildings, blocks and streets. These forms of mutual support from below were the only ones capable of making a difference for those already trapped by socio-economic inequalities, who were, and still are, the most vulnerable to and affected by the pandemic (see also Burke, Chapter 2).

These initiatives were crucial in complementing the institutional actions prescribed by the national government and by local authorities, which invested a substantial part of the public budget to support those most in need. In this regard, Italy might be seen as a good example in addressing both the medical and the socio-economic consequences of the COVID-19 pandemic (Horton 2020a). Yet a critical dimension is in the incapacity of government, at all levels, to develop the operative integration of social and medical actions grounded in community participation as a form of care and the promotion of equity.

In the summer of 2020, as transmission of COVID-19 slowed down, local and national institutions developed emergency plans in order to be adequately prepared for a possible second wave of the pandemic (as occurred a few months later). Such plans were mainly designed to enhance the capacity of medical services to treat patients, to store equipment for testing and treatment, and to ensure a proper supply of personal protective equipment. In other words, preparedness was again tailored on pathology rather than on the wider reality of which pathology is part. By stripping COVID-19 of its social dimensions, again, institutional preparedness ended up limiting its effective responsiveness. No attention was given to those dynamics that made resilient specific local contexts, i.e. community participation. The crucial role of social relations is the main issue that was exposed by the COVID-19 pandemic. Yet Italian institutions have not been able so far to consider them as part of any form of preparedness.

In anthropological terms, preparedness should be seen as a means by which a specific social order is produced, especially in a critical time in which habitual forms of relatedness are compromised and need to be rethought. The post COVID-19 scenario cannot be imagined as a return to a previous normality, as if the impact of the pandemic might leave no trace in our conscience and social arrangements. Clearly, we have to talk of new forms of normalisation, by which a new social order becomes embodied and can promote our unproblematic being-in-the-world. In order to avoid that such a process of re-normalisation ends up in naturalising the medicalisation and criminalisation of sociality, we must engage in forms of creative social relatedness to produce new forms of sociality capable of sustaining a meaningful collective existence. For this reason, we need to include the promotion of those forms of social relatedness that have proved protective in our institutional responses to the pandemic. If we reduce preparedness merely to the adoption of protective individual behaviours, we are stripping the person of its constitutive social dimension. As anthropology has long taught us, by focusing on the body, cultural practice articulates broader social and political issues. This is precisely why it is crucial to work beyond the sole adoption of protective individual behaviours and towards the idea of designing forms of protective social relatedness.

Primary healthcare as a space for integrated action

Institutional action on COVID-19 has not valued community participation as a resource in dealing with the emergency, despite its crucial role in giving birth to adaptive forms of sociality. Such a lack stems in part from having relegated institutional action to the hospital level, without drawing on the network of community-based primary care services, the only component of the health system capable of proximate contact with local neighbourhoods and their inhabitants. As already discussed above, primary healthcare (PHC) has been severely undermined over the last decades by processes of underfinancing and cultural devaluation (Geddes da Filicaia 2020). Yet PHC represents the only articulation of the NHS capable of producing forms of participation and mutual trust between institutional actors and people.

This is not intended to diminish the decisive role that hospital settings have played in treating people affected by COVID-19; this would be both ungenerous and inaccurate. Rather, it highlights that the healthcare system is culturally calibrated on values that do not take into account the proximity of services to local neighbourhoods, the only context in which it would be possible to create a proactive synergy between institutions and people's agency.

Again COVID-19 seems to play a pedagogic role in making manifest the limitation and contradictions of our social reality, shedding light on its fault lines, a critical situation that unveils those implicit processes that inform our social reality.

A different approach for future preparedness

By dividing medical action from social support, and by formulating the latter mainly in a top-down manner centred on individuals, Italy ended up limiting its institutional capacity to manage the local configuration of the pandemic. The focus of Italy's response was mainly on the virus, SARS-CoV-2, rather than on the disease, COVID-19. The current challenge is related to the possibility of grounding medical and social services with a view of health as a cultural construct that requires the participation of people to define their needs. This must be socially produced, and this can only occur through the constitutive relations that people have with the social circumstances of their life in a given context. Unless we are capable of taking into account the constitutive social dimensions of medical reality, we are bound to a permanent state of emergency.

Future preparedness, in other words, should not be reduced to the adequate storage of medical supplies. It should rather take advantage of the lessons we are learning in the current global predicament. On the one hand, we need a global perspective capable of looking at health as a common global good, and we need to strengthen an approach that looks at the mutual involvement of the contexts we imagine as local, with awareness that one's own interests coincide with the promotion of those of others. On the other hand, we need to place as central community involvement and participation (Rajan et al. 2020), with the aim of considering people as actors in the process of health promotion, avoiding their reduction to a 'mere population' (in Foucauldian terms) crushed by top-down measures and incapable of generating their active valorisation (Loewenson et al. 2020). To do so, we need a culture of health and healthcare capable of creating conceptual and political room for local participatory action in local services.

As anthropologists, we know well that communities are not entities but forms of relatedness rooted in the ongoing symbolic processes of belonging. Institutions should accommodate and rely on forms of symbolic belonging that emerge at the grassroots level (especially if they proved to be resilient in facing the critical circumstances produced by the pandemic). Otherwise, when community participation is most needed, we run the risk of having no community to rely on. Social policy should complement medical reasoning in designing emergency plans for future preparedness, bearing in mind the symbolic performance of institutional activity. Our challenge today relates to the ability to create organisational settings capable of overcoming those cultural fragmentations that reduce care to disease treatment, while they strip health of those social relationships on which we might act for its promotion (Wilkinson and Kleinman 2016).

Conclusion

The COVID-19 pandemic has laid bare the many strains that Italy's healthcare system has amassed over past decades. Yet we have shown how analysis cannot be reduced to the mere impact of austerity measures: we also need to address the broader cultural assumptions at the core of medical and public health policy. As we have shown for the Italian context, in order to design an effective preparedness, we need an institutional culture capable of considering health as a cultural construct to be socially generated, where participation is the means to operationalise both: people's involvement in defining their best interest, and their engagement in transformative actions.

Quite timely, on 26 September 2020 *The Lancet* chief editor, Richard Horton (2020b), claimed that we should look at COVID-19 as a syndemic rather than a pandemic. In introducing the concept of syndemic, Merrill Singer (2009) referred to the constitutive social embeddedness of any given biological reality, and their complex articulations at the local as well as global level. Along such a line of reasoning, in this chapter we have showed the local emergence of COVID-19 in Italy, arguing for a finer approach capable of addressing its social articulation at the local level. Likewise, we have tried to show how to translate the outcome of such a theoretical approach in designing institutional responses capable of taking into proper account the constitutive social dimensions of COVID-19.

The concept of syndemic is most welcome if it helps to drive institutional reasoning towards the appreciation of human agency and responsibility in medical reality, and coherently of public health interventions as cultural practices by which a specific social order is produced, and, by focusing on the body, naturalised. The way we approach the present critical situation related to COVID-19 will inevitably have a deep impact on the way we represent ourselves, social relations and the global scenario – in a nutshell, the very meaning of humanity.

References

Basu, Sanjay, Megan A. Carney and Nora J. Kenworthy. 2017. 'Ten years after the financial crisis: The long reach of austerity and its global impacts on health'. *Social Science & Medicine* 187: 203–7.
Biehl, Joao and Adriana Petryna, eds. 2013. *When People Come First. Critical studies in global health*. Princeton, NJ: Princeton University Press.
De Ceukelaire, Wim and Chiara Bodini. 2020. 'We need strong public health care to contain the global corona pandemic'. *International Journal of Health Services* https://doi.org/10.1177/0020731420916725.
Farmer, Paul, Jim Kim, Arthur Kleinman and Matthew Basilico, eds. 2013. *Reimagining Global Health: An introduction*. Berkeley. CA: University of California Press.
Geddes da Filicaia, Marco. 2020. *La sanità ai tempi del coronavirus*. Rome, Italy: Il Pensiero Scientifico Editore.
Giuffrida, Angela and Sarah Boseley. 2020. 'Italy's pandemic plan "old and inadequate", Covid report finds'. *The Guardian*, 13 August 2020. Accessed 15 August 2020. https://www.theguardian.com/world/2020/aug/13/italy-pandemic-plan-was-old-and-inadequate-covid-report-finds.
Horton, Richard. 2020a. *The COVID-19 Catastrophe: What's gone wrong and how to stop it happening again*. Cambridge, UK: Polity Press.
Horton, Richard. 2020b. 'Offline: COVID-19 is not a pandemic'. *The Lancet* 396: 874. doi: https://doi.org/10.1016/S0140-6736(20)32000-6.
Kearney, Michael. 1995. 'The local and the global: The anthropology of globalization and transnationalism'. *Annual Review of Anthropology* 24: 547–65.
Kleinman, Arthur and James L. Watson. 2006. *SARS in China: Prelude to pandemic?* Stanford, CA: Stanford University Press.
Loewenson, Rene, Kirsten Accoe, Nitin Bajpai, Kent Buse, Thilagawathi Abi Deivanayagam, Leslie London, Claudio A Méndez, et al. 2020. 'Reclaiming comprehensive public health'. *BMJ Global Health* 5(9): e003886. https://doi.org/10.1136/bmjgh-2020-003886.
Marinoni, Guido. 2020. Radio 24 Mattino interview. Accessed 27 December 2020. https://www.radio24.ilsole24ore.com/programmi/24mattino-le-interviste/puntata/la-verita-dietro-numeri-062053-ADZv26H.
Ministry of Health. 2020. 'Nuovo coronavirus'. Last modified 27 December 2020. Accessed 27 December 2020. http://www.salute.gov.it/portale/nuovocoronavirus/homeNuovo Coronavirus.jsp.
Napier, A. David and Edward F. Fischer. 2020. 'The culture of health and sickness'. *Le Monde Diplomatique*. Accessed 27 December 2020. https://mondediplo.com/2020/07/04uganda.
Napier, A. David, Clyde Ancarno, Beverley Butler, Joseph Calabrese, Angel Chater et al. 2014. 'Culture and health'. *The Lancet* 384(9954):1607–39.
Packard, Randall. 2016. *A History of Global Health: Interventions into the lives of other peoples*. Baltimore, MD: Johns Hopkins University Press.
Raffaetà, Roberta. 2020. 'Another day in dystopia. Italy in the time of COVID-19'. *Medical Anthropology: Cross-Cultural Studies in Health and Illness* 39(5): 371–3. https://www.tandfonline.com/doi/full/10.1080/01459740.2020.1746300.
Rajan, Dheepa, Kira Koch, Katja Rohrer, Csongor Bajnoczki, Anna Socha, Maike Voss, Marjolaine Nicod, Valery Ridde and Justin Koonin. 2020. 'Governance of the Covid-19 response: A call for more inclusive and transparent decision-making'. *BMJ Global Health* 5(5): e002655. https://doi.org/10.1136/bmjgh-2020-002655.
Richards, Paul. 2016. *Ebola: How a people's science helped end an epidemic*. London: Zed Books Ltd.
Singer, Merrill. 2009. *An Introduction to Syndemics: A critical systems approach to public and community health*. San Francisco, CA: John Wiley & Sons.
Villa, Simone, Andrea Lombardi, Davide Mangioni, Giorgio Bozzi, Alessandra Bandera, Andrea Gori and Mario C. Raviglione. 2020. 'The COVID-19 Pandemic preparedness … or lack thereof: From China to Italy'. *Global Health & Medicine* 2(2): 73–7. https://doi.org/10.35772/ghm.2020.01016.
Wilkinson, Iain and Arthur Kleinman. 2016. *A Passion for Society. How we think about human suffering*. Berkeley, CA: University of California Press.

Index

Adalet ve Kalkınma Partisi (AKP), Turkey
   mishandling of pandemic by 13, 162–4, 170, 175
   moralist discourse on pandemic by 13, 163, 165–6, 175
   suppression of critical voices by 165–6, 175–6
   violation of secularism clause by 167
Adler-Lazarowitz, Chanah 385–6, 392–6, 402–3n4
Agamben, Giorgio 29, 129–30, 142, 429
Ali, Ahmet 12, 132–3
Amazonian rainforest 429–30
Ambedkar, B.R. 141, 203
Andrejevic, Mark 345, 347
'anonymous care' 30–1, 42
anthropology of care 29, 41–2 See also biopolitics of pandemic
apartheid 10, 47
   structural legacies of 48, 55–6, 60–1
Australia 9, 50
   Melbourne 8, 14
   use of armed forces in 58, 60
authoritarianism 81, 173
   COVID-19-related 4, 38, 165, 185, 190
Avishai, Orit 389, 392

Bacchi, Carol 206, 208
Bailey, F.G. 68–9, 79, 82–3, 85
Bangladesh 8
   catastrophic consequences of lockdown in 281–2
   dependence on informal economy in 282–3, 285, 287–9
   government stimulus/support package 286, 288
   police enforcement of lockdown in 284–6, 288–9, 291–2, 294
   population of 281–2
   See also Dhaka, impact of lockdown on adolescents/youth in
Băsescu, Traian 152–3
biodiversity 437, 439
bioethics and notions of vulnerability 15, 17, 119, 123, 262, 271–5
   lack of power as main criterion 272–3, 284, 292, 295
   See also COVID-19 amplification of vulnerability; healthcare: triaged access to; COVID-19 'risk groups', designation of

biopolitics of pandemic
   Cuban approach 29–30, 37, 41–2
   'make live and let die' approach 21, 128–31, 137, 142–3, 249
   Roma responses 147, 153
   in UK 109, 119, 447
   See also Foucault, Michel: concept of biopolitics
Black, Asian and Minority Ethnic (BAME) communities 12, 120–1, 129, 140, 143, 319
   disproportionate infection/death rates among 108–9, 111–14, 116, 131, 319
   inherent racism of acronym 111, 131, 140
#BlackLivesMatter (BLM) 12, 62, 108, 129
#BlackLivesMatter uprisings, LA 91, 95–6, 108, 113
   abolitionist views of 92, 97, 100–1, 104
   link with disparities of COVID-19 99, 102, 105
   radical Black founders of 92–3
   use of armed forces/curfews against 58–9, 64n4, 94, 101–2
   white support for 102
   See also Floyd, George, murder of; Movement for Black Lives; racism, systemic; underlying conditions of COVID-19: police brutality
Black radical tradition, US 93, 102
Bolsonaro, Jair
   negationist stand on COVID-19 244–5, 247–9, 251, 256
   positive test for COVID-19 6
   survival of the fittest philosophy 244, 248, 253, 256
Bosak, Krzysztof 77–8
Brazil
   as COVID-19 epicentre 4, 6–7
   decline of Public Health System (SUS) in 246, 248, 251
   emergency aid 254
   favelas of 1, 50, 56
   as international centre of medical research 249–50
   Workers' Party of 245–6, 251
   See also disability support, impact of COVID-19 on; syndemic: COVID-19 as; Zika virus
Breman, Jan 137–8
Briggs, Charles 2, 33–4, 37, 69, 71, 85

Brotherton, P. Sean 29–30, 33–4
Bulgaria 148, 154, 158

cancer 20, 239, 329
  impact of COVID-19 on screening and treatment of 15, 233–4, 308, 341n2
  normalising of 30, 34
Cape Town 50, 61
  Anti-Land Invasion Unit activities 59
carceral state 98–9, 101, 104–5
Carreño, Hiram 261, 267
caste-based structural violence 128, 136, 140–1
  'shroud stealer' as allegory for 12, 132–6, 142–3
  See also viral vagility of prejudice: and Indian caste system
caste system, India
  and imposition of *cordon sanitaire* 141–2, 413
  and practice of untouchability 12, 131, 135, 139–41, 203, 205
  Scheduled Castes (SC) 131–2, 138, 140, 204, 209
  Scheduled Tribes (ST) 132, 140
  and tropes of purity and pollution 140–1, 203, 218
  upper caste prejudice and 12, 139–41
  See also Dalit, India
Castro, Fidel 30, 33–4
Castro, Raul 34, 38
Chile 36, 58, 266–7, 271
Chimudu, Simukai 71, 411
China 11, 19, 354, 411
  donation of masks, respirators from 35
  See also Wuhan
cholera 2, 35–6, 184, 249, 412
  conspiracy theories 71
chronic disease
  care infrastructure for 10, 15, 30, 34, 326–7, 329–30, 337–8
  impact of COVID-19 on care 2, 11, 28, 47, 244, 249, 256, 273, 324, 331–2, 338–9
  link between inequality and 11, 28, 51, 110, 119, 129, 318
  mobile technologies as support mechanism for 333–4, 344, 346
  See also Denmark's universal healthcare system: focus on chronic care; syndemic: framework on chronic disease
  See also comorbidities; cancer; diabetes; heart disease
citizen surveillance 10, 47, 49 *See also* Cuban state systems of surveillance/control
citizenship 3, 402
  aspirational vision of 71
  biological 29, 149, 189, 192
  compromised 205
  contested discourses about 185–7
  digital 355
  limitations of 13, 205
  neoliberal 143
  preferential access to 118
  See also COVID-19 amplification of vulnerability: lack/denial of citizenship and

Cold War 57, 148, 415
colonial/imperial legacy 12, 55, 75, 411
  health of black/ethnic minority communities as 108–10, 122
  notions of ideational superiority as 109, 111, 119, 121
  racism/racial inequality as 11–12, 64, 70, 98, 108, 122
  See also racial hierarchies, post-colonial continuation of
colonialism
  afterlife of 108–9, 111, 113, 115, 119–20, 122–3
  as multispecies process 436
Comănescu, Denisa 151–2
communal boundaries in public health crises 153–4, 159
  scapegoating within 185, 187–92
  See also xenophobia: COVID-19 related
community
  participation in health promotion 451–4
  support/solidarity during COVID-19 8, 10, 103–4, 215, 225–8, 245, 255, 350
  See also Cuban responses to COVID-19: relational care through social networks/*socios*
comorbidities 11, 20, 261, 264–5, 270–3, 275, 317
  multimorbidity 328, 338
conspiratorial theorising/thinking 69–70, 83
  medical 70–1, 73, 84–5
  See also COVID-19 conspiracy theories
Corrupted Nanny State 83–4
COVID-19
  anthropological insights into 2–4, 11, 19–21, 109, 356, 381, 451–2
  biomedical discourses on 19, 73, 175, 386, 402, 414, 432–3, 444, 448–50
  denialism 48, 69, 80
  human visualisation of 432
  'microbiopolitics' of 430, 433–4
  as portal to rethinking healthcare 3, 28
  'stealth' nature of 4, 18
  timeline 5–7
  See also biopolitics of pandemic; 'outbreak narratives'; underlying conditions of COVID-19
COVID-19 amplification of vulnerability 2, 14, 37
  adolescents and youth and 225, 228–30, 233–7, 239, 295
  female sex workers and 225, 228, 230, 237
  lack/denial of citizenship and 223–4, 234–5, 238–40
  people living with HIV and 225, 230–3, 236
  transwomen and 225, 230, 235, 237
  waste pickers and 215
  women and 227–30, 233, 237–9
  See also health inequalities; inequalities exposed by COVID-19; sexual and reproductive health rights, Indonesia; waste pickers, India
COVID-19 configurations of shame and blame 2, 11, 15, 71, 449
  nonhumans and 18, 414, 434–6

references to 'Chinese virus' 72, 432, 443
on social media 13, 49, 79, 147, 151–2
See also COVID-19, designated 'risk groups': blaming/stigmatisation as focal point of; LGBTQI+ communities: blaming of; scapegoating
COVID-19 conspiracy theories
anti-Semitic tropes 72, 77
around 5G networks 72
boundaries between fact and fiction 84–5
debunking approach to 72–3, 174
'deep state' 10–11, 68, 73–4, 79–80, 83–4
in Ireland 68, 74–7, 85
in Poland 77–8, 85
link with identity/belonging 70, 78–9
see also QAnon; social media: spreading of misinformation via; Trump, Donald: conspiracy-mongering/spreading of disinformation by; vaccines, conspiracy theories around
COVID-19 deaths 3, 6–7, 17, 41, 49–50, 91, 303
among black/ethnic minorities 11–12, 28, 93, 98–9, 103, 105, 131, 267
conspiracy theories around 75–6, 248
of healthcare workers 115–16, 118, 319
in India 137, 139
in Italy 5, 57, 164, 318, 444, 446
in Latin America 244, 248–9, 260–1, 266–7, 257
underreporting of 20, 248, 260
See also Black, Asian and Minority Ethnic communities: disproportionate infection/death rates among; Turkey: COVID-19 infection rates/deaths in
COVID-19, designated 'risk groups' 2, 7, 9, 11, 252
blaming/stigmatisation as focal point of 15, 262, 267–8, 271, 273–5
link between inequality and 50, 98, 108, 112, 118, 123, 233, 252–3, 255
COVID-19 improvisational strategies, US/UK HCWs 303, 307, 320
addressing workforce gaps 308
altering triage processes 16, 308, 310
creative use of ventilators 305, 313–15, 317
and faultlines of inequality 303, 318–19
implementing telemedicine 310
informal information networks 305, 316–17
infrastructural 306, 308–10
as life-saving technique 303, 316–17
prioritising cancer treatments 308
for risk reduction 303, 305, 310, 314–15
suspending non-elective surgeries 308, 310
using and reusing PPE 306–7, 311–13, 315–16
See also healthcare workers (HCWs) US/UK, challenges facing
COVIDIndiaTrack policy analysis 206, 208–9, 212
bureaucratic accountability 215, 219
inclusion and exclusion criteria 207
recognition of vulnerabilities 209–10
Cresswell, Tim 283, 294–5
criminalisation of COVID-19 regulations 14, 37, 60, 62, 64n1, 445, 450, 452

Cuba
impact of US trade embargo on 33–5, 40
shift to bureaucratic socialism in 34
during Special Period 29, 33, 38–40, 43n3
tourism in 28, 34–5, 42
Cuba, international humanitarian tradition of 29–30
Henry Reeve Brigade 36–7, 43n4
Cuban responses to COVID-19 27, 32, 37
creative attitudes to *resolver* 28, 39, 42–3
humour in context of 38–9
lessons from previous pandemics 31–2, 41
relational care through social networks/ *socios* 28–9, 31, 40, 42–3n2
See also Cuban state systems of surveillance/control
Cuban Revolution 28, 30, 32, 34, 38–9
Cuban socialist public health system 8, 28–9, 37
mobilisation of 32–3, 41–2
National Action Plan for Epidemics 32–3
primary health care system 30, 32, 35
See also biopolitics of pandemic: Cuban approach
Cuban state systems of surveillance/control 8, 33, 36–7, 41, 57
Pesquisador Virtual app 7, 27
role of MEF programme in 33
tensions around/criticism of 8, 27, 31, 33, 37

Dalit, India
as confrontational identity 131
impact of COVID-19 pandemic on 138–40
as political force 132
prejudice against 12, 131, 135, 140–1, 143–4n2, 204
Danish Heart Foundation 328, 331
debility 14, 20
as 'durational death' 218–19
massification of 10, 47
Deleuze, Gilles 218, 429, 434
Delhi 16, 50, 132–3
dengue 11, 20, 222, 250
Cuban response to 28, 31, 35–6
dengue haemorrhagic fever (DHF) 31, 35
Denisova, Anastasia 364–5
Denmark, lockdown in 5, 324
disrupted social care of seniors during 337–40
impact on people living with congenital heart disease 17, 326–8, 330–2
patient-driven online diabetes communities during 333–7
National Board of Health hospital guidelines on 325–7, 330–1, 340
Denmark's universal healthcare system 17
focus on chronic care/*kronikere* 326–7, 329–30, 340
inequalities within 327, 330, 337
and informal 'carescapes' 326–7, 330–1, 334–6, 340–41
KRAM health initiatives 328–9
Derrida, Jacques
concept of 'hauntology' 48, 55, 61–2
Deshpande, Ashwini 138, 376

Dhaka, impact of lockdown on adolescents/
youth in
   emotional distress and anxiety 283–5,
290–1, 294
   insecurity and hunger as greatest fear 284,
286–7, 292, 294
   intersecting vulnerabilities 15, 282–3, 287,
293–5
   lack of state support 286–7
   plight of street peddlers 9, 15, 282,
284
   relational networks as survival
strategy 283, 287, 289, 294
   solace of religion 292–3
   See also power relations: and discourses of
intersectionality; structural violence:
COVID-19 deepening of
diabetes 15, 34, 119, 244, 255, 261, 273
   as disease of poverty 63, 99, 265–6
   genetic basis of 263
   See also Denmark, lockdown in: patient-
driven online diabetes communities
during
Dickey, Sara 367–8
Din İşleri Yüksek Kurulu 168–9
disability support, impact of COVID-19 on 14,
17, 246, 252–3
   and coordination of care networks 254–5,
257–8
Diyanet, Turkey
   condemnation of non-
heteronormativity 171–4, 176
   controversial moralistic discourses of 163,
167
   critique of neoliberal world order 168–70
   intervention in COVID-19 debate 13,
162–3, 168–70
   as political tool 163, 165–7, 175
domestic violence 167, 260, 275 See also
intimate partner violence
Doron, Assa 362–3
Douglas, Mary 384, 413, 423
   analysis of anomaly and danger 18, 386,
394, 402
   and notion of 'secular' cleanliness 390
Duterte, Rodrigo 431–3

Ebola epidemic 2, 10–11, 28, 32, 36, 55, 244,
292, 414
   militarisation of response to 57
   scapegoating of Peul migrants during 13,
183–4
Erbaş, Ali 162, 165, 171–3
Erdoğan, Recep Tayyip 162, 164, 167, 173–6
Esposito, Roberto 130–1
essential workers 119, 356, 368
   and higher risk of infection 7, 9, 12, 94, 98,
102, 444
   See also frontline workers
eugenics 149, 245, 262, 264, 267, 274
European Union (EU) 121
   collaborative preparations for
COVID-19 109, 118, 123n4
   health workers in UK 12, 116, 122
   poverty levels in 356
   Romanian attempts to join 149
   See also United Kingdom: post-Brexit
isolationism of
evictions See under housing insecurity

Façade or Cardboard State 83–4
Facebook 54, 60, 261, 339, 362
   chronic care support groups on 328, 331,
333–7
   launch of 'care emoji' 344
   and political protest 93, 96
   #SafeHands/#HealthyAtHome
hashtags 349–50
   spread of conspiracy theories via 67–8, 75,
77
   See also social media
'fake news' 76, 79, 144n6
Farmer, Paul 12, 30, 71, 109, 283
fatwa 167, 176n4
Fauci, Anthony 80–1
Faye, Sylvain 181, 183, 190–1
feminism
   equation with immorality 167
   religious 392–4
Ferrer, Barbara 98–9
Floyd, George, murder of 96, 123n1
   'I can't breathe' movement 60, 91, 129
   Minneapolis protests against 91–2
   as spark for anti-racism protests 12, 58–9,
62, 93, 96, 101–2, 104, 108
   See also #BlackLivesMatter; Movement for
Black Lives
food insecurity 11, 38, 50, 63, 265, 282, 287
   emergency food distribution, LA 103–4
   See also hunger; waste-pickers, India: food
insecurity/fear of hunger among
Foucault, Michel 49, 267, 388
   concept of biopolitics 29–30, 128–9, 144n1
   See also biopolitics of pandemic
France 5, 60, 150, 164, 182, 226
Franklin, Sarah 117
   concept of 'nostalgic nationalism' 12, 109,
113, 118, 121, 123
Frederiksen, Mette 324, 326, 339
frontline SRHR workers 222–3, 227–8, 231–2,
235, 238
   and holistic engagement with clients 224–6
frontline workers 1, 57, 94, 212, 352, 374
   See also healthcare workers: frontline

Gates, Bill 67, 81
Geddes da Filicaia, Marco 446, 452
Germany 5–6, 77, 117
Goffman, Erving 48, 52, 153
Gómez, Carolina 33, 275
Graber, Nils 30, 41
Guardian, The 112–14
Guattari, Félix 218, 429, 434
Guinea 13, 57, 183–4, 191

H1N1 epidemics 2, 11, 73, 63, 243, 250
   segregation of Roma during 13, 147,
153–5, 157
Habermas, Jürgen 48, 52–3
Haiti 31, 36, 60, 71
halachic family purity laws (FPL), Israel 389
   changes in niddah laws 389, 392, 397

historic contestation over 388, 392–3
interplay between risks and dangers 384, 386, 394–5, 397–8, 400–2
See also women's *mikveh* crisis, Israel
Haraway, Donna 413, 428, 433
Harrison, Mark 411–12, 414
Harriss-White, Barbara 202–3, 205
Hartman, Saidiya
notion of 'afterlife of slavery' 109, 111, 119
Hastrup, Kirsten 69, 84
Havana, Cuba 9, 39–40
health inequalities
connection with structural racism 12–14, 94–5, 99, 108, 110, 113, 153–7, 356
everyday/systemic 210, 212, 214–15, 219
exposed by COVID-19 1–2, 95–9, 108, 110, 113–14, 122, 212, 318
lack of state accountability for 174, 206, 265, 273–4
See also Denmark's universal healthcare system: inequalities within
healthcare 17
triaged access to 15–16, 308, 310
uneven/limited access to 1–2, 14, 94–5, 97, 99, 103–4, 153, 156
See also health inequalities; Mexico: extreme triage guidelines in; public healthcare systems
healthcare workers (HCWs) 6, 16, 36, 156, 324, 353
Danish home/auxiliary 330, 338
frontline 12, 16, 305–6, 312
in Turkey 164–5,
See also frontline SRHR workers
healthcare workers US/UK, challenges facing
constantly changing recommendations 309–13
inequality 318–19
medical uncertainty/lack of knowledge 303, 305–7, 316
shortage of PPE 5, 12, 16, 40, 109, 113–14, 116–18, 139, 306, 312–13, 315–16, 318
shortage of ventilators 313–14
stress and anxiety 304, 310, 312, 314, 316
See also COVID-19 improvisational strategies, US/UK HCWs
heart disease 15, 99, 119, 244, 255, 274
congenital heart defects (CHDs) 327–8, 330–3
hypertension 40, 63, 261, 273, 429
Helmond, Anne 345, 347
herd immunity *See* immunity: herd
Herring, D. Ann 2–3, 243
Hirsch, Afua 110, 119
HIV/AIDS 2, 10–11, 28, 47, 50–1, 63
conspiracy theories around 71, 73
Cuban response to 31, 57
feminisation of 224
See also COVID-19 amplification of vulnerability: people living with HIV and
Horton, Richard 444, 451, 454
Hossain, Md Shahadat 281, 286
housing insecurity 11, 14, 103, 282
and evictions 59, 61

Hungary 154, 158
hunger 9–10, 47, 52, 55, 63, 136–7, 139, 169, 212, 281, 294–5
Crusade Against Hunger, Mexico 265
See also food insecurity
hydroxychloroquinine 305, 416
Bolsonaro's promotion of 247, 251
Trump's promotion of 73

ICT 'fantasies of caregiving' during pandemic 17, 347–8, 357
in context of digital divide/inequality 17, 346, 348, 353–6, 358
in context of physical distancing 344, 346, 349–50, 356
COVID-19 Solidarity Response Fund 352–3
exploitation of care rhetoric 345, 347–50, 353–5
facilitation of digital surveillance 345, 353, 358
gatekeeping strategies 351–2
notion of community connectedness 350, 357
partnerships with health organisations 350–3, 357
promotion of 'digital wellness'/ wellbeing 348, 355–7
See also social media; YouTube
identity
ethnic 148
imagined 109
national 119–22
relational 111, 120
territorialisation of 189–90
See also COVID-19 conspiracy theories: link with identity/belonging
immunity
biosocial 422–3
herd 128, 249, 423
partial 410, 415–16
See also Rollback Malaria campaign: link between ITNs and acquired immunity
India
1918 flu pandemic in 132–4
growth of ICT in 362–4
healthcare landscape in 137–8, 144n5
middle-class reliance on domestic help in 367–8, 370–2, 377–9
new middle class in 142, 363
See also caste system, India
India, lockdown in 5, 8
and challenge to traditional gender roles 17–18, 365, 368–9, 370–1, 372–3, 378, 381–2
dehumanising impact of 12, 15, 140–2
Hindu fundamentalist views on 139–41
impact on stranded migrant workers 14, 21, 136–8, 366–7, 374–5
impact on working mothers 376–81
loss of jobs/livelihoods due to 368, 373–4
media discourse on 138–9, 144n6
middle class solidarity around 10, 137–8, 142, 144n3, 374–5
and public distribution system (ration cards) 213, 216–17

See also biopolitics of pandemic: 'make live and let die' approach; COVIDIndiaTrack analysis; sanitation workers, India; waste-picking communities, India
inequalities exposed by COVID-19 38
   class 47, 50, 52, 55, 128, 137, 239, 253, 256–7, 267, 293, 368
   gender 18, 49–50, 55, 128, 293, 295, 369
   justification of 286, 434
   sexual and reproductive health 2, 14, 223–4, 226, 238
   socio-economic 2, 9, 50, 97–8, 103, 138–9, 253
   spatial 7, 14, 48, 50–1, 59, 140–41
   See also health inequalities; racial inequalities exposed by COVID-19; structural inequality
Information and Communication Technologies (ICTs) 344
   commodification of personal data by 345, 347, 353–4
   and transnational care collectives 346
   See also ICT 'fantasies of caregiving' during pandemic
intimate partner violence 49, 51, 237, 239
   See also domestic violence
Ireland 68, 74, 85
   challenges to lockdown restrictions in 75–6
Italy, COVID-19 pandemic in 57, 63, 155–6, 305, 308, 337, 340, 354
   and contradictory public messages 443–4
   Cuban medical support for 37
   lack of preparedness of NHS for 5, 19, 317, 324, 443, 446–8
   and role of social/cultural articulation at local level 448–52, 454
   romanticisation of 10, 144n3, 374
   See also Lombardy region as first 'red zone'

Jakarta 222, 227, 230–1, 233, 235
Jeffrey, Robin 362–3
job insecurity 95, 104, 284, 287 *See also* unemployment
Jones, Alex 79–80

Khoza, Collins 60, 62
King, Rodney 60, 95
Koca, Fahrettin 162, 164, 174, 176n2
Kyela district, Tanzania 19, 410, 423
   beliefs about malaria in 417
   colonial health education in 416–17
   multispecies co-existences in, acceptance of 418–21
   See also malaria

LaFrance, Adrienne 80, 82
Lakoff, Andrew 4, 243, 258
Langstrup, Henriette 326, 329
LGBTQI+ communities 231, 236
   blaming of 13, 163, 167, 170–1, 173–6
   See also Diyanet, Turkey: condemnation of non-heteronormativity
Liberia 57, 183, 191
Livingston, Julie 15–16, 30, 306, 318–19
logic of separation 19
   anthropocentricity of 413

at centre of malaria control 414–15, 417, 421
   and 'contagionist' view of infection 413
   and puncturing of multispecies and social relationships 410–11, 414, 421, 423
   See also One Health responses to COVID-19
Lombardy region as first 'red zone' 8, 37, 443, 447
   Bergamo 5, 15, 67, 444–6
   and overwhelming of hospitals 5, 19, 443, 445
London 1, 50, 115–16, 118
   Nightingale hospitals 309
'Long COVID'
   #CountLongCovid support group 20
López-Gatell Ramírez, Hugo 260–1, 268
Los Angeles
   healthcare system 94–5, 97, 100, 103–5
   Police Department (LAPD) 92, 94–5, 100–101 *See also* police brutality and racism, US
Lula *See* Silva, Luis Ignácio
Lynteris, Christos 10, 109, 118, 411–12, 414

Madrid *See* Spain
malaria 15, 19, 73, 244
   Anopheles mosquito as vector of 411–12, 415, 417, 421
   endemicity of 410–12
   failure of GMEP treatment for 415–16
   rebound effect 415–16, 421–2
   See also Kyela district, Tanzania; logic of separation: at centre of malaria control; Rollback Malaria campaign
Malawi 57, 307
Malaysia 10, 58
Mandetta, Luis Henrique 246–7
Mantini-Briggs, Clara 33–4, 37
Martin, Trayvon 92–3
memes 18, 362
   anthropological perspective on 364–5, 376, 381–2
   derogatory/racist 147, 151–3
   Indian lockdown in 368–76
MERS 11, 184, 319
Mexico 15
   extreme triage guidelines 262, 270–2, 274
   impact of NAFTA on food systems 264–5
   informal economy of 260, 267
   genetic strength linked to mestizaje 262–3, 266–7
   government's war against obesity in 261–2, 265, 268–9, 274
   militarised response to pandemic in 58, 272–3
   obsession with diets and foodways 262, 264–5
   Spanish colonisation of 262, 264
   undertesting/underreporting of COVID-19 in 260
   See also obesity
Mexico City, slums of 50, 56
microbes 19
   divergence between local and biomedical knowledge of 433

INDEX   461

human relationships with 10, 409, 413, 430–3, 448
  Pasteurian notions of 428–9, 431–2
  usefulness of 432–3
Mignolo, Walter 120, 412
migrant workers, impact of pandemic on 14, 58
  UK 114, 118, 123n5
  See also India, lockdown in: impact on stranded migrant workers; Senegalese emigrants
militarisation of pandemics 9–10, 50, 52–3, 56–8, 71, 105 *See also under* South Africa, lockdown in; Mexico
Ministry of Health (MH), Israel 387–8
  lockdown guidelines 393–4
  sanitation standards for *mikveh* 390, 391–2, 395, 397, 399
Ministry of Religious Services (MRS), Israel 389, 391, 396
  on use of *mikvehs* during lockdown 388, 393–5, 398–401
Modi, Narendra 5, 366, 370–1, 380–1
Mokgopa, Kneo 62
Moore, Ronnie 75, 78
Mossialos, Elias 116–17
Movement for Black Lives (M4BL) 92–4, 102
multispecies perspective 422, 431, 438
  as ecological necessity 19, 421, 428, 430
  incompatibility of logic of separation with 410, 415, 421, 423
  and notion of 'biophilia' 430, 437
  and relationship between humans and nonhumans 409, 411, 427–9, 438–40
  See also 'outbreak narratives': and anxieties about nonhuman life
Mumbai 1, 137, 286, 366–7, 377

National Council Against Discrimination (CNCD), Romania 152–3
National Health Service (NHS), UK
  coloniality of 109, 113, 115–16, 121
  dropping of Test and Trace system 117
  ethnic patterning of care provision in 109, 112–13, 115–16, 118, 122
  high vacancy/low retention rates of staff 304
  lack of PPE and testing in 16, 109, 113–14, 116–18
  and notions of 'heroism' of health/care workers 113–14
  underfunding of 114, 117, 304
  See also COVID-19 improvisational strategies, US/UK HCWs; Public Health England
Necula, Ciprian 151–2
neoliberal austerity policies 341
  undermining of health systems by 4, 15, 110, 244, 246, 257, 447–8, 454
neoliberalism 128, 138
  effect on Mexican food systems 264–5
  See also Diyanet, Turkey: critique of neoliberal world order
New York 1, 50
  changing care practices in 305, 309, 317
  as first epicentre of US pandemic 6, 8, 16, 271, 305

nostalgic nationalism *See* Franklin, Sarah: concept of 'nostalgic nationalism'
Nyamnjoh, Francis 186–8, 191

obesity 265–6, 268, 269, 275
  genetic and epigenetic approaches to 119, 262–4, 266–7
  risk of death of COVID due to 261–2
  and stigmatisation of fatness 262, 268–70, 271, 273–4
  See also Mexico: government's war against obesity in
O'Doherty, Gemma 74–6
One Health responses to COVID-19 409, 411, 422–3
'outbreak narratives' 2, 411
  and anxieties about nonhuman life 413–14, 422–3

Packard, Randall 412, 414–15, 421, 450
Paxson, Heather 430–2
Pesquisador Virtual app 7–8
Philippines 347–8, 430–3, 435, 439
  botanic boom in 436–8
  ostrich internet sensation 427–9
  study of bats in 435
physical distancing *See* social distancing
Piotrokowski, Malka 385–6, 392, 400
Poland 68, 77–8, 85, 148
Poleykett, Branwyn 10, 109, 118
police brutality and abuse 10, 15, 47, 76, 139
  in South Africa 51, 55–6, 59–62
  See also under underlying conditions of COVID-19
police brutality and racism, US 58–60, 91–2
  Los Angeles 92–6, 100–1, 104–5
  as public health crisis 99, 101
  See also Black Lives Matter; 1965 Watts Rebellion
political Islam 163, 167
  as threat to public health 13, 168, 175–6
polydemics 411
  and concept of 'interconnected diversity' 412–13, 423
pluriversal 410, 412, 415, 421–3
poverty 11
  dehumanisation/depredation of 12, 60–2, 133–6, 140, 143
  and homelessness 10, 47, 56, 63, 138, 206, 233, 356, 449
  impact of COVID-19 on 138–9
  spatialisation of 48
  systemic/chronic 10, 47
  See also underlying conditions of COVID-19: poverty and discrimination as
power relations 203
  and discourses of intersectionality 219, 283–4, 295
  of epidemiological control 118
  human-nonhuman 439
  sexuality as dense transfer point of 388
Premchand, Munshi 134–6, 143
primary healthcare 413, 452
primary healthcare, COVID-19 overburdening of
  in Brazil 250, 255
  in Indonesia 227–30, 232, 234, 238–9

in Italy 443, 446–7
in UK's NHS 446–7, 452
See also under Cuban socialist public health system
Puar, Jasbir K. 218–19
Public Health England (PHE) 110, 112–13, 119
public health initiatives 3–5, 8–9, 261–2
　tensions between religion and 384, 386–7, 401–2
　See also women's *mikveh* crisis, Israel
public healthcare systems 15, 41
　challenges to/lack of preparedness of 4, 6, 16, 18, 63, 78
　impact of market-oriented reforms on 19
　See also Cuban socialist public health system; Denmark's universal healthcare system; National Health Service, UK

QAnon 80, 82
quarantine 91, 142, 153–5, 163, 245, 253, 256, 393, 413
　social media platforms and 353–4
quarantine enforcement 2, 4–5, 8–10, 412
　in Cuba 32, 37, 41, 57
　in Romania 152, 157–8
　in Senegal 183
　in South Africa 57
　in Vietnam 41

rabbinic authority, Israel
　Fertility in Light of Halacha (FLOH) 387, 396, 400, 402
　gendered challenges to 18, 385–6, 388, 292–3, 401–2
　and restructuring of worship and sociality during pandemic 384–5, 393
　women scholars/rabbanit 18, 385–7, 392–3, 395, 403n2
　See also halachic family purity laws, Israel; women's *mikveh* crisis, Israel: interaction between rabbinic discourse and public health
racial capitalism 64, 98–9, 102, 104–5
racial discrimination *See* racism
racial hierarchies, post-colonial continuation of 10, 12, 47, 99, 109, 111, 119, 121, 141, 367, 413
racial inequalities exposed by COVID-19 2–3
　in South Africa 48, 50, 55–6, 60, 62
　in UK 11, 108, 110
　in US 11–12, 28, 91–3, 98
　See also #BlackLivesMatter: link with disparities of COVID-19
racism 2, 11, 21, 53, 55, 60, 62, 120, 413
　scapegoating as form of 72, 153
　systemic 63, 94, 97, 99, 120, 122, 129, 157
　See also #BlackLivesMatter; colonial/imperial legacy: racism/racial inequality as; health inequalities: connection with structural racism; memes: derogatory/racist
Ramaphosa, Cyril 5, 49, 60, 62
Robinson, Cedric 99, 102
Rollback Malaria (RBM) campaign
　insecticide-treated mosquito nets (ITNs) 410, 415–20, 423
　link between ITNs and acquired immunity 421–2
Roma
　dehumanisation of 150
　ethnic identity of 148
　human trafficking case 158
　impact of measles epidemic on 13, 147, 153, 155–7, 159
　negative stereotyping of 148–52, 156, 159
　pre-COVID segregation and marginalisation of 149–50, 153–6
　resistance to assimilation policies 148
　transnational mobility of 147–9
　See also memes: derogatory/racist; structural violence: against Roma
Romanian lockdown measures 159
　and 'civil disobedience' of Roma 13, 157–9
　and institutionalisation of racism 13, 143, 147, 151–2, 157–8
　in Suceava 159n2
　See also biopolitics of pandemic: Roma responses
Rosenberg, Charles E. 412–13
Rosenfeld, David 98–9
Rousseff, Dilma 246, 250–1
Roy, Arundhati 3, 28

Sahni, Rohini 202–4
Sanders, Andrew 75, 78
sanitation workers, India
　increased risk of COVID-19 for 201, 212
　lack of protective equipment for 201, 205
SARS-COV-1 virus 2, 11, 16, 73, 184, 414
SARS-COV-2 virus 1, 5, 18, 27, 67, 72, 81, 128, 130–1, 141–2, 366, 412, 448, 453
　See also COVID-19
scapegoating 11, 13
　of Roma 149, 153
　of returning Senegalese emigrants 183, 185, 187, 189–92, 449
　See also Ebola epidemic: scapegoating of Peul migrants during; racism: scapegoating as form of
Scorza, D'Artagnan 96–7
self-isolation 8, 324
　and 'at risk' groups 2, 17, 324, 327, 335, 339–40
　enforced 55–6
　limited capacity for 2, 4, 10, 14, 36, 42, 98, 128, 190
　See also under social exclusion
Senegalese emigrants 181
　local reactions to returning 9, 13, 182–3, 190
　role in economy/local livelihoods 187–9
　See also scapegoating: of returning Senegalese emigrants
sexual and reproductive health rights (SRHR), Indonesia 2, 14
　access to safe abortion 224, 227, 229, 238
　barriers to accessing free healthcare 224, 234–7, 239
　ethnographic research on 224–7
　gender imbalance 226
　low capacity/under-investment of GOI in 223–4, 227, 238–9

maternal mortality rate 223–4, 227
reproductive cancer screening 233
rising private sector costs 229–31
STI and HIV prevention and
    treatment 230–3, 235, 237,
    239–40n3
unmet contraception needs 223, 227–31,
    236–8
youth programmes 228–30, 233–4
See also COVID-19 amplification of
    vulnerability; frontline SRHR workers
Shadow State 83–4
Shankan, V. Kalyan 202–4
Sierra Leone 57, 183, 191, 296
Silva, Luis Ignácio 245–6
Simpkin, Victoria L. 116–17
Singer, Merrill 266, 283, 365, 454
Slovakia 148, 158
social contract, ruptures in 70, 82
social distancing 1–2, 4, 8–9, 27, 39, 54, 69,
    304, 413
  difficulties with/criticisms of 48–9, 74–5,
    98, 190, 255, 318
  enforced 56
  impact on SRH care 224, 231, 233
  impact on work/livelihoods 235, 253–7
  as threat to civil liberty/basic rights 80,
    245, 247
  See also under social exclusion
social exclusion 109, 122
  dehumanisation of 143
  geopolitical discourses 184, 186–7
  self-isolation/social distancing as form
    of 12, 128–32, 136–7, 139–40, 285–6,
    356
social injustice 28, 53, 118
  faced by young slum-dwellers 283, 296
  historic 131, 272, 274–5
  racialised 93, 95
social media
  and facilitation of work from home 17,
    254, 362
  hate speech on 173
  as scapegoating/blaming mechanism 183
  spreading of misinformation via 37, 68, 75,
    77, 351–2
  as technology of support 10, 17–18, 20, 40,
    55, 96, 157, 205
  as tool for social analysis 183, 185, 189
  See also COVID-19 configurations of shame
    and blame: on social media; Facebook;
    ICT 'fantasies of caregiving' during
    pandemic
sociality 328–9, 410
  new modes of 60, 384–5, 450, 452
solid waste management (SWM), India 203
  informal system as backbone of 203–4, 208
  kabaadi system 208–9
  Municipal Solid Waste Management
    (MSWM) 208
  See also waste pickers, India
Solis, Hilda 99, 101
Solís, Patricio 261, 267
South Africa
  scale and speed of viral spread in 49–50,
    56

South Africa, lockdown in
  apartheid-style militarisation of 47–52,
    55–6, 58, 60–1, 63
  constraints/prohibitions under 48–9
  disproportionate impact on informal
    settlements of 1, 5, 10, 47, 50–1,
    59–61
  massification of surveillance under 47, 49,
    55
South African Social Security Agency (SASSA)
  COVID-19 grant 51
South Korea 10, 171
Soviet Union 33, 77
Spain 1, 5, 8, 16, 182, 324, 337, 435
Spanish flu *See* H1N1 epidemics
state power 3
  and enforcement of lockdowns 4, 8–9, 28,
    36, 41, 48, 50, 52, 54, 56, 58
  moralist discourses and 163
  problematic expressions of 83–5
  and technologies of surveillance 10, 57,
    60–1, 63, 67, 105, 153, 155
  See also COVID-19 conspiracy theories:
    'deep state'; South Africa, lockdown in:
    massification of surveillance under
Stevenson, Lisa 30, 42
stigmatising power of infection 11
  and designated 'risk groups' 2, 123, 324,
    328, 330
  LGBTQI+ 11, 171
  in poorest strata of society 215–17
stratified livability 2, 4, 21
Street, Alice 306, 319
structural inequality 15, 56, 123, 141–2, 257
  link between white supremacy and 91–2,
    97–8
  See also chronic disease: link between
    inequality and
structural violence
  COVID-19 deepening of 11–12, 51, 55, 98,
    283, 293, 295
  extension to nonhumans 439
  against Roma 149, 155, 157–8
  See also caste-based structural violence
structural vulnerability 11, 15, 98, 157, 293,
    307 *See also* bioethics and notions of
    vulnerability; COVID-19 amplification of
    vulnerability
Swedlund, Alan C. 2–3, 243
swine flu *See* H1N1 epidemics
syndemic
  COVID-19 as 11, 21, 243–4, 428, 454
  framework on chronic disease 265–6

Tadiar, Neferti Xina M. 357–8
  notion of fantasy production 347–8, 353
Țăndărei, Romania 147, 150–3, 157–8
Taylor, Breonna 60, 96
Thiam, Jamil 182–3
Tismăneanu, Vladimir 151–2
tourism, impact of COVID on 8–9, 28, 31–2
Trump, Donald
  armed enforcement of curfew regulations
    by 59–60
  conspiracy-mongering/spreading of
    disinformation by 39, 73, 77, 79–81, 432

crackdown on foreign trade by 35, 40
downplaying of virus by 6, 80, 247
endorsement by far-right of 79–81
positive COVID-19 test 6
tuberculosis (TB) 10, 30, 47, 51, 63, 412
Turkey 116
  COVID-19 infection rates/deaths in 162, 165, 175–6n1
  criminalisation of hate speech in 171–3
  export of PPE equipment from 170, 177n5
  2016 failed coup attempt 165, 167
  militarised response to pandemic in 58
  veracity of COVID-19 statistics in 164, 176n2
  See also Adalet ve Kalkınma Partisi, Turkey; Diyanet, Turkey; political Islam
Turkish Medical Association (TTB) 164, 175

underlying conditions of COVID-19 2, 17, 20
  police brutality/violence 15, 56, 91–2, 99, 275, 284–6, 291–2
  poverty and racial discrimination 13–15, 21, 28, 42, 50–1, 63, 94, 97–9, 110, 119, 257
unemployment 51, 110, 257, 267
  COVID-19 deepening of 10–11, 29, 52, 55, 63, 102–3, 138, 258n7
United Kingdom (UK) 5–7, 10, 60, 63
  post-Brexit isolationism of 12, 109, 113, 115–18
  See also Black, Asian and Minority Ethnic communities: disproportionate death rates among; health inequalities: connection with systemic racism; National Health Service, UK
United Nations 10
  International Children's Education Fund (UNICEF) 281–2, 351
urbanisation, link with pandemics 29, 205, 429
US
  anti-lockdown protests in 81–2
  COVID-19 infection rates in 4, 6–8, 91, 131, 304
  generational inequities in 28
  Helms-Burton Act 35, 40
  movements for prison abolition in 92, 101, 104
  sustained faith in American Dream 79–81
  2008 foreclosure crisis 79
  See also Los Angeles; New York; police brutality, US; Trump, Donald

vaccination/immunisation 250, 331, 413, 422–3, 428, 431
  hesitancy in orthodox Jewish communities 387
  against HPV 234
  against malaria 422
  against MMR 156–7
vaccines, conspiracy theories around 69, 72, 74–5, 81
  Big Pharma tropes 77, 81–3
vaccines, COVID-19 244
  development of/race for 1, 6, 50, 57, 67–8, 130, 352–3

possible contribution of digital platforms to 357
  rollouts of 1, 72
van Dijck, Jose 345, 347
Vaughan, Megan 414, 417
Venezuela 35, 71
Vietnam 4, 9, 41, 117
viral vagility of prejudice 128–9, 131
  and Indian caste system 132, 141–2
viruses 10, 19–20, 409, 430
  as ancient life forms 411, 448
  mutation of 429
  as quasi-species 431
  zoonotic 18, 413–14, 422, 429, 434

Wahl-Jorgensen, Karin 347, 349
Wald, Patricia 411, 413–14
waste pickers, India 14, 201–2
  as backbone of MSWM 203–4, 208, 219
  conflict with private players 203, 205
  discrimination against/stigmatisation of 202–3, 205, 214–17
  food insecurity/fear of hunger among 201, 205–6, 212–14, 216–17
  harassment from state institutions 204
  inability to access healthcare 210, 212–15
  issuing of identity cards to 209–11, 217
  legal recognition of 203, 208–11
  loss of income due to lockdown 201, 205, 213, 216
  migrant labour among 204–5
  ragpickers 204, 209–11
  and sexual division of labour 204, 220n7
Waters, John 75–6
1965 Watts Rebellion 95–6
WhatsApp *See* memes; social media
white supremacy *See* structural inequality: link between white supremacy and
Whiteford, Linda M. 8, 31, 36
whiteness 111, 120, 122
women's *mikveh* crisis, Israel
  evidence-based halachic statement on 394–7, 400–1
  Facebook discussions on 388, 393–4, 397–400
  and interaction between rabbinic discourse and public health 18, 385–6, 388, 391–2, 397, 401–2
  medical anthropological perspective on 387–8
  and micro-politics of spousal intimacy 285–6, 396, 400–1
  and negotiability of halacha 392, 397–8, 402
  and risk of COVID-19 infection 384, 386, 393–4, 397, 399
  Zoom panel discussions on 385–6, 388
  See also Ministry of Religious Services, Israel; public health initiatives: tensions between religion and
World Bank 50, 139, 189, 223, 243, 286
World Health Organization (WHO) 5, 10, 109, 114, 154, 164, 223, 243
  recommendations to treat/contain pandemic 17, 244, 247, 352, 414, 445
  social media partnerships with 350–2

Wuhan 5, 8, 16, 18, 37, 72, 305, 337, 432
  Huanan Seafood Market in 18

xenophobia 56
  COVID-19 related 153, 186, 190–2
  See also scapegoating

Yogyakarta 222, 227, 230–1, 235
YouTube 17, 75, 157, 345–6, 348, 351
'At Home #WithMe' campaign 349–50, 353

Zika virus 11, 35, 244–5, 258n1
  and children with congenital Zika syndrome 14, 249–50, 251–2, 258n1, 5
  vulnerability of survivors 252–3
Zimbabwe 52, 71, 116
Zimmerman, George 92–3